COMPREHENSIVE GERIATRIC ASSESSMENT

COMPREHENSIVE GERIATRIC ASSESSMENT

Dan Osterweil, MD, MSEd, CMD

Professor of Medicine & Geriatrics, UCLA School of Medicine
Research Association, UCLA Borun Center for Gerontological Research
Los Angeles

Kenneth Brummel-Smith, MD

Professor of Family Medicine
Oregon Health Sciences University
Bain Chair, Providence Center on Aging

John C. Beck, MD

Professor of Medicine-Emeritus, UCLA School of Medicine
Los Angeles

McGRAW-HILL

Medical Publishing Division

New York / St. Louis / San Francisco / Auckland / Bogotá / Caracas
Lisbon / London / Madrid / Mexico City / Milan / Montreal
New Delhi / San Juan / Singapore / Sydney / Tokyo / Toronto

McGraw-Hill

A Division of The **McGraw·Hill** *Companies*

Comprehensive Geriatric Assessment

1234567890 DOCDOC 09876543210

ISBN 0-07-134725-9

This book was set in Times Ten by The PRD Group, Inc.
The editors were Susan Noujaim and Barbara Holton.
The production supervisor was Catherine Saggese.
The cover designer was Aimee Nordin.
The index was prepared by Jerry Ralya

R. R. Donnelley & Sons was printer and binder.

This book is printed on acid-free paper.

Library of Congress Cataloging-in-Publication Data

Geriatric assessment / editors, Dan Osterweil, Kenneth Brummel-Smith,
John Beck.
     p.; cm.
   Includes bibliographical references and index.
   ISBN 0-07-134725-9
   1. Aged–Diseases–Diagnosis. 2. Health   status   indicators. 3.
Medical screening. I.
  Osterweil, Dan. II. Beck, John C., 1924-
  [DNLM: 1. Geriatric Assessment. WT 30 G36871 2001]
  RC953.G46 2001
  618.97'075–dc21

                                             99-087542

CONTRIBUTORS

Linda Abbey, MD
Associate Professor of General Medicine
Medical College of Virginia
Virginia Commonwealth University

Cathy A. Alessi, MD
Associate Professor
UCLA Multicampus Program in Geriatric
    Medicine & Gerontology
Geriatric Research, Education and Clinical
    Center
VA Greater Los Angeles Healthcare System,
    Sepulveda

Mario Mendez Ashla, MD, PhD
Director, Neurobehavior Unit
VA Great Los Angeles Healthcare System
Professor, Neurology and Psychiatry &
    Biobehavioral Sciences
UCLA, Los Angeles

Carol M. Ashton, MD, MPH
Director
Houston Center for Quality of Care and
    Utilization Studies:
A VA Health Services Research & Development
    Field Program
Professor of Medicine
Baylor College of Medicine

Carol Banyas, MD
Director of Geriatric Psychiatry
California Pacific Medical Center
San Francisco

Barbara M. Bates-Jensen, PhD, RN, CWOCN
Assistant Professor of Nursing
University of Southern California

Peter A. Boling, MD
Professor of Medicine
Medical College of Virginia
Virginia Commonwealth University

Kenneth Brummel-Smith, MD
Professor of Family Medicine
Oregon Health Sciences University
Bain Chair, Providence Center on Aging

Kerry P. Burnight, PhD
Assistant Clinical Professor
Program in Geriatric Medicine
University of California, Irvine
College of Medicine

Richard Camicioli, MD
Associate Professor
Department of Medicine
Division of Neurology
University of Alberta

JoAnn Damron-Rodriguez, PhD
Associate Professor
School of Public Policy & Social Research
UCLA
Associate Director, Evaluation & Education
Geriatric Research Evaluation and Clinical
    Center
VA Greater Los Angeles Healthcare System

Susan J. Denman, MD, CMD
Associate Professor of Medicine
Chief, Section of Geriatric Medicine
Temple University Hospital and School of
    Medicine
SVP, Medical Affairs
Philadelphia Geriatric Center

Maggie A. Donius, RN, MN
Gerontology Clinical Nurse Specialist
Providence Benedictine Nursing Center
Assistant Professor, School of Nursing
Oregon Health Sciences University

Rebecca D. Elon, MD, MPH
Medical Director
North Arundel Senior Care
Associate Professor of Medicine
Johns Hopkins University School of Medicine

Bruce A. Ferrell, MD
Associate Professor
UCLA School of Medicine
Division of Geriatrics

Thomas E. Finucane, MD
Associate Professor of Medicine
Division of Geriatric Medicine & Gerontology
    and Bioethics Institute
Johns Hopkins University School of Medicine

Joseph Francis, MD, MPH
Chief Medical Officer, Mid-South Healthcare
    Network
Department of Veterans Affairs
Nashville, TN

Janet C. Frank, DrPH
Assistant Director for Academic Programs in
    Geriatric Medicine & Gerontology
UCLA

Meghan B. Gerety, MD
Associate Chief of Staff/Geriatrics & Extended
    Care
South Texas Veterans Health Care System
Professor, Department of Medicine
University of Texas Health Science Center in
    San Antonio

Melanie W. Gironda, PhD, MSW
Lecturer
Department of Social Welfare
School of Public Policy and Social Research
UCLA

Mary K. Goldstein, MD, MSc
Associate Professor of Medicine
Center for Primary Care and Outcomes
    Research
Stanford University
Senior Research Associate
VA Palo Alto Health Care System

C. Bree Johnston, MD, MPH
Assistant Clinical Professor of Medicine
University of California, San Francisco
Program Director, UCSF Fellowship in Geriatric
    Medicine
Director, Graduate Medical Education
VA Medical Center, San Francisco

Marshall B. Kapp, JD, MPH
Frederick A. White Distinguished Professor of
    Service
Departments of Community Health and
    Psychiatry and Office of Geriatric
    Medicine & Gerontology
Wright State University School of Medicine

Jeffrey Kaye, MD
Professor of Neurology
Director, Aging and Alzheimer's Disease Center
Oregon Health Sciences University
Portland Veterans Affairs Medical Center

Mary Jane Koren, MD, MPH
Vice President
Director of Health Care Program
Fan Fox & Leslie R. Samuels Foundation

Ira M. Lesser, MD
Professor, Department of Psychiatry &
    Biobehavioral Sciences
UCLA School of Medicine
Director, Psychiatry Residency Program
Harbor-UCLA Medical Center

John F. Loome, MD
Clinical Instructor
Departments of Internal Medicine &
    Geriatrics & Gerontology
Johns Hopkins University School of Medicine
Associate Medical Director
North Arundel Senior Care
Severna Park, Maryland

James Lubben, DSW, MPH
Professor of Social Welfare & Urban Planning
UCLA School of Public Policy and Social
    Research

Carol M. Mangione, MD, MSPH
Associate Professor of Medicine
Division of General Internal Medicine & Health
    Services Research
UCLA School of Medicine

Richard A. Marottoli, MD, MPH
Senior Research Associate
VA Connecticut Healthcare System
West Haven, CT
Associate Professor of Medicine
Yale University School of Medicine

Donald E. Morgan, PhD
Vice President
Clinical Research & Medical Affairs
Decibel Instruments, Inc.
Fremont, CA

Laura Mosqueda, MD
Director of Geriatrics
Associate Clinical Professor of Family Medicine
University of California, Irvine
College of Medicine

Marcia G. Ory, MPH, PhD
Chief, Behavioral Medicine & Public Health
National Institute on Aging
National Institutes of Health
Bethesda, MD

Joseph G. Ouslander, MD
Professor of Medicine
Director, Division of Geriatric Medicine &
    Gerontology
Vice President of Professional Services
Wesley Woods Center for Emory University
Director, Atlanta VA Rehabilitation Research &
    Development Center

Robert A. Pearlman, MD, MPH
Professor, Departments of Medicine and
    Medical History & Ethics
University of Washington
Veteran Affairs Puget Sound Health Care
    System

Cheryl Phillips, MD, CMD
Medical Director, Skilled Nursing and Chronic
    Care
Sutter Health Center
Sacramento, CA

David B. Reuben, MD
Chief, Division of Geriatrics
Director, Multicampus Program in Geriatric
    Medicine & Gerontology
Professor of Medicine
UCLA

Laurence Z. Rubenstein, MD, MPH
Professor of Geriatric Medicine
UCLA School of Medicine
Director, Geriatric Research Education and
    Clinical Center (GRECC)
Sepulveda VA Medical Center

Mindel Spiegel, MD, MPH
Medical Consultant
Health Facilities Division
Los Angeles County Department of Health
  Services

George Triadafilopoulos, MD
Professor of Medicine
Stanford University School of Medicine
Chief, Gastroenterology Section
VA Palo Alto Health Care System

Anita M. Woods, PhD
Program Director
Center of Excellence in Geriatrics
Huffington Center on Aging
Baylor College of Medicine
Assistant Professor
Department of Medicine and Department of
  Family and Community Medicine
Baylor College of Medicine

Geriatric assessment is the heart and soul of geriatrics.

When geriatrics entered its renaissance in the late 1970s, directors of fledgling geriatrics training programs were confronted, first and foremost, with the most natural of all questions. What, if any, is the contribution geriatrics can make to the well-being of older patients? This was a more or less polite way of asking why a specialty of geriatrics was needed at all. Such confrontational questions were in the minds of those caring for elders as they began to analyze the problems and needs of the patients they were asked to see. Referrals were few in number at first despite an increasingly aged population. This was clear evidence of the skepticism with which the emerging discipline was viewed by medical and surgical colleagues, house officers, students, patients and their families.

The answer was found in the teachings of the many esteemed British geriatricians and the few pioneers in academic geriatrics in the United States. They emphasized the difference between caring and curing, between disease and functional status, between tional Oslerian diagnose-and-treat medicine and the simultaneous management of multiple diseases, between medicine acting competently alone and medicine as part of an interdisciplinary effort. From this series of contrasts comprehensive geriatric assessment (CGA) emerged, as a response to the remarkable complexity presented by elders. Thus, CGA was primarily a systematic effort to organize the extensive database that must be acquired in order to properly manage an elderly patient with complex, interacting problems.

By the early 1980s, geriatricians, nurses, social workers and other health professionals had come together to define the essential components of CGA. It remained for a geriatrician fresh out of the Robert Wood Johnson Clinical Scholars Program, too young to be afraid to tackle a really big clinical problem, to design and carry out a randomized clinical trial comparing CGA on a special geriatrics unit with usual care on a teaching medical service. The report of this study by Laurence Rubenstein and his colleagues galvanized the adolescent specialty of geriatrics and added CGA to the medical lexicon.

Three years later, in 1987, the NIH held a consensus conference on CGA. Its report defined CGA; outlined its goals, structures and processes; described its essential components; and stressed requirements that the resources and strengths of the patient be listed, the need for services be assessed, and a coordinated care plan be developed. Careful follow-up was identified as a key to success since the care plan must be modified continually to take into account changes in the patient's condition and variable responses to therapy. In other words, CGA from the beginning was judged to be useful only if it was embedded in the continuing process of care of elders. The report also suggested areas for future research. Highlighted were studies of the effectiveness of CGA in many different settings, examination of the contribution of each of its components, a closer look at a number of additional outcomes, evaluation of different approaches to implementation of the care plan, rules for targeting CGA to the patients who would benefit the most, and improvements in the standardization and accuracy of measurement tools. In the subsequent 13 years to the present, a vast literature has been created, reporting work in these areas of investigation. As a result, the authors of this book come to their task armed with a quite impressive body of knowledge. Thus, publication of this volume is timely.

We can be more specific about the themes of the past decade of research on CGA. Physicians, nurses, social workers, therapists and nutritionists have reported about each discipline's contribution to CGA. Studies have examined the use of CGA in the hospital, the clinic, the office, the home and the nursing facility. Others have focused on CGA's role in fee-for-service medicine, the managed care organization, the HMO, the Social HMO, the PACE and vertically integrated long-term-care systems. Still others have tested less comprehensive variants of geriatric assessment with the goal of reducing cost while maintaining utility. Targeting has continued to attract intensive study, particularly in terms of screening methods to select from the greater population of elders those with the risk factors for functional decline that signal the need for CGA and aggressive, carefully aimed interventions.

As the field has matured, some degree of consensus has emerged regarding many, but not all, aspects of geriatric assessment. Geriatricians have come to understand that CGA, while demonstrably improving health outcomes, is not a panacea on its own. It is simply a valuable beginning of the process of enlightened care of elders.

The greatest obstacle to achieving optimal care of the elderly patient is often at the transition between the team performing the CGA and the primary care physician (PCP). If the PCP is part of the team, there is no problem. However, if the CGA is performed as a consultation, special care must be taken in transmitting the findings and recommendations to the PCP. Proper implementation may require attempts to influence both the PCP and the patient. For the former, telephone contact, in addition to a written consultation report and recommendations, buttressed by key literature references, appears to increase compliance. It is also helpful to share the consultation report and recommendations with the patient and to take steps to empower the patient to discuss openly with the PCP his/her wishes regarding implementation of the recommendations.

Geriatrics is principally concerned with long-term care. CGA is the *sine qua non* in meeting the objective of improved long-term care. Therefore, this volume should be of great value to all health care professionals caring for elderly patients. The field of CGA is still in a growth phase. Thus, even as the first edition of this volume comes to publication, I would express the hope that a second edition be planned for the not-too-distant future, when it may be hoped the indications for and utility of CGA will have become more firmly established.

David H. Solomon, M.D.
UCLA School of Medicine
Los Angeles, CA
The RAND Corporation
Santa Monica, CA

Comprehensive geriatric assessment (CGA) was developed in the early 1970s and has proliferated since that time. Conceptually, it borrowed heavily from the methodologies of rehabilitation. It is of interest historically that the report of the Technical Committee on Health Services of the 1981 White House Conference on Aging recommends combining annual assessments with preventive services.

Various settings and formats for CGA have been reported including inpatient geriatric evaluation units, inpatient geriatric consultation, ambulatory geriatric assessment clinics and in-home assessment programs. Most reports of effectiveness have been institution-based, and randomized controlled studies have demonstrated important benefits, the most dramatic of which were first documented in in-hospital programs. However, even in academic settings, the assessment process, settings for CGA, persons targeted and the personnel involved have not been uniform. Some effectiveness studies have demonstrated significant benefits including improvements in diagnostic accuracy, placement, functional status, affect, cognition and survival, as well as reduction in medications, use of hospital services, nursing home days, and overall medical costs. Each of these benefits has not been demonstrated in every study. The inconsistencies of findings have been postulated as due to the following limitations: (1) basic flaws in study design; (2) small sample sizes; (3) homogenous settings of patient populations such as in the Department of Veterans Affairs or in academic medical centers where many of the studies have been done; (4) selection criteria for study populations; (5) patient gender; (6) different levels and types of care in control groups, ranging from usual care by attending professionals to enhanced care similar to CGA; (7) adherence of participants and/or their providers; and, most recently (8) the training and continuing competence of the professional responsible for the process. Recent evidence has suggested that this is a critical factor in obtaining positive outcomes.

In addition, there have been differences in the interventions which make comparisons of reported studies difficult. These include: the timing of the intervention; variable patient lengths of stay for delivery of the intervention in hospital settings; assessment approaches such as geriatric assessment units as compared with consultation teams; strategies aimed at restorative treatment as contrasted with prevention of functional decline; and the interven-

tion strategies themselves. Some studies have offered recommendations only, while others have implemented recommendations, and
still others have provided specialized follow-up care.

These controversies were resolved except for the in-home assessment setting by a meta-analysis reported in 1993. This analysis
clearly demonstrated that CGA with strong long-term management
is effective for improving survival and function in elders. Most
recently, one of us, with colleagues, has completed an updated
meta-analysis of randomized trials of preventive home visits.
Among 870 papers, 13 randomized trials meeting *a priori* inclu-
sionary criteria were identified. Favorable effects were shown on
mortality, nursing home admissions, and functional status outcomes. Intervention programs including three components were
significantly associated with more favorable outcomes. These included (1) the use of multidimensional geriatric assessment as the
initial evaluation method; (2) giving recommendations to elders;
and (3) extended follow-up of the intervention with subsequent
home visits.

The issue of targeting the multidimensional assessment process
remains controversial, in part, because of the conceptual expansion
of the process to include the objective of prevention of loss of
independence. The initial objective of CGA was to identify elders
at high risk and develop programs combining rehabilitation or
tertiary prevention and improved care coordination. The whole
process focused primarily on the special needs of very frail elders,
who because of the complexity of the clinical presentations and
needs, required a special approach to their assessment and care,
usually not available in most standard settings.

When assessment is primarily targeted at identification of risk
factors for functional decline and the development of intervention
programs to prevent or delay impairment, there is now compelling
evidence that these efforts need to be addressed in low risk elders.
It has been shown that for high risk elders preventive assessments
and interventions have no favorable effects on outcomes and, under
certain circumstances, might have unfavorable effects. Further
studies identifying those predictive criteria for identifying elders
who would clearly benefit from either of these assessment strategies
are needed.

Geriatrics has focused primarily on the management of acute
and chronic conditions in frail elders with less emphasis on promotion of health and prevention of disease than in younger populations including children. The growing body of knowledge about
disease/problem prevention in later life suggests a valid basis for
strengthening efforts in preventive geriatrics. Assessment of risk
factors is clearly an important element of such a strategy.

It is important to emphasize that intervention effects such as
CGA are often diluted when applied to large-scale community

programs in the real world. Standardizing the multiple steps in CGA outside the research setting is difficult, and subtle changes in the intervention often result in lower levels of effectiveness. This ongoing monitoring of community programs of this type is an essential element for successful outcomes.

In the early phases of the evolution of American geriatrics and gerontology, CGA was defined by the 1987 National Institute of Health Consensus Development Conference as being "a multidisciplinary evaluation in which the multiple problems of older persons are uncovered, described, and explained, if possible, and in which the resources and strengths of the person are catalogued, need for services assessed, and a coordinated care plan developed to focus interventions on the person's problems. At that time it was viewed as being truly multidisciplinary, with many health professionals each contributing their special knowledge and skills to the process. With the emerging cost constraints, increased interest in cost effectiveness as well as practicability, the composition of the assessment team changed. In many instances only one health professional type is involved, calling upon other health professionals as need arises. Simultaneously, the term multidimensional assessment came into usage, and today CGA and multidimensional assessment are used interchangeably.

Other terminology, such as "interdisciplinary" and "multidisciplinary" are used interchangeably as well. Recognizing the semantic difference, the reader may find it used as interdisciplinary in particular settings and multidisciplinary in others. This may indicate process differences rather than conceptual differences. In sites where team members are present most of the time (i.e., a nursing home with a medical staff model) the practice may involve frequent face-to-face meetings of all specialties involved in the client's care; while in others (i.e., acute hospital, office) they will communicate differently (phone, notes); the input by all team members plays a role in the decision-making process carried out usually by one representative of the team.

Our implied definition of long-term care throughout the volume is a broad one and includes any aspect of the care of elders that is provided over a long period of time. It implies that this care may occur in many settings and that an effective coordination of the care across these various settings is an essential component.

The editors embarked on the monumental task of describing the process and skills required to conduct a CGA throughout the continuum of long-term care. The design takes into account the changes in the practice of medicine and the increased pace, calling for time efficiency, while maintaining quality.

Originally we envisioned an innovative format utilizing color-coded text with sidebar margin boxes and illustrations, allowing the busy reader to access and retrieve information quickly so it could be implemented in practice. This process started with the California Geriatric Education Center project whose objective had been to improve the knowledge and skills of medical directors in long-term care institutions. The Medical Directors' Guide, which was published in a binder format, attracted the attention of publishers in the field of aging. In 1995, we were approached by a new publisher, a parternship venture created by a non-profit organization and a proprietary publisher. While none of us was preparing to write another text, we were lured into the project by the appealing promise of creating a flagship of a "new generation of publications" utilizing an exciting format, and teaching skills rather than being just another textbook. Our enthusiasm enabled us to convince an impressive list of the best in the field to produce this manuscript. Almost two years later, when we were near the end of the process, the publisher declared itself bankrupt. The remaining partners of the venture withheld the manuscript for over a year despite a clear contract guaranteeing the return of the manuscript. More than three years from the inception of this project, we finally received the manuscript. Although we realized enough time had elapsed to necessitate starting all over again, we rejected the thought of abandoning the project—out of respect for the contributors' hard work and a sense of responsibility to you, the reader, who was seeking out this kind of information. After almost five years, the longest time any of us has spent writing a book the publication of this first edition brings this saga to a bittersweet ending.

The present format is a compromise we had to make, abandoning the illustration and color-coding for a more traditional format. Recognizing that CGA is a work in progress requiring constant updating to fill in the gaps in our knowledge, we are grateful to the contributors for their overwhelming response and willingness to rewrite the chapters to make them current.

The editors were able to recruit Mary Bail at the inception of this project. She had just completed playing a major role as the Managing Editor of the Journal of the American Geriatrics Society under David H. Solomon's leadership. The qualities which she displayed during that tenure period were carried through the difficult management task related to this volume. The editors acknowledge that without her guidance and assistance, this volume would not have been published. We are grateful for this valuable contribution.

Above all we are thankful to our patients throughout our careers and our mentors and trainees who have enriched our knowledge and experience, allowing us the privilege of editing this text.

Dan Osterweil
Kenneth Brummel-Smith
John C. Beck

Contents

SECTION I: GENERAL ISSUES AND IMPLICATIONS FOR USE OF ASSESSMENT TOOLS

SECTION II: A: ASSESSMENT TOOLS AND THEIR APPLICATIONS

SECTION II: B: COMMON PROBLEMS

GENERAL ISSUES AND COMPREHENSIVE APPROACH TO ASSESSMENT OF ELDERS

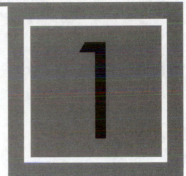

REBECCA ELON / CHERYL PHILLIPS / JOHN F. LOOME / SUSAN DENMAN / ANITA WOODS

INTRODUCTION

The Importance of Comprehensive Assessment in Caring for Elders

Comprehensive assessment is a clinical approach for assisting elders to achieve their best possible health and highest level of function. For elders with chronic illness and functional impairment, comprehensive assessment provides the information that is essential in formulating clinical recommendations and plans of care. In addition to evaluating a person's medical status, a comprehensive assessment evaluates realms outside of the traditional medical purview, such as the following:

1. A person's preference for what sort of care they might prefer in various situations.
2. His or her functional capabilities and disabilities.
3. The financial resources available to purchase care.
4. Whether or not family members are available to provide assistance at home.

The Agency for Health Care Policy and Research (AHCPR) was renamed in December 1999.
This agency is now known as the Agency for Healthcare Research and Quality (AHRQ).

5. The mental or emotional strengths or weaknesses that can influence a person's health and level of functioning.

An expanded clinical approach is necessary to accurately define the important issues and create a plan focused on health, well-being, and functional capabilities.

The traditional approach to medical evaluation focuses on establishing the correct diagnoses so that the most appropriate, state-of-the-art treatments can be applied. The implicit goal is to fix or cure the problem.

In contrast to the traditional model that first establishes exact diagnoses, the comprehensive assessment involves setting goals and agendas before every diagnostic possibility is explored. In this way, the evaluation and treatment can become tailored to meet the needs of each person. This individualized, patient-centered focus enables health care providers to work more effectively to achieve desired outcomes.

Interdisciplinary Team Concept

The collection of information is the first step in clinical decision making. Health care providers are taught to gather information in a very structured format. Disciplines such as medicine, nursing, psychology, social work, occupational therapy, physical therapy, and speech-language therapy, all have their own standardized structured approaches to information gathering and clinical decision making. Physicians learn to take a history, perform a physical examination, and based upon the information gathered, to construct a list of possible disease entities that might be causing the patient's symptoms (the differential diagnosis). Laboratory studies including body fluid analysis, radiologic or other imaging studies, pathologic tissue examinations, and numerous basal or stimulated measures of physiologic performance may be ordered to further define and clarify which of the various diagnostic possibilities is causing the patient's symptoms. This is the core concept of the medical approach to clinical decision making: a patient presents with a symptom; the physician gathers the relevant information from the history, the physical exam, and the laboratory studies to make a diagnosis; the diagnosis leads to a therapeutic plan; and the goal of the treatment is to cure the underlying disease in order to return the patient to a state of health.

When the underlying disease process is chronic, the goals of the clinical process may change dramatically. Often, the goal in chronic illness is to improve the quality of life and attain the patient's highest possible level of functioning, physically, cognitively, emotionally, and/or socially. The goals can be to relieve symptoms, with less emphasis directed to determining the exact diagnosis. For end-stage conditions, the goals can be to maintain comfort and dignity or achieve a peaceful and meaningful death. As chronic illness becomes increasingly prevalent in the population, the "diagnose–treat–cure" paradigm becomes an inadequate model for clinical decision making.

Traditional medical education ignores the realities of the population with chronic illnesses and functional impairments. Medical students are not well educated in assessing functional ability or working effectively as team members with other health care disciplines. For example, if maximizing function is the goal for the patient, a very detailed analysis of the social support network becomes a critical part of the clinical information necessary to achieve the best outcomes. The underlying medical diagnosis may have secondary importance. The traditional physician's medical history includes only a cursory investigation into the social support system. The assessment performed by a social worker could adequately elucidate the patient's support status and define areas for intervention. In addition, functional capacity may be highly dependent on a person's cognitive abilities. Defining areas of cognitive strength and weaknesses may be more important than determining the etiology of the dementia for many individuals. Defining the potential impact of deficits on function can become more important than the actual deficits themselves. Neuropsychological testing can contribute to formulating an effective plan for compensating for the deficits. When function is limited by mobility or self-care deficits, a physiatrist or physical or occupational therapist may provide the important evaluations of physical function and environmental barriers to help create an appropriate therapeutic plan (see Chapter 2).

Treatment of elders with functional deficits due to chronic illness requires the skills of multiple disciplines. A multidisciplinary approach implies that many different disciplines are involved. An interdisciplinary approach implies that different disciplines are working together in a coordinated fashion to achieve patient-centered goals. In today's cost-conscious environment, a large number of team members may not be justifiable for every frail elder's care. Therefore, individual health care practitioners must be knowledgeable in areas that go beyond the boundaries of their specific disciplines. A multidimensional approach can be performed by one or two health care providers, but draws from a large number of different clinical disciplines. Social workers must understand the relevance of medical issues. Physicians must understand the relevance of social issues in constructing a treatment plan. Nurses must understand the person's progress in therapy. Therapists must understand nursing issues to maximize a person's progress. Each discipline must acquire a breadth of knowledge that exceeds the traditional scope of their training. Each health care provider must also know when more in-depth analysis requiring a referral or formal consultation from another discipline is in order. Health care providers who lack either breadth of knowledge across disciplines or depth of knowledge in their specific discipline will be unable to provide adequate care for elders with chronic illness and functional impairment.

Health status, physical capacity, cognitive ability, mood and behavior, social support, and the environment can all contribute to the treatment goals and outcomes for a person with chronic illness and functional impairment. The assessment tools presented in this book will help health care providers to gather information that may be outside of their discipline-specific training or gather it in a way that is more useful in addressing the clinical issues in chronic illness. These tools offer a structure for the systematic collection of information that can help health care providers of various backgrounds evaluate common problems of elders and develop an appropriate plan of care.

This text is not intended to supplant the traditional approaches to clinical information gathering and clinical decision making that are specific to the various clinical disciplines, but rather to help a broad array of health care providers gather information in a manner that should translate into the relevant maximum clinical benefit for elders with chronic illness.

DEMOGRAPHICS OF AGING— THE IMPERATIVE

The demand for chronic health services is fueled by the burgeoning growth in the numbers of older Americans. In 1991, 12.5 percent of the U.S. population of 252 million was 65 years or older. The rate of population growth from 1980 to 1991 for the total population was 11.3 percent. This compares to a growth rate of 24.2 percent for the over-65 years group and a remarkable 41 percent growth rate for the over-85 years group. It is anticipated that by the year 2030, there will be 65 million Americans over 65 years of age, 20 percent of the total population. These numbers will strain the health care delivery system and challenge us to develop more effective means of managing chronic illnesses and disabilities. The fastest growing over-85 cohort is the heaviest user of nursing home care. In 1985, 22 percent of the people in this age group resided in nursing homes.[1] The 1.3 million nursing home residents in 1985 represented a 200 percent increase since 1963. Between 1985 and 1993, the number of nursing home residents rose to 1.7 million people. The early rapid growth rate is related to the enactment of Medicare and Medicaid legislation in 1995. Subsequently, the rate of growth of the nursing home population slowed to 17 percent from 1977 to 1985; and between 1992 and 1993, the number of nursing home beds increased by only 1 percent. There are approximately 16,700 nursing homes with 1.8 million residents at any one time in the United States.[2] There is a wide range in the estimates of the number of assisted-living facilities nationwide due to various interpretations of what constitutes one. One estimate at the beginning of 1998 put the number at 11,472 facilities, with approximately 650,500 beds and 558,400 residents.[3] The growth of assisted-living facilities in the 1990s contributed to the decreased growth in nursing home beds, providing alternatives for elders requiring activities of daily living (ADL) support.

Figure 1-1 illustrates an estimate of the number of elders who will need long-term care services in the next several decades.[4] In 1994, it was estimated that three quarters of older Americans who needed help performing 3 or more activities of daily living currently lived in the community rather than in a residential setting. The U.S. Senate Special Committee on Aging estimated that 80 percent of people age 65 years and older have one or more chronic illnesses. Approximately 40 percent report disability from chronic illness. The health care of most people with chronic illness and disability will be delivered in community and home health care settings. Although it is anticipated that the need for nursing home beds will grow in the coming decade, the variety of levels of care provided will also continue to expand.[5] These currently include assisted living, traditional nursing home care, subacute (also called post-acute care), subacute and skilled nursing facility for rehabilitation, respite care, and inpatient hospice care. Whereas the chronic nursing home stay has not changed, the length of stay in acute hospitals and post-acute care skilled nursing facilities has shortened. A greater variety

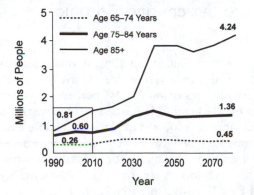

FIGURE 1-1   Projected growth in the number of nursing facility residents. *Source:* U.S. Bureau of the Census, 1986 Statistical Abstract of the United States.

and number of community-based health care services will be necessary. Although home health services consume the smallest percentage of personal health care expenditure, they represent the highest rate of growth. From 1988 to 1996, expenditures increased an average of 31 percent annually from approximately $2 billion to $17 billion. The rise in spending is attributed to the increase in the number of beneficiaries receiving home health services rather than higher payments per visit.[6] Because of the growth in the number of older Americans, increasing numbers of people with chronic illnesses and disabilities are anticipated. Although rates of age-adjusted disability have diminished in recent years, the longevity gain is still divided into years of active life expectancy and dependent life expectancy. The death rates for the two leading causes of mortality, cardiovascular and cerebrovascular diseases, have declined for the older population. As the incidence of acute stroke and its mortality decline, the prevalence of stroke survivors is increasing. Comprehensive geriatric assessment is essential to minimize disability and prevent further morbidity by targeting persons for rehabilitation services and primary, secondary, and tertiary prevention strategies.

The most significant causes of morbidity in the older population, such as arthritis and dementia, often lead to physical or cognitive disability requiring long-term care services. It is estimated that 50 percent of those 65 years and older have arthritis and that a third or more of those 85 years and older suffer from dementia. Comprehensive assessment is an essential part of the health care for older adults with physical or cognitive impairment, or both.

CURRENT SYSTEMS OF CARE

Acute Care System and Chronic Care System

When Medicare was enacted in 1965, it was intended to provide access to the health care system for elderly and disabled Americans.[7, 8] Currently approximately 98 percent of older Americans are covered by Medicare. Medicare Part A covers hospitalization costs. Participants are required to pay a deductible and copayment. If skilled home care services or skilled nursing home services are needed after an acute hospitalization, Medicare provides limited benefits in these realms. A comparison of the benefits of Medicare Part A and Part B is illustrated in Table 1-1.

Participation in Medicare Part B is voluntary and requires the payment of monthly fee for coverage. Virtually all but a few percent of older Americans with the automatic Medicare Part A benefit,

TABLE 1-1. COMPARISON OF MEDICARE PART A AND MEDICARE PART B

	MEDICARE PART A	MEDICARE PART B
Financing	From the special Medicare portion of the Social Security tax, which is accrued into the Hospital Insurance Trust Fund.	From general tax revenues (75%) and by premiums paid by enrollees (25%). The current premium is $43.80/month.
Reimbursement	Payments from this fund are made to providers through selected private insurance companies (Medicare Intermediaries). Payment to hospitals is based on a prospective payment system based on classification AT DISCHARGE of the diagnostic related group for which the person was ADMITTED (with exceptions for surgical procedures, etc.). Payment to home-care services and nursing homes is based on modified costs with limits based on average costs.	Funds are disbursed from the Medicare Supplemental Trust Fund via carriers. There is a yearly $100 deductible on Part B services and most services require a 20% copayment. Reimbursement is as follows: Physicians: payments based on Medicare fee schedule: RVUs including physician work, malpractice, and office expense components × base rate per RVU in $ = fee schedule. Physicians must either accept fee schedule and bill Medicare carrier directly, or bill patient an amount equal to no more than 115% of Medicare fee schedule. Clinical laboratory: mostly based on set fee schedule (no deductible for patient). Home-health care: (ONLY if no Part A with no deductible)—Modified charges. Outpatient hospital: Modified cost-based reimbursement.
Eligibility	Aged (65 and over) OR blind or disabled and receiving Social Security or Railroad Retirement for 24 months OR end-stage renal disease (dialysis or transplant) AND have, either directly or through a spouse, paid Social Security taxes for a specified number of quarters and eligible for Social Security benefits. (NOTE: Others 65 and over can pay premium to get Medicare [currently $311/month for Part A] and Medicare is SECONDARY to other insurance plans if person continues to work.)	All who qualify for Part A are enrolled in Part B—but must pay premium of $43.80 to remain enrolled.
Benefits	Medicare Part A reimburses for most hospital and hospice care and some home and skilled nursing care.	Medical physician services Mental health services (with 50% copayment) Outpatient PT/OT (with cap of $720/yr) Outpatient laboratory and radiology Durable medical equipment Ambulance services Speech and language therapy Pneumococcal and influenza immunizations

Abbreviations: OT, occupational therapy, PT, physical therapy, and RVUs, relative value units.

Reprinted with permission from the American Geriatrics Society.

TABLE 1-2. COVERAGE FOR SERVICES UNDER THE MEDICARE PROGRAM, PART A, HOSPITAL INSURANCE, 1997		
COVERAGE	SERVICES INCLUDED	CONDITIONS THAT MUST BE MET
Inpatient general hospital care	Semiprivate room, special units, laboratory, x-ray, medication, supplies, blood (except for first 3 units), meals, nursing (not private duty)	Care ordered by physician; care can be provided only in hospital for stay approved by peer-review organization
Inpatient skilled nursing care in a certified nursing facility	Semiprivate room, rehabilitation services, meals, nursing, medications, use of appliances	Most follow within 30 days of a 3-day-or-longer hospital stay, for a condition related to reason for NF admission; care ordered by physician; care approved by Medicare intermediary
Home-health care	Part-time skilled nursing, PT, ST, OT; part-time home-health aide and medical equipment also covered if skilled nursing, PT, ST needed	Be homebound and require intermittent (up to 21 days) skilled nursing, PT, ST, ordered by physician and approved by Medicare intermediary
Hospice care	Inpatient and outpatient nursing, physician, drugs, PT, ST, OT, homemaker, counseling, inpatient respite (5 days or less) care, medical and social services	Patient certified by a physician as "terminally" ill; patient chooses hospice over standard Medicare benefits for terminal illness

Abbreviations: NF, nursing facility, OT, occupational therapy, PT, physical therapy, and ST, speech therapy.

Reprinted with permission from the American Geriatrics Society.

which accompanies the Social Security benefit, also sign up for the voluntary Part B coverage. Part B pays for physician services and other items (see Tables 1-2 and 1-3).

Over the years since Medicare's enactment, various preventive services have been added to its coverage. Vaccinations currently recommended for elders, such as the pneumococcal vaccine and influenza vaccine, are covered services. Annual mammography, Pap smears, colorectal cancer screening, bone densitometry, diabetic supplies, and education have all been designated covered services in recent years (see Tables 1-3 and 1-4 for lists of services and their coverage).

Despite some progress in adding preventive services to Medicare's coverage and despite limited coverage for post-acute skilled care in the home or nursing home, Medicare remains a principal form of insurance coverage for acute care needs. That is to say, Medicare pays for hospitalization cost for acute illnesses, for some services immediately following hospitalization, and for physician services in the clinic, hospital emergency room, or nursing home setting.

In 1997, Congress authorized several new options for Medicare recipients, including a limited medical savings account plan, a private fee-for-service plan, and a provider sponsored organization

TABLE 1-3.   COVERAGE FOR SERVICES UNDER THE MEDICARE PROGRAM, PART B, MEDICAL INSURANCE, 1997

COVERAGE[a]	SERVICES INCLUDED	CONDITIONS THAT MUST BE MET
Physician services	Medical and surgical services, diagnostic procedures, radiology, pathology, drugs and biologicals that cannot be self-administered	Care medically necessary for diagnosis and management of acute or chronic illness; care approved by Medicare carrier; may be delivered in hospital, office, or clinic, nursing facility, home visit
Mental health services	Outpatient therapy for mental illness by physician, psychologist, or in comprehensive rehabilitation outpatient setting	As above
Hospital outpatient services	Ambulatory surgery services incident to services of physician, diagnostic tests (laboratory, x-ray), ED, hospital-based medical supplies	Care approved by Medicare carrier
Independent laboratory	Clinical diagnostic laboratory	Care ordered by physician
Independent physical or occupational therapy	Rehabilitative outpatient therapy	Care ordered by physician
Durable medical equipment	Wheelchairs, oxygen equipment (but not oxygen)	For use in home; to serve a medical purpose for people who are sick or injured

Abbreviation: ED, emergency department.

[a]Beneficiaries must pay a monthly premium of $43.80 per month for coverage.

Reprinted with permission from the American Geriatrics Society.

TABLE 1-4.   ADDITIONAL SERVICES NOT COVERED BY MEDICARE

Acupuncture
Chronic, ongoing home care services
Chronic, long-term nursing home services
Cosmetic surgery
Dental care
Hearing services
Hospital care over 210 days of a benefit period
Mental health services (outpatient services require a 50% copayment)
Prescription drugs that are self-administered
Preventive foot care except for patients with diseases such as diabetes or peripheral vascular disease
Routine eye care or eye glasses
Routine (preventive) history and physical examinations (most screening tests are covered)

Modified with permission of the American Geriatrics Society.

(PSO) or preferred provider (PPO) plan. The impact of the diversification of Medicare remains to be seen. In 1998, many managed care companies withdrew their Medicare products, leaving seniors with fewer choices among the remaining Medicare HMO plans. Many elders resumed their traditional Medicare benefit, resulting in greater out-of-pocket expenses for Medi-gap policies or prescription drugs that are not covered under traditional Medicare.

None of the old or new Medicare products covers much of the cost of the long-term care or chronic care services required by people who need some human assistance every day just to live their daily lives. Most of the human assistance provided to disabled people comes from family members or friends. This is known as the *informal support system.* When the disabled person's needs exceed or exhaust their informal support system or when the disabled person lacks an informal support system, the *formal support system* is called upon to provide services. The formal support system is typically referred to in terms of services provided in the community, *community-based long-term care,* or to a person living in an institution, *institutional long-term care* (Tables 1-5 and 1-6). The term "long-term care" generally refers to the medical, nursing, social, and personal care services required by individuals with chronic illness and functional disabilities (see Chapters 9 and 26).

TABLE 1-5. INFORMAL AND FORMAL SYSTEMS OF CARE

Informal system
  Family, friends
Formal system—Community-based care
  Care management
  Home health aide for personal care
  Chore services/homemaker services
  Meals on Wheels
  Congregate meal sites
  Home delivery of groceries, medications, etc.
  Respite care services
  Day care services
  Skilled nursing, physical therapy, occupational therapy, and speech-
    language therapy
  Home medical visits
  Home laboratory, x-ray, and other diagnostic services
Formal system—Institutional care
  Nursing homes
  Board and care homes
  Foster homes
  Residential care facilities
  Chronic psychiatric facilities

TABLE 1-6. EXAMPLES OF HOME AND COMMUNITY-BASED SERVICES	
SERVICE	DESCRIPTION
Care management	Assists beneficiaries in getting medical, social, educational, and other services.
Personal care	Included bathing, dressing, ambulation, feeding, grooing, and some household services such as meal preparation and shopping.
Adult day care	Includes personal care and supervision and may include physical, occupational, and speech therapies. Also provides socialization and recreational activities adapted to compensate for any physical or mental impairments.
Respite care	Provides relief to the primary caregiver of a chronically ill or disabled beneficiary. By providing services in the beneficiary's or provider's home or in other settings, respite care allows the primary caregiver to be absent for a time.
Homemaker	Assists beneficiaries with general household activities and may include cleaning, laundry, meal planning, grocery shopping, meal preparation, transportation to medical services, and bill paying.

From GAO Report, 1995.[2]

Although all but a few percent of older Americans have Medicare that provides protection for the majority of acute care costs, only a few percent of older Americans have long-term care insurance that provides protection against nursing home or home care costs. Although many private insurance policies, HMOs, and Medicare provide coverage for some nursing home and home care costs, these are generally post-acute in focus and quite limited in scope and duration. For example, Medicare pays less than 5 percent of all nursing home costs. In 1991, 43 percent of all nursing home care was paid for privately, as an out-of-pocket expense. Similarly, most older disabled people find they must pay privately out-of-pocket for the services that they need to stay at home. Even if there are the monetary resources to pay for in home assistance, it is difficult to find individuals willing or able to provide the service. People who are impoverished to the point of qualifying for the social welfare medical system, Medicaid, may have some home care services provided. Since Medicaid is a joint federal–state program, availability of services and monetary limits for qualifying for services vary greatly from state to state. In the climate of deficit

TABLE 1-7. SOURCES OF PAYMENT FOR SERVICES

Acute care
  Medicare, Medigap, private insurance, copayments and deductibles, and Medicaid
Long-term care[a]
  Private pay, Older Americans Act Programs, local governmental programs, private charitable sources, Medicaid, long-term care insurance, and Medicare (post-acute)

[a]See Chapter 26 for coverage.

reduction, the services offered by a state's Medicaid program or by the federal Medicare program today may not be available in the future. The Older Americans Act through the federal Administration on Aging and the states' Area Agencies on Aging provide some long-term care services to community-dwelling elders, but these programs are also at risk for significant budgetary pruning in the future.

Some funding for community-based long-term care services also comes from other local governmental sources, private religious, and not-for-profit organizations. Although acute medical services (hospital fees and physician fees) are usually paid for by one or two insurers (Medicare, Medigap, Medicaid, or private insurer), long-term care services are paid for by a patchwork of multiple resources, with out-of-pocket private pay being the largest category and informal caregiving network shouldering the most significant burden (Tables 1-7 and 1-8).

For every one disabled elder living in a nursing home in the United States, there are three equally disabled people who are still living in the community. The major difference between the two groups is the scope and integrity of their respective informal support systems. Although most people indicate that they would rather receive care in their own homes than in an institutional setting, the current system of reimbursement favors institutionalization.

Institutional Care

Prior to the passage of the Social Security Act in the 1930s, older, infirm people who did not have family to care for them typically ended up in alms houses. One of the initial provisions of the Social Security Act was that the payments received by older Americans under the act could not be used to pay for services from a public institution. This led to private enterprises that offered to care for older, infirm people in exchange for receiving their social security check. The private enterprise of providing care for older, infirm

TABLE 1-8. MAJOR FEDERAL PROGRAMS SUPPORTING LONG-TERM CARE SERVICES FOR ELDERS AND PERSONS WITH DISABILITIES			
PROGRAM	OBJECTIVES	ADMINISTRATION	LONG-TERM CARE SERVICES
Medicaid/Title XIX of the Social Security Act	To pay for medical assistance for certain low-income persons	Federal: HCFA/HHS State: State Medicaid Agency	Nursing home care, home and community-based health and social services, facilities for persons with mental retardation, chronic care hospitals
Medicare/Title XVIII of the Social Security Act	To pay for acute medical care for the aged and selected disabled	Federal: HCFA/HHS State: None	Home health visits, limited skilled nursing facility care
Older Americans Act	To foster development of a comprehensive and coordinated service system to serve elders	Federal Administration on Aging/Office of Human Development, HHS State: State Agency on Aging	Nutrition services, home and community-based social services, protective services, and long-term care ombudsman
Rehabilitation Act	To promote and support vocational rehabilitation and independent living services for the disabled	Federal: Office of Special Education and Rehabilitative Services/Department of Education State: State Vocational Rehabilitation Agencies	Rehabilitation services, attendant and personal care, centers for independent living
Social Services Block Grant/Title XX of the Social Security Act	To assist families and individuals in maintaining self-sufficiency and independence	Federal: Office of Human Development Services, HHS State: State Social Services or Human Resources Agency; other state agencies may administer part of Title XX funds for certain groups; for example, State Agency on Aging	Services provided at the states' discretion, may include long-term care

Adapted from GAO/HEHS-95-109.

people began an exponential growth after the passage of the Medicare and Medicaid legislation in 1965. Although Medicaid was intended to provide medical services to the poor, it soon became a major payer source for people who needed institutional long-term care services by paying the nursing home bill for people who exhausted their resources and became impoverished by paying for their care. Today almost three quarters of the nursing homes in the United States are proprietary, profit-making enterprises, yet they receive almost half of their revenues from public Medicaid sources.

Nursing homes have dual roles of providing a home-like environment for the older infirm resident and providing professional services, that is, the personal care, psychological care, religious/spiritual care, and nursing and medical services required by the resident. On the one hand, the nursing home strives to substitute for a person's home. On the other hand, it is a health care institution. Some nursing homes failed to fulfill either role adequately, leading to newspaper exposes, congressional hearings, and the formation of citizen advocacy groups for nursing home reform in the 1970s. With the advent of the Medicare prospective payment system to hospitals in the 1980s, there was incentive and pressure to discharge older patients more quickly from the hospital into less costly settings such as the nursing home. The higher medical acuity and needs of the nursing home patients coming from the hospital settings led many nursing homes to reexamine the medical care being delivered to their patients and residents. In the 1990s, many nursing homes decided to increase the level of medical and nursing service they provided in the formation of "subacute care" units. These units accept patients who require medical and nursing services, but at a less intense acuity than provided in an acute hospital. For example, patients needing intravenous antibiotics, analgesia, anticoagulation, parenteral nutrition, extensive wound care, or rehabilitative therapies can be appropriately cared for in a subacute unit. The development of such units has been driven by market forces, with managed care organizations seeking the lowest per diem cost and the nursing homes seeking the highest per diem reimbursement. Managed care organizations allowed patients to be directly admitted to a subacute unit from the community or emergency room in lieu of hospitalization to decrease the cost of treating such conditions as deep vein thrombosis, pneumonia, or urinary tract infection. Subacute care challenges the nursing home's basic balance between being a home for the long-stay residents versus being a medical institution for its short-stay patients.

In 1998, the prospective payment system (PPS) for Medicare Part A skilled nursing care caused some subacute units to close and others to actively change their case mix to maintain profitability. The long-term impact of PPS on subacute care remains to be seen.

In 1982, Congress directed the Health Care Financing Administration (HFCA) to undertake a study of how to improve the quality of nursing home care through improved regulation of the nursing home industry. The Institute of Medicine was given the responsibility of conducting a study and making recommendations to HCFA. The recommendations were published in 1986 and served as a blueprint for regulatory reform legislation that was passed in 1987. A major component of this legislation was the requirement that all persons admitted to a nursing home would undergo a comprehensive, standardized, assessment of their functional, cognitive, social, medical, and nursing needs at the time of admission in order to have an adequate database from which to generate an individualized plan of care. The standardized assessment tool, known as the Minimum Data Set (MDS), is now used nationwide to determine reimbursement categories under PPS, as well as clinical care planning (see Chapter 9).[9-19] When specific problems are identified, the MDS then triggers the use of one of the following resident assessment protocols (RAP) that guide follow-up and care planning.

1. Activities
2. Feeding tubes
3. ADL function/rehab potential
4. Physical restraints
5. Behavior problem
6. Psychotropic drug use
7. Cognitive loss/dementia
8. Pressure ulcers
9. Communication
10. Psychosocial well-being
11. Dehydration/fluid maintenance
12. Mood state
13. Delirium
14. Nutritional status
15. Dental care
16. Urinary incontinence and indwelling catheter
17. Falls
18. Visual function

Multiple factors contribute to the difficulty of multidimensional assessment. First, simple point-in-time measurements are impossible given the functional status changes that can occur day-to-day. Second, with cognitive impairments so prevalent in the nursing home self-report measurements are unreliable. Last, information necessary to complete such a tool is found across many sources i.e., medical records, licensed nurses, nursing assistants, the residents themselves, and the residents' families. Studies addressing the reliability of the MDS across settings as a research tool reveal mixed results.[9-19]

The emphasis on the minimum data set reflects the fact that the collection of accurate comprehensive information is the first step to providing high quality care to older patients with multiple conditions and functional limitations.[20] Accurate assessment is also the first step to payment for post-acute care under the Medicare Prospective Payment System.

Two critical areas for the assessment of nursing home residents are the determination of the resident's capacity to understand and make decisions and the documentation regarding his or her desires for intensity of treatment (see Chapters 24 and 25). Both of these require significant input and participation on the part of the primary care provider. Since the determination of capacity significantly affects all other aspects of care planning, it should be made with a thoughtful, measurable process. Bedside mental status testing, tools such as the Folstein Mini-Mental Status Exam or the Short Portable Mental Status Exam (see Chapter 3 and Appendix #s 29 and 41), can screen for the presence of cognitive impairment but cannot determine decision-making capacity.[21] Even moderately demented individuals may be able to participate in some decision making, articulating their preferences and desires. The assessment should include whether or not individuals can understand the issue being discussed, weigh the options in terms of their values, and communicate their understanding and preferences back to the interviewer. Such discussions, as well as related diagnoses that contribute to lack of capacity, need to be documented in the medical record. Discussions concerning advance directives should extend beyond cardiopulmonary resuscitation, to include the resident's/ family's wishes regarding issues such as artificial hydration and nutrition and hospitalization. For patients with end-stage disease such discussions may also include desired intensity of treatment for such "treatable" conditions as urinary tract infections, pneumonia, and dehydration. These discussions allow the physician, patient, and family to talk openly about the dying process and their fears and beliefs. It is also important to remember that such discussions are not limited to the admission, but often need to be readdressed at times of acute illness and functional decline (see Chapter 25).

Assessment of the nursing home resident actually begins prior to admission.[22] Information regarding the individual's functional status and medical and nursing needs is submitted with the application for admission to determine eligibility for services, often referred to as the "level of care determination." This process typically also includes results of TB screening (PPD or chest x-ray). Federal law also requires that applicants for admission to the nursing home be assessed for the presence of active psychiatric disease or mental retardation. This is known as the PASAR (pre-admission screening and referral) process. It is intended to identify individuals who may not be appropriate for care in a nursing home because of special needs.

Once the individual is admitted to the nursing home, the nursing staff perform an assessment of vital signs, weight, skin integrity, functional capacity, and bowel and bladder function. Initial orders for medications and treatments are typically transcribed by the nurses from hospital discharge summaries or clinic notes accompanying the individual. Most nursing facilities require the physician's history and physical examination (H&P) to be performed within 48 hours after admission, although in postacute units admitting patients with higher medical acuity, same day H&Ps may be necessary. The postacute care patient may require an assessment that is more comparable to an acute hospital or rehabilitation patient than a long-stay nursing home resident (see Chapter 9).

Home Care

In the nineteenth century and into the early twentieth century, medical care in the home was the rule rather than the exception (see Chapter 8). Hospitals were places where people went to die. Rates of hospital-acquired infection were high. Surgical techniques were crude. The physician could take most of the diagnostic and therapeutic equipment into the home. Transporting an ill patient to a hospital was problematic and once the patients arrived, there was not a great deal more that could be done for the person in the hospital setting than could have been done in the home.

Advances in medical technology led to a dramatic shift in the location of care in the twentieth century. As diagnostic techniques such as body fluid analysis, ECG, and x-ray and other imaging techniques progressed, the patient needed to be brought to the center where these interventions were available. As drug therapies, intravenous therapies, and surgical techniques became more sophisticated, acutely ill patients could benefit from the vast resources of the modern hospital. Ambulance transportation with emergency medical technicians allowed for diagnostic and therapeutic interventions to begin prior to arrival at the hospital.

With the dramatic increase in the number of older Americans with functional impairment, for whom transport to the doctors office or hospital may be problematic, excessively burdensome, and costly, home-based care is regaining its place in American medicine. Many of the diagnostic techniques once only available in the hospital can now be brought into a person's home (e.g., blood and body fluid analysis, x-ray, ultrasound, and ECG). Therapies, which a decade ago were rare or unheard of in the home setting, are now common place (e.g., intravenous antibiotics, analgesia, parenteral nutrition, hemodialysis, peritoneal dialysis, and chronic ventilator support).

Hospice care, in which the focus is on comfort and dignity of the dying patient and family support, allowing people to die in the comfort of their own homes without the high technology intervention of the hospital, is becoming increasingly common.

There are two separate forces driving the increase in home care services. One force is the rejection of high technology interventions for the terminally ill and for those with end stage, incurable diseases. For these people, home care provides a focus on quality of remaining life in familiar surroundings with family, friends, and pets. The other force driving use of home care services is the demand to decrease hospital length of stay and utilization. Because it may be less expensive to deliver therapies such as intervenous antibiotics in the home setting, managed care organizations increasingly utilize the high technology side of home care as a cost control mechanism.

Despite the growth in home care services covered by Medicare, Medicaid, and private insurers, it must be remembered that 75 percent of all care delivered in the home is done by informal, unpaid family or friends of the impaired person without support from public funding sources. New models of community-based care are emerging to support the informal care network or substitute for it.

COMMUNITY-BASED LONG-TERM CARE MODELS

Program of All-Inclusive Care of the Elderly (PACE)

PACE began in San Francisco's Chinatown as the "On Lok" Program in the early 1970s.[23, 24] The purpose of the present PACE demonstration model is to provide comprehensive primary, specialty, acute and long-term care in a community-based setting. The focus is to maintain function and allow older frail people to remain in their homes and community. Participants must meet state nursing home eligibility criteria, that is, dependence in one or more activities of daily living (ADLs) such as feeding, ambulation, bathing, dressing, grooming, and toileting coupled with medical and/or nursing needs. In 1997, the average PACE enrollee was 80 years old, dependent in 2.9 ADLs, had 8.1 medical diagnoses, and stayed in the program 3 years (death is the usual reason for discharge). Reimbursement is based on capitated, pooled dollars from Medicare, based on the average annual per capita cost (AAPCC), and a Medicaid rate that is negotiated with each state. Individuals who are ineligible for Medicaid can pay privately for that portion of the capitated reimbursement. As of May 1998, there were 12 PACE sites fully operational in the United States, and nearly three times that number in development. With the passing of the 1997 Balanced Budget Act, Congress allowed PACE to become a recognized federal provider program rather than a demonstration project, allowing more sites to apply for funding.

PACE is a unique managed care program in that it serves only frail, older adults. Participants are enrolled for life (in contrast to other community-based programs that disenroll participants if they move to institutional care), and the care is provided through a tightly integrated interdisciplinary team process. Assessment is, therefore, critical to determine initial eligibility, as well as to provide the basis for a care plan and to track the functional status of the participant. PACE participants undergo a comprehensive assessment at the time of enrollment, on a quarterly basis, and annually. Episodic care is also provided, as needed, in the primary care clinic. The areas of assessment include nursing, medicine, rehabilitation services, social services, podiatry, dental, audiology, nutrition, and psychiatry.

Early in the replication project, On Lok saw the need for consistent data across all PACE sites. This data would be used to track overall program performance, assist in site and program management, and provide sites with comparative information for program evaluation and quality management. In addition to extensive utilization review, this data set, called "DataPace," tracks the following clinical and functional information over time: (1) average number of medical conditions; (2) percentage of patients needing assistance with bathing, feeding, dressing, transfering, grooming, walking, and toileting; and (3) average number of medications per enrollee per month.

Specific clinical data are also collected. The prevalence of particular diagnoses or conditions is based on annual assessment. The ten most common conditions for PACE enrollees, based on 1993 data were the following.

1. Diseases of the eye (53%)
2. Hypertension (52%)
3. Arthritis (50%)
4. Dementia (42%)
5. Cerebral vascular disease (35%)
6. Coronary artery disease (30%)
7. Peripheral vascular disease (25%)
8. Diabetes mellitus (25%)
9. Diseases of the ear (24%)
10. Depression/anxiety (23%)

The nursing evaluation provides a comprehensive review of the participant, including demographic data, medications, advance directives, behaviors, use of assistive devices and ADLs and IADLs (instrumental activities of daily living such as the use of transportation, shopping, cooking, cleaning, use the telephone and managing financial matters), use of assistive devices, and behaviors. As the PACE replication program continues to grow, such multicenter data will be invaluable for tracking functional changes in frail elders over time.

Assisted Living

Assisted living represents a broad array of service and settings meant to bridge the gap between total independent living and institutional care. In a housing service model, services typically include hotel-like options such as house cleaning, transportation, meals, and minimal ADL assistance (bathing, dressing, grooming). At the other end of the spectrum, a nursing home replacement model will often include ADL and IADL services, medication management, skin care, and ostomy and catheter care. Services are often "menu" driven, based on the client's needs and wishes. Although congregate areas are often used for meals and activities, the majority of individuals have private living quarters with their own belongings and a home-like atmosphere.

Such options of care are becoming increasingly popular with elders as they provide an option to nursing homes, and allow for more privacy and autonomy. Although room and board costs are usually less expensive than institutional long-term care, adding menu-driven services often make the overall costs comparable. Services are flexible and staff can fill multiple roles. Assisted-living settings are typically not as tightly regulated by outside agencies and may vary significantly. Although state and local regulations do exist, they are much broader in interpretation and usually safety based (i.e., fire codes, codes addressing whether or not residents can safely leave the building) or provide standards that attempt to specify whether or not a resident actually requires skilled nursing services that exceed the capacity of the assisted living staff (e.g., complicated wound care, infectious diseases that require isolation, IVs, etc.). When residents can no longer transfer, or require a feeding tube, or develop a stage 3 pressure lesion, they frequently must move to a skilled nursing facility or return home for in-home nursing care. Although resident safety has been the reasoning behind many of these regulations, residents may be prohibited from aging or dying in their chosen residential assisted-living setting.

In part, because of the lack of regulation, there is also an absence of a standardized assessment processes industry-wide. Most assisted-living facilities have a form that is required upon admission that identifies the following.

1. Medical problems
2. Allergies
3. Infectious disease
4. Medications
5. ADL capabilities
6. IADL capabilities
7. Cognitive status
8. Decision-making capacity

Most require a physical examination by a physician at the time of admission, but few do regularly scheduled reassessments. Several assisted-living centers have developed resident assessment tools that provide cumulative scoring for activities of daily living, instrumental activities of daily living, and cognitive status measures that can be tracked over time. This can be used to compare a resident's functional change over time as well as to compare entire populations within the facility (see Appendix #3).

Continuing Care Retirement Communities

Continuing care retirement communities (CCRCs) provide a unique approach to meeting the needs of elders as they age and require varying levels of service. In exchange for an entry fee and a monthly maintenance fee, the CCRC provides housing, social services, and nursing care that ranges from limited assessments in the independent section, to 24-hour nursing in the skilled nursing facility.[25] Levels of care built into the model span the spectrum from independent apartments or cottages with a congregate meal package to full-service skilled nursing beds. One study found that when compared to a community cohort, CCRC residents were more likely to be female, older, better educated, and had increased financial resources.[25] The goal of the CCRC model has been that of "aging in place," if not in one's own home, at least within the CCRC community. It is also in the CCRC's best interest to provide needed services that allow residents to stay in more independent settings and minimize the reliance on the few skilled nursing beds.

Regulations, as with more traditional assisted-living models, tend to be based on safety codes and assurances that residents do not require skilled nursing care more appropriately delivered in a nursing home. There is no formal assessment process in the industry. Typically, CCRCs have an enrollment screen that requires a physician history and physical exam and summary of present needs, including use of assistive devices, reliance on caregivers, or other in-home therapies. Most centers do not require annual or periodic assessment, but rely on the resident's expression of needs and the staff's ability to meet them to determine the appropriate "level of care." When conflict arises between the resident's desire for one level of care and the staff's perception of needs, the decisions are usually then based on the resident's primary care physician's assessment of service needs. This, along with relevant safety code issues (e.g., whether or not the resident can leave the building unassisted), determines the appropriate level. Some CCRCs have had rules regulating the use of assistive devices, such as walkers and wheelchairs, in the "independent side" of the community. This has recently been challenged through the Americans with Disability Act (ADA), which requires "reasonable accommodations for those persons with handicaps." Many centers have difficulty balancing "reasonable accommodation" and strict fire code regulations for congregate housing.

Social Health Maintenance Organization

The Social Health Maintenance Organization (SHMO) began in 1984 as a Health Care Financing Administration (HCFA) demonstration project involving four not-for-profit HMOs.[26] The purpose was to test models of community-based care to see if long-term care benefits could be delivered in a managed care setting. Seniors are enrolled in the program and the provider groups are reimbursed 100 percent of what it would cost HCFA in the fee-for-service market (based on the AAPCC). In comparison, Medicare risk HMOs receive 95 percent of the AAPCC. In exchange for the increased reimbursement, the SHMO providers have an expanded benefits package that typically includes drugs, eyeglasses, as well as long-term care benefits such as home health, personal care, skilled nursing, and therapy services. These benefits have historically been limited to $1,000 per month or $10,000 per year. The SHMO model differs from PACE in that enrollees are usually less frail and those persons requiring extended long-term care benefits would need to disenroll or pay out of pocket when their long-term care benefits are exhausted. The SHMO program, however, does offer a unique option for those individuals less frail or who need long-term-type care on a short-term basis. The second phase, SHMO II, consists of six sites selected in 1995, with a focus on rural care and end-stage renal disease. Comprehensive geriatric assessment is a new component of the SHMO II demonstration project.

Various models of capitated care and Medicare risk contracts have emerged as potential cost-saving models. Medicare and Medicaid waiver programs are emerging to test innovations in provision of and reimbursement for services. In one such model in the nursing home setting, an insurance company contracts with physicians to work with a nurse practitioner with the overall goal of improving the quality of medical care and reducing acute hospital utilization by providing more assessments and on-going medical management in the nursing home. This model is being implemented as a demonstration program at selected sites and will undergo evaluation of its cost effectiveness and quality of care.

Demonstration programs such as PACE and SHMOs can provide benefit for relatively small groups of older persons. There is, however, a great need to reach a larger population more effectively with current payor systems. The vertical integration of care utilizing existing payor systems is embraced by the National Chronic Care Consortium (NCCC). NCCC member organizations represent a variety of acute and chronic health care networks that have formed to meet the needs of older Americans as they move through the complex health care system. The goal of this organization is to provide a variety of models of integrated care systems across the continuum of acute and chronic health care settings. The movement of the health care delivery system to integrate acute and chronic services necessitates the availability of interdisciplinary assessments.

Integrated information systems are considered an essential component of integrated service systems. High quality care cannot occur without comprehensive assessment data available at all sites of care.

Comprehensive geriatric assessment programs are critically important to the process of matching care needs with appropriate support services to achieve the best outcome for a growing older population. It is clear that comprehensive assessment services will be essential to identify the most appropriate treatment plans to achieve optimal clinical outcomes for frail older Americans.

TEAM MEMBERS IN ASSESSMENT

Multidimensional geriatric evaluation can be performed in many different settings including the person's home, outpatient clinics, inpatient units, and nursing homes. Because the problems of elders are often complex and chronic, a broad base of knowledge and skills is required for the comprehensive assessment.

The basic unit for providing this care is an interdisciplinary team consisting of health care professionals from a variety of disciplines. The composition of these teams can vary by the circumstances and the site in which this evaluation process is taking place.

The terms "multidisciplinary" and "interdisciplinary" are often used interchangeably to describe this assessment approach; however, the distinctions between the two have been well documented.[27, 28]

A multidisciplinary assessment team is a group of health care providers sharing patient assessment information, but tending to work *independently* of one another in developing and implementing treatment plans. The interdisciplinary team is distinguished by the considerable amount of collaboration and coordination occurring among team members. Interacting both formally and informally, interdisciplinary team members work *interdependently*.

Each interdisciplinary team member contributes a unique body of knowledge and area of expertise to the patient assessments. Findings are shared among team members to obtain a biopsychosocial understanding of patients and their needs, their health problems, and their resources. This information is used to generate coordinated plans, which define the overall treatment goals and the role of each team member in working to accomplish them. Interdisciplinary teams also recognize that coordinated work demands attention to process goals, such as monitoring and evaluating relationships among team members and the quality of team functioning.

The spectrum between the loose network of consultants in a multidiscplinary team and the tightly integrated health care providers in an interdisciplinary team is wide and offers opportunities for innovation and customization of elder care across a range of practice settings. The interdisciplinary team model, in contrast to other models, highlights the following processes.

1. Integrated clinical care resulting from coordinated decision making and management, division of labor around common goals, shared responsibility for patient outcomes, and the ongoing evaluation of goals and outcomes.
2. Open and frequent communication that invites participation of the patient, family, and community in the diagnosis and management of health problems and which is encouraged and supported at the highest levels of the health care organization.
3. Training in team concepts that focuses on collaboration, communication, conflict resolution, flexibility in problem solving, role definition, and the changing nature of leadership.
4. Respect for the other team members as demonstrated by an open-minded attitude, the ability to acknowledge the contributions of others, and a valuing of diversity.[29]

There is a wide range of providers who play a role in the health care of the older adult. In an interdisciplinary team, the levels and areas of responsibility must be clearly established. The interdisciplinary team model is seen as an ideal approach to comprehensive geriatric assessment. Assessment information is used to generate team goals for overall outcomes and to delineate how different disciplines will work together to create desired outcomes. Interventions can be implemented either individually or collectively and progress evaluated in an ongoing manner. The team takes responsibility for program effectiveness and leadership functions are shared. The interpretations of various components of this assessment, and the implementation of the plan, require health care providers who are trained in normal aging and the care of the frail elderly.

Geriatric interdisciplinary teams traditionally refer to "core" teams consisting of a physician, nurse, and social worker, as well as to "extended" teams that include providers whose expertise is called upon for specific cases or who are required by statute in settings such as nursing homes.[26] There has recently been great interest in the concept of the "virtual" interdisciplinary team in which the communication is often by e-mail or other electronic means.

Nurses

There are several levels of nursing education ranging from licensed vocational nurse (LVN) training, diploma programs, the associate degree (AA), the bachelor of science in nursing (BSN), to the master's (MS) and doctoral programs (DNSc, ND, or PhD). Vocational nurses receive up to 12 months of basic nursing skills training and are often recent high school graduates. LVNs are considered "nurse technicians" and practice under the supervision of a registered nurse (RN) or physician. They must pass a national licensing examination.

Most diploma programs are 24-months long and involve in-hospital teaching and training. The baccalaureate program is a 4-year university-based curriculum including course work in nursing science, communication, decision-making, and patient care. Most associate degrees are completed within 3 years and programs are offered primarily through community colleges. The graduates of these three programs are considered somewhat equivalent in their training and must take a licensing exam to become registered nurses (RNs).

Increasing numbers of nurses are completing advanced degrees. Master's education involves specialization in such area as adult or child health, gerontology, women's health, and mental health. Doctoral programs prepare nurses to become faculty members, administrators, and researchers in the field of nursing.

Nurse Practitioners

All candidates who enter the 2-year graduate program have training and work experience as registered nurses. The program emphasizes health assessment and health promotion skills, performance of histories and physicals in outpatient settings, and the consideration of the overall biopsychosocial model and well being of the patients. Nurse practitioners (NP) are trained to diagnose and manage common acute outpatient conditions and common stable chronic conditions. There are different fields of specialization including family, adults, women's health, and geriatric nurse practitioners (GNP). GNPs usually work very closely with primary care physicians or geriatricians. Graduates earn an MS degree, pass a board examination for advanced practice nursing, and receive certification to practice.

Physicians

Physician training begins with a bachelor's degree from a 4-year college or university following the completion of required "pre-med" classes in chemistry, biology, physics, and mathematics. Medical school usually consists of 2 years of course work followed by 2 years of clinical experience, although revisions of the curriculum to facilitate earlier clinical exposure are being implemented in many medical schools across the country.

The clinical years include required clerkships in surgery, internal medicine, ob/gyn, pediatrics, psychiatry, neurology, and family medicine. Elective clerkships include more advanced work in areas of specialization such as geriatrics. Students develop clinical, diagnostic and therapeutic skills, and are taught about disease risk factors and prevention. After graduation, most physicians enter intensive post-graduate residency training, which lasts a minimum of 3 years.

Geriatricians

These physicians are board certified in internal medicine or family medicine and have either completed a 1- to 3-year, post-graduate fellowship training program in geriatric medicine or have passed an examination granting them a certificate of added qualification (CAQ) in geriatrics. The CAQ examinations have been offered by the combined boards of the American Board of Family Practice and the American Board of Internal Medicine for primary care physicians, and by the American Board of Psychiatry for psychiatrists.

Physician Assistants

Physician assistants (PAs) practice medicine with the supervision of licensed physicians. They are educated in specially designed 2-year PA programs located at medical colleges and universities. The first year is based on classroom learning of medical sciences and the second year is predominantly spent on outpatient clinical rotations. Most PAs have a bachelor's degree and over 4 years of health care experience before entering a PA program. Many PA programs are offering Master's Degree level training. After graduation, PAs must pass a national certifying examination before they can begin to practice. To maintain certification, they must complete 100 hours of continuing medical education every 2 years and take a recertification exam every 6 years. PAs provide a broad range of medical services that would otherwise be provided by physicians.

Social Workers

Social work students can receive either a baccalaureate degree in social welfare (BSW) or a master's degree (MSW). Increasing numbers of graduate schools in social work are offering a concentration in gerontology. Candidates with a master's degree who wish to become licensed clinical social workers (LCSW) must complete a required 3200 supervised hours of work experience and complete course work in three subject areas: reporting child abuse, human sexuality, and chemical dependency. LCSW licensing is a state-regulated procedure. This licensing permits social workers to bill insurance companies for their services.

Social workers are trained to enable patients and their families to obtain social services; provide counseling and psychotherapy to individuals and groups; to advocate for the individuals who are neglected, vulnerable, and/or indigent; and to serve as care managers and hospital discharge planners.

Psychologists

Students may enter a 4-year graduate training program leading to a doctorate (PhD., PsyD) after completing a baccalaureate program at a college or university. An internship year in an American Psychological Association accredited training program must be completed for graduation. Licensing as a clinical psychologist differs from state to state. Clinical psychologists are highly trained in the assessment, treatment, and management of mental disorders as well as in psychotherapy with individuals, groups, and families. Most doctoral programs include course work in gerontology and clinical experiences with older adults.

Pharmacists

Pharmacist education includes 2–3 years of pre-pharmacy coursework similar to pre-med curricula. Pharmacy School coursework includes basic science such as chemistry, physiology, anatomy, and biochemistry, as well as pathophysiology, pharmacology and pharmaceutics. The fifth and sixth year are mainly clerkships with exposure to a variety of inpatient, outpatient and community experiences. The majority of schools now offer a Doctorate in Pharmacy degree (PharmD) as the standard degree.

Postgraduate residencies and fellowships, such as in Geriatrics, offer specialization opportunities. States require a licensure exam and most require internship hours before licensure as a registered pharmacist. Continuing education is required by most states.

Occupational Therapist

The occupational therapist (OT) must complete a baccalaureate program with upper division courses in human development, activity intervention, and psychological issues, typically followed by a 6-month clinical clerkship. Master's programs are also available. OTs must take an accreditation examination after completing the program. They teach or reteach people everyday skills necessary to function at home, school, work, or in the community. OTs help patients regain abilities and adjust to functional changes.

Physical Therapist

Most physical therapy (PT) programs are offered at the master's degree level, with baccalaureate programs transitioning into master's level accreditation. The master's in physical therapy (MPT) requires 2 to 3 years to complete and includes course work in kinesiology, physiology, and patient management skills. There are a few doctoral programs in the country.

Role of Interdisciplinary Team Members

Once the training, knowledge, and skills of the various disciplines are understood by individual team members, a greater understanding of each member's role can evolve. One activity that assists the team's progress toward this understanding is the shared development of a role map. Role maps help clarify the competencies and expectations of each team member and define the function of each member within their specific team structure and clinical environment.

Each discipline is represented by a circle, and circles overlap with others. The functions of each role are listed within the circle. In the part of the circle that does not overlap with other circles are those clinical responsibilities that only the specific discipline involved assumes. In other words, that team member is solely accountable for these functions. In areas where two or more circles overlap, clinical responsibilities might be performed by any one of the disciplines or be jointly addressed by two or more providers.[29] Thus, in the role map shown in Figure 1-2, a geriatric assessment team is depicted as it might operate within an outpatient clinic.

In a nursing home setting, the roles might shift, with a GNP taking primary responsibility for many of the physician functions under supervision of a medical director. The process of role mapping results in clarification of roles and progress toward enhanced patient care outcomes. Clear role definitions also contribute to

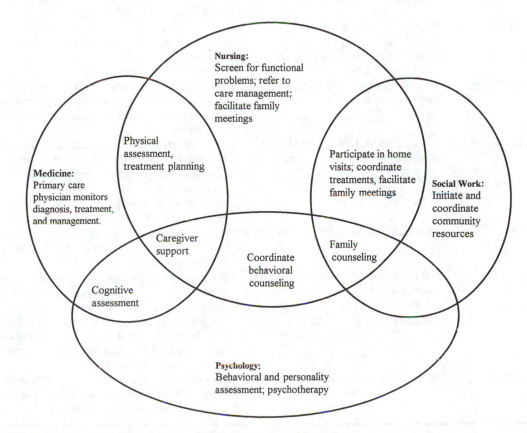

FIGURE 1-2   The Roles of the Interdisciplinary Team Members

better role modeling for trainees who are working with an interdisciplinary team. Trainees thrive when ambiguity is reduced in the clinical care setting (see Table 1-9 for a more detailed description of discipline-specific education and skills).

Performance of comprehensive geriatric assessment requires skills that are beyond the scope of traditional training found in

TABLE 1-9. QUALIFICATIONS AND SKILLS OF THE TEAM		
DISCIPLINE	QUALIFICATIONS	SKILLS
Dentist	DDS, state license	Preventative care; periodontistry experience helpful; tolerance and good interpersonal skills
Nurse practitioner	Master's prepared with certificate in gerontology	History and physical evaluation; knowledge of geriatric rating scales, geriatric prescribing; leadership and communication skills
Occupational therapist (OT)	Registered, licensed, certificate in aging preferred	Knowledge of assessment in frail elderly, geriatric rating/tools, scales relevant to OT such as MMSE, GDS, ADL, document regulations
Office clerk	High school education Preferable—college graduate	Computer literacy, communication skills, knowledge of state and federal regulations
Pharmacist	Pharm D, licensed with special training in aging	Knowledge of the physiology of aging; pharmacodynamics and good interpersonal skills
Physical therapist	Licensed, some certificate in aging/gerontology preferred	Knowledge of assessment in frail elderly, normal aging, geriatric assessment tools (i.e., Tinetti); familiar with HCFA documentation regulations
Physician	Physician with II\A/FP training Preferred fellowship in geriatrics	Comprehensive geriatric assessment, including assessment of cognitive and affective disorders: geriatric prescribing practices; good interpersonal skills
Podiatrist	DPM, state license	Preventative care, surgical skills and privileges; experience with diabetes and wound care
Psychiatrist	Physicians, geropsychiatric training	Geropsychiatric evaluation, cognitive and affective, psychopharmacology, geriatric prescribing, good interperonal skills
Psychologist	PhD, training in psychology of aging or neuropsychology	Group and individual psychotherapy, psychological testing, relevant assessment scales
Social worker	LCSW/MWS/MFCC with training in gerontology	Assessment of normal aging, knowledge of assessing cognitive and affective disorders in elders, knowledge of state and federal regulations, coordination of community resources for continuity of care
Speech therapist	Master's degree, licensed, training in aging preferred	Knowledge of communication in cognitively impaired individuals; knowledge in assessment of swallowing, mental status

TABLE 1-10. THE GERIATRIC TEAM

Core Team
  Physician
  Nurse
  Social worker
Members of the Extended Geriatric Team
  Clinical Pharmacist
  Psychiatrist
  Psychologist
  Neurologist
  Urologist
  Occupational therapist
  Physical therapist
  Dietitian
  Dentist
  Podiatrist
  Surgeon

most professional schools. Table 1-10 describes the tasks of the "core" disciplines in various settings where multidimensional, geriatric assessment is carried out. Again, assigning tasks to disciplines can vary from region to region according to state laws that govern licensing of these professionals. It can also vary depending on payor sources (i.e. fee-for-services versus managed care); some laws require physician involvement whereas others encourage utilizing physician "extenders" such as physician assistants (PAs) and nurse practitioners (NPs) as a cost-cutting measure. The disciplines listed are just some of those that could carry out these tasks.

Viewing the roles of different practitioners by the setting in which they practice reveals the evolving nature of the functions for each discipline. Table 1-11 describes the accountability of assessment components by site. (As noted earlier, role function for various practitioners can vary by setting). Nurse practitioners (NPs) require, in addition to the appropriate state license of an RN, standardized procedures regarding practices with physicians that allow NPs to perform assessment and interventions that overlap with the physician's function. The NPs operate under their own licenses and in collaboration with physicians.

Other practitioners include nurses who are licensed by the state board. In nursing homes, however, regulatory standards are often overinterpreted, thus unnecessarily restricting the nurse's scope of practice compared to their peers in clinics and hospital settings. In the nursing home setting most of the assessment and care is provided by nursing staff utilizing the minimal data set

TABLE 1-11. ACCOUNTABILITY OF ASSESSMENT COMPONENTS BY SITE

	SITE			
TASK OR ROLE	HOME	CLINIC	NURSING HOME	INPATIENT/REHAB
Functional assessment	RN, NP, OT	NP, OT	RN	OT, PT
Mental status	Social worker, RN	Social worker, physicians	Social worker	Physicians, PhD
Psychosocial	RN, Social worker	NP, Social worker	Social worker	Social worker
History and physical	RN, NP, physicians	PA, NP, physicians	Physicians, PA, NP	Physicians
Verify eligibility	Nurse	Clerk	Clerk	Clerk
Coordination	Nurse, clerk, social worker	Clerk, social worker	Nurse	Nurse

Abbreviations: RN, registered nurse; NP, nurse practitioner; OT, occupational therapist; PT, physical therapist; PhD, clinical psychologist; and PA, physician assistant.

(MDS), a federally mandated framework addressing 18 domains of resident function. Although the MDS is a great improvement over the prior years, where no standards for assessment were available, this format lacks specific guidelines for nursing home staff to competently complete the evaluation in a valid and reliable fashion.[30] The team as a unit is responsible for developing and coordinating the patient care plan, which is updated quarterly (see Chapter 9).

The physician's role in the nursing home includes initial evaluation and subsequent services, monthly for the first 90 days, and then every 60 days or more frequently as needed. The only formal guidelines for standards of physician care are provided by the Health Care Financing Administration's requirements for documentation and billing.[31] Physicians' input into the MDS and care plan is through admission notes and when permanent change of resident status occurs. Note that postacute units, or units designated as distinct parts from the nursing home which provide skilled nursing care for Medicare residents, are mandated to review progress of the residents and to determine eligibility for services under the program. These evaluations occur periodically and include all team members and the unit's medical director.[32] The clinical pharmacist has a specifically delineated role in the hospital and nursing home, being in charge of dispensing medications, providing information regarding dosage and substitutions to the practitioners, policy making, and oversight of drug regimens. In the nursing home, a pharmacy consultant is mandated by federal law to review charts and comment on the appropriateness of prescribed medication.[33] In many systems of care, pharmacists have been awarded permission to order laboratory tests that are necessary for appropriate monitoring of drug use.

The role of mental health providers had been expanded following the legislative implementation in 1991 of the Omnibus Budget Reconciliation Act.[34] That legislation contained new federal rules requiring evaluation of specific diagnosis and target behaviors prior to prescribing psychoactive drugs to nursing home residents, and reimbursement brought more psychiatrists and clinical psychologists to practice in institutional long-term care.

In Table 1-12, the descriptions of the roles of team members in the inpatient unit are illustrated. The team on the inpatient unit varies according to designation and site.[35-38] In academic and/or Veterans Administration (VA) settings where resources have been allocated for special geriatric units, the consultation team or the unit team consists of an attending physician, a geriatric fellow (trainee), a nurse coordinator who often is a clinical nurse specialist, and a social worker. By the nature of the institution, all other disciplines are available as needed. The goal of the team is to identify rehabilitation goals and discharge disposition.

In private, nonacademic centers, the care manager or discharge planner is charged with the responsibility of assisting in the dis-

TABLE 1-12. ROLE OF GERIATRIC TEAM IN A HOSPITAL UNIT		
HEALTH CARE PROVIDER		RESPONSIBILITY
Physician/ geriatrician	Team leader	Review of evaluation, specific parts of examination, problems lists, and initial intervention
Nurse	Independent	Functional assessment, patient education
Social worker	Independent	Discharge planning, psychosocial assessment, community resources
Psychologist	Independent	Mental status, psychological assessments
Dietitian	Independent	Nutritional assessment, diet plan, patient education
Occupational therapist	Independent	ADLs, IADLs, adaptive devices, environment evaluation
Physical therapist	Independent	Mobility, balance, pain management
Speech therapist	Independent	Communication, swallowing, evaluation and management

Abbreviations: ADL, activities of daily living; IADL, instrumental activities of daily living.

TABLE 1-13. THE ROLE OF THE TEAM IN THE OUTPATIENT SETTING		
HEALTH CARE PROVIDER		RESPONSIBILITY
Physician	IM/FP/Geriatrics-trained	History, physical, mental status, order laboratory tests, monitor therapy, communicate with physicians, conference leader
Nurse	RN/NP/Nurse specialist	Nursing assessment, home visits, coordinate care plan
Social worker groups	LCSW	Liaison with family and community agencies, elder's family advocate
Geropsychiatrist	Physicians	Psychiatric consultation, psychopharmacologic management
Clinical psychologist	PhD	Psychotherapy, caregivers, supportive care
Neuropsychologist	PhD	Neuropsychological testing
Pharmacist	PharmD	Patient education, monitor compliance and changes

charge process. This often requires liaisons with family, community services such as home health and durable medical equipment suppliers, as well as other institutions. In these settings, the physician often delegates to care managers functions associated with patients although he or she remains responsible for implementation of the care plan.

In Table 1-13, are descriptions of professional roles in the outpatient setting, and Table 1-14 describes the role of the NP and PA. In view of their expanded role in the health care delivery system, the American College of Physicians developed a policy statement regarding NP and PA roles.[39] NP statements and physician policy differ, however, on the degree of independence of NPs. Whereas physicians see the NPs' role as physician extenders functioning under physician supervision, NPs view themselves as independent practitioners who are accountable to their patients.[40] NPs and PAs can be critical to team success, usually are closely supervised by the physician member with greater professional autonomy developing as knowledge and skills improve.

In the outpatient setting, geriatric teams exist only in specialized units, usually in academic centers, private, not-for-profit community hospitals and VA medical centers. In this setting, the core team consists of a physician and a nurse who carry out most of the assessments, deferring to other members of the experienced team

TABLE 1-14.   POTENTIAL ROLES OF NURSE PRACTITIONERS AND PHYSICIAN ASSISTANTS

Clinical
  Primary care in conjunction with physician
  Admission and readmission assessment
  Periodic functional and medical assessments
  Management of subacute problems
  Discharge planning from acute hospital
  Organize and participate in special clinics for demands, incontinence, and falls
  Liaison with family
Administrative
  Participate in interdisciplinary team meeting
  Participate in nursing and medical staff committees and meetings
  Assist in the development of policies and procedures and protocols
  Assist in the employee health program
  Quality assurance activities
Education
  Presentation to patients and families
  Undergraduate and postgraduate led programs for nursing and medical students
Research
  Implement data collection
  Independent research

specialized tasks on a consultation basis. Attempts to train staff in a private medical office to carry out parts of geriatric assessment have been described.[41] The more often called-upon disciplines include physical and occupational therapy for assessment of rehabilitation potential and requests for assistance in management.

Social workers serve as care managers and often as mental health providers. Psychiatrists and/or psychologists provide diagnostic evaluation in newly diagnosed and more complicated cases of affective and cognitive problems, and often engage in ongoing management. Utilizing the services of neuropsychologists depends on the knowledge and skill of the physician or other team members to make use of the information. These data can often be of benefit in the diagnosis of a dementing illness with atypical presentation and in planning of management of the disorder to emphasize the patient's cognitive strengths and minimize the weaknesses.

Elders are frequently concerned about their feet. With this in mind, podiatric assessment and management is an integral part of ambulatory care and is equally as important in the institutional long-term care setting. Podiatrists have a limited role in the acute hospital and are significantly underutilized in the home care environment. Individuals with disorders such as diabetic ulcers, arterioocclusive disease, and gait and balance disorders may benefit from a podiatrist's input.

Dentistry is another vastly underutilized discipline in geriatrics, despite the variety of oral pathology in elders and the potential benefits from assessment and management.[42] The need for an annual dental examination for the prevention of periodontal disease, reconstructive dentistry, and regular general dentistry is on the rise with the increase in the number of dentulous elders.[43] Dentists and oral hygienists share the task for preventative care. Interventional reconstructive dentistry is reserved for general dentists and dental subspecialists.

In order for geriatric patients to reap the benefits of appropriate interdisciplinary health care, geriatric education must be integrated throughout the course work and clinical rotations in health professions schools. The ideal goal would be to have students from multiple disciplines taught didactically by multiple faculty members and in clinical settings by an interdisciplinary clinical geriatric team.

Many authors have already noted what is lacking in traditional health professional education and what necessary skills are not being taught. Some of these obstacles are noted in a recent publication by the U.S. Department of Health and Human Services titled *A National Agenda for Geriatric Education: White Papers* (1995).[44] The paper's conclusions are as follows.

1. Health care professionals currently working with elders have rarely received any formal education regarding interdisciplinary care and yet are expected to work collaboratively and function as interdisciplinary team members.
2. Most health and social service professionals lack a knowledge and experiential base in interdisciplinary functioning, gerontology, and geriatrics.
3. The complex health care needs of frail elders and the increasing complexity of health care delivery systems demand knowledge, skills, and expertise that no one discipline can adequately provide.
4. Under current health care reimbursement systems, there is no provision for services rendered by an interdisciplinary team of professionals. Fees are set for individual health professional services with no incentive for interdisciplinary care.
5. There is a paucity of rigorous scientific literature about outcomes or interdisciplinary approaches to geriatric team education and practice.

Changes must be introduced into the curricula of all health care providers in order to meet the needs of appropriate, comprehensive geriatric assessment and care. The strength of any curriculum is its grounding in both classroom and clinical education. The principles of teamwork emphasize group skills with the consistent acknowledgment of the importance of interpersonal communication skills.

The concepts of feedback, role negotiation, conflict analysis and resolution, interactive problem identification, and creative problem solving, along with evaluation of team functioning and outcomes are key factors in team building. They must first be taught in a classroom and then applied in a clinical setting so that they become conscious behaviors at the individual level and are performed in relation to other health care providers. Learning the language, jargon, metaphors, nouns, values, and culture of a team is critical to becoming an integral, productive member of the team.

SUMMARY

Comprehensive assessment is often necessary to accurately define an older person's problems, develop interventions, and serve as a baseline against which to measure outcomes of treatment. Because of the complexity of geriatric care, dedicated teams of geriatric care providers are often needed to complete the assessment. Teams focus on the person's functional limitations, cognition, affect, and social needs, not just the medical diagnoses with which the patient is living. With the marked increase in numbers of elders predicted to be seen in the next few decades, the acute care orientation of traditional medical care, and changes in health care financing, the need for comprehensive geriatric assessment should rise in the future.

REFERENCES

1. Cohen RA, VanNostrand JF. Trends in the Health of Older Americans: United States, 1994. National Center for Health Statistics. *Vital Health Stat.* 1995;3(30):
2. *Nursing Home Trends, 1987 and 1996.* (Publication Number 99-0032). Silver Spring, MD: AHCPR Publications Clearinghouse,
3. Myers Research Institute, Menorah Park Center for the Aging. A National Study of Assisted Living for the Frail Elderly. Beachwood, OH, April, 1999.
4. US Bureau of the Census, 1986 Statistical Abstract of the United States.
5. Burton J. The evolution of nursing homes into comprehensive geriatrics centers: a perspective. *J Am Geriatr Soc.* 1994;42:794–796.
6. *Access to Home Health Services under Medicare's Interim Payment*

The Editors gratefully acknowledge the input of Diane E. Tobias, Pharm D, and Michelle Arling, RPh.

System. Issue Brief No. 744, National Health Policy Forum. Washington, DC: The George Washington University, July, 1999.

7. DeLew N. The first 30 years of Medicare and Medicaid. *JAMA*. 1995; 274:262–267.

8. Vladeck BC, King KM. Medicare at 30: Preparing for the Future. *JAMA*. 1995;274:259–262.

9. Hawes C, Morris J, Phillips C, Mor V, Fries B, Nonemaker S. Reliability estimates for the minimum data set for nursing home resident assessment and care screening (MDS). *Gerontologist*. 1995;35(2): 172–178.

10. Morris J, Hawes C, Fries B, et al. Designing the national resident assessment instrument for nursing homes. *Gerontologist*. 1990;30(3): 293–302.

11. Ouslander JG. The Resident Assessment Instrument (RAI): promise and pitfalls. *J Am Geriatr Soc*. 1997;45:975–976.

12. Hawes C, Mor V, Phillips CD, et al. The OBRA-87 Nursing Home Regulations and implementation of the Resident Assessment Instrument: effects on process quality. *J Am Geriatr Soc*. 1997;45:977–985.

13. Phillips CD, Morris JN, Hawes C, et al. Association of the Resident Assessment Instrument (RAI) with changes in function, cognition, and psychosocial status. *J Am Geriatr Soc*. 1997;45:986–993.

14. Fries BE, Hawes C, Morris, JN, et al. Effect of the National Resident Assessment Instrument on selected health conditions and problems. *J Am Geriatr Soc*. 1997;45:994–1001.

15. Mor V, Intrator O, Fries BE, et al. Changes in hospitalization associated with introducing the Resident Assessment Instrument. *J Am Geriatr Soc*. 1997;45:1002–1010.

16. Morris JN, Nonemaker S, Murphy K, et al. A commitment to change: revision of HCFA's RAI. *J Am Geriatr Soc*. 1997;45:1011–1016.

17. Morris JN, Fries BE, Steel K, et al. Comprehensive clinical assessment in community setting: applicability of the MDS-HC. *J Am Geriatr Soc*. 1997;45:1017–1024.

18. Uman GC. Where's Gertrude? *J Am Geriatr Soc*. 1997;45:1025–1026.

19. Schnelle JF. Can nursing homes use the MDS to improve quality? *J Am Geriatr Soc*. 1997;45:1027–1028.

20. Ouslander J. Maximizing the minimum data set. *J Am Geriatr Soc*. 1994;42:1212–1213.

21. Markson L, Kern D, Annas, G, Glantz L. Physician assessment of patient competence. *J Am Geriatr Soc*. 1994;42:1074–1080.

22. Ouslander J, Osterweil D. Physician evaluation and management of nursing home residents. *Ann Int Med*. 1994;121:584–592.

23. Branch LG, Coulam RF, Zimmerman YA. The PACE evaluation: initial findings. *Gerontologist*. 1995;35:349–359.

24. Shen J, Iversen A. PACE: a capitated model towards long-term care. *Henry Ford Hosp Med J*. 1992;40(1, 2):41–44.

25. Ruchlin H, Morris S, Morris J. Resident medical care utilization patterns in continuing care retirement communities. *Health Care Finan Rev*. 1993;14(4):151–168.

26. Leutz W, Hallfors D. Lessons from social HMO marketing, Institute for Health Policy. Brandeis University, Dec. 1993: Supported by the

Health Care Financing Administration under Cooperative Agreement 99-C-98526/1-08.

27. Baldwin DC. *The Role of Interdisciplinary Education and Teamwork in Primary Care and Health Reform.* Rockville, MD: Health Professions Bureau, Health Resources and Services Administration, U.S. Department of Health and Human Services; 1994.

28. Zeiss AM, Steffen AM. Interdisciplinary health care teams: the basic unit of geriatric care. In Cartensen LL, Edelstein BA, Dombrand L, eds. *The Handbook of Clinical Gerontology.* Newbury Park, California: Sage Publications, Ltd., 1996;423–450.

29. Grant RW, Finnocchio LJ, and the California Primary Care Consortium Subcommittee on Interdisciplinary Collaboration. *Interdisciplinary Collaborative Teams in Primary Care: A Model Curriculum and Resource Guide.* San Francisco, CA: Pew Health Professions Commission; 1995.

30. Kane RL, Ouslander JG, Abrass IB, eds. *Essentials of Clinical Geriatrics,* 3rd ed. New York: McGraw-Hill; 1995:516–523.

31. Rapp K, Rapp MP. A guide to the improved reimbursement codes. *NH Practitioner.* 1994;May/June:34–35.

32. Smith RL, Osterweil D. The medical director in hospital-based transitional care units. *Clin Geriatr Med.* 1995;11(2):373–389.

33. Health Care Financing Administration. *Interpretive Guidelines.* 483.60, 1:1, 1988, 6324 Security Blvd., Baltimore, MD 21207.

34. The Omnibus Budget Reconciliation Act, *Federal Register.* 1987; 56(187):48865–48921.

35. McVey LS, Becker RM, Saltz CC, et al. Effect of a geriatric consultation team on functional status of elderly hospitalized patients. *Ann Int Med.* 1989;110(1):79–84.

36. Landefeld CS, Palmer RM, Kresevie DM, et al. A randomized trial of care in a hospital medical unit especially designed to improve the functional outcomes of acutely ill older patients. *N Engl J Med.* 1995;332(20):1338–1344,

37. Thomas DR, Brahan R, Haywood BP. Inpatient community-based geriatric assessment reduces subsequent mortality. *J Am Geriatr Soc.* 1993;41:101–104.

38. Rubenstein LZ, Josephson KR, Wieland D, et al. Effectiveness of a geriatric evaluation unit. *N Engl J Med.* 1984;3211:1664–1670.

39. American College of Physicians. Position paper, physician assistants and nurse practitioners. *Ann Int Med.* 1994;121(9):714–716.

40. Maffie-Lee J, Cadegan D, Geronomo M. Physician assistants and nurse practitioners. *Ann Int Med.* 1995;123(3):237.

41. Moore AA, Siu AL. Screening for common problems in ambulatory elderly: clinical confirmation of a screening instrument. *Am J Med* 1996;100(4):438–443.

42. Ettinger RL. Oral care for the homebound and institutionalized. *Clin Geriatr Med.* 1992;8(3):659–672.

43. Burt BA. Epidemiology of dental diseases in the elderly. *Clin Geriatr Med.* 1992;8(3):447–459.

44. U.S. Department of Human Services. *A National Agenda for Geriatric Education: White Papers.* Washington, DC: 1995.

HEALTH STATUS AND PHYSICAL CAPACITY

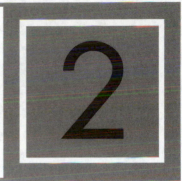

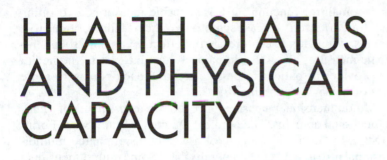

MEGHAN B. GERETY

Health-related quality of life (HRQOL) has come to be a familiar concept to many health care providers and researchers. These measures include self-report, proxy-report, observer-administered, and performance-based tests. When added to "hard" measures of health, such as laboratory tests or clinical condition, health-related quality of life provides supplemental information regarding the effects of illness or therapy on the "function" of the individual in the context of his or her environment. A myriad of health status, or HRQOL, instruments exist and have been reviewed extensively.[1–3] Measures of HRQOL have become almost standard in clinical trials comparing therapies and in cohort studies of aging.

The theoretic advantages of adding these measures are numerous. Given an equal effectiveness of two therapies in controlling disease, one may choose the therapy that has the most positive (or least negative) effect on quality of life. As many HRQOL measures use self-report as the basis of assessment, these measures allow the patient to have a "voice" in the experimental literature. Over the last two decades, this patient-centered perspective has become a more prominent feature in the evaluation of aging, health, disease, and therapy.

Ware and others agree that the concept of HRQOL is multidimensional. Essential domains include physical, emotional, social, role functioning, and bodily pain.[4] In recent years, there has been a proliferation of measures of function, or HRQOL, that are domain-, disease-, or person-specific. Domain-specific measures, such as the physical performance-based measures, tell us most about a

41

single domain of function. Disease-specific measures, like rating scales for Parkinson's disease symptoms or heart failure, often cross domains of function to capture the full effects of an illness. Patient-specific measures allow the domain of most interest to the health care provider or patient to be selected and each person to serve as his or her own denominator.[5]

Multidimensional measures incorporate assessments of multiple functional domains. The Medical Outcomes Study Short Form-36 (MOS-SF 36) is an example of a widely disseminated multidimensional instrument[6] (see Appendix #40). Some multidimensional measures, like the Sickness Impact Profile, aggregate domains into a single score, or a "snapshot," of health-related function.[7] To the extent that they describe the overall impact of specific conditions, multidimensional measures allow the effects of disabilities, illnesses, or therapies to be compared to one another. Measures with an aggregate score can be used not only for comparison but also for cost-effectiveness analysis.

Not surprisingly, information from the recipient's perspective may be at odds with other outcomes. In risk reduction therapy, primary goals are "hard outcomes," such as control of blood pressure, and consequent reduction in stroke and cardiovascular events. In the context of risk reduction, HRQOL measures inform us about the functional costs and benefits of therapy. If adverse outcomes are reduced *and* HRQOL improves, then the functional cost–benefit equation is positive. If HRQOL declines in the face of reduced adverse outcomes, we are informed about the real trade-offs of therapy. This information assists the health care provider in selecting therapy and gives the recipient of care information about effects on daily functioning.

In other therapeutic contexts, information from HRQOL measures should be interpreted differently. Many therapies for disabled or chronically ill persons are not aimed at cure, but at improving function.[8] Joint replacement for intractable pain or surgical or medical therapy for prostatism cannot be judged successful unless they improve function. This function-promoting context is where self- or observer-reported measures of HRQOL are the most difficult to interpret. The problems inherent in self- or observer-reported HRQOL have spawned an interest in performance-based measures of functioning. Measuring "real function," by having the recipient of care perform the task, seemed that it might avoid some of the problems listed as follows.

- *Respondent differences:* Results systematically differ when the respondent is the recipient, the caregiver, or the health care provider. Where, therefore, is truth? Whose report will we rely on to make our judgments?[9–11]

- *Domain differences and overlap:* Function measured in different domains can produce different results. How do we decide which domain deserves the most attention? When domains are evaluated statistically, they overlap. Analyses of multidimensional instruments show modest but significant correlation between psychological and physical function and cognitive and affective function, particularly in frail elders.[12–14] As health care providers, we intuitively understand these interrelationships. Yet, how can we assess "true" function if results are significantly affected by intellectual ability, education, affective function, acculturation, and experience? How can we tease apart the domain to target?
- *Interpreting aggregate scores:* When a single score is produced from multiple domains, the resulting snapshot may have little meaning to the health care provider. An identical score can be derived from many patterns of deficits. How does this aggregate score translate into useful clinical information?
- *Disease activity versus HRQOL:* Results reflecting disease activity and HRQOL may be discordant. If the person's FEV_1 is low and wheezing is heard, yet he or she describes improved HRQOL, which do we believe?
- *Actual versus typical functional capacity:* Responses to HRQOL measures vary by question format. Are we asking the participant to estimate ability (can you), typical performance (do you), or estimated capacity (could you)?
- *Causal pathways to disability:* These are often clouded by multidimensional measures. As health care providers we wish to treat. When diminished function is present, what type of intervention or combination of interventions should we provide? As health care providers, we are much more comfortable with physical- and disease-oriented interventions than with psychosocial. In fact, we may feel psychosocial interventions are outside of our expertise.

EMERGENCE OF PERFORMANCE-BASED MEASURES OF FUNCTION

Broadly defined, a performance-based measure is a test where a participant (or a patient) performs a movement, behavior, or task according to a standardized protocol that is scored by an observer. Simple examination techniques have always used performance-based approaches. Assessment of speech, vision, gait, grasp, strength, and endurance (climbing stairs, etc.) have been a part of

Broadly defined, a performance-based measure is a test where a participant (or a patient) performs a movement, behavior, or task according to a standardized protocol that is scored by an observer.

physical examination as long as it has been routine in the practice of medicine.

The earliest performance-based measures emerged as estimates of physiologic function, rehabilitation progress, and service prediction. Simple tests like the Master's Step Test and climbing flights of stairs served as measures of cardiovascular fitness before exercise ergometry. In the 1960s, multiple observer ratings of function were developed for use in rehabilitation settings. The most famous of these is the Barthel Index,[15] where a physical therapist judges upper and lower extremity function and mobility. The score describes the therapist's observations over a period of days. These ratings were used to document progress toward independence and predict the need for prosthetic devices (see Appendix #4 and Chapter 5).

In the last two decades, there have been dramatic changes in performance-based measures. Many measures emphasize an entire functional action, rather than its component parts. In the past, flexibility of the shoulder joint would have been evaluated using standard goniometry to measure the six motions of the shoulder. Newer techniques employ integrated functional motions. The person may be asked to place his or her palms together, extend the elbows, lift the joined hands over the head, and then, behind the back. Changing to a functional approach has advantages. First, fewer observations are required. Second, the observer has the opportunity to evaluate the elbow, hand, and wrist simultaneously. Functional limitations that affect upper extremity activities (e.g., putting on a shirt, washing one's back, or changing an overhead light bulb) often involve the entire arm–shoulder–neck complex. Functional evaluation makes deficits in this complex more easily apparent than a one-by-one joint evaluation.

In many cases, administration and scoring of performance-based instruments are standardized. This allows trained lay personnel to assist in patient assessment. Research has now shown that many performance-based measures can detect between-person differences (distinguishing impairment from independence) and within-person change (change over time). Perhaps most importantly, research over the last decade helped us understand the utility of performance-based measures. Relationships of performance-based functional tests to disease, disability, and risk of functional decline and adverse events, such as falls, have been explored.

A HIERARCHICAL MODEL OF PHYSICAL FUNCTION

When selecting a performance-based measure of function, rules that are used to choose any functional status measure apply.[16]

Margin notes

The earliest performance-based measures emerged as estimates of physiologic function, rehabilitation progress, and service prediction.

Many measures emphasize an entire "functional" action, rather than its component parts.

Research has now shown that many performance-based measures can detect between-person differences (distinguishing impairment from independence) and within-person change (change over time).

Relationships of performance-based functional tests to disease, disability, and risk of functional decline and adverse events such as falls have been explored.

Does the selected measure take a comprehensive picture of the desired area of function? Is the scope or range of function applicable for the target population? Is the area of function relevant to the target population? Is it reliable, valid, and acceptable to the participant?

Like self-report measures, performance-based measures each have their own unique characteristics. Each taps a specific range of function and is susceptible to ceiling or floor effects. A measure of physical function capable of measuring the endurance of a master athlete is unlikely to function well with frail elders, who will have scores that cluster at the lowest end of endurance (floor effects). Conversely, when well elders are assessed with measures designed to measure lower levels of function, they are likely to cluster at the maximum end of the scoring range (ceiling effects). Before choosing a performance-based measure for clinical or research use, the spectrum of function in the target population or person must be determined and a suitable instrument chosen.

Figure 2-1 shows a hierarchical model of physical function developed at a workshop on performance-based measures of function sponsored by the National Institute on Aging in May 1993. This model is *not* meant to substitute for existing models of disability.[17] Specifically, for the purposes of this chapter, this model serves to demonstrate the spectrum of physical function available to be tapped by various performance-based instruments. This model approaches physical function as a series of increasingly integrated steps, beginning with basic components and progressing through

When selecting a performance-based measure of function, rules that are used to choose any functional status measure apply.

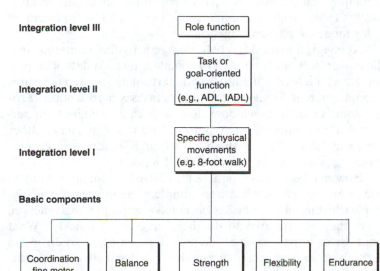

FIGURE 2-1 Hierarchy of physical function. ADL, activities of daily living; IADL instrumental activities of daily living.

additional levels, each increasingly integrating physical and non-physical function. At the very bottom of the model are the basic components (strength, balance, coordination, flexibility, and endurance). These basic components cannot be conceived of as functional "tasks." Instead, these are the requisite building blocks that, when put together, allow performance of specific physical movements and goal-oriented functional tasks.

At each subsequent level, the components of physical function become more integrated with one another and with nonphysical elements of function. Integration level I comprises "specific physical movements." These specific movements have at least three properties. First, they require integration of the underlying basic components to create a movement sequence. For example, reaching requires integration of strength, coordination, flexibility, and balance. Deficits in any one of the basic components can impair reaching capacity. Second, specific physical movements are component parts of other actions. In fact, human factors analysis of activities of daily living (ADLs) has identified at least 11 movements common to many tasks. These include: lift/lower, push/pull, hold/carry/suspend, rotate, side to side, hand to hand, fold/drop/throw, lean/reach, bend/stoop, and sit/stand and lift.[18] Third, these specific physical movements are relatively "over-learned" behaviors, that is, they can be performed with little conscious effort.

These characteristics of "specific physical movements" support their place in the hierarchy of physical function. They are predominantly physical, although their performance is somewhat influenced by nonphysical parameters such as cognition, habit, and motivation.[19-21] Table 2-1 gives examples of activities and their placement in this model of physical function.

At integration level II, goal-oriented activities, numerous specific movements are combined to complete tasks as described previously. At this level, difficulties with performance-based measures become apparent. What constellation of tasks comprise housekeeping? Some tasks, (e.g., window cleaning, carpet cleaning) are performed infrequently by many persons and never by some. Other tasks, such as dusting, washing dishes, and laundry, can be performed satisfactorily in many different ways.

How can these tasks be studied? Will we look for appropriately sequenced movements? Time to complete the dusting chore? Do people who dust or wash dishes faster have better physical function, or are they acculturated to do these tasks more quickly? What about errors in performance? Who will judge when an error has taken place? Indeed, recent work using timed and error-rated measures of activities of daily living shows wide variation in time *and* number of "errors" while performing ADLs in independent, cognitively intact persons.[22] This suggests that neither time nor "error rating" may be relevant parameters for these tasks.

TABLE 2-1. EXAMPLES OF PHYSICAL ACTIVITIES AND THEIR LEVEL OF INTEGRATION			
BASIC COMPONENTS	SPECIFIC PHYSICAL MOVEMENTS	TASK- or GOAL-ORIENTED ACTIVITIES	ROLE-RELATED ACTIVITIES
Strength	Bridge	Groom	Occupational activities
Balance	Reposition oneself	Dress	Volunteer activities
Coordination	Roll side to side	Bathe	Creative productivity
Flexibility	Walk	Rise from chair and walk	Recreation
Endurance	Stances, wide, narrow, and tandem	Toileting	Parental activities
	Chair rise/stand to sit	Locomote place to place	Family activities
	Supine to sit/sit to supine	Shopping, errands	Community activities
	Transfers	Cooking, meal preparation	Caregiving activities
	Climb/descend	House or yard work	Socialization
	Turn/pivot	Manage medications	
	Carry	Use transportation	
	Reach	Manage money	
	Bend/stoop/crouch/kneel	Climb stairs to get somewhere	
	Grip/grasp	Walk to a specific destination	
	Manipulate small objects	Do laundry	
	Foot tapping	Use telephone	

Occasionally, the distinctions between levels II and III are blurred. Are walking across a small room or walking one half mile goal-directed activities or specific physical movements? Table 2-1 clearly plants walking in level 2, yet walking by itself may be a goal-directed activity (e.g., to get somewhere, to obtain exercise). Thus, the levels in the proposed model of physical function overlap to some degree, as do levels in self- or proxy-reports of function. Finally, the goal-oriented level of function has been repeatedly demonstrated to be affected by nonphysical parameters. Cognition, motivation, gender, affect, illness, culture, education, and socioeconomic status all affect performance of goal-oriented activities.[12, 23–28]

EVOLUTION OF PERFORMANCE-BASED INSTRUMENTS OF FUNCTION

Performance-based measures have not evolved following a model of physical function. Instead, it is the results of performance-based tests that informed the model.[29] These tests evolved to *describe* the presence or absence of functional impairment in populations[26, 30–34]; identify risk factors that *predict* adverse events, for example, falls,[34] mortality,[32, 35] hip fracture, incident disability, or nursing home placement,[15, 32, 35–38]; or as outcome measures used to *evaluate* change in function or therapeutic efficacy.[39–42]

Some instruments measure a broad spectrum of physical function whereas others may focus on only one level or a single task.

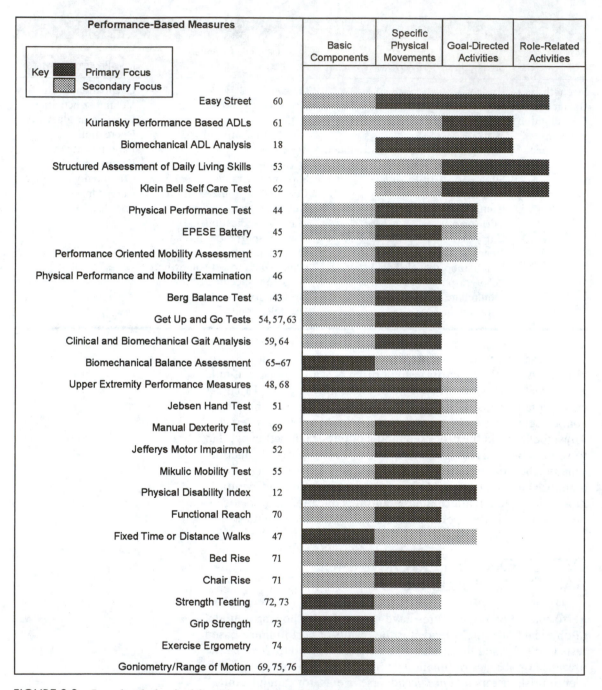

FIGURE 2-2   Levels of physical function measured by instruments.

Figure 2-2 is intended to serve as a guide to the level of function assessed by performance-based instruments. Some measures have been evaluated in healthy community-dwelling elders[43-45] and others have been designed specifically for frail elders.[12, 46] Others are intended to evaluate populations that have minimal to moderate disability.[47-59] No single measure taps all levels of function and is suitable for any population. How, then, should the health care provider apply these performance-based measures? The best approach will be one which, while keeping in mind the model of physical function, also takes into account the natural history of disability.

PERFORMANCE-BASED MEASURES AND THE DISABLEMENT PROCESS

The disablement process is extremely complex. Multiple models have been proposed and are well summarized in an article by Verbrugge and Jette.[17] The following discussion is not intended to be a comprehensive discussion of the disablement process; rather, it highlights aspects of this process relevant to measuring physical function.

A differential pattern of health outcomes is seen across the older age groups. Risk of mortality is relatively higher in the young-old, whereas risk of disability and institutionalization is relatively greater in the old-old.[77, 78] Thus, for the young-old, disease-oriented interventions may be best suited to prevent morbidity and mortality. In the old-old, those already functionally impaired, or at high risk for disability, interventions should emphasize detection of early disability and prevention of progression. In this context, performance-based measures offer a great deal of promise.

To understand the utility of performance-based measures in disability detection and prevention, it is essential to understand what is known about the evolution of function in old age. Recent epidemiologic information has added greatly to the understanding of the evolution of disability. Several sources of data, the Longitudinal Study on Aging (LSOA), Established Populations for Epidemiologic Study of the Elderly (EPESE), Cardiovascular Health Study, and the Framingham Study provide information about self-report and performance-based assessments of function.[25-27, 31, 79, 80] Analyses of self-report data from these studies show a consistent pattern.

Functional decline appears to progress in an hierarchical pattern. Limitations in upper or lower body specific physical movements or vigorous physical activities precede dependence in daily living tasks. Poor performance of activities such as reaching, car-

For what purpose will the instrument be used? What areas of physical function are to be measured? Does the range of physical function measured by the instrument match the range of function of the patient population?

rying, lifting, stooping, prolonged standing, or walking one quarter a mile may identify persons at high risk of functional decline.[25, 27, 80] Moreover, a dose–response effect is present. Odds of future disability are increased as impairment worsens.[32, 81] To put this in perspective, mobility impaired persons have a 16 percent chance of developing ADL dependence over a 2-year period.[82, 83] Poor performance of specific bodily movements is not only useful in predicting functional decline but also in identifying persons at risk for adverse clinical events such as falls. Impairments in gait, balance, and lower extremity strength have all been identified as risk factors for falls.[34]

Fitting the Performance-Based Measures into the Disablement Process

The natural history of disability supports the importance of tests of balance, gait, mobility, and upper extremity movements as methods to identify persons at high risk for disability. Detection, however, is not enough. What intervention will we apply once risk is identified? The etiology of mobility impairment is undoubtedly multifactorial. Substantial evidence suggests that both the total numbers and types of disease, particularly cerebrovascular disease, arthritis, angina, atherosclerosis, and claudication play a role in mobility impairment.[27, 80, 81, 84, 85] Disease, however is a relatively weak predictor, with maximum relative risk only reaching 3.3 (95%, CI = 2.2, 5.0) when the number of chronic conditions exceeds five.[27, 77] Thus, disease management, while important, cannot be the only focus of disability prevention.

In the old-old, those already functionally impaired, or at high risk for disability, interventions should emphasize detection of early disability and prevention of progression.

Disuse may play both initiation and maintenance roles in functional limitation. This is suggested by the protective effects of physical activity[81, 86] and the relative weakness and reduced cardiovascular fitness of those who are functionally impaired compared to independent persons.[21, 80, 87] Intervention studies clearly demonstrate that both weakness and diminished aerobic capacity are reversible.[86, 88–90] In frailer persons, interventions affect not only the basic components of physical function but also specific physical movements such as walking and climbing stairs.[90] Importantly, interventions that incorporate strength, balance, gait, or aerobic training have recently been shown to be successful in preventing falls.[91] Whether these interventions can also reduce the risk of functional decline is not known.

In summary, we know that identifiable limitations in physical function are important risk factors for both adverse clinical events and functional decline. Interventions that improve physical function can prevent falls and have the potential to minimize functional decline. As health care providers, we must know how best to identify persons who are at risk or already impaired and to match their limitations to an appropriate intervention.

SELECTING A PERFORMANCE-BASED MEASURE OF FUNCTION

Selection of performance-based measures for use in clinical practice should be dictated by criteria similar to those used to select a measure for research. The instrument should be feasible to use in the clinical setting and acceptable to the recipient of care and staff. It should be valid and reliable. When selecting a measure, the health care provider should consider several questions. For what purpose will the instrument be used? What areas of physical function are to be measured? Does the range of physical function measured by the instrument match the range of function of the patient population?

The natural history of disability supports the importance of tests of balance, gait, mobility, and upper extremity movements as methods to identify persons at high risk for disability.

Purpose

Performance-based instruments, like other health status assessments, can be useful for several purposes. They may serve to *discriminate* persons with functional limitations or neuromuscular deficits from those who do not. Ability to identify specific neuromuscular deficits (weakness, poor balance, etc.) or specific functional deficits (trouble transferring, or ambulating, etc.) is particularly important in selecting interventions to maintain or restore function.

Performance-based measures are useful to *predict* risk of adverse clinical events such as falls or subsequent functional disability. Some instruments, particularly those that assess task- or goal-oriented functional tasks, can also be of assistance in determining services necessary for the care of the patient or establishing an appropriate level of care. Last, performance-based instruments have the potential to *evaluate* change over time. Many measures of strength, range of motion, and endurance are sensitive to change. Relatively few instruments that measure balance, specific physical movements, or goal-oriented tasks, however, have been formally evaluated with respect to sensitivity to change. Thus, although these measures are particularly useful to predict risk and identify deficits, they should not routinely be applied to assess change. Table 2-2 provides a list of performance-based measures and their respective applications. Instruments that are brief, portable, and suitable for use in clinical practice are shown.

TABLE 2-2. USES OF PERFORMANCE-BASED MEASURES OF PHYSICAL FUNCTION

Identify Neuromuscular Defects
  Strength
    Manual Muscle Testing[94]
    Hand Held Dynamometry[12, 95, 96]
    Isokinetic, Isometric Evaluation[72, 99]
  Balance
    Berg Balance Test[100 a]
    Clinical and Biomechanical Gait Analysis[59, 64]
    Performance Oriented Mobility Assessment[34, 36, 37 a,b]
    Physical Performance and Mobility Exam[46 a,b]
    Physical Disability Index[12, 39 a]
    Serial Stances[102 b]
    EPESE Battery[32, 45, 101 a,b]
    Clinical and Biomechanical Bed Rise[12, 71]
    Clinical and Biomechanical Chair Rise[58, 97, 98]
    Functional Reach[49, 104 b]
    Get up and Go Test[54, 57, 63 a,b]
  Flexibility/Range of Motion
    Goniometry[75, 76, 105]
    Arthritis Performance Measure[106 a]
    Jebsen Hand Test[51]
    Upper Extremity Performance Measure[48]
    Functional Reach[49, 104 b]
    Physical Disability Index[12, 39 a]
    Jeffreys Motor Impairment Battery[52]
    Mikulic Mobility Test[55]
    Get up and Go Test[54, 57, 63 a,b]
  Coordination/Fine Motor Skills
    Jebsen Hand Test[51]
    Arthritis Performance Test[107]
    Quantitative Upper Extremity Function[68]
    TEMPA (Upper Extremity Function in Elderly)[108]
    Manual Dexterity Test[56, 109 a,b]
    Performance Oriented Mobility Assessment[34, 36, 37 a]
    Jeffreys Motor Impairment Battery[52]
    Structured Assessment of Daily Living Skills[53]
    Physical Performance Test[38 a,b]
    Klein Bell Self Care Test[62]
    EPESE Battery[32, 45, 101 a,b]
  Endurance
    Two, six, and twelve minute walking tests[42, 47, 110 b]
    Exercise Ergometry[111]
  Mobility
    Get up and Go Test[54, 57, 63 a,b]
    Performance Oriented Mobility Assessment[34, 36, 37 a,b]
    Jeffreys Motor Impairment Battery[52]
    Mikulic Mobility Test[55]

Mobility (cont'd)
    Timed Walks[72, 92, 93 b]
    Physical Disability Index[12, 39 a]
    Clinical and Biomechanical Chair Rise[58, 97, 98]
    Clinical and Biomechanical Bed Rise[12, 71]
    Physical Performance Test[38 a]
    Clinical and Biomechanical Gait Analysis[59, 64]
    Gait speed[92]
    Physical Performance and Mobility Exam[46 a,b]
    EPESE Battery[32, 45, 101 a,b]
Predict Adverse Events
  Falls
    Isokinetic, Isometric Strength Assessment
    Clinical and Biomechanical Gait Analysis[59, 64]
    Biomechanical Balance Assessment[103]
    Performance Oriented Mobility Assessment[34, 36, 37 a,b]
    Physical Performance and Mobility Exam[46 a,b]
    Berg Balance Test[100 a]
    Serial Stances[102 b]
    Functional Reach[49, 104]
    Get up and Go Test[54, 57, 63 a]
    Biomechanical Gait Analysis[59]
    Performance Oriented Mobility Assessment[34, 36, 37 a]
    Physical Performance Test[38 a]
    Physical Disability Index[12, 39 a]
  Incident Functional Disability
    Performance Oriented Mobility Assessment[34, 36, 37 a,b]
    EPESE Battery[32, 45, 101 a,b]
    Physical Performance and Mobility Exam[46 a,b]
    Functional Reach[49, 104 b]
    Get up and Go Test[54, 57, 63 a,b]
    Jebsen Hand Test[51]
    Physical Disability Index[12, 39 a]
    Manual Dexterity Test[56, 109 a,b]
    Physical Performance Test[38 a,b]
Predict Service Need, Level of Care
    EPESE Battery[32, 45, 101 a,b]
    Mikulic Mobility Test[55]
    Manual Dexterity Test[56, 109 a,b]
    Structured Assessment of Daily Living Skills[53]
    Klein Bell Self Care Test[62]
    Easy Street[60]
    Biomechanical ADL Evaluation[18]
    Kuriansky Performance ADLs[61]
    Performance Oriented Mobility Assessment[34, 36, 37 a,b]
Discriminate Independence/Impairment
    Virtually all tests

[a]Multifunction or multilevel tests with aggregate scores.

[b]Portable, suitable for clinical use.

Measurement Area

Instruments should be selected to measure the area of physical function that is of interest. Fall risk assessment, for example, should emphasize strength, balance, and gait. Table 2-3 describes the principal measurement areas of each instrument. Scanning Table 2-3, it is easy to see that many measures focus on a single area of physical function, whereas others include multiple areas of function. Some primarily focus on basic components of physical function (Figure 2-2), whereas others indirectly assess basic components through observation of integrated specific physical movements such as serial stances, reaching, and so forth. Balance and mobility are represented in at least 12 measures.

Level of Function

How then, should one choose among these instruments? Many can simply be excluded because they require complex equipment (biomechanical measures) and are reserved for research purposes. Instruments that focus primarily on the basic components of function are useful to assess each individual component, but provide little information about the role of each component in functional limitation. To identify deficits that may be contributing to limitations in functional tasks or events such as falls, instruments that focus on specific physical movements may be more useful. For example, the Performance Oriented Mobility Assessment (POMA)[37] assesses balance by observing the patient sit, rise from a chair, walk, and turn (see Appendix #36). Weakness can be indicated by unsteady chair rise or use of arms to rise. Wide-based stance or gait can signal weakness or poor balance. Abnormal gait characteristics can indicate poor proprioception, poor cerebellar function, and trunk or lower extremity weakness. Although each of these deficits could be assessed directly, the POMA takes fewer than 5 minutes, and assesses the role of the underlying components of physical function within the context of ambulation (where most falls occur). Further deficits identified by the POMA are easily understood by the patient and are readily translated into a rehabilitation program by a therapist. Figure 2-3 illustrates the relative utility of performance-based instruments by level of physical function (see Chapter 23).

Target Population

An additional consideration in selecting instruments is the match between the range of function captured by the instrument and the

TABLE 2-3. PRINCIPAL MEASUREMENT AREAS OF PERFORMANCE-BASED MEASURES

PERFORMANCE-BASED INSTRUMENT	REFERENCES	PRINCIPAL MEASUREMENT AREAS
Goniometry (Passive Range of Motion)	75, 76, 10	Range of motion
Isometric Strength Testing	72, 73	Strength
Biomechanical Gait Analysis	59	Gait quality
Two, six, and twelve minute walking tests[a]	47	Endurance
Chair Rise[a]	58, 98	Balance and mobility
Biomechanical Bed Rise Analysis	71	Balance and mobility
Biomechanical Chair Rise Analysis	97, 112	Balance and mobility
Williams Manual Dexterity Test[a]	113, 114	Hand strength and function
Arthritis Performance Measure	107	Upper extremity range of motion and function
Upper Extremity Function Test	48, 68	Upper extremity strength, range of motion, multiple functions
Jebsen Hand Test	51	Upper extremity range of motion and function
Manual Dexterity and Strength	69	Upper extremity range of motion and function
Functional Reach[a]	70, 115	Balance
Biomechanical Static and Dynamic Balance	103, 116	Balance
Serial Stances Balance Tests	102	Balance
Berg Balance Scale	43	Balance and mobility
EPESE Lower Extremity Battery[a]	32	Lower extremity strength, balance and mobility
Get Up and Go Test[a]	54, 57, 63	Balance and mobility
Physical Performance and Mobility Exam[a]	46	Balance and mobility
Quantitative Clinical Gait Analysis	64	Clinical observations of gait quality
EPESE Performance Based Battery	45	Upper extremity coordination, manual dexterity, lower extremity strength, balance and mobility
Physical Disability Index	12	Upper and lower extremity strength, range of motion, balance, bed mobility and locomotion
Performance Oriented Mobility Assessment[a]	37	Balance, mobility, foot coordination and manual dexterity
Physical Performance Test[a]	44	Upper and lower extremity function, manual dexterity, gait, climb, and simulated eating
Mikulic Mobility Test	55	Upper and lower extremity range of motion, balance, bed mobility and locomotion
Jeffreys Motor Impairment Battery	52	Upper and lower extremity strength, range of motion, manual dexterity, stoop, balance, step up and down, ambulation
Biomechanical ADL analysis	18	Qualitative assessment of performance of daily living tasks
Klein Bell Self Care Test	62	Observed performance of some activities of daily living tasks
Structured Assessment of Independent Living Skills	53	Upper and lower extremity function, manual dexterity, simulated activities of daily living and instrumental activities of daily living tasks

[a]Portable, brief, and suitable for clinical practice.

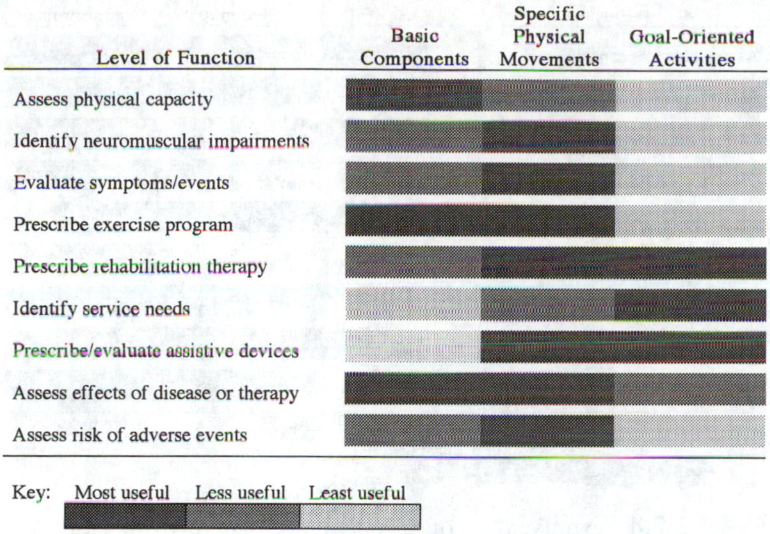

Level of Function	Basic Components	Specific Physical Movements	Goal-Oriented Activities
Assess physical capacity			
Identify neuromuscular impairments			
Evaluate symptoms/events			
Prescribe exercise program			
Prescribe rehabilitation therapy			
Identify service needs			
Prescribe/evaluate assistive devices			
Assess effects of disease or therapy			
Assess risk of adverse events			

Key: Most useful   Less useful   Least useful

FIGURE 2-3   Application of physical performance measures by level of function.

range of function in the target population. Many measures that assess specific physical movements or goal-oriented tasks are designed for frail or ill elders. If applied to fit or well elders, scores will cluster at the highest range of functioning (ceiling effects) and fail to discriminate differences among individuals. The MacArthur Studies of Successful Aging used the EPESE battery to study a select cohort of high functioning persons over the age of 70 years.[45] Marked ceiling effects were found in the mobility scale. This battery, which requires sustaining serial stances for 10 seconds, five chair rises, and a short walk, did not tax the capacity of these well subjects sufficiently to detect differences between individuals.

In most cases, the need to assess elders with performance-based instruments will arise when an event such as a fall has occurred, the patient or caregiver or physician perceive limitations or change in function, or to prescribe assistive devices, rehabilitation, or exercise programs. Figure 2-4 illustrates the relative utility applications of performance-based assessments in fit, sedentary, and compromised people. Physicians whose practices contain many patients who are compromised or are of very advanced age may wish to routinely incorporate assessments of mobility and balance, such as the POMA (see Appendix #36),[37] the EPESE battery,[45] Physical Performance and Mobility Examination,[46] or Get Up and Go.[54] These assessments are brief, estimate risk of falls and functional decline, and identify specific neuromuscular deficits that can be targeted by rehabilitation or safety training.

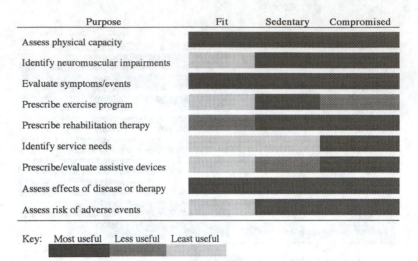

Purpose	Fit	Sedentary	Compromised

Assess physical capacity

Identify neuromuscular impairments

Evaluate symptoms/events

Prescribe exercise program

Prescribe rehabilitation therapy

Identify service needs

Prescribe/evaluate assistive devices

Assess effects of disease or therapy

Assess risk of adverse events

Key: Most useful   Less useful   Least useful

FIGURE 2-4   Application of physical performance measures by patient population.

Reliability and Validity

In this chapter, only performance-based instruments that have been shown to be reliable are presented (i.e., have similar results when readministered by the same rater under similar conditions). Of note, multilevel or multifunction performance-based scales that have an aggregate score (shown in Table 2-2) have exceptionally high test–retest or inter-rater reliabilities, often with correlation coefficients in the 0.85 to 0.95 range. This is not unique to the performance-based measures. Chances for agreement are always higher with a summary scale than with item-by item evaluation. When evaluated item by item, reliability falls.

The MacArthur battery evaluating high functioning elders showed test–retest reliabilities that varied from 0.6 to 0.71 for each item.[117] Other instruments listed in this chapter all have test–retest and inter-rater reliabilities for individual items in the 0.60 to 0.85 range. Does this mean that the performance-based tests have not fulfilled the hopes of greater precision than the self-report measures? Perhaps. They appear to be no more and no less reliable than self-report measures.

Carefully done reliability studies show that high-tech biomechanical measures of range of motion, strength, balance, and endurance have higher test–retest reliability than clinical measures. The farther one gets from the laboratory, however, the lower reliabilities become.[118] Even in the laboratory, inter-rater agreement is lower than test–retest agreement. This suggests that both rater *and* testing conditions influence performance. This is no surprise. Virtually all performance-based measures are susceptible to varying subject motivation, fatigue, interpretation of instructions, and minor changes in testing conditions.[92–119]

These cautions should not discourage the health care provider from using these measures. Appropriate care, however, must be taken in training personnel to administer the examination. Precise instructions, standardized encouragement, and careful recording techniques should be emphasized. Testing conditions should be kept as similar as possible from one person to another and from one point in time to another. For example, the same hallway should be used for gait speed assessment and the same chair for chair rises. Visual and auditory distractions should be minimized. Important for the health care provider, these precautions are most necessary when planning to use test results to compare one person to another, or to monitor the effects of therapy in a single person. If a one-time assessment is planned only to identify deficits or assess risk, elaborate precautions taken to ensure reproducibility may not be necessary.

Are the performance-based measures valid? In general, evaluation of validity has shown the performance-based tests to have properties similar to self-report instruments.[3] They discriminate impaired from independent people, detect abnormalities in neuro-musculoskeletal function (help build a differential diagnosis for disease), predict adverse events, and measure change in persons. The uses of these instruments is vast. Table 2-3 gives citations that substantiate their validity.

PERFORMANCE-BASED VERSUS SELF-REPORT MEASURES

Are performance-based measures a "more accurate representation" of physical capacity than self-report measures? Perhaps. Some of the problems inherent with self- or observer-reports of function are reduced, others are not. Differences in reports of function from the patient and caregiver (respondent bias) are eliminated by witnessing the participant actually perform the task. Performance-based measures do not more clearly reflect "true capacity" or "usual performance" than do self-report measures. Even if the person performs the task independently in the examining room, he or she may not do so at home. Standard equipment and encouragement in the testing situation can produce markedly different results than in the home situation.

Do performance-based measures capture a more pure picture of physical function than self-report measures? Sometimes. When responding to a self-report instrument, the person integrates many factors into a response (cognition, affect, cultural expectations, self-efficacy, etc.). When testing at less integrated levels of physical function, that is, basic components and specific physical movements, performance-based measures may indeed approximate physiologic function. Two-, six-, and twelve-minute walk tests are closely related to measures of maximum oxygen consumption.[72, 92, 93] In weaker people, chair rise and gait speed are closely correlated with lower extremity strength. With stronger people, the relationship between these tasks and strength weakens, as the task no longer represents maximum effort.[40]

Biomechanical measures of balance have been viewed as a valid representation of physiologic function, yet, these do not always correlate highly with clinical measures of balance, particularly in frailer populations.[65] As clinical measures of balance have been shown to predict falls and functional decline, one may be wiser in choosing the clinical measures for patient assessment.

When performance-based measures of function are compared to those obtained by self-report, considerable differences are seen.[11, 120] It may have been naive to assume that one method of measurement was more accurate than the other in the complex concept of physical function. The model of physical function illustrated in Figure 2-1 can assist us in determining when to apply performance-based versus self-report measures of function. Lower levels of physical function are the least influenced by nonphysical parameters. Performance-based measures may have the greatest utility at lower levels of integration. Indeed, there are no valid or reliable self-report measures for the basic components. Performance-based assessments appear to be the best method of measuring strength, balance, coordination, flexibility, and endurance.

At the level of specific physical movements, the method of ascertainment should fit the clinical situation. These can be measured using direct observation or self- or proxy-report. Each of these methods has been shown to discriminate deficit from independence and predict future disability. Goal-, task-, or role-oriented activities are harder to link to any single physiologic function.[93] Cooking, eating, and grooming are routines that are highly individualized and heavily influenced by cultural or social norms. Performance-based tasks assessing these daily living activities may place individuals whose habits differ from the testing scheme at a disadvantage. Because of substantial input by nonphysical factors, performance-based assessment of these activities would be a poor choice for a health care provider wishing to measure physical capacity. Instead, self- or proxy-report may be the best method of measurement.

Particularly at the levels of basic components and specific physical movements, performance-based measures have certain advantages. First, performance-based measures provide specific etiologic information. Neuromuscular deficits that contribute to functional limitation can be directly observed and identified. Next, performance-based measures can serve as the foundation of a therapeutic plan. Identified deficits can be targeted by individually tailored interventions. Last, the performance-based measures can often provide an objective evaluation of the effect of therapy on the underlying deficits.

It is not possible to say whether or not performance-based measures are superior to self-report measures. They are reliable, valid, discriminate ability from disability, and predict adverse events. They provide important supplemental information to self-report and assist in the identification of specific neuromuscular deficits and selection of treatment modalities, particularly in the area of falls prevention and rehabilitation.

SUMMARY

In summary, performance-based measures are and will continue to be important parts of the clinical and research repertoire. This chapter presents a model of physical function and illustrates how the performance-based measures fit in that model. The reader is provided with a guide to the specific assessments made in numerous performance-based measures and their use in patient assessment. Comparisons of the performance-based assessments with self-report measures are summarized. Discrepancies among forms of measurement are viewed as providing valuable supplemental information rather than contradiction. Finally, uses of performance-based measures in practice are presented.

REFERENCES

1. Kirschner B, Guyatt G. A methodologic framework for assessing health indices. *J Chron Dis.* 1985;38:27–36.
2. Wagner EH, LaCroix A, Grothaus LC, Hecht JA. Responsiveness of health status measures to change among older adults. *J Am Geriatr Soc.* 1993;41:241–248.
3. Guayatt GH, Feeny DH, Patrick DL. Measuring health-related quality of life. *Ann Intern Med.* 1993;118:622–629.
4. Ware JE. Standards for validating health measures: definition and content. *J Chron Dis.* 1987;40:473–480.
5. MacKenzie CR, Charlson ME, DiGioia D, Kelly K. A patient-specific measure of change in maximal function. *Arch Intern Med.* 1986;146:1325–1329.

6. Ware JE, Sherbourne CD. The MOS 36-item Short-Form Health Survey (SF-36). *Med Care.* 1992;30:473–483.

7. Bergner M, Bobbitt R, Carter W, Gilson B. The Sickness Impact Profile: development and final revision of a health status measure. *Med Care.* 1981;19:787–805.

8. Deyo RA. Measuring functional outcomes in the therapeutic trials for chronic disease. *Cont Clin Trials.* 1984;5:223–240.

9. Pinholt EM, Kroenke K, Hanley JF, Kussman MJ, Twyman PL, Carpenter JL. Functional assessment of the elderly. *Arch Intern Med.* 1987;147:484–488.

10. Elam JT, Beaver T, Derwi D. Comparison of sources of functional report with observed functional ability of frail older persons. *Gerontologist.* 1989;29(suppl):30A.

11. Reuben DB, Valle LA, Hays RD, Siu AL. Measuring physical function in community-dwelling older persons: a comparison of self-administered, interviewer-administered, and performance-based measures. *J Am Geriatr Soc.* 1995;43:17–23.

12. Gerety MB, Mulrow CD, Tuley MR, et al. Development and validation of a physical performance instrument for the functionally impaired elderly: the physical disability index (PDI). *J Gerontol.* 1993;48:M33–M38.

13. Gerety MB, Mulrow CD, Cornell JE, et al. The Sickness Impact Profile for Nurisng Homes (SIP-NH). *J Gerontol.* 1994;49:M2–M8.

14. Stewart AL, Greenfield S, Hays RD, et al. Functional status and well-being of patients with chronic conditions: results from the Medical Outcomes Study. *JAMA.* 1989;262:907–913.

15. Mahoney FI, Barthel DW. Functional evaluation: The Barthel Index. *Md State Med J.* 1965;14:61–65.

16. Deyo RA, Inui T. Toward clinical applications of health science measures: sensitivity of scales to clinically important changes. *Health Serv Res.* 1984;19:275–289.

17. Verbrugge LM, Jette AM. The disablement process. *Soc Sci Med.* 1994;38:1–14.

18. Cherrie CM, Czaja SJ, Weber RA. Older adults and daily living task profiles. *Hum Factors.* 1993;32(5):537–549.

19. Guyatt GH, Pugsley SO, Sullivan MJ, et al. Effect of encouragement on walking test performance. *Thorax.* 1984;39:818–822.

20. Myers AM, Huddy L. Evaluating physical capabilities in the elderly: the relationship between ADL self-assessments and basic abilities. *Can J Aging.* 1985;4:189–200.

21. Williams ME, Hornberger JC. A quantitative method of assessing persons at risk for increasing long term care services. *J Chron Dis.* 1984;37:705–711.

22. Gerety MB, Mulrow CD, Hazuda HP, et al. Comparisons of variability in performance-based vs. self-report measures of function. Preliminary results from an aging bi-ethnic cohort. *J Am Geriatr Soc.* 1994;42:A80.

23. Boult C, Kane RL, Louis TA, Boult L, McCaffrey D. Chronic conditions that lead to functional limitation in the elderly. *J Gerontol.* 1994;49:M28–M36.

24. Harris RE, Mion LC, Patterson MB, Frengley JD. Severe illness in older patients: the association between depressive disorders and functional dependency during the recovery phase. *J Am Geriatr Soc.* 1988;36:890–900.

25. Harris T, Kovar MG, Suzman R, Kleinman JC, Feldman JJ. Longitudinal study of physical ability in the oldest old. *Am J Pub Health.* 1989;79:698–702.

26. Jette AM, Pinsky JL, Branch LG, Wolf PA, Feinleib M. The Framingham Disability Study: physical disability among community-dwelling survivors of stroke. *J Clin Epidemiol.* 1988;41:719–726.

27. Johnson RJ, Wolinsky FD. The structure of health status among older adults: disease, disability, functional limitation, and perceived health. *J Health Soc Behav.* 1993;34:105–121.

28. Kelly-Hayes M, Jette AM, Wolf PA, D'Agostino RB, Odell PM. Functional limitations and disability among elders in the Framingham Study. *Am J Pub Health.* 1992;82:841–845.

29. Guralnik JM, Branch LG, Cummings SR, Curb JD. Physical performance measures in aging research. *J Gerontol.* 1989;44(5):M141–M146.

30. Andersen LB. Blood pressure, physical fitness and physical activity in 17-year-old Danish adolescents. *J Gen Intern Med.* 1994;236:323–329.

31. Cornoni-Huntley JC, Foley DJ, White LR, et al. Epidemiology of disability in the oldest old: methodologic issues and preliminary findings. *Milbank Q.* 1985;63:350–376.

32. Guralnik JM, Ferrucci L, Simonsick EM, Salive ME, Wallace RB. Lower-extremity function in persons over the age of 70 years as a predictor of subsequent disability. *N Engl J Med.* 1995;332:556–561.

33. Ferrucci L, Guralnik JM, Baroni A, Tesi G, Antonini E, Marchionni N. Value of combined assessment of physical health and functional status in community-dwelling aged: a prospective study in Florence, Italy. *J Gerontol.* 1991;46:M52–M56.

34. Tinetti M, Soeechly M, Ginter S. Risk factors for falls among elderly persons living in the community. *N Engl J Med.* 1988;319:1701–1707.

35. Guralnik JM, Ferrucci L, Simonsick EM, Salive ME, Wallace RB. Lower-extremity function in persons over the age of 70 years as a predictor of subsequent disability. *N Engl J Med.* 1995;332:556–561.

36. Tinetti ME, Ginter SF. Identifying mobility dysfunction in elderly patients. Standard neuromuscular examination or direct assessment. *JAMA.* 1988;259:1190–1193.

37. Tinetti ME. Performance-oriented assessment of mobility problems in elderly patients. *J Am Geriatr Soc.* 1986;34:119–126.

38. Reuben DB, Siu AL, Kimpau S. The predictive validity of self-report and performance-based measures of function and health. *J Gerontol.* 1992;47:M106–M110.

39. Mulrow CD, Gerety MB, Kanten D, et al. A randomized trial of physical rehabilitation for very frail nursing home residents. *JAMA.* 1994;271:519–524.

40. Judge JO, Underwood M, Gennosa T. Exercise to improve gait velocity in older persons. *Arch Phys Med Rehabil.* 1993;74:400–406.

41. Brown M, Holloszy JO. Effects of a low intensity exercise program on selected physical performance characteristics of 60- to 71- year olds. *Aging.* 1991;3:129–139.

42. Guyatt GH. Use of the six-minute walk test as an outcome in clinical trials of heart failure. *Heart Failure.* 1987;211–220.

43. Berg K, Wood-Dauphinee S, Williams JI, Gayton D. Measurement of balance in the elderly: preliminary development of an instrument. *Physiotherapy Canada.* 1989;41:304–311.

44. Reuben DB, Siu AL. An objective measure of physical function of elderly outpatients: the physical performance test. *J Am Geriatr Soc.* 1990;38:1105–1109.

45. Seeman TE, Berkman LF, Charpentier PA, Blazer DG, Albert MS, Tinetti ME. Behavioral and psychosocial predictors of physical performance: Macarthur studies of successful aging. *J Gerontol.* 1995;50:M177–M183.

46. Winograd CH, Lemsky CM, Nevitt MC, et al. Development of a physical performance and mobility examination. *J Am Geriatr Soc.* 1994;42:743–749.

47. Butland RJA, Pang J, Gross ER, Woodcock AA, Geddes DM. Two-, six-, and twelve-minute walking tests in respiratory disease. *BMJ.* 1981;283:1007–1008.

48. Desrosiers J, Hebert R, Dutil E, Bravo G. Development and reliability of an upper extremity function test for the elderly: the TEMPA. *Can J Occupational Therap* 60(1):9–16, 1993;

49. Duncan PW, Studenski S, Chandler J, Prescott B. Functional reach: predictive validity in a sample of elderly male veterans. *J Gerontol.* 1992;47:M93–M98.

50. Falconer J, Hughes SL, Naughton BJ, Singer S, Chang RW, Sinacore JM. Self report and performance based hand function tests as correlates of dependency in the elderly. *J Am Geriatr Soc.* 1991;39: 695–699.

51. Jebsen RH, Taylor N, Trieschmann RB, Trotter MJ, Howard LA. An objective and standardized test of hand function. *Arch Phys Med Rehabil.* 1969;50:311–319.

52. Jefferys M, Millard JB, Hyman M, Warren MD. A set of test for measuring motor impairment in prevalence studies. *J Chron Dis.* 1969;22:303–319.

53. Mahurin RK, DeBettignies BH, Pirozzolo FJ. Structured assessment of independent living skills: preliminary report of a performance measure of functional abilities in dementia. *J Gerontol.* 1991;46: P58–P66.

54. Mathias S, Nayak ESL, Isaacs B. Balance in elderly patients: the "Get up and go test." *Arch Phys Med Rehabil.* 1986;67:387–388.

55. Mikulic MA, Griffith ER, Jebsen RH: Clinical applications of a standardized mobility test. *Arch Phys Med Rehabil.* 1976;57: 143–146.

56. Ostwald S, Snowdon D, Rysavy S, Keenan N, Kane R. Manual dexterity as a correlate of dependency in the elderly. *J Am Geriatr Soc.* 1989;37:963–969.

57. Podsiadlo D, Richardson S. The timed "up and go," a test of basic mobility for older persons. *J Am Geriatr Soc.* 1991;39:142–148.

58. Weiner DK, Long R, Hughes MA, Chandler J, Studenski S. When older adults face the chair-rise challenge. A study of chair height availability and height-modified chair-rise performance in the elderly. *J Am Geriatr Soc.* 1993;41:6–10.

59. Wolfson L, Whipple R, Amerman P, Tobin JN. Gait assessment in the elderly: a gait abnormality rating scale and its relation to falls. *J Gerontol.* 1990;45:M12–M19.

60. Dix A. Life on easy street—rehabilitation. *Nurs Times.* 1992;88: 26–29.

61. Kuriansky J, Gurland B. The performance test of activities of daily living. *Int J Aging Hum Dev.* 1976;7:343–352.

62. Klein RM, Bell B. Self-care skills: behavioural measurement with the Klein-Bell scale. *Arch Phys Med Rehabil.* 1982;63:335–338.

63. Nayak ESL, Babell A, Simons MA. Measurement of gait and balance in the elderly. *J Am Geriatr Soc.* 1982;30:516–520.

64. Robinson JL, Smidt GL. Quantitiative gait evaluation in the clinic. *Phys Ther.* 1981;61:351–353.

65. Thapa PB, Gideon P, Fought RL, Kormicki M, Ray WA. Comparison of clinical and biomechanical measures of balance and mobility in elderly nursing home residents. *J Am Geriatr Soc.* 1994;42: 493–500.

66. Lichtenstein MJ, Burger C, Shields SL, Shiavi RG. Comparison of biomechanics platform measures of balance and videotaped measures of gait with a clinical mobility scale in elderly women. *J Gerontol.* 1990;45:M49–M54.

67. Wolfson L, Whipple R, Derby CA, et al. A dynamic posturography study of balance in healthy elderly. *Neurology.* 1992;42:2069–2075.

68. Carroll D. A quantitative test of upper extremity function. *J Chron Dis.* 1965;18:479–491.

69. Young VL, Pin P, Kraemer BA, Gould RB, Nemergut L, Pellowski M. Fluctuation in grip and pinch strength among normal subjects. *J Hand Surg.* 1989;14A:125–129.

70. Weiner DK, Duncan PW, Chandler J, Studenski SA. Functional reach: a marker of physical frailty. *J Am Geriatr Soc.* 1992;40: 203–207.

71. Alexander NB, Fry-Welch DK, Ward ME, Folkmier LC. Quantitative assessment of bed rise difficulty in young and elderly women. *J Am Geriatr Soc.* 1992;40:685–691.

72. Buchner DM, Hornbrook MC, Kutner NG, et al. Development of the common data base for the FICSIT trials. *J Am Geriatr Soc.* 1993;41:297–308.

73. Jones RE. Reliability of muscle strength testing under varying motivational conditions. *J A P T A* 1995;42:240–243.

74. American College of Sports Medicine. *Guidelines for Exercise Testing and Prescription.* Philadelphia: Lea & Febiger; 1986.

75. Fiebert I, Fuhri JR, Dahling New M. Elbow, forearm, and wrist passive range of motion in persons aged sixty and older. *Physi Occupational Therap Geriatr.* 1992;10:1732.

76. James B, Parker AW. Active and passive mobility of lower limb joints in elderly men and women. *Am J Phys Med Rehab.* 1989; 68:162–166.

77. Guralnik JM, LaCroix AZ, Branch LG, Kasl SV, Wallace RB. Morbidity and disability in older persons in the years prior to death. *Am J Pub Health.* 1991;81(4):443–447.

78. Wolinsky FD, Johnson RJ. Perceived health status and mortality among older men and women. *J Gerontol.* 1992;47(6):S304–S312.

79. Fitti JE, Kovar MG. The supplemental on aging to the 1984 National Interview Survey. In: *Vital and Health Statistics of the National Center for Health Statistics, Series 1. No. 21.* Hyattsville, MD. DHHS Publication No. (PHS 87-1323); 1987.

80. Fried LP, Ettinger WH, Lind B, Newman AB, Gardin J, Cardiovascular Health Study Research Group. Physical disability in older adults: a physiological approach. *J Clin Epidemiol.* 1994;47:747–760.

81. Guralnik JM, LaCroix AZ, Abbott RD, et al. Maintaining mobility in late life. I. Demographic characteristics and chronic conditions. *Am J Epidemiol.* 1993;137:845–847.

82. Wolinsky FD, Callahan CM, Fitzgerald JF, Johnson RJ. Changes in functional status and the risks of subsequent nursing home placement and death. *J Gerontol.* 1993;48:S94–101.

83. Miller B, Prohaska T, Mermelstein R, Van Nostrand J. Changes in functional status and the risk of institutionalization and death. In: National Center for Health Statistics, ed. *Vital and Health Statistics: Health Data on Older Americans: United States, 1993.* Hyattsville, MD: U.S. Department of Health and Human Services; 1993:41–47.

84. Boult C, Kane RL, Louis TA, McCaffrey D. Chronic conditions that lead to functional limitation in the elderly. *J Gerontol.* 1994; 49:M28–M36.

85. Guralnik JM, LaCroix AZ, Everett DF, Kovar MG. Aging in the eighties: the prevalence of comorbidity and its association with disability. In: *Advance Data from Vital and Health Statistics of the National Center for Health Statistics.* Hyattsville, MD. National Center for Health Statistics; 1989

86. Buchner DM, Beresford SA, Larson EB, LaCroix AZ, Wagner EH. Effects of physical activity on health status in older adults. II. Intervention studies. *Ann Rev Public Health.* 1992;13:469–488.

87. German PS, Fried LP. Prevention and the elderly: public health issues and strategies. *Ann Rev Public Health.* 1989;10:319–332.

88. Posner JD, Gorman KM, Windsor-Landsberg L, et al. Low to moderate intensity endurance training in older adults: physiological responses after four months. *J Am Geriatr Soc.* 1992;40:1–7.

90. Fiatarone MA, O'Neill EF, Ryan ND, et al. Exercise training and nutritional supplementation for physical frailty in very elderly people. *N Engl J Med.* 1994;330:1769–1765.

91. Tinetti ME, Baker DI, McAvay G, et al. A multifactorial intervention to reduce the risk of falling among elderly people living in the community. *N Engl J Med.* 1994;331:821–827.

92. Cunningham DA. Determinants of self-selected walking pace across ages 19–66. *J Gerontol.* 1982;37:560–564.

93. Cress ME, Schechtman KB, Mulrow CD, Fiatarone MA, Gerety MB, Buchner DM. Relationship between physical performance and self-perceived physical function. *J Am Geriatr Soc.* 1995;43:93–101.

94. Bohannon RW. Manual muscle test scores and dynamometer test scores of knee extension strength. *Arch Phys Med Rehabil.* 1986; 67:390–392.

95. Marino M, Nicholas JA, Gleim GW, Rosenthal P, Nicholas J. The efficacy of manual assessment of muscle strength using a new device. *Am J Sports Med.* 1982;10:360–364.

96. van der Ploeg RJ, Fidler V, Oosterhuis HJ. Hand-held myometry: reference values. *J Neuro, Neurosurg Psychiatry.* 1991;54:244–247.

97. Alexander NB, Schultz W. Rising from a chair: effects of age and functional ability on performance biomechanics. *J Gerontol.* 1991; 46:M91–M99.

98. Ikeda ER, Schenkman ML, Riley PO, Hodge WA. Influence of age on dynamics of rising from a chair. *Phys Ther.* 1991;71:473–481.

99. Bemben MG, Massey BH, Bemben DA, Misner JE, Boileau RA. Isometric muscle force production as a function of age in healthy 20- to 74-year old men. *Med Sci Sports Exerc.* 1991;23:1302–1310.

100. Berg KO, Wood-Dauphinee SL, Williams JI. Measuring balance in the elderly: Validation of an instrument. *Can J Public Health.* 1992;S2:S7–S11.

101. Guralnik JM, Simonsick EM, Ferrucci L, et al. A short physical performance battery assessing lower extremity function: association with self-reported disability and prediction of mortality and nursing home admission. *J Gerontol.* 1994;49:M85–M94.

102. Stribley RF, Albers JW, Tourtellotte WW, Cockrell JL. A quantitative study of stance in normal subjects. *Arch Phys Med Rehabil.* 1975;55:74–80.

103. Judge JO, Lindsey C, Underwood M, Winsemius D. Balance improvements in older women: effects of exercise training. *Phys Ther.* 1993;73:254–262.

104. Weiner DK, Duncan PW, Chandler J, Studenski SA. Functional reach: a marker of physical frailty. *J Am Geriatr Soc.* 1992;40:203–27.

105. American Academy of Orthopedic Surgeons. *Joint motion: Method of measuring and recording,* 1993. Purpose and principles of measuring joint motion p. 1–14. in The Clinical Measurement of Joint Motion. Greene WB, Heckman JK eds. American Academy of Orthopedic Surgeons, Rosemont, IL, 1994.

106. Fries JF, Spitz PW, Kraines RG, Holman HR. Measurement of patient outcome in arthritis. *Arthr Rheum.* 1980;23:137–145.

107. Pincus T, Brooks RH, Callahan LF. Reliability of grip strength, walking time and button test performed according to a standard protocol. *J Rheumatol.* 1991;18:997–1000.

108. Edwards MM. The reliability and validity of self-report activities of daily living scales. *Can J Occupational Therap* 57(5):273–8, 1990;

109. Williams ME. Identifying the older person likely to require long-term care services. *J Am Geriatr Soc.* 1987;35:761–766.

110. Lipkin DP, Scriven AJ, Crake T, Poole-Wilson PA. Six minute walking test for assessing exercise capacity in chronic heart failure. *BMJ.* 1986;292:653–655.

111. Bunc V. A simple method for estimating aerobic fitness. *Ergonomics.* 1994;37:159–165.

112. Schultz AB, Alexander NB, Ashton-Miller JA. Biomechanical analyses of rising from a chair. *J Biomech.* 1992;25:1383–1391.

113. Williams ME, Gaylord SA, McGaghie WC. Timed manual performance in a community dwelling elderly population. *J Am Geriatr Soc.* 1990;38:1120–1126.

114. Keram S, Williams ME. Quantifying the ease or difficulty older persons experience in opening medication containers. *J Am Geriatr Soc.* 1988;36:198–201.

115. Duncan PW, Weiner DK, Chandler J, Studenski S. Functional reach: a new clinical measure of balance. *J Gerontol.* 1990;45:M192–M197.

116. Luchies CW, Alexander NB, Schultz AB, Ashton-Miller J. Stepping responses of young and old adults to postural disturbances: kinematics. *J Am Geriatr Soc.* 1994;42:506–512.

117. Seeman TE, Charpentier PA, Berkman LF, et al. Predicting changes in physical performance in a high-functioning elderly cohort: Macarthur studies of successful aging. *J Gerontol.* 1994;49:M97–108.

118. Smith LA, Branch LG, Scherr PA, et al. Short-term variablility of measures of physical function in older people. *J Am Geriatr Soc.* 1990;38:993–998.

119. Willmont M. The effect of a vinyl floor surface and a carpeted floor surface upon walking in elderly hospital inpatients. *Age Ageing.* 1986;15:119–120.

120. Myers AM, Holliday PJ, Harvey KA, Hutchinson KS. Functional performance measures: are they superior to self-assessments? *J Gerontol.* 1993;48:M196–M206.

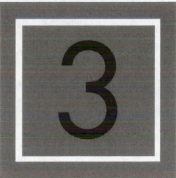

COGNITIVE FUNCTION, MOOD, AND BEHAVIOR ASSESSMENTS

MARIO MENDEZ ASHLA

Cognitive deficits, mood disorders, and other behavioral disturbances are common among elders. To assess these behaviors, the health care provider must develop some proficiency or familiarity with the neuropsychiatric assessment of older individuals. For example, the health care provider needs the neuropsychiatric assessment to distinguish the cognitive changes of dementia from those associated with delirium, depression, or "normal" aging. This assessment may disclose the behavioral syndromes associated with strokes, mass lesions, and other focal brain dysfunction. Moreover, in dementia and related disorders, investigators and clinicians use the neuropsychiatric assessment to follow the course of the illness and to evaluate the results of therapy.

The purpose of this chapter is to provide the health care provider with a foundation in the assessment of cognitive function, mood, and behavior in elders. The emphasis is on developing proficiency in the mental status history and examination. This chapter also discusses and compares the commonly used rating scales, interviews, and brief inventories that may supplement the mental status examination. Some elders require referral for neuropsychological testing. This chapter includes sufficient descriptions of neuropsychological tests and batteries so that the health care provider can interpret the neuropsychologist's report.

The neuropsychiatric assessment of elders ranges from a screening mental status examination to a formal neuropsychological evaluation. As part of the general clinical evaluation, geriatricians, neurologists, psychiatrists, psychologists, social workers, therapists, and others can perform a screening mental status assessment in about 15 minutes. On this screening examination, health care providers must be able to recognize abnormalities requiring referral for further testing. An extended mental status examination is necessary when recipients of care have behavioral complaints, such as memory difficulty, confusional behavior, personality change, or depressive symptomatology. In addition, a broad range of cognitive and behavioral rating scales are available for confirmation and quantification of the person's mental status. The choice of rating scale depends on the specific goals of the evaluation; however, it is recommended that the health care provider gain familiarity with a limited number of widely used scales, such as the Mini-Mental State Examination (MMSE) (see Appendix #29), the Mattis Dementia Rating Scale (MDRS), the Brief Psychiatric Rating Scale (BPRS), the Beck Depression Inventory (BDI) (see Appendix #5), and the Geriatric Depression Scale (GDS) (see Appendix #16). Finally, health care providers should request neuropsychological testing when an extensive and in-depth evaluation is desired. This testing requires greater time and effort than do "bedside" mental status examinations or rating scales. In the clinical setting, neuropsychological testing is preferably reserved for specific indications (e.g., in evaluating potentially mild deficits, in obtaining detailed and functional assessment as for competency determination, or helping to differentiate specific conditions such as dementia versus depression). Table 3-1 outlines the use of tests in clinical practice research. It also addresses the question of when to refer a person for more specialized assistance.

Five characteristics of behavioral evaluation in elders may affect the neuropsychiatric assessment and need further discussion at the outset. First, aging itself results in behavioral changes, and the range of "normality" broadens with age. It may be difficult to distinguish disease from the behavioral changes of normal aging. Second, age-associated decreases in psychomotor speed disproportionately affect some cognitive measures as opposed to others. Thus, performance IQ declines with normal aging in comparison to verbal IQ, and other time-dependent mental tasks are performed less efficiently. Third, psychometric scores are not entirely comparable between the elderly and the young. Even after age-adjustment, there is a cohort effect due to differences in generational experiences and education. Fourth, compared to younger people, elders may not be as open to neuropsychiatric assessment and may be more easily threatened by it. The examiner can reduce defensiveness by spending considerable time explaining the purpose and nature of the examination. Fifth, elders have physical difficulties that can affect the neuropsychiatric assessment. Changes

TABLE 3-1. LEVELS OF COGNITIVE ASSESSMENT			
LEVEL	EXAMPLES	WHO ADMINISTERS	NEXT STEP, IF ABNORMAL
Screening	MMSE, SPMSQ	Trained health care provider	In-depth mental status testing
Extensive examination	See Table 3-2	Physicians, psychiatric nurse practitioner	Determine need for structured rating scales
Rating Scales, structured interviews	ADAS, BCRS, GDS, BDS, CCSE, MDRS, CDR, CERAD, CIBI, GERRI	Psychiatrist, neurologist, psychometrician, research personnel	Determine need for neuropsychological testing
Neuropsychological testing	WAIS, WAIS-R, Halstead-Reitan Battery, Luria Battery, WMS	Neuropsychologist	Repeat after treatment or for follow-up

Abbreviations: MMSE, Mini-Mental Status Examination; SPMSQ, Short Portable Mental Status Questionnaire; ADAS, Alzheimer's Disease Assessment Scale; BCRS, Brief Cognitive Rating Scale; GDS, Global Deterioration Scale; BDS, Blessed Dementia Scale; CCSE, Cognitive Capacity Screening Examination; MDRS, Mattis Dementia Rating Scale; CDR, Clinical Dementia Rating Scale; CERAD, Consortium to Establish a Registry for Alzheimer's Disease; CIBI, Clinicial Interview-Based Impression; GERRI, Geriatric Evaluation by Relative's Rating; WAIS and WAIS-R, Wechsler Adult Intelligence Scale (Revised); and WMS, Wechsler Memory Scale.

in vision, hearing, sleep patterns, and health status, as well as drug effects, can affect cognition, mood, and behavior.

This chapter is composed of four sections. The first section describes the neurosychiatric history and the mental status examinations. Clinicians should become skillful in both the screening and the extended mental status examination.[1,2] The second section, gives concrete examples of common clinical problems in the neuropsychiatric assessment of elders. The rest of the chapter is a reference source of testing instruments for health care providers. Sections three and four are essentially a compendium of rating scales and neuropsychological tests[3,4,5] The third section involves cognitive functions, and the fourth involves mood and behavior. Health care providers should focus on learning a few of the commonly used scales and when to refer for neuropsychological testing.

THE MENTAL STATUS HISTORY AND EXAMINATION

Initial History and Interview

Every neuropsychiatric assessment begins with a history and interview. The examiner must first put the patient at ease and establish rapport. The interviewer listens attentively, letting the patient talk, and minimizes interruptions or distractions. Note-taking does not interfere with listening, and eye contact is intermittent rather than prolonged. The interviewer may need to probe with open-ended questions, using "echoing" and other facilatory comments judiciously. The interviewer searches for the underlying emotions and areas of concern, attempts to view things from the patient's perspective, and expresses an awareness of the nature and extent of the patient's feelings. Cognitive deficits or behavioral disorders can interfere with the patient's ability to provide history, and the examiner must also interview family members or friends.

The mental status history includes an evaluation of specific behavioral symptoms, a behavioral review of symptoms, and a history of neuropsychiatric disorders. The examiner asks the patient to describe his or her specific behavioral difficulties (e.g., problems forgetting recently learned information, word-finding difficulty, or getting lost in familiar surroundings). The review of symptoms includes questions about activities of daily living (e.g., impaired driving, inability to balance his or her checkbook, or decreased personal hygiene). The past history inquires into prior strokes, psychiatric disturbances, head trauma, and other neurologic disorders. Finally, the patient's education, sociocultural background, primary language, and handedness as an index of cerebral dominance are relevant to the interpretation of the neuropsychiatric assessment.

> The pattern of cognitive deficits indicates delirium, dementia, or focal neuropsychiatric deficits.

Mental Status Examinations

The mental status examination evaluates 12 areas: arousal and orientation; general behavior and mood; psychomotor speed and activity; attention; language; memory; perceptual skills and constructions; praxis; computational skills; executive concepts; executive operations; and speech, language, and thought processes (Table 3-2). Most health care providers can perform a brief screening examination, which includes one or two representative tasks in each of these 12 mental status areas, in about 15 minutes. The recommended screening tasks follow in this section; the remaining tasks are part of a more extended mental status examination, which may take 45 minutes to several hours to complete. Although designed to be performed at the bedside, mental status testing is optimal in a quiet room with few distractions. The only equipment required are unruled, white paper and pencil. An additional principle in mental status testing is that proficiency in some cognitive areas, such as attention and language, are a prerequisite for adequate performance in others, such as memory and perception.

TABLE 3-2. ELEMENTS OF THE MENTAL STATUS EXAMINATION

Arousal and orientation
  Response to verbal or physical stimulation
  Orientation to time, place, person
General behavior and mood
  Appearance, attitude, personality, and affect and mood
Psychomotor speed and activity
  Physical activity and movements
Attention
  Digit span test and digit reversal test
  "A" Vigilance Test
Language
  Fluency, auditory comprehension, repetition, and confrontational
    naming
Memory
  Word List Learning
Perceptual skills
  Constructional tasks
Praxis
  Buccofacial and upper limb ideomotor movements
Information management
  Calculations
Judgement, insight, and abstraction
  Awareness of understanding of illness
  Proverb interpretation
Executive functions
  Goal-directed behavior
  Luria Three-Step Hand Sequence
Speech, language, and thought processes
  Delusions and hallucinations

AROUSAL AND ORIENTATION

An adequate state of arousal is a prerequisite to other cognitive functions (see also Chapters 20 and 21). Arousal is the state of awareness or responsiveness to environmental stimuli. States of arousal depend on the degree of stimulation required to maintain it. States of arousal include alertness, wakefulness, lethargy, clouding of consciousness, sleep, obtundation, stupor, and coma. Patients with abnormal arousal may need vigorous stimulation to maintain a conversation, fall asleep easily, are unaware of environmental events, and are unresponsive to verbal or physical stimulation. Disorders of arousal arise from brain stem lesions, bihemispheric metabolic or structural disturbances, or disorders causing increased intracranial pressure. A persistent vegetative state is a disorder of arousal from bihemispheric damage, and an akinetic mute state is

Arousal originates in the ascending reticular activating system in the upper brain stem and is mediated by both cerebral hemispheres.

In addition to disturbances of arousal, disorientation may also occur from disturbances of attention and memory.

a disorder of arousal from upper brain stem and medial frontal lesions. These disorders are distinct from catatonia, which may include mutism, posturing, waxy flexibility, and stereotypical movements.

A disturbance of arousal is usually evident on initial patient presentation. If a disturbance of arousal is suspected, the examiner evaluates the patient's response to verbal and, if necessary, physical stimulation. The examination also assesses whether or not the patient has spontaneous movements, maintains the eyes open, or visually tracks stimuli. Further assessment of the "sensorium" includes a determination of orientation for time, place, and person. The most common disorientation occurs to time, that is, day of the week, date, month, year, and season. Normal participants are orientated to within 2 days of the day and date. The next most common disorientation occurs to place, that is, specific floor or building, clinic or hospital, city, county, and state. The least common disorientation occurs to person, that is, the loss or personal identity, and usually indicates a psychiatric as opposed to neurologic disorder. The **Face-Hands Test** may test an element of arousal or awareness. In this test, the examiner touches the patient on the hands and cheek simultaneously in 10 trials (4 contralateral, 4 ipsilateral, 2 symmetric). On the last 4 non-symmetric trials, an error in recognizing where the patient was touched suggests dementia or another neurologic disease (see Chapter 21).

GENERAL BEHAVIOR AND MOOD

The patient's general behavior can provide important diagnostic clues. A brief consideration of general behavior includes attention to the patient's appearance, attitude, personality, affect, and mood. For example, a slovenly appearance with poor personal hygiene can reflect psychosis, depression, apathy, and many other behavioral disturbances. Dementia patients often fail to match their clothes or dress in multiple layers. Specific findings such as neglect of one side of the body can indicate a focal hemispheric insult.

The examiner determines the patient's attitude toward the examination. Patients may be cooperative, indifferent, interested in the interview, or hostile. The examination of a violent or agitated patient is particularly important. In a violent patient, express concern over the safety of that patient and others and ask the patient directly whether it is safe to remove restraints. Always use a calm, nonthreatening tone of voice. Never examine the patient alone, however, and leave the interview room door open. The examiner sits so that he or she can exit the room unimpeded if necessary.

During the examination, the interviewer appraises the patient's personality, affect, and mood. Personality refers to habitual patterns of behavior and is composed of character traits or dispositions to behave in a particular manner. Personality assessment can reveal personality disorders or frontal lobe or temporal lobe personality changes. Affect refers to the expression of emotion, and mood refers to the patient's emotional state. Characteristics of affect and mood include type, intensity, lability, reactivity, appropriateness, degree of empathy, and degree of apathy. Major mood states, such as depression, manifest affective changes such as sad appearance, poor eye contact, tearfulness, withdrawal from interaction, and so forth. A depressive mood is also evident from verbal behavior such as expressions of guilt, self-deprecation, hopelessness, and suicidal ideation. Affect and mood changes occur with mania (euphoria, expansiveness, grandiosity), agitation (anger, outbursts), anxiety (trembling, sweating, cold clammy hands, worry), and others.

PSYCHOMOTOR SPEED AND ACTIVITY

Psychomotor speed is one of the most important cognitive functions, but it is often difficult to formally assess. Other than observation of the latency and speed of response, the patient's physical activity and movements can reflect psychomotor speed or another neuropsychiatric disorder. There may be bradykinesia, decreased expressiveness, fidgetiness and inability to sit still, hand wringing stereotypical movements or mannerisms, and tremors or other movement disorders. Causes of decreased psychomotor speed and activity include delirium, dementia, depression, parkinsonism, frontal lobe disease, or catatonia. Causes of increased psychomotor speed and activity include delirium, agitation, anxiety, mania, psychosis, akithisia, or hyperthyroidism.

ATTENTION

Attention is the ability to concentrate awareness or to focus mental activity on one thing to the exclusion of others. Elements of attention include selectivity and the ability to sustain (vigilance), divide, and shift attention. Patients with abnormal attention have difficulty concentrating, impersistence, ease of distraction, and increased vulnerability to interference. Attention requires the ascending reticular activating system in the upper brain stem, the reticular nucleus of the thalamus for modulating sensory input, prefrontal cortex for complex attention, and parietal cortex for shifting attention. Abnormal attention is the hallmark of delirium, the most common cause of behavioral disturbance among hospitalized elderly patients. (See Chapter 20).

Bedside tests of attention include serial recitation tasks, continuous performance tasks, and alternating sequence tasks. The most

Attention is a prerequisite for other cognitive abilities.

common serial recitation task is the **Digit Span Test.** The examiner speaks a digit one per second in a clear voice and asks the patient to repeat the sequence. If the patient can correctly repeat three digits, the examiner presents four digits, and then five digits, until the patient incorrectly repeats a string of digits twice. A normal performance is a forward digit span of 7 ± 2, regardless of age. This task can be performed in a verbal or nonverbal **Sequence Span Test.** The examiner asks the patient to serially tap four blocks (or objects or spots) in the same sequence as presented by the examiner. The test can be done with or without verbal counting, hence has the advantage of a nonverbal presentation. In the reverse digit span, the patient repeats digits in reverse order, beginning with the last number. Elders have a modest decline in the reverse digit span but normally, can reverse a string of three or more digits. A more difficult serial recitation is the **Serial 7's Test.** The examiner asks the patient to subtract by 7 beginning with the number 100 (e.g., 93, 86, 79, 72, 65, etc.). Mathematical competence is required for this task. If this test is too difficult, the examiner can do the **Serial 3's Test,** that is, subtract by 3s beginning with the number 20. Other common serial reversal tasks include spelling "world" backwards, reciting the months of the year in reverse order beginning with December, or reciting the days of the week backwards.

A different set of tasks require continuous performance. In the **A Test,** the examiner recites a list of 30 or more random letters and instructs the patients to tap on a table each time they hear the letter "A." An abnormal performance includes any errors of omission where the patient fails to tap for an "A" or errors of commission where the patient taps for a letter other than "A." The examiner can administer this task in written form, either by asking the patient to cross out the letter "A" in a written paragraph, or on a piece of paper, with 60 random letters scattered on the page (Figure 3-1).

A final group of complex attentional tasks are the alternating sequence tasks. These test response inhibition and are also measures of executive abilities. In the alternate tapping task, the exam-

B E I F H E H F E G I C H E I C B D A C H F B E D A C D A F C I H C F E B A F E A C F C H B D C F G H E

C A H E F A C D C F E H B F C A D E H A E I E G D E G H B C A G C I E H C I E F H I C D B C G F D E B A

E B C A F C B E H F A E F E G C H G D E H B A E G D A C H E B A E D G C D A F C B I F E A D C B E A C G

C D G A C H E F B C A F E A B F C H D E F C G A C B E D C F A H E H E F D I C H B I E B C A H C D E F B

A C B C G B I E H A C A F C I C A B E G F B E F A E A B G C G F A C D B E B C H F E A D H C A I E F E G

E D H B C A D G E A D F E B E I G A C G E D A C H G E D C A B A E F B C H D A C G B E H C D F E H A I E

FIGURE 3-1 "A" cross-out attention test.

punctuation and subsequently to compose and write one sentence of his or her own.

Right–left disorientation and finger agnosia are specific naming disturbances that can indicate a left angular gyrus lesion. The examiner asks the patient to identify body parts on the left and right side of both the patient's body and the examiner's body. For finger naming, ask the patient to point to named fingers or to state, with occluded vision, the number of fingers between two fingers touched by the examiner.

MEMORY

Memory has multiple dimensions. These include primary memory (immediate recall or short-term memory), working memory (manipulation of primary memory), secondary memory (new learning or recent memory), and tertiary memory (retrieval of remote information). Health care providers use primary memory and immediate recall synonymously with attention and test them with the digit span and similar tests. Working memory is synonymous with mental control and includes previously described tests of serial reversal. In memory disorders, what the examiner is most concerned with are disturbances in new learning and in the retrieval of remote information. The term amnesia refers to difficulty learning new information. It is usually antegrade or on-going but also encompasses retrograde amnesia for events that occurred just before a cerebral insult. Amnesia implies injury to the limbic system, either both hippocampi in the temporal lobes or the midline limbic structures. Vebral amnesia may be more impaired with injury in left hemispheric limbic structures, and visual memory with lesions in right hemispheric limbic structures. Amnesia results from dementia, head trauma, strokes and other lesions involving limbic structures, Korsakoff's psychosis, epilepsy, and anoxic injury to the hippocampi.

The examination of memory begins with the assessment of orientation, the ability of the patient to provide history, and his or her knowledge of current events. A common way to assess verbal memory is a word list learning task. For the screening examination, a list of three or four words may suffice; however, for the more extended examination, a list of eight or ten words, with multiple repetitions, is preferable (Table 3-4). In the three to four word tests, the examiner repeats the word list until the patient is able to repeat the words on his or her own and, subsequently, asks him or her to recall the words after a 3-minute delay with distraction. Normal individuals learn all the words. The examiner screens visual memory by evaluating delayed recall for three or four figures previously drawn by the patient or three or four items previously

Health care providers often use the term "short-term" memory incorrectly to designate secondary memory.

	Immediate Repetitions				15-Minute Delayed Recall	Recognition	
	Trial 1	Trial 2	Trial 3	Trial 4		Category Cue	Multiple Choice
Cabbage	_____	_____	_____	_____	_____	_____	_____
Table	_____	_____	_____	_____	_____	_____	_____
Dog	_____	_____	_____	_____	_____	_____	_____
Chevrolet	_____	_____	_____	_____	_____	_____	_____
Baseball	_____	_____	_____	_____	_____	_____	_____
Rose	_____	_____	_____	_____	_____	_____	_____
Belt	_____	_____	_____	_____	_____	_____	_____
Blue	_____	_____	_____	_____	_____	_____	_____
TOTALS:	_____	_____	_____	_____		_____	_____

TABLE 3-4. WORD LIST LEARNING

In the 8–10 word tests, the examiner reads a list and asks the patient to immediately recall as many words as possible from the list. The examiner repeats this process up to 4 times. After an interval of 15 or more minutes, during which time the patient's attention is diverted to other tasks, the examiner tests the patient's spontaneous recall of the 8 words. Normal individuals learn most of the list after three or four repetitions and spontaneously recall two thirds or more of the words on delayed recall. The examiner then checks recognition memory and retrieval by giving categorical and multiple choice clues for the words that are not recalled. Normal elders recognize all of the 8 words.

hidden in the room. Finally, the examiner assesses remote memory by asking the patient to recall three or four past public events that have occurred during the individual's lifetime. Alternatively, the patient must recognize photographs of famous people or recall the names of television programs. The main difficulty in interpreting remote memory tasks is determining the extent to which the past information was acquired in the first place.

Perceptual Skills and Constructions

Adequate visual acuity and visual fields are a prerequisite for visual constructional tasks.

Perceptual disturbances are a sensitive indicator of brain disease, particularly those involving the occipital cortex and parietal cortex in the right hemisphere. Complex visual processing processes include form discrimination, figure–ground discrimination, visual synthesis, spatial frequency analysis, color discrimination, depth perception, spatial analysis, and movement detection. Specific disorders include visual agnosia (inability to visually recognize objects despite intact primary visual functions), abnormal facial discrimination, prosopagnosia (inability to recognize familiar faces), color agnosia and achromatopsia, abnormal point localization, simultanagnosia (inability to visually attend to more than one item at a time), and topographagnosia (inability to spatially orient in the environment).

On the baseline mental status examination, the easiest way to screen for complex visual disturbances is through constructional tasks such as drawings (Figure 3-2). The examiner asks the patient

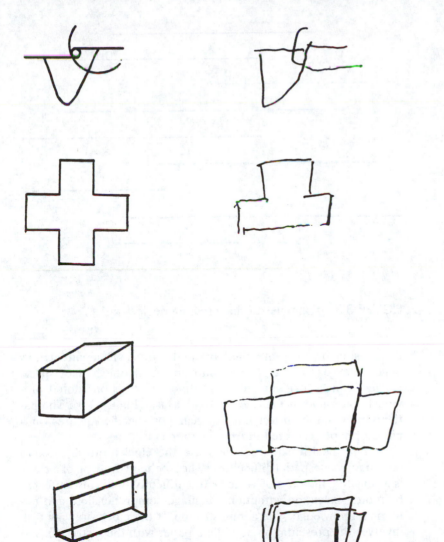

FIGURE 3-2   Examples of drawings to copy.

to copy a simple 2-dimensional figure such as a triangle, a complex 2-dimensional figure such as overlapping pentagons, a 3-dimensional figure such as a box, and the face of a clock. These drawings can show abnormal spatial relationships, absence of detail, stimulus-boundedness (closing-in and drawing over the master copy), loss of 3-dimensional perspective, or neglect of one part of the drawing.

Hemispatial neglect is a unique indicator of unilateral visuospatial dysfunction. In this disorder, patients are unable to attend to one side of their body or space, usually the left side. The predomi-

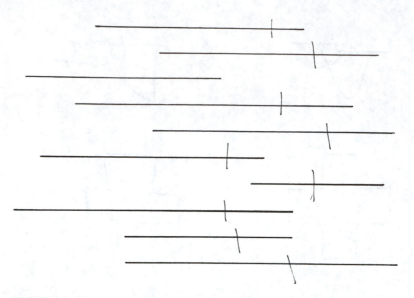

FIGURE 3-3   Examples of line crossing neglect tasks.

nant lesion involves the right parietal cortex. The patient may neglect sensory input or avoid movement in one half of space. Neglect can be evident on the routine constructions noted previously on a line or figure cancellation task (Figure 3-3). The patients must either bisect lines or scan for specified figures on a piece of paper centered in front of them.

Many health care providers use the clock drawing task to screen for visuospatial difficulties.[7] The freehand drawing of a clock is a sensitive measure of visuospatial difficulty but is also affected by motor execution, attention, language comprehension, and numerical knowledge. The administration of the clock drawing task involves the presentation of a blank paper with the instructions to "draw a clock." After the initial clock drawing attempt, the examiner instructs the patient, both orally and in writing, to indicate the time as "ten after eleven." (Figure 3-4). There are many scoring systems for distinguishing normal elderly participants from those with early dementia (Appendix #8).

PRAXIS

Praxis is the integration and performance of learned, complex motor acts. Ideomotor apraxia is a disturbance of these motor acts despite the presence of normal elementary motor, sensory, and language functions. Moreover, the patient with apraxia may be able to spontaneously perform the motor act. The examiner asks the patient to pretend to use an object and to demonstrate symbolic

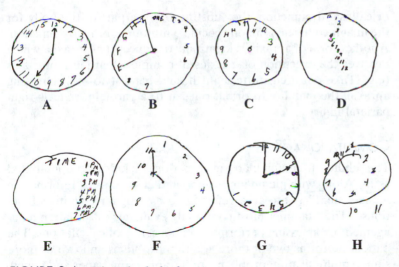

FIGURE 3-4   Disturbed clocks.

gestures. The screening examination includes at least one task of buccofacial movements and of both upper limbs, first the dominant hand and then the nondominant hand (Table 3-5). If the patient fails to perform the move on verbal command, then examiner pantomimes the motor act and asks the patient to try again. The inability to perform the movement reflects left parietal, left frontal,

	USE OF OBJECTS	SYMBOLIC GESTURES	OTHER
Buccofacial	Blow out match	Stick out tongue	Whistle
	Suck on straw	Blow a kiss	Show teeth
	Sniff flowers	Wink	Lick lips
Upper limb	Brush teeth	Salute	Snap fingers
	Comb hair	Wave	Touch ear
	Flip coin	Hitchhike	Hold up thumb,
	Cut paper	Thumbs-up sign	pinkie
	Hammering	Make a fist	
	Sawing	"Stop"sign	
	Turn knob	"V" sign	
		Beckon	
Lower limb	Kick ball	Figure eight	—
	Put out cigarette		
Whole body	Swing bat	Bow	Stand or sit
	Sweep	Stand like boxer	Turn around

TABLE 3-5.   PRAXIS BATTERY

Source: Lezak, MD. *Neurosychological Assessment,* 3rd ed. Oxford University Press, 1993, p. 679.

or callosal dysfunction; the substitution of a part of the body for the imagined object is a non specific symptom of brain dysfunction. Another form of apraxia is ideational or conceptual apraxia, which involves the execution of a series of complex, learned motor acts (e.g., Take out a cigarette, light it, and hand it to me). Dressing apraxia, the inability to orient oneself to a garment, reflects right parietal injury.

COMPUTATIONAL SKILLS

The ability to manipulate information includes computational skills. Along with judgment, insight, and abstraction, "information management" is the area referred to as "higher cognitive functions." The examiner most commonly evaluates information management by assessing performance on a series of calculations. The patient performs two or more addition problems and two or more simple multiplication problems, preferably using paper and pencil. A written assessment allows for a greater process interpretation of the actual steps used to solve the calculation problems. Primary anarithmetia, or a disturbed numerical ability usually from a left angular gyrus lesion, is only one form of acalculia. Other forms of acalculia include aphasic acalculia due to a disturbance of the comprehension of symbols and spatial acalculia due to a disturbance of the placement of numbers in a calculation.

Anarithmetia may occur with right-left disorientation, finger agnosia, acalculia, and agraphia as part of Gerstmann's syndrome.

EXECUTIVE CONCEPTS: JUDGMENT, INSIGHT, AND ABSTRACTION

Judgment reflects the presence or absence of logic and reasoning. Along with information management, judgment and reasoning account for a large part of "intelligence." It is very difficult to test a patient's judgment; responses to questions such as "what would you do if you saw a fire in a theater?" are unreliable. In everyday life, good judgment is the presence of personally and socially appropriate goals, strategies, and procedures, and the best assessment of judgment are examples or observations of behavior from the patient's daily life. One form of judgment is insight, or the awareness and understanding of illness. Patients may have anosognosia or denial of illness, anisodiaphoria or decreased appreciation of illness, and *la belle indifference*, or a flat disinterest in their illness.

The ability to abstract is a related feature that is disturbed in dementia, psychosis, and other neuropsychiatric conditions. The examiner asks the patient to interpret similarities, idioms, and proverbs. Patients with brain lesions are often unable to extract abstract meaning and respond with concrete interpretations. Examples of similarities include orange–banana, lie–mistake, poem–statue, watch–ruler, and child–midget. Common idioms include the meaning of "level-headed," "narrow-minded," and "warm-hearted." Examples of proverbs include relatively familiar ones such as "People who live in glass houses shouldn't throw stones." Unfamiliar proverbs are preferable, since their interpretation requires novel ways of thinking (see Chapter 21).

EXECUTIVE OPERATIONS

Executive functions deal with strategic planning and follow-through. They include the ability and impetus to formulate long-range goals, the steps and program to meet those goals, the motivation to act on those steps, and the ability to monitor and reassess progress in attaining those goals. Related functions that are more easily testable include verbal and design fluency, set-shifting, motor programming, and response inhibition. The prefrontal cortex and the connections through the caudate nuclei are the main source of executive functions. Lesions of the dorsolateral frontal cortex can produce decreased goal-oriented behavior, decreased verbal and design fluency, decreased set-shifting, and impaired motor programming with perseverations or impersistence. Lesions of the orbitofrontal region can produce decreased goal-oriented behaviors, personal disinhibition, and social inappropriateness. Lesions of the medial frontal lobe can produce apathy, aspontaneity, and decreased verbal output. There is no sharp separation of these manifestations; most patients have mixtures of these symptoms.

The mental status evaluation of executive functions is difficult, and the tests are generally insensitive. The history provides the most important information including a change in personality with decreased goal-directed behavior, disinhibition, and apathy and disengagement. The mental status tests corroborate the historical evidence of altered executive functions. Furthermore, the patient's planning strategy can be evident in a process interpretation of his or her drawings and the way he or she performs other tasks.

Four types of mental status tasks are helpful. First, there is a decline in verbal and design fluency. In addition to the verbal fluency tasks noted during language testing, there is a decline in the number of free form designs per minute. Second, the examiner evaluates the ability to change set. For example, the previously described alternate tapping task is a test of set changing as well as of attention. Third, the examiner evaluates motor programming. The patient must reproduce a simple rhythm that the examiner taps out of the table. The patient must also copy alternating programs such as a series of "m" and "n" letters, continuing the pattern to the end of the page (Figure 3-5). Disturbances include perseveration of one of the letters or impersistence. Another test of motor programming involves the **Luria Three-Step Hand**

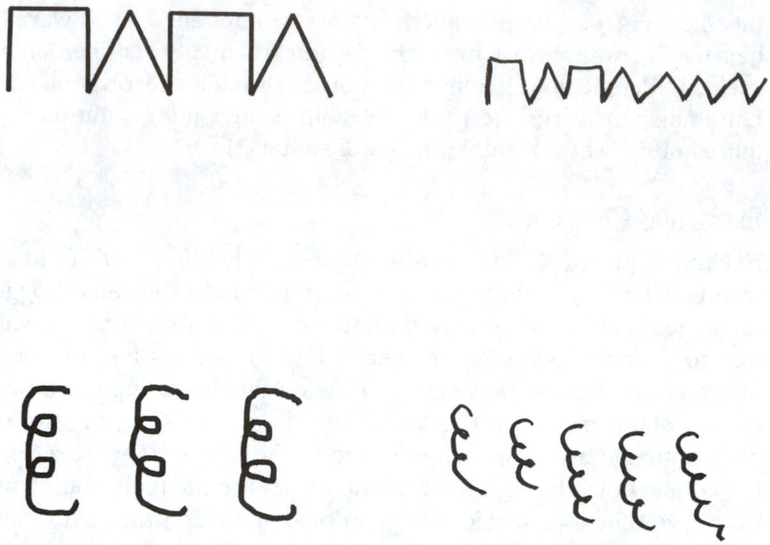

FIGURE 3-5   Alternating programs: m's and n's and spirals.

Sequence or Slap–Side–Fist. The examiner first demonstrates this task. The patient must then reproduce the sequence within five trials and repeat it five times without error. Finally, the examiner evaluates the patient's ability to inhibit responses. For example, the patient must copy a pattern, such as spiral loops, continuing the pattern to the end of the page (Figure 3-5). Disturbances include perseveration of one of the letters or impersistence. The **Go No–Go Test** is a test of response inhibition as well as of attention. Furthermore, the patient may manifest stimulus-bound behavior such as the compulsion to imitate the examiner's movements or to utilize ambient objects.

SPEECH, LANGUAGE, AND THOUGHT PROCESSES

By observing speech processes, the examiner can make deductions about patients' thought processes. Characteristics of speech include rate, quantity, loudness, and the presence of blocking, clanging, or repetitions. Pressured speech is very rapid, profuse, and urgent and suggests mania. In the presence of normal hearing, loud speech may indicate agitation or anxiety. Blocking, or brief interruptions in mid-sentence, can occur with auditory hallucinations. Clanging, or associations based on speech sounds, occur in some psychotic patients. Repetition of the patient's own syllables (stuttering, logoclonia), words (palilalia), or phrases or of the examiner's words or phrases (echolalia) can mean perseveration, a primary reiterative speech disorder, or an aphasia.

Like speech processes, observation of language lead to deductions about thought processes. Characteristics of language discourse include coherence, clarity, relatedness, and the presence of neologisms or idiosyncratic words, phrases, or grammar. Poorly coherent and unintelligible discourse occurs in delirium and schizophrenia. Disordered relatedness such as circumstantiality (circuitous answers), tangentiality (side-tracked), flight of ideas, and loose associations suggest psychosis, mania, and some personality disorders. Idiosyncratic phrases and neologisms (made-up words used with a specific meaning) can occur in schizophrenic word salad.

Other important observations are the presence of delusions, special preoccupations, overvalued ideas, impaired reality testing, paranoia, and suicidal or homicidal ideation. Evaluate the patient for anxieties, phobias or unrealistic fears, ruminations, and obsessions. Paranoid ideation manifests as feelings of persecution, self-reference, and suspiciousness. Delusions are fixed false beliefs not explained by the patient's sociocultural background. Schneiderian First Rank Symptoms are delusions of thought broadcasting, thought withdrawal, and thought insertion. Overvalued ideas are potentially credible but exaggerated and immutable notions held by the patient. Bizarre or unusual logic further suggests impaired reality testing. Finally, the interviewer should assess the patient for thoughts that suggest that the patient is a danger to self or to others.

> In a psychotic patient, the interviewer communicates an understanding that the patient believes a delusion to be true, without endorsing the delusion.

Thought processes can reflect hallucinations and illusions. These are abnormal perceptions that occur in the absence of external sensory input, and illusions are altered perceptions that are based on a genuine sensory input. Hallucinations can involve any modality. With dementia and delirium, they are more common in the visual sphere and are often formed animate and lilliputian figures. In an elder, these visual hallucinations can occur in association with cognitive impairment and ophthalmologic disease (i.e., visual hallucinations of Bonnet). Auditory hallucinations are common in psychotic individuals and can form part of the patient's delusional belief. Derealization and depersonalization are part of the spectrum of disturbed perceptions. Derealization is a feeling that the environment is unreal, strange, or alien, and depersonalization is the feeling about oneself.

CLINICAL EXAMPLES OF PROBLEMS IN NEUROPSYCHIATRIC ASSESSMENT

"Normal" Aging

Age-associated changes in the brain can result in mild changes in cognition.[4, 8] Both longitudinal and cross-sectional studies have

TABLE 3-6. NEUROPSYCHIATRIC FEATURES OF NORMAL AGING

Tonic underarousal and decreased sensory processing
Slowed neuronal processing and increased stimulus persistence
Decreased complex, divided, and sustained attention
Interference from redundant or irrelevant material
Accentuation of certain personality traits
  Decreased excitability and impulsivity; more cautious
  Disengagement and fewer risk goal-oriented behaviors
  Decreased flexibility and tolerance for change
Classical aging pattern of intelligence
  Preserved crystalized intelligence (employing old information in old solutions)
  Decreased fluid inteligence (novel approaches, new information, new solutions)
  Relatively stable verbal IQ
  Progressive decline in performance IQ
Language has richer narrative style and decreased active naming
Decreased primary and working memory
Decreased retrieval of stored memory
Decreased perception and increased spatial segmentation

shown a decline in the speed of neuronal processing, selective attention, memory, and certain aspects of higher cognitive function (Table 3-6). These changes are not inevitable or universal. There is a great deal of individual difference, and about a third of persons age 80 to 85 years continue to perform like younger people. Cognitive changes occur at different rates for different cognitive functions and are usually not evident until age 75 years or older. Because of these age-associated changes, the interpretation of mental status tasks, rating scales, and neuropsychological tests in elders must be done with caution. Many instruments have age-stratified norms; although, there are few tests with norms for persons over age 75 years. On the mental status examination, normal aging can particularly differ from mild dementia by disproportionately decreased performance on timed performance tests, preserved orientation and simple digit span, relatively preserved verbal free recall and visual memory, and adequate constructions. On neuropsychological tests, the pattern of normal aging includes a greater decline in performance IQ versus verbal IQ and decreased "fluid" (e.g., novel solutions) versus "crystalized" (old solutions) intelligence.

    Mild cognitive impairments refer to these subtle alterations in cognition that can occur with normal aging.[9] There is controversy over whether these "impairments" are significant enough to adversely affect daily functioning. For example, age-associated memory impairment (AAMI) is a debated entity characterized by mild dysfunction from age-related memory difficulty.[10] Subscribers to the concept of AAMI describe retrieval difficulty, which improves with recognition and cueing; disproportionate declines in visuospatial memory; and difficulty with working memory. The diagnosis of AAMI or a mild cognitive impairment requires documentation of an otherwise adequate intellectual background on intelligence tests and the absence of dementia on mental status scales. Of greater importance is the differentiation of memory declines as a function of normal aging versus early dementia.[8] On the verbal list learning tasks, the most significant distinctions are the greater severity of memory difficulty and the greater problems in responding to memory cues in dementia as compared to normal aging. In sum, the extended mental status examination, with occasional referral for more in-depth neuropsychological testing, is critical in differentiating age-related cognitive changes from dementia.

Competency

Competence is a legal term that refers to an individual's ability to make rational, informed decisions concerning oneself or one's property (see Chapter 24).[11] Health care providers who care for elders may need to assess behavior for evidence of incapacitation. Most of this assessment involves a review of behavioral history and observations. The primary elements of mental competency include an awareness of the nature of the situation, a factual understanding of the issue, and an ability to manipulate information rationally to reach a decision. Can the person care for himself or herself at home? Is the person aware of his or her current medical status? Is he or she able to rationally discuss issues and arrive at a decision? In order to reach a conclusion on competency, the court requires the results of mental status and neuropsychological testing along with medical observations and an evaluation of the person's ability to perform activities of daily living. An extended mental status examination and cognitive mental status scales can substitute for neuropsychological testing when patients cannot tolerate or perform the testing.

Delirium Versus Dementia

The two most common neurobehavioral disorders in elders are delirium and dementia (see also Chapters 20 and 21).[12, 13] Mental status examination, rating scales, and neuropsychological tests are important in distinguishing between these two clinical disorders (Table 3-7). Although both conditions have multiple cognitive deficits, the pattern of impairments differentiates the two disorders.

TABLE 3-7. DEMENTIA VERSUS DELIRIUM		
Onset	Insidious	Acute
Duration	Months–years	Hours–days
Fluctuations	Constant	Prominent, abnormal day–night cycle
Kineses	Normal–lethargy	Abnormal movement, lethargy–agitated
Attention	Normal–moderately abnormal	Prominently abnormal
Memory	Abnormal	Normal when registers
Speech/language	Anomic or worse	Dysarthric/misnaming
Speech content	Empty or sparse	Confused (incoherent)
Perceptual	Normal–moderately abnormal	Prominently abnormal
EEG[a]	Normal–moderately slow	Diffusely slow

[a]Electroencephalogram.

Delirium is a more acute disorder with prominent attentional deficits. Patients with delirium also have disorganized thinking, altered level of consciousness, and perceptual disturbances. Gross swings in attention, arousal, or both occur unpredictably and irregularly and become worse at night. Recent memory is disrupted in large part by to the decreased registration caused by attentional problems. Dementia, on the other hand, is a more chronic compromise in three or more areas of cognitive function in the absence of delirium. Memory loss is a major symptom of dementia and constitutes a true amnesia with inability to incorporate new, well-registered information. Health care providers cannot reliably make the diagnosis of dementia in the presence of delirium. Moreover, one of the main risk factors for delirium in elders, is the presence of dementia. The mental status examination is the usual tool for distinguishing the fluctuating attentional deficits and confusional behavior of delirium from the memory, language, and other cognitive changes of dementia.

Depression Versus Dementia

The differentiation of dementia from depression in elders is often quite difficult (Table 3-8).[13, 14] In general, affective symptoms are more prominent with depression than with dementia, and depressed patients have a more discrete time course of their illness. The neuropsychiatric interview, depression scales, and even the

TABLE 3-8. DEPRESSIVE PSEUDODEMENTIA

Affective symptoms and/or a history of prior depression
Discrete course with subacute onset
MMSE > 21 and HAM-D > 21
The patient emphasizes cognitive deficits
Variably disturbed "effortful" cognition without focal deficits
More comparable recent and remote memory loss
More comparable impairment of verbal and performance skills
Normal neurologic examination, neuroimaging, and P300 evoked responses
Antidepressant drugs result in improvement rather than delirium

Abbreviations: MMSE, Mini-Mental Status Examination; HAM-D, Hamilton Depression Scale.

Minnesota Multiphasic Personality Inventory (MMPI-2) can help in distinguishing the cognitive changes of depression in elders from those of AD or a related disorder. Depressed patients do better on cognitive scales such as the MMSE, but do poorly on depression scales such as the Hamilton Depression Scale (HAM-D).[3] Depressed patients have particular difficulty with effortful cognitive tasks and give many "I don't know" responses on mental status testing. Ultimately, the differentiation of depression and dementia in elders may be so difficult that a trial of antidepressant therapy is initiated to distinguish between the two disorders.

Differential Diagnosis of the Dementias

Dementing illnesses include those that have a predominant cortical profile of cognitive deficits and those that have a predominant frontal–subcortical profile (Table 3-9). This dichotomy is based more on the pattern or mental status changes than on a neuropathologic distinction. "Cortical dementias" have amnesia, aphasia, apraxia, and higher cortical disturbances. AD exemplifies a cortical dementia with major involvement of cortical association areas. Most other dementias have a predominant "frontal–subcortical" profile from involvement of frontal–subcortical circuits in the basal ganglia, thalamus, and subcortical white matter. The dementia of AIDS exemplifies a frontal–subcortical disorder with disease in the cerebral white matter. Frontal–subcortical dementias feature slowed mental processing, difficulty in memory retrieval, increased prominence of affective disturbances, relative sparing of language, and the presence of movement disorders. The mental status examination as well as the pattern of cognitive deficits on neuropsycho-

Table 3-9. Predominant Cortical Versus Frontal-Subcortical Dementia		
	Cortical	Frontal-Subcortical
Psychomotor speed	Normal	Slow
Complex attention	Normal	Abnormal
Executive function	Normal to abnormal	Abnormal
Information management	Abnormal sequential steps	Abnormal for complex
Memory	Amnesia	Abnormal retrieval
Communication	Aphasia; decreased verbal fluency	Dysarthria; decreased verbal fluency
Visuospatial	Abnormal	Abnormal
Affect	Unconcern; disinhibition	Apathy; depression
Motor	Normal	Abnormal movements, gait, or tone

logical testing can lead to a cortical–frontal–subcortical distinction and facilitate the differential diagnosis of dementia (see Chapter 21).

Neuropsychiatric Manifestations of Alzheimer's Disease

Most AD patients develop neuropsychiatric symptoms.[16] Behavioral disturbances cause great distress to caregivers and other concerned individuals, and are the most frequent reason for the hospitalization of AD patients. Their memory loss and other cognitive impairments interact to predispose them to delusions. They may incorrectly feel that people are stealing from them (the delusion of theft), that a deceased relative continues to interact with them, that an intruder is living in their home (phantom boarder syndrome), or that their caregiver or guardian is an impostor that has been replaced by a malevolent double (Capgras syndrome). A paranoia pervades many of these delusions. Furthermore, AD patients are predisposed to agitation, aggressive behaviors, and hallucinations. The Neuropsychiatric Inventory (NPI) and other scales are useful in assessing these symptoms in AD patients. Other AD patients are depressed, but this depression can go undetected if it is masked by cognitive impairments or by other behavioral difficulties. The BDI, the Cornell Scale of Depression in Dementia, and others can aid in the evaluation of depression among demented patients.[3, 5]

COMPENDIUM OF INSTRUMENTS FOR ASSESSING COGNITIVE FUNCTION

Scales, Interviews, and Brief Inventories

Scales, interviews, and brief inventories screen for cognitive deficits and corroborate and quantify the mental status examination. Most of these scales focus on the evaluation of dementia or delirium. They are also useful for identifying specific cognitive impairment and screening patients for more detailed neuropsychological assessment. Many scales assess the severity of cognitive dysfunction. Quantification of the mental status examination enables the patient to be monitored over time and facilitates the evaluation of response to therapies. In addition, the use of these structured instruments helps communicate the cognitive status to other health care providers.

There are many differences between mental status scales, interviews, and brief inventories. Although most rating scales involve mental status testing and scoring by professionals, these scales vary in their coverage of cognitive areas, their comprehensiveness, and their sensitivity to subtle or early cognitive changes. The instrument's brevity greatly increases its clinical utility. Professional interviews or inventories gather information by a series of structured inquiries or by list of questions, respectively. Many scales are combinations of mental status testing and professional interviews or inventories [e.g., the Blessed Dementia Scale (BDS) and the Alzheimer's Disease Rating Scale (ADAS)]. Finally, ratings scales differ in their sensitivity to the effects of age, education, and sociocultural background.

In selecting among the different mental status scales, the health care provider considers the strengths and weaknesses of the instrument. In addition to its form and ease of administration, strengths and weakness depend on the instrument's sensitivity to cognitive disturbances, validity, reliability, and whether or not it has been normed for elders.[17] Most scales lack specificity for etiologic diagnoses but are sufficiently sensitive to identify persons with cognitive deficits. The validity is the degree to which an instrument actually measures what it is supposed to measure. Among the pertinent measures of validity are criterion validity (agreement with an external criteria such as clinicopathologic correlation or a neuropsychological test scores), concurrent validity (agreement with another mental status scale), predictive validity (agreement with a predicted outcome), content validity (items reflect the cognitive areas), and face validity (appearance of measuring what it claims to measure). Reliability is the degree to which an instrument gives consistent

An excellent reliability is consistent with a Pearson r coefficient of 0.85 or greater or a kappa coefficient of 0.75 or greater, and a poor reliability is about 0.5 or less.

results. Measures of reliability include inter-rater reliability, test–retest reliability, alternate-half and split-half reliability, and measures of internal consistency.

There is a plethora of cognitive rating scales. The most widely used cognitive scale is the Mini-Mental State Examination (MMSE).[18] It is strongly recommended because of the extensive experience with this instrument and the familiarity of many health care providers with the MMSE score. The Mattis Dementia Rating Scale (MDRS) and the Blessed Dementia Scale (BDS) are two other widely used scales for the assessment of dementia patients.[19, 20] The MDRS is particularly valuable because it is the rating scale equivalent of the extended mental status examination, and the BDS scores correlate with the number of neuritic plaques in the neocortex in AD. A fourth recommended scale is the Short Portable Mental Status Questionnaire (SPMSQ).[21] The SPMSQ is useful when a very brief scale is desired (see Chapter 21). Furthermore, the Clinical Dementia Rating (CDR) Scale is a very useful scale for retrospective or chart ratings when the patient is not available.[22] This section gives brief descriptions of ten of the most commonly used cognitive scales with generally acceptable reliability and validity (Table 3-10). Instruments that include both cognitive items and behavioral or mood items occur in this section if they are predominately cognitive scales, the rest are in the following section on behavioral and mood scales. Where available, the discussion includes information on the use of the instrument in the elderly.

- *Alzheimer's Disease Assessment Scale (ADAS):*[5] This 21-item scale includes a cognitive examination (11 items) and a behavioral rating scale (10 items) of changes associated with AD. The purpose of the ADAS is to monitor patients diagnosed with AD and to assess their response to therapy. The cognitive examination evaluates memory, language, constructions, praxis, and orientation. The behavioral rating scale evaluates appetite changes, delusions, depression, distractibility, hallucinations, motor activity, pacing, tearfulness, tremors, and uncooperativeness. Examiners score most items on the ADAS on a scale of 1, mild change, to 5, marked change, and complete the test in about 45 minutes. In addition to acceptable inter-rater and test–retest reliability, the ADAS has concurrent validity with the Blessed Dementia Scale. Although it is not a diagnostic instrument, the ADAS can discriminate AD patients from normal elders, and it is sensitive to cognitive and behavioral changes in AD patients over time.
- *Brief Cognitive Rating Scale (BCRS) and the Global Deterioration Scale:*[5] The BCRS is also a 2-part scale, with mental status questions and a structured interview, developed to

		TABLE 3-10. PREDOMINATELY COGNITIVE SCALES, INTERVIEWS, AND INVENTORIES		
SCALE	TYPE	NUMBER OF ITEMS	TIME (MINUTES)	ADVANTAGES AND DISADVANTAGES
ADAS	Two parts: mental status examination and behavioral interview	21	45	Sensitive to changes over time; Not a diagnostic scale
BCRS	Two parts: mental status examination and behavioral interview	8	30	Yields a Global Deterioration Score; Uncertain reliability; Weak language items
BDS	Two parts: mental status examination and behavioral scale	50	20	Correlated with number of neuritic plaques; Contains an informant interview
CDR	Overall staging	6	Variable	Brief cognitive, functional, behavioral scale; Not a thorough examination; Memory loaded
CERAD	Structured examination and interview	Variable	Variable	Comprehensive, structured examination; Lengthy, includes forms of BDS and HAM-D
GERRI	Caregiver rating	49	Variable	Discriminates dementia severity; Relies on caregiver assessments
MDRS	Mental status examination	144	< 45	Can distinguish mild cognitive impairment; Uses screening approach to save time
MMSE	Mental status examination	30	5–10	Brief, easy to administer; Language dependent, many attention items
NBRS	Mental status examination	28	40	Designed for head-injured; May underestimate mood, behavioral change
NCSE	Mental status examination	10	20	Uses screening approach to save time; Not widely used; needs specific materials
SPMSQ	Mental status examination	10	5 (sec)	Brief and reliable; Misses mild deficits

Abbreviations: ADAS, Alzheimer's Disease Assessment Scale; BCRS, Brief Cognitive Rating Scale; BDS, Blessed Dementia Scale; CDR, Clinical Dementia Rating Scale; CERAD, Consortium to Establish a Registry for Alzheimer's Disease; GERRI, Geriatric Evolution by Relative's Rating; MDRS, Mattis Dementia Rating Scale; MMSE, Mini-Mental Status Examination; NBRS, Neurobehavioral Rating Scale; NCSE, Neurobehavioral Cognitive Status Examination; SPMSQ, Short Portable Mental Status Questionnaire.

assess dementia severity. The mental status examination evaluates five axes consisting of concentration and calculating ability, recent memory, remote memory, orientation, and functioning and self-care. The second part evaluates language, motor function, and mood. The examiner grades each area on a 7-point scale where 1 represents no cognitive decline and 7 represents very severe cognitive decline. The average of the five mental status axes is the Global Deterioration Scale, a measure of the level of severity of the dementia. (See Appendix #20). The Global Deterioration Scale

In AD, the BDS scores correlate with dementia progression, the numbers of neuritic plaques in the brains on autopsy, and the levels of brain choline acetyltransferase.

score is most dependent on memory impairment, less dependent on psychiatric symptoms and functional impairment, and least affected by language deficits. The BCRS lacks good reliability studies, but it has predictive validity. One criticism of this instrument in AD is that the axes do not deteriorate at a similar rate.

- *Blessed Dementia Scale (BDS):*[20] This widely used test is a third 2-part scale consisting of a rating scale assessing the functional status as reported by informants (the Blessed Dementia Rating Scale) and a mental status examination (the Information–Memory–Concentration Test). The purpose of the BDS is to follow and diagnose dementia. Investigators and health care providers most often use the two parts of this 50-item scale separately. The Blessed Dementia Rating Scale measures performance of activities of daily living and is composed of cognitive, personality, apathy, and basic self-care factors. In the absence of an informant, medical records and alternate sources can supply information for this scale. Scores of 4 to 9 indicate mild impairment and scores of 10 or more indicate moderate to severe impairment. The Information–Memory–Concentration Test has led to a brief 6-item mental status screening test, the Blessed Orientation–Memory–Concentration Test. This brief test has orientation items and gives points for failures. The Blessed Orientation–Memory–Concentration Test has high test–retest reliability, and scores greater than 10 are consistent with dementia. The entire BDS has high reliability and validity as does the Blessed Orientation–Memory–Concentration Test.

- *Clinical Dementia Rating Scale (CDR):*[22] The CDR is a global rating scale for staging patients diagnosed with dementia (Table 3-11). The CDR evaluates cognitive, behavioral, and functional aspects of dementia. The CDR also measures a broad range of severity of impairment, and a more recent addition extends the CDR by two additional severity scores. Rather than a mental status examination or inventory, the rater simply makes a judgment on six categories based on all the information available. Consequently, the CDR can be applied retrospectively to medical records. The CDR has good inter-rater reliability in staging dementia, and the validity of the CDR is reflected in its correlation with the BDS and other mental status scales. On clinicopathologic correlation, however, the CDR reliably identifies only AD patients with CDR scores of 2.0 or greater. The scoring system for the CDR is somewhat complicated and heavily dependent on the memory scores (see

	Healthy CDR 0	Questionable Dementia CDR 0.5	Mild Dementia CDR 1.0	Moderate Dementia CDR 2.0	Severe Dementia CDR 3.0
Memory	No memory loss or slight inconstant forgetfulness	Consistent slight forgetfulness; partial recollection of events; "benign" forgetfulness	Moderate memory loss, more marked for recent events; defect interferes with everyday activities	Severe memory loss; only highly learned material retained; new material rapidly lost	Severe memory loss; only fragments remain
Orientation	Fully oriented	Fully oriented except for slight difficulty with time relationships	Moderate difficulty with time relationships; oriented for place at examination; may may have geographical disorientation elsewhere	Severe difficulty with time relationships; usually disoriented in time; often to place	Oriented to person only
Judgment and problem solving	Solves every day problems well; judgment good in relation to past performance	Only doubtful impairment in solving problems similarities, differences	Moderate difficulty in handling complex problems; social judgment usually maintained	Severely impaired in handling problems, similarities, differences; social judgment usually impaired	Unable to make judgments or solve problems
Community affairs	Independent function at usual level in job, shopping, business and financial affairs, and volunteer and social groups	Slight impairment in these impairment activities	Unable to function independently at these activities though may still be engaged in some; may still appear normal to casual inspection	No pretense of independent function outside of home	No pretense of independent function outside of home
Home and hobbies	Life at home, hobbies, intellectual interests well maintained	Life at home, hobbies, intellectual interests well maintained or only slightly impaired	Mild but definite impairment of function at home; more difficult chores abandoned; more complicated hobbies and interests abandoned	Only simple chores preserved; very restricted interests, poorly sustained	No significant function at home outside of own room
Personal care	Fully capable self-care	Fully capable self-care	Needs occasional prompting	Requires assistance in dressing, hygiene, keeping of personal effects	Requires much help with personal care; frequent incontinence

If memory equals 0, the CDR is either 0 or 0.5 if there are scores of ≥ 1.0 in two or more other categories. If memory equals 0.5, the CDR is either 0.5 or 1.0 if there are scores of ≥ 1.0 in three or more other categories (excluding personal care). Otherwise, the CDR equals that of memory, unless the sum of the number of other category items scored on each side of memory is two or more, then the CDR equals the score of the majority of other categories.

Reprinted, with permission, from Hughes et al. A new clinical scale for the staging of dementia. *Br J Psychiatry* 1982;140:566–572.

Table 3-11 for details of the scoring system and Appendix #41).

- *Geriatric Evaluation by Relative's Rating (GERRI):*[5] The purpose of the GERRI is to rate the severity of impairment of elderly patients with cognitive difficulty. Caregivers use a 5-point scale to rate patients on 49 items covering not only cognitive symptoms but also other behaviors observable in the home. There are three item clusters: cognitive function (21 items), social functioning (18 items), and mood (10 items). The GERRI has inter-rater reliability, and, except for mood items, discriminates between three levels of dementia severity. Despite the advantages of caregiver reports of patients in their homes, untrained caregivers may not give objective assessments.

The total MDRS score correlates with measures of cerebral blood flow in AD patients.

- *Mattis Dementia Rating Scale (MDRS):*[19] This instrument can discriminate mildly impaired AD patients from normal participants. It is composed of five subtests: attention, initiation and perseveration, construction, conceptual, and memory. In elderly patients, initiation and perseveration and memory are the subtests that correlate best with functional level. The overall cognitive score yields a maximum of 144 points. Normal elders with a mean age of 75 years score 137 ± 7. The administration of the MDRS starts with difficult items and proceeds with easier items only if the answers to the initial items were incorrect. The MDRS has good split-half and test–retest reliability. The five subtests can give a profile of cognitive weaknesses; however, the MDRS does not examine language or calculations. The instrument requires 30 to 45 minutes to complete. A revision of the MDRS, the Extended Scale for Dementia, adds new items and separates out the orientation items. In distinguishing dementia patients from normal elders, the Extended Scale increases the sensitivity and specificity of the MDRS to over 90 percent.

- *Mini-Mental State Examination (MMSE):*[18, 23, 24] This popular 30-item instrument is used to screen for cognitive deficits, aid in the diagnosis of dementia, and quantify the severity of cognitive impairments (see Appendix #29). The MMSE evaluates orientation, registration of information, attention and calculation, recall, language, and constructions. It has three main factors: verbal functions, memory abilities, and construction. A total score of 23 or less suggests dementia; however, the MMSE is dependent on the age and education of the patient. Scores as low as 18 may be normal in persons over 85 years of age and lacking a grade school education. The MMSE takes only 5 to 10 minutes to administer and score. The MMSE has high inter-rater and test–retest reliability and has demonstrated validity when correlated with scores on the Wechsler Adult Intelligence Scale (WAIS). Although it is not specific for dementia, the best use of the MMSE is in measuring and following the severity of AD. The three word recall is the most sensitive to dementia followed by orientation to date and the drawing of the intersecting pentagons. The MMSE is less sensitive for patients with mild cognitive impairment, a frontal–subcortical dementia, focal cognitive deficits, or medical conditions with cognitive impairments. Moreover, some demented patients can achieve scores as high as 30. Other problems with the test include the heavy language dependency, although the MMSE lacks verbal fluency items, and the fact that spelling the word "world" backwards, is not equivalent to the serial 7s task as claimed by some.

- *Neurobehavioral Rating Scale (NBRS)*:[5] This 28-item scale measures mood and behavior as well as cognition. The original purpose of the NBRS was the assessment of head-injured patients, but it is potentially useful for dementia and other conditions. Each item receives a scale score of 0 to 6 based on patient observation. The NBRS yields six factor scores that are applicable to demented patients as well as those with head-injuries. In addition to the length of the test, which takes about 40 minutes to complete, another disadvantage is that the NBRS often underestimates the presence of mood or behavioral disturbances. Investigators developed the NBRS for head-trauma patients but have since used this scale for dementia patients as well.

- *Neurobehavioral Cognitive Status Examination (NCSE)*:[5] This instrument is a semi-structured mental status examination. The NCSE generates a subscore for each of 10 areas: orientation, attention, comprehension, repetition, naming, memory, calculation, visuoconstructive skills, similarities, and judgment. The NCSE uses specific testing material and, similar to the MDRS, if a patient correctly answers the earlier, more difficult items, the rest of the items in the section are skipped. The NCSE takes about 20 minutes to complete. Reliability and validity testing are not as extensive as for the MDRS or the MMSE.

- *Short Portable Mental Status Questionnaire (SPMSQ)*:[21] This is a very brief mental status inventory composed of ten questions that evaluate orientation (7 items), concentration (serial threes test), and remote memory (current and immediate past presidents) (see Appendix #41). Most of the variance is due to three items: the date of birth, the previous president, and the day of the week. For young or middle-aged adults, a score of 3 to 8 indicates moderate cognitive impairment and 9 to 10 is severe. The average number correct drops from 7.8 to 6.05 from the ages of 65–69 to 85–89 years. The SPMSQ has high test–retest reliability and internal consistency, and norms take education and race into account. SPMSQ scores correlate with measures of cortical and subcortical brain metabolism. Its great strength is its great brevity. Like the MMSE, the SPMSQ is more accurate in identifying moderately or severely impaired patients but is a poor instrument for detecting mild cognitive impairment or early dementia.

Standardized Neuropsychological Tests

Neuropsychological assessment with psychometrician administered, standardized testing is useful in distinguishing normal from impaired cognitive function and in characterizing cognitive symptoms.[3,5] These tests require referral to a neuropsychological testing service and are not performed in the usual clinical setting. They are most useful in detecting patients with mild cognitive deficits not evident on the less sensitive mental status examination and rating scales. Neuropsychological testing is also important where there is a need for a thorough analysis of cognitive function. This includes the quantification of cognitive deficits, definition of the underlying mechanisms, and identification of residual strengths. This characterization of cognition can assist in diagnosis and brain localization, and some tests distinguish between two or three diseases. Without other clinical information, however, neuropsychological testing cannot diagnose causative diseases or etiology.

There are several general concepts of neuropsychological assessment. First, these are formal tests. They have standardized administration and scoring by trained psychometricians; have undergone significant testing, item analysis, and reliability and validity determinations; and have normative values for different populations. Second, there is no single, best neuropsychological test or battery of tests. Multiple cognitive functions can affect performance on each test, hence the value of a battery approach with neuropsychological interpretation of the profile on the entire battery. Third, a flexible, "process" approach is important in testing and interpretation. Rather than a fixed, predetermined battery, testing can start with a broad survey using tests of intermediate difficulty, which dictate the choice of further tests based on the cognitive deficits. In addition the "process approach" includes observing the steps and strategy used in performing the cognitive tasks. Fourth, the patient's age, education, sociocultural background, and gender can affect test performance. Psychologists have attempted to construct "culture-fair" tests, and gender effects are generally minor (e.g., women may do better on tests of verbal memory than men). Very old age and very high or low educational levels have highly significant effects on neuropsychological tests, yet normative data is frequently lacking. Finally, psychiatric status affects test performance and interpretation. Anxiety, depression, and motivation impair performance on effort-demanding tasks most and have less effect on tests of overlearned skills.

This section discusses several tests that are of potential value in the assessment of the elderly (Table 3-12). There are many other neuropsychological tests available and more extensive compendiums of these tests are published.[3, 5] The health care provider must be sufficiently familiar with the common neuropsychological tests so as to be able to evaluate a neuropsychological report.

Neuropsychological Batteries

Wechsler Adult Intelligence Scale (WAIS) and **Wechsler Adult Intelligence Scale-Revised (WAIS-R)**.[3, 5] The WAIS/WAIS-R is actually a test battery composed of a heterogeneous group of 11

TABLE 3-12. SAMPLE NEUROPSYCHOLOGICAL BATTERY FOR DEMENTIA EVALUATION

MMSE = Mini-Mental State Examination
General Behaviior and Mood
 GDS = Geriatric Depression Scale
 NPI = Neuropsychiatric Inventory
Language
 W-V = WAIS-R Verbal Subscale
 LNG = Language and Speech Battery
 BNT = Boston Naming Test
 VFT = Verbal Fluency Test (FAS and Categories)
Memory
 CVL = California Verbal Learning Test
 W-L = Wechsler Memory Scale–Logical Memory
 CFT = Rey-Osterrieth Complex Figure Recall
Perceptual
 CFT = Rey-Osterrieth Complex Figure Copy
 CVT = Complex Visual Screening Tasks
Attention and Executive Functions
 TMK = Trailmaking A and B
 W-D = WAIS-R Digit Symbol Subtest

Performed by a neuropsychologist or a trained psychometrician in about 3 hours.

Disproportionate impairment of the Verbal Scale on the WAIS/WAIS-R is associated with left hemisphere damage with aphasia.

subtests organized into verbal and performance scales. Although the WAIS was not originally designed for the assessment of cognitive disorders, the extensive experience and large normative data with the WAIS provides a basis for interpreting the tests in relation to cognitive changes. The Verbal Subtests include information, comprehension, similarities, arithmetic, digit span, and vocabulary. The Performance Scale includes digit symbol, picture completion, picture arrangement, block design, and object assembly. The Verbal Scale reflects retention of previously acquired information. Although the Performance Scale emphasizes visuospatial capacity and visuomotor speed on relatively novel problems. The Performance Scale is less dependent on formal education; it is more sensitive to normal aging. The WAIS/WAIS-R scores are scaled for this age effect. For example, a lower raw score at age 70 to 74 years gives the same scaled score as a higher raw score at age 16 to 17 years. General indicators of cognitive impairment include an increased Verbal-Performance discrepancy over 15 points and increased inter-test "scatter" of subtest scores. Furthermore, the pattern of subtest scores is informative as to the type of disturbance.

The **Halstead-Reitan Neuropsychological Battery**[3, 5] is composed of five original tests specifically designed to assess cognitive dysfunction. It includes the **Category Test** (discerning the principle embedded in arrangements of figures and shapes), the **Tactual Performance Test** (placing different shaped blocks without vision), the **Rhythm Test** from **Seashore Test of Musical Talent** (judging the similarity of auditory rhythmic pattern), the **Speech Sound Perception Test** (identifying spoken nonsense syllables), and the **Finger Oscillation Test** (tapping a mechanic counter as fast as possible). The Halstead-Reitan Battery yields seven scores from which an Impairment Index is derived by adding the number of defective scores and dividing by 7. Frequent additions to these five tests include the **Trailmaking Test;** modifications of the **Aphasia Screening Test** of Halstead and Wepman; a somatosensory examination of finger gnosis, graphesthesia, stereognosis, and double simultaneous stimulation; grip strength on a dynamometer, and the **Wechsler Memory Scale (WMS).** The Halstead-Reitan Battery distinguishes patients with and without brain damage; however, it is not based on current knowledge of the organization of behavior in the brain. Moreover, this battery is not helpful in differentiating psychiatric from neurologic disorders.

Like the Halstead-Reitan Battery, the **Luria Nebraska Neuropsychological Battery**[3, 5] proposes to distinguish patients with and without brain injury. In contrast to the Halstead-Reitan Battery, the Luria-Nebraska Battery incorporates principles of brain–behavior relationships as proposed by Alexander Luria. The Luria-Nebraska includes the following scales: motor, rhythm, tactile, visual, oral language, writing, reading, arithmetic, memory, and intellectual. An additional scale consists of the items drawn from the other scales found to be maximally sensitive to brain dysfunction. In addition, there are right and left hemisphere scales, reflecting items that measure unilateral sensorimotor function. The battery yields a profile of transformed standard scores after correction for age and education. The complex motor skills developed by Luria are particularly innovative and are least redundant with other neuro-psychological tests. Although the Luria-Nebraska Battery has its adherents, it is not sufficiently sensitive to detect subtle deficits, and there is insufficient normative data.

The **Consortium to Establish a Registry for Alzheimer's Disease (CERAD)**[5] investigators have agreed on an extensive battery of mental status tests, scales, and examinations to assess patients with AD. The purpose of the battery is to provide sufficient information to diagnose AD. The CERAD formalizes the mental status examination in semistructured interviews and contains items on verbal fluency, word list memory, constructional praxis, and word list recognition. The CERAD incorporates a short form of the BDS Rating Scale portion consisting of 11 items each phrased positively, a modified form of the MMSE, and the HAM-D. Some investigators use parts of the CERAD as an entry battery for dementia patients. The total CERAD also incorporates the medical history, neurologic and physical examinations, and laboratory findings. The total CERAD has variable inter-rater and test–retest reliability. Recently, the CERAD group introduced a Behavioral Rating Scale for dementia that is representative of the CERAD battery.

INFORMATION PROCESSING TECHNIQUES

Cognitive techniques that depend on the flow of information are becoming more important in the assessment of patients. They generally depend on timed tasks such as reaction time measures.[5] Using Donder's techniques for the evaluation of complex reaction times, the examiner can determine the cognitive decision time by subtracting basic motor reaction time. Event-related responses are another method to access this flow of information.

ATTENTION

The **Continuous Performance Task** is useful to assess sustained attention or vigilance.[5] Similar to the bedside mental status "A" Test, the continuous performance measures involve attending to a series of visual stimuli, such as letters, occurring over a specific interval; the patient responds whenever a target letter appears, or when it appears in a sequence (e.g., "A" only when followed by

"B"). These tests involve the use of computerized stimuli and timed, standardized scoring. Normal adults correctly identify over 80 percent of targets. Other attentional tests include formalized **Sequence Span Tests** using four blocks on a board. There are norms for this test and a version for elders. An important timed test of attentional interference is the previously mentioned **Trailmaking Test,** which measures the time required to draw a line between scattered circles (Figure 3-6). On part A of the Trailmaking Test, the patient must draw a line connecting a series of randomly arrayed numbers in numerical sequence (1, 2, 3, etc.). On part B, the patient

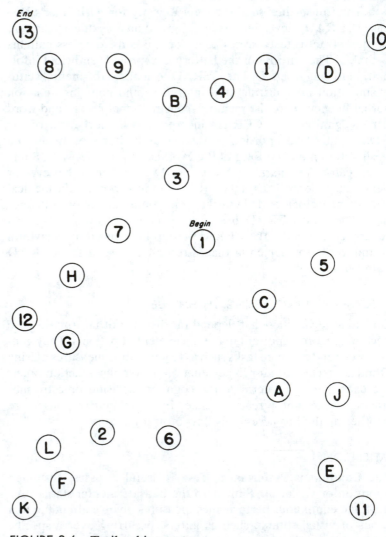

FIGURE 3-6   Trailmaking tests.
The score is the time in seconds to correctly complete each test.

must draw a line connecting numbers and letters in alternating sequence, that is, 1 to A then 2 to B then 3 to C, and so forth. The Trailmaking Tests are also important measures of executive functions.

LANGUAGE TESTS

The **Boston Diagnostic Aphasia Examination** and the **Western Aphasia Battery** are two batteries that examine the different elements of language based on a neurologic representation of language in the brain.[3, 5] These two batteries have aged norms and have proven validity in characterizing the aphasias and other language-related disorders. The **Token Test** is another commonly used language test, which involves increasingly complex commands regarding small tokens. The Token Test is easy to use at the bedside and is useful in identifying early comprehension difficulty. The **Boston Naming Test (BNT)** is a sensitive confrontational naming test that presents a series of 60 line drawings of increasing difficulty. Since patients may misname the line drawings due to visuospatial patterns, the BNT test includes conceptual and phonemic cueing trials. There are established, aged norms. In addition, there is a shorter, alternative version of the BNT consisting of 15 items. Normal elderly individuals name at least 14 of the 15 items on the modified BNT. The **Peabody Picture Vocabulary Test** is an additional test that evaluates the comprehension of single words.

MEMORY TESTS

The **Wechsler Memory Scale (WMS)** and the **Wechsler Memory Scale-Revised (WMS-R)** are commonly used batteries of memory measures similar to the WAIS and WAIS-R.[3, 5] The entire WMS is not the best memory test for evaluating elders, although subtests such as the paired-associate learning and logical memory tests may be useful. Among its shortcomings, the WMS-R battery greatly focuses on attention and immediate recall. Memory tests in elders need to focus on an assessment of delayed recall in order to distinguish dementia and other brain disorders. Another problem is the combination of verbal and visual tests in an overall memory quotient (MQ). In elders, this obscures the fact that there is a significant decline in visual but not in verbal material. Similar to the WAIS, aged norms on the WMS/WMS-R MQ for people 70 to 74 years old are up to 50 percent lower than for those 25 to 34 years old.[25]

Verbal word-list learning tests, such as the **Rey Auditory Verbal Learning Test,** the **California Verbal Learning Test,** and the **Buschke-Fuld Selective Reminding Test** are good measures of recent verbal memory and new learning in elders. These tests provide a list of 15, 16, or 12 words, respectively, which are repeatedly rehearsed by the patient either in their entirety or selectively, that is, only those words not recalled on the immediately preceding trial are presented. The patient then attends to an interference task or verbal list. Subsequently, after a delay, the patient must recall the words. When spontaneous recall is impaired, the examiner tests recognition by cueing the patient or having the patient identity the words from a list or in a short paragraph. These tests allow for the evaluation of various aspects of memory including learning curve, sensitivity to interference, amount of new learning, recognition and retrieval, and others. In general, young adults miss only 1 or 2 words; older adults over the age of 70 years normally learn about 80 percent after rehearsal and retain about 70 percent of the learned words on delayed recall.

Several other memory tests evaluate visual memory, implicit learning, working memory, and everyday memory. The most commonly used visual memory test is the **Rey-Osterrieth Complex Figure Test (CFT)** (Figure 3–7). The CFT is approximately equivalently difficult as the verbal list learning tests but has an added constructional component. The patient must copy a complex design containing 36 scorable elements and must reproduce it after a delay. Normal adults can correctly copy an average of 22 out of 36 scorable elements of the design with little loss after delays of up to 1 hour. The norms for older adults, however, gradually decrease in proportion to age. The neuropsychologist can test implicit procedural memory using special techniques such as the pursuit rotor task and

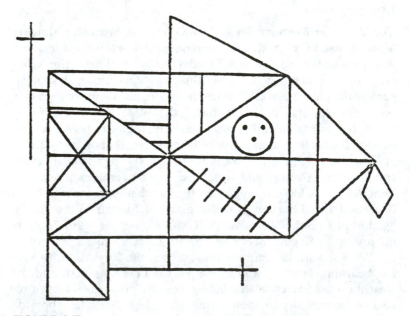

FIGURE 3-7   Rey-Osterrieth Complex Figure Test.

mirror writing. The **Brown-Peterson Test** is a measure of working memory involving consonant trigrams followed by a distraction task, such as counting backwards from a number. The patient must recall the trigrams immediately after the distracter task. The **Sternberg Paradigm** is a second working memory test. It involves learning sets of stimuli containing different numbers of items. The patient is then presented with one probe stimulus at a time and asked to decide whether or not it is a member of the original set. Decision time increases as a function of the set size and is proportionately more prolonged in elders at a given set size. A final test of everyday memory is the **Rivermead Behavioural Memory Test.** This instrument has good validity and reliability for detecting common, practical memory problems but is less sensitive for mild memory problems, compared to other memory tests.

PERCEPTUAL TESTS

Many tests that have already been mentioned have visuospatial properties such as the **WAIS-R Block Design** and **Object Assembly** subtests.[3, 5] On the **Rey-Osterrieth CFT** copy, patients with right hemisphere lesions have a disturbed overall configuration with a disorderly basic form, and patients with left hemisphere lesions tend to omit internal details (Figure 3-7). Figure–ground tasks, in which visual information is incomplete or ambiguous, are useful for detecting more subtle visuospatial disturbances. The Gollin Incomplete Figures and the Moody Figures are common examples of fragmented visual tasks (Figure 3-8). Other ambiguous stimuli include the **Southern California Figure–Ground Test** of overlapping figures, the **Poppelreuter Embedded Figures Task** of superimposed line drawings of common objects, and the identification of pictures of objects photographed from unusual perspectives. A useful test of visual synthesis is the **Hooper Visual Organization Test** (Figure 3-8). This test presents 30 cards with drawings of cut-up objects. Patients must mentally assemble the fragments and then name the objects. A normal score for young or middle-aged adults is 25 or above, but drops to 22 or above for those over the age of 70 years. Another sensitive test is the **Benton Judgment of Line Orientation Test.** The patient must match the orientation of a test line to another line in an array of 11 lines. An "abnormal" score of less than 25 out of 30 occurs in 11 percent of those over the age of 70 years.

    Several tests are available for auditory perception. In the previously mentioned **Seashore Tests of Musical Talent,** the patient must discriminate measures of timbre and pitch. In the **Environmental Sounds Test,** the patient must identify the source of a common sound by pointing to a picture of the sound source. In

Right parietal lesions are associated with difficulty with figure–ground tasks, embedded or overlapping figures, facial discrimination, visual synthesis, dressing praxis, and visuospatial localization.

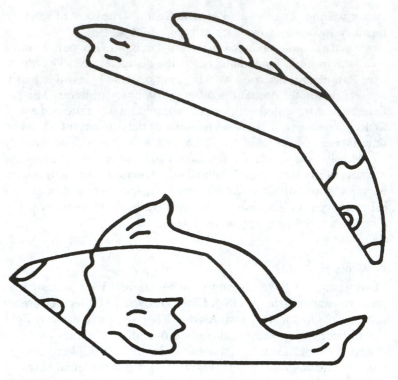

FIGURE 3-8   Example of Hooper Visual Organization Test.

the **Dichotic Listening Test** of interhemispheric processing, the patient listens to different auditory stimuli presented separately to each ear. The normally higher suppression of left-sided input reflects the dominance of the left hemisphere for speech perception.

CALCULATIONS

The **Wide Range Achievement Examination** has an arithmetic subtest that provides an extensive examination and has normative data for up to 64 years of age.[3,5] The **WAIS-R Arithmetic Subtest** contains numerical problems that are delivered orally. Consequently, patients may fail the WAIS-R problems because of attentional or language problems. In addition to the ability to manipulate knowledge, calculations require an ability to perform a sequence of operations, memory for basic tables, semantic knowledge, and spatial concepts (for written calculations).

EXECUTIVE TESTS

Many tests that have already been mentioned have executive properties including the **WAIS-R Digit Symbol** and **Similarities Sub-**

tests, the **Controlled Oral Word Association Test,** the **Categories Test** from the Halstead-Reitan Battery, the **Trailmaking Test,** and many of the Luria tasks in the **Luria-Nebraska Battery.**[3, 5] The **Stroop Test** is a measure of response inhibition and interference. In this test, the patient first reads as quickly as possible 100 color words and then names the colors of 100 colored dots. In the third, interference condition, the patient must name the color of 100 color words, each of which is printed in a color other than the one spelled by the letters. The **Wisconsin Card Sort Test** is an executive test that assesses the ability to discern a strategy and shift their response. The patient must sort 64 cards on the basis of four stimulus cards containing geometric forms of different numbers, colors, and shapes. The patient must deduce the sorting principle from the examiner's response to each placement, that is, right or wrong. After ten consecutive cards have been correctly sorted, the examiner shifts the principle of sorting, and the patient must shift to this new strategy. The **Porteus Mazes** is a test of planning and sequencing abilities. Patients trace paths through different mazes of escalating levels of complexity. The **Raven Progressive Matrices** and the **Colored Progressive Matrices** are other tests of planning and sequencing involving visual reasoning. The patient must choose the correct visual stimulus that completes a visual pattern with a missing part. Similar to the Porteus Mazes, these tests also reflect visuospatial abilities. A final test is the **Visual-Verbal Test,** a measure of abstraction and shifting comparable to the Categories Test. The patient must sort cards containing four stimuli, three of which share one attribute.

On the Wisconsin Card Sort Test, patients with frontal lobe lesions achieve fewer categories and make more perseverative errors than patients with lesions elsewhere in the brain.

COMPENDIUM OF INSTRUMENTS FOR ASSESSING MOOD AND BEHAVIOR

Scales, Interviews, and Brief Inventories

There are many rating scales that assess mood and behavior. These scales may evaluate a broad range of psychiatric behaviors or focus on a specific psychiatric disturbance, such as depression. Their purpose is to help in clinical diagnosis, monitor for change, and assess behavioral severity. Although the included mood and behavior scales have at least acceptable reliability and validity, they are not as reliable or valid as cognitive rating scales or neuropsychological testing. The best mood and behavior scales are completely structured interviews. Other scales are based on semistructured psychiatric interviews or an open interview and the interviewer's impression, and, hence, are heavily dependent on the psychiatric expertise of the interviewer. Still other of these instruments are

Compared to the young, elders are less forthcoming in reporting mood and behavior symptoms on self-report inventories.

self-rating scales where the individual reports his or her subjective feelings. Many patients have poor insight into their thoughts or emotions, others are uncooperative, and some may elaborate or highlight their symptoms. Other inventories query family members or persons familiar with the patient, for example, the Geriatric Evaluation by Relative's Rating Instrument (GERRI). Despite these limitations, mood and behavior scales may be the only practical way to document and quantify a behavioral problem.

General Mood and Behavior Scales

This section discusses ten of the most commonly used general behavioral rating scales in elders (Table 3-13). The recommended scales are the Brief Psychiatric Rating Scale (BPRS), because of the extensive experience with this instrument, and the Neuropsychi-

	Table 3-13.	General Mood and Behavior Scales			
Scale	Type	Number of Items	Time (minutes)	Advantages and Disadvantages
Behav AD	Interviewer ratings	25	Variable	Assess neuropsychiatric symptoms in Alzheimer's disease; Heavy on delusions, weak on other behavior
BPRS	Interviewer ratings	16	Variable	Brief overall rating of psychopathology; Little information on specific behaviors
CBRS	Caregiver questionnaire	117	Variable	Comprehensive behavioral and functional; Lengthy; Caregiver dependent
GAF	Inteviewer ratings		Variable	Primarily a broad functional assessment; Does not assess discrete behaviors
GMS	Semi-structured interview	100–200	< 60	Psychiatric and cognitive symptoms in aged; Requires well-trained interviewer
GRS	Caregiver rating	31	Variable	Correlates with severity of impairment; Applies to more impaired inpatients only
NPI	Semi-structured interview	10+	Variable	Evaluates many behavior in AD; Severity and frequency of behavior; Uses screening strategy
PSE	Semi-structured interview	140	60	Strong in evaluation of psychotic symptoms; Requires a trained clinician
SCAG	Interview, mental status examination	18	Variable	Useful for drug trials in elderly; Misses symptoms; Much interpretation left to rater
SCID	Structured interview, examination	Variable	> 90	Comprehensive DSM-based interview; Can limit to modules; Needs trained clinician

Abbreviations: Behav AD, Behavioral Pathology in Alzheimers Disease Rating Scale; BPRS, Brief Psychiatric Rating Scale; CBRS, Cognitive Behavior Rating Scales; GAF, Global Assessment of Functioning; GMS, Geriatric Mental State Schedule; GRS, Geriatric Rating Scale; NPI, Neuropsychiatric Inventory; GMS, Geriatric Mental State Schedule; PSE, Present State Examination; SCAG, Sandoz Clinical Assessment-Geriatric, and SCID, Structured Clinical Interview from DSM.

atric Inventory (NPI), because of its ability to evaluate a broad range of behaviors in neuropsychiatric conditions.[26, 27] Many scales have both cognitive and behavioral items. This section includes those mixed scales with a greater emphasis on mood and behavior than on cognitive impairments.

The **Behavioral Pathology in Alzheimer's Disease Rating Scale (Behav-AD)**[5] was developed to assess neuropsychiatric symptoms in patients with AD. The Behav-AD evaluates delusions, paranoid ideation, hallucinations, aggression, activity, affective state, anxiety and phobias, and disturbances in circadian rhythms. The interviewer rates each of 25 items on a 4-point scale, based on information obtained from caregivers and from clinical observations. In addition to being dependent on history and rater expertise, the Behav-AD emphasizes delusions but lacks sufficient items on mood, agitation, and other neuropsychiatric manifestations of AD.

The **Brief Psychiatric Rating Scale (BPRS)**[26] is a 16-item instrument used to document and quantify the results of an open-ended psychiatric interview. A psychiatrist or psychologist rates psychiatric symptoms, such as anxiety, hostility, affect, guilt, and orientation on a 7-point Likert scale from absent to extremely severe. Analysis of the BPRS in elders reveals five main factors: withdrawn depression, agitation, cognitive dysfunction, hostile-suspiciousness, and psychotic distortion. The main advantages of the BPRS are that it is brief, provides a quantitative score of global psychopathology, and is useful in monitoring treatment. The subscales are less reliable and valid than the total score, and the BPRS provides little information on specific behaviors.

The **Cognitive Behavior Rating Scales (CBRS)**[5] is a 117-item questionnaire that assesses nine areas of functioning: language deficits, apraxia, disorientation, agitation, need for routine, depression, higher cognitive deficits, memory disorder, and dementia. The CBRS also includes questions on educational and occupational background, current social situation, and activities of daily living. Caregivers use a 5-point scale to rate items based on the patient's behavior. The CBRS has particularly high test–retest reliability. Ratings of the dementia patient are higher than for those from normal participants on all scales except depression. The CBRS is too long for routine clinical use, however, and it relies heavily on the impressions of caregivers, who may not be able to make objective observations.

The **Global Assessment of Functioning Scale (GAF)**[5] is a revision of the **Global Assessment Scale** and focuses on rating Axis V of the DSM. After a semistructured interview, the GAF provides a quantified index of overall current functioning. Although the GAF depends on social and occupational impairment, it is discussed here because it also includes clinical symptoms. The interviewer assigns patients two numbers from 1 (no symptoms) to 100 for current status and for the highest functioning status in the past year. The interpretation of the GAF scale is dependent on assessing the effects of both functional status and clinical symptoms and does not allow for an assessment of discrete behaviors.

The **Geriatric Mental State Schedule (GMS)**[5] is a semistructured interview that examines psychopathology in elders. Trained interviewers present 100 questions and another 100 are available as needed. These questions cover patient reports, examiner observations, mental status questions, and the Face-Hands Test. Important factors include depression, anxiety, somatic concerns, depersonalization, retarded speech, no insight, nonsocial speech, impaired memory, cortical dysfunction, and disorientation. The GMS has good inter-rater reliability and adequately explores both psychiatric and cognitive disturbances. The average GMS interview takes less than 1 hour.

The 31-item **Geriatric Rating Scale (GRS)**[5] primarily assesses function in elders. Similar to the GAF, the GRS includes behavioral items as well as functional items. Nonprofessionals rate inpatients' problems on such items as eating, toileting, self-direction, and sociability using a severity scale of 0 to 2. The GRS has three main factors: withdrawal and apathy, antisocial disruptive behavior, and deficits in activities of daily living. The GRS is reliable, and high scores correlate with severity of impairment. It is not applicable for assessing less impaired outpatients.

The **Neuropsychiatric Inventory (NPI)**[27] is similar to the Behav-AD. The purpose of the NPI is to assess neuropsychiatric disturbances in dementia patients. The interviewer obtains information from a caregiver on frequency and severity of symptoms in ten domains: delusions, hallucinations, dysphoria, anxiety, agitation and aggression, euphoria, disinhibition, irritability and lability, apathy, and aberrant motor activity. A screening strategy minimizes administration time; only behavioral domains with positive response to screening questions require further examination. Studies demonstrate the content and concurrent validity as well as interrater, test–retest, and internal consistency reliability. In dementia patients, the NPI has the advantage of evaluating a wide range of psychopathology. The differentiation between severity and frequency of behavioral changes is also clinically useful.

The **Present State Examination (PSE) and Schedules for Clinical Assessment in Neuropsychiatry (SCAN)**[5] is a semistructured interview that focuses on psychiatric symptoms and functioning in the month preceding the interview. The PSE combines structured questions on 140 items with open-end questions exploring psychiatric symptoms. Like the DIS, the PSE leads to computer generated (CATEGO) diagnoses based on the ICD classifications. The PSE has its greatest strength in the evaluation of psychotic symptoms. The SCAN is an extension of the PSE and includes other elements that can give a patient's present state, present episode, and "lifetime ever." The PSE requires a trained health care provider for administration and takes approximately 1 hour to administer. It may be too long for many uses.

Investigators use the **Sandoz Clinical Assessment-Geriatric (SCAG)**[5] primarily for drug trials in elderly patients. The instrument uses 18 subscales to assess uncooperativeness, unsociability, mood changes, self-care, appetite, and cognition. More items deal with behavioral disturbances than with cognition, and there are four major factors: agitation and irritability, mood and depression, cognitive dysfunction, and withdrawal. The interviewer scores each item on a 7-point scale based on observations of the patient. Despite the lack of standardized administration, the SCAG has excellent reliability and validity. It can differentiate elderly patients with severe dementia or depression from normal participants. The range of behavioral, functional, and cognitive items is also useful in evaluating the effects of medications. The SCAG does not assess other symptoms that might be affected by medications, such as sleep problems and the presence of hallucinations. Furthermore, much interpretation is left to the rater since the ratings require a trained examiner.

The **Structured Clinical Interview from DSM (SCID),**[9] like the PSE and the Schedule for Affective Disorders and Schizophrenia (SADS), is a semistructured interview designed for administration by a trained examiner. It differs in that it is based on diagnostic criteria from the DSM. Health care providers can use the entire SCID or just parts or modules of it. The SCID has two parts, one for Axis I disorders and another for Axis II personality disorders. At the start of a SCID interview, the interviewer obtains an overview of the present illness, chief complaint, and past episodes of major psychopathology before systematically asking about specific symptoms. After an overview, the interviewer can move to modules that cover mania, psychosis, depression, substance abuse, somatization disorders, eating disorders, and adjustment disorders. The SCID interview also includes the GAF Scale. The SCID has acceptable test–retest reliabilities for lifetime diagnoses for patients but poor reliability for nonpatients. One advantage of the SCID is the presence of many open-ended questions so that patients can describe symptoms in their own words. Other advantages are the way it leads the interviewer thorough Axis I diagnostic criteria and the fact that the interview can be limited to relevant modules. The interviewer must be a competent examiner, preferably a psychiatrist, and the Axis I part of the SCID takes about 60 to 90 minutes to complete.

SPECIFIC MOOD AND BEHAVIOR SCALES

These scales focus on a particular behavior rather than a broad psychiatric sample. The majority of these scales assess depression, but there are anxiety scales as well as agitation scales (Table 3-14). The recommended scales are the Beck Depression Inventory (BDI) and the Geriatric Depression Scale (GDS) for assessing depression and the Beck Anxiety Inventory (BDI) for assessing anxiety.[28, 29, 30] The popular HAM-D may have too many somatic items for assessing depression in elders or in demented patients. This review includes ten of the most commonly used specific scales, interviews, and brief inventories.

TABLE 3-14.   SPECIFIC MOOD AND BEHAVIOR SCALES

SCALE	TYPE	NUMBER OF ITEMS	TIME (MINUTES)	ADVANTAGES AND DISADVANTAGES
Depression				
BDI	Self-report inventory	21	30	Correlates with psychiatrist's diagnosis; False positives with physical disabilities
Cornell	Caregiver inventory	19	Variable	Valuable for depression in dementia; Dementia itself may count for some items
HAM-D	Interviewer ratings	17 or 21	Variable	Sensitive to depression changes over time; Heavy loading on physical symptoms
GDS	Interviewer ratings	30	Variable	Specifically designed for elderly; Not as valid for cognitively impaired
Zung	Self-report inventory	20	< 45	False positives among the elderly; Mild but frequent symptoms may score high
Anxiety and Agitation				
BAI	Self-report inventory	21	Variable	Applicable to elderly; Weak correlation with HAM-A and STAI
CMAI	Interviewer ratings	29	Variable	Best scale for agitation in dementia; Frequency and state dependent
HAM-A	Interviewer ratings	14	30	Rates severity of anxiety; Heavy loading on physical
OAD	Interviewer ratings	16+	< 10	Excellent general agitation instrument; Includes additional intervention items
STAI	Self-report inventory	20	Variable	Measures both state and trait anxiety

Abbreviations: BDI, Beck Depression Inventory; Cornell, Cornell Scale of Depression in Dementia; HAM-D, Hamilton Depression Scale; GDS, Geriatric Depression Scale; Zung, Zung Self-Rating Scale for Depression; BAI, Beck Anxiety Inventory; CMAI, Cohen-Mansfield Agitation Scale; HAM-A, Hamilton Anxiety Scale; OAS, Overt Aggression Scale; and STAI, State-Trait Anxiety Inventory.

The **Beck Depression Inventory (BDI)**[28] is one of the most widely used self-report inventories for current depression (see Appendix #5). The patient answers the 21 items of the BDI on a continuum of severity from 0, "I don't feel sad," to 3, "I am so sad or unhappy that I can't stand it." The BDI focuses on the cognitive symptoms of depression, such as pessimism and diminished self-esteem, and 7 items assess physical symptoms. The BDI has adequate test–retest and split-half reliability that includes non-depressed and depressed elderly patients. It correlates well with a psychiatrist's ratings of depression. The BDI is useful for screening for depression in elders, assessing the severity of depression, and monitoring mood changes over time. False positive scores can occur in individuals with physical disabilities.

The specific purpose of the **Cornell Scale of Depression in Dementia (Cornell)**[5] is the assessment of depression in patients with dementia, (see Appendix #13). The Cornell has subsections on depressive symptoms including mood related signs, behavioral disturbances, physical signs, cyclic functions, and ideational disturbance. A caregiver rates the 19 items of the Cornell as 0 (absent), 1 (mild or intermittent), or 2 (severe). The scale has acceptable reliability, is sensitive to mood changes in dementia patients, and has concurrent validity with the research diagnostic criteria for depression. In assessing dementia patients, this scale has the advantages of being designed specifically to elicit information from caregivers with brief confirmatory observations of the patient. Several of the items, however, could be produced by dementia syndromes even in the absence of a mood disorder.

The **Hamilton Depression Scale (HAM-D)**[3,5] (see Appendix #21) is the most widely used depression scale and the "gold standard" for other depression scales. The interviewer evaluation is based on a semistructured interview. The original purpose of the HAM-D was to measure the severity of depression in patients already diagnosed with depression. It has items on psychomotor retardation, insomnia, mood, and insight. The HAM-D has 17 items (some versions have 21) with ratings along a continuum of 0 to 4 or 0 to 2 intensity and frequency within the past few days. The HAM-D allows the assessment of individuals who could not complete a self-report inventory. The HAM-D is useful for monitoring a depressed state over time and for evaluating the effects of treatment, but it is less effective for the diagnosis of depression. Weaknesses of the HAM-D include an overemphasis on somatic, neuro-vegetative symptoms (nine items reflect concern over physical symptoms) and an underemphasis on mood, affective, and cognitive changes of depression. In elderly depressed patients, the HAM-D over-reports changes in psychomotor activity and cognitive com-

Several forms of the HAM-D exist with different numbers of symptom ratings.

plaints, and the HAM-D is unreliable in patients with dementia, particularly given its emphasis of physical symptoms. One variant of the HAM-D, the Montgomery-Asberg Depression Rating Scale, omits many somatic or psychomotor symptoms and adds measures for sadness, inner tension, reduced sleep, lassitude, pessimism, and suicidal thoughts. The HAM-D and its close variants do not have standardized questions but depend on the skill of the interviewer to collect the information and to make rating decisions.

The specific purpose of the **Geriatric Depression Scale (GDS)**[29] is to rate depression in the elderly (see Appendix #16). The GDS avoids the emphasis on physical symptoms present in the HAM-D and uses items with ecological validity for elders. The GDS is a self-report inventory of 30 yes to no questions. Scores of 0 to 10 are normal, scores of 11 or higher yield a sensitivity of 84 percent and a specificity of 95 percent for depression in elders, and scores of 14 or higher yield a sensitivity of 80 percent and a specificity of 100 percent for depression. The GDS correlates with RDC depression and can differentiate physically ill depressed from physically ill nondepressed elders, but it may not be appropriate for those with cognitive impairment or dementia.

After the BDI, the **Zung Self-Rating Scale for Depression**[5] is the most popular self-report inventory of depression. The Zung has 20 items similar to those of the BDI. The interviewer rates each item on frequency of occurrence on a scale ranging from 1 to 4, a "little of the time" to "most of the time." Symptoms that occur frequently but may not be severe may receive a high rating, and this scale may not be sensitive to changes in depression over time. Elders have higher Zung score and endorse more items reflecting physical symptoms. The Zung overclassifies nondepressed elderly participants as depressed and is limited in distinguishing depression in older patients. In sum, the Zung may not be appropriate for assessing depression in those over 70 years of age.

The **Beck Anxiety Inventory (BAI)**[30] is a self-report anxiety inventory similar to the BDI (Table 3-15). This 21-item questionnaire has two factors: fourteen items reflect somatic symptoms and 7 reflect cognitive symptoms associated with anxiety. The BAI assesses frequency of anxiety symptoms over 1 week and minimizes their relationship with depression. Patients rate the severity of each symptom on a 4-point scale from "Not at all" to "I could barely stand it." It has good internal consistency, test–retest reliability, and convergent and discriminant validity, but correlates modestly (in the 0.5 range) with the HAM-A and STAI. Self-reported anxious symptoms differentiate elderly medical and psychiatric outpatients, but two symptoms, "fear of the worst happening" and "unsteady," account for most of the differentiation between the two groups.

Instruments that measure situational anxiety or agitation are highly state dependent with high low test–retest reliability.

TABLE 3-15. BECK ANXIETY INVENTORY

1. Numbness or tingling
2. Feeling hot
3. Wobbling in legs
4. Unable to relax
5. Fear of the worst happening
6. Dizzy or lightheaded
7. Heart pounding or racing
8. Unsteady
9. Terrified
10. Nervous
11. Feelings of choking
12. Hands trembling
13. Shaky
14. Fear of losing control
15. Difficulty breathing
16. Fear of dying
17. Scared
18. Indigestion
19. Faint
20. Face flushed
21. Sweating (not due to heat)

Reprinted, with permission, from Steer RA, Willman M, Kay PA, Beck AT. Differentiating elderly medical and psychiatric outpatients with the Beck Anxiety Inventory. *Assessment* 1994;4:345–351.

Agitation is a common management problem in dementia. The **Cohen-Mansfield Agitation Scale (CMAI)**[31] measures agitation as defined by inappropriate, abusive, or aggressive verbal or motor activity that is not explained by needs or confusion. The CMAI consists of 29 agitated behaviors rated on a 7-point frequency scale with 7 representing a behavior that is exhibited several times in a day. Factor analysis of ratings on nursing home residents reveal three factors: verbal and physical aggressive behavior, physically nonaggressive behavior such as pacing and restlessness, and verbally agitated behaviors such as screaming or repetitive requests for attention. This instrument may be the best scale for the assessment of agitation in both demented and nondemented elderly patients.

Similar to the HAM-D for depression, the **Hamilton Anxiety (HAM-A)**[5] is the most widely used scale for measuring anxiety. After an open clinical interview, the examiner rates patients with anxiety syndromes on 14 items according to their severity. The HAM-A is a very reliable and valid instrument. It is intended for rating the severity of anxiety rather than for the diagnosis of anxiety disorders and is not useful for measuring generalized anxiety in other psychiatric or medical illnesses. Furthermore, it resembles the HAM-D in it bias toward somatic experiences and in its need for trained clinician raters.

The **Overt Aggression Scale (OAS)**[31] documents aggressive behaviors based on observable criteria and recorded by hospital staff or other observers. The OAS divides observed aggressive behaviors into four categories: verbal aggression, physical aggression against objects, physical aggression against self, and physical aggression against others. Within each of these categories, descriptive statements define four levels of severity. As an additional indicator or severity, the OAS records the therapeutic interventions used in response to each aggressive episode. The OAS has high inter-rater reliability and is useful for assessing aggression in chronically hospitalized patients including individual patterns of aggression, week-to-week fluctuations, and response to interventions.

The **State-Trait Anxiety Inventory (STAI)**[5] measure is a brief self-report inventory that differentiates between state anxiety, which may be experienced in specific situations, and trait anxiety, which is the relatively stable anxiety-proneness experienced by the patient. The 20 items are short descriptive statements. For state anxiety, the patient responds to the items on a 4-point intensity scale of how he or she feels at the moment. For trait anxiety, the patient responds to the items on a 4-point frequency scale of how he or she generally feels. The STAI may be useful in elders, but, compared to other instruments, there is less information on the feasibility and value of the STAI in older people.

Standardized Personality and Projective Tests

There are few mood and behavior psychometric instruments that are widely used or applicable to older people.[3, 5] The **Minnesota Multiphasic Personality Inventory (MMPI/MMPI-2)** is the most popular personality inventory. The MMPI is a 566-item questionnaire originally developed in the early 1940s to measure clinical personality disorders and to aid in diagnosis. It evolved beyond its original clinical intent to become an instrument for determining personality traits. The MMPI includes three validity scales designed to assess test-taking attitude. These validity scales are useful in assessing for malingering or embellishment. The MMPI-2, introduced in 1989, updates the items of the MMPI and relies on a broader, more representative cross-section of the U.S. population (although biased towards higher education and socioeconomic status). Some psychologists continue to use the original MMPI positing that the experience with the MMPI may not be transferable to the MMPI-2. The interpretation of the MMPI and MMPI-2 scales involves a configural interpretation of the pattern or profile of scale scores usually based on the two highest scale scores. The use of additional scales beyond the original Clinical Scales can contribute to the configural interpretation. Moreover, reliable computer software is available for interpreting the MMPI/MMPI-2.

There is limited information on the use of other standardized tests of mood and behavior in elders. These tests are primarily personality inventories or projective tests. The **Millon Clinical Multiaxial Inventory (MCMI)** is a 175-item personality inventory consisting of true or false questions. The MCMI has 11 scales based on DSM personality disorders. In addition, it has a validity scale and nine scales designed to assess Axis I disorders. Although there is much less data on the MCMI compared to the MMPI/MMPI-2, this instrument is shorter, grounded in current psychiatric terminology, and is frequently updated. Other quantitative personality inventories are infrequently used in elders. Projective tests are relatively unstructured instruments that permit conclusions about personality based on the interpretation of ambiguous stimuli. Important projective tests include the **Rorschach Test, Apperception Tests (Thematic, Gerontological, Senior),** the **Holtzman Inkblot Test,** and the interpretation of the **Bender-Gestalt, Figure Drawing, and Sentence Completion.** In general, these projective tests lack reliability and validity and rely heavily on the examiner's interpretation. Two projective tests that specifically target elders are the Gerontological Apperception Test and the Senior Apperception Test. These two tests are rarely used and consist of 14 or 16 cards, respectively, of elders in common life situations. The patient must give a story about each of the cards.

REFERENCES

1. Strub RL, Black FW. *The Mental Status Examination in Neurology.* 3rd ed. Philadelphia: FA Davis; 1993.
2. Trzepacz PT, Baker RW. *The Psychiatric Mental Status Examination.* New York: Oxford University Press; 1993.
3. Spreen O, Strauss E. *A Compendium of Neuropsychological Tests. Administration, Norms, and Commentary.* 2nd ed. New York: Oxford University Press; 1998.
4. La Rue A. *Aging and Neuropsychological Assessment.* New York: Plenum Press; 1992.
5. Lezak MD. *Neuropsychological Assessment.* 3rd ed. New York: Oxford University Press; 1993.
6. Benson DF. *Aphasia, Alexia, and Agraphia.* New York: Churchill Livingstone; 1979.

7. Mendez MF, Ala T, Underwood KL. Development of scoring criteria for the clock drawing task in Alzheimer's disease. *J Am Geriatr Soc.* 1992;40:1095–1099.

8. Christensen J, Hadzi-Pavlovic D, Jacomb P. The psychometric differentiation of dementia from normal aging: a meta-analysis. *Psychol Assess.* 1991;3:147–155.

9. American Psychiatric Association. *Diagnostic and Statistical Manual of Mental Disorders.* 4th ed. DSM-IV. Washington DC: American Psychiatric Association; 1994.

10. Larrabee GJ, McEntee WJ. Age-associated memory impairment: sorting out the controversies. *Neurology.* 1995;45:611–614.

11. Freedman M, Stuss DT, Gordon M. Assessment of competency: the role of neurobehavioral deficits. *Ann Intern Med.* 1991;115:203–208.

12. Mendez MF. Delirium. In: Bradley WG, Daroff RB, Fenichel GM, Marsden CD, eds. *Neurology in Clinical Practice.* 3rd ed. Boston: Butterworth-Heinemann; 2000;25–36.

13. Coffey CE, Cummings JL. *Textbook of Geriatric Neuropsychiatry.* Washington, DC: The American Psychiatric Press; 1994.

14. Yesavage JA. Differential diagnosis between depression and dementia. *Am J Med.* 1993;94:23S–28S.

15. Lamberty GJ, Bieliauskus LA. Distinguishing between depression and dementia in the elderly: a review of neuropsychological findings. *Arch Clin Neuropsychol.* 1993;8:149–170.

16. Cummings JL, Benson DF. *Dementia: A Clinical Approach.* 2nd ed. Boston: Butterworths; 1992.

17. Gifford DR, Cummings JL. Evaluating dementia screening tests: methodologic standards to rate their performance. *Neurology.* 1999; 52:224–227.

18. Folstein M, Folstein SE, McHugh PR. "Mini-Mental State": a practical method for grading the cognitive state of patients for the clinician. *J Psychiatr Res.* 1975;12:189–198.

19. Mattis S. Dementia Rating Scale. Odessa, FL: Psychological Assessment Resources; 1988.

20. Blessed G, Tomlinson BE, Roth M. The association between quantitative measures of dementia and of senile changes in the cerebral gray matter of elderly patients. *Br J Psychiatry.* 1968;114:797–811.

21. Pfeiffer E. A short portable mental status questionnaire for the assessment of organic brain deficits in elderly patients. *J Am Geriatr Soc.* 1975;23:433–441.

22. Hughes CP, Berg L, Danzinger WL, Coben LA, Martin RL. A new clinical scale for the staging of dementia. *Br J Psychiatry.* 1982;140: 566–572.

23. Tombaugh TN, McIntyre NJ. The Mini-Mental State Examination: a comprehensive review. *J Am Geriatr Soc.* 1992;40:922–935.

24. Crum RM, Anthony JC, Bassett SS, Folstein MF. Population-based norms for the Mini-Mental State Examination by age and education level. *JAMA.* 1993;269:2386–2391.

25. Ivnik RJ, Malec JF, Smith GE, et al. Mayo's older Americans normative studies: WMS-R norms for ages 56–97. *Clin Neuropsychologist.* 1992;6:1–30.

26. Overall J, Gorham D. Brief Psychiatric Rating Scale. *Psychol Rep.* 1962;10:79.
27. Cummings JL, Mega M, Gray K, Rosenberg-Thompson S, Carusi DA, Gornbein J. The Neuropsychiatric Inventory: comprehensive assessment of psychopathology in dementia. *Neurology.* 1994;44:2308–2314.
28. Beck AT. *Beck Depression Inventory: Manual.* San Antonio, TX: Psychological Corporation; 1987.
29. Yesavage JA. Geriatric depression scale. *Psychopharmacol Bull.* 1988;24:709.
30. Steer RA, Williman M, Kay PA, Beck AT. Differentiating elderly medical and psychiatric outpatients with the Beck Anxiety Inventory. *Assessment.* 1994;4:345–351.
31. Kluger A, Ferris SH. Scales for the assessment of Alzheimer's disease. *Psychiatr Clin North Am.* 1991;14:309–326.

SOCIAL SUPPORT NETWORKS

JAMES LUBBEN / MELANIE GIRONDA

Whereas routine health examinations increasingly inquire about past and present smoking behavior, similar inquiry regarding an elderly person's social support network remains rare. Research evidence indicates, however, that social isolation can be as detrimental to health as smoking in terms of a health risk,[1-4] so health risk appraisals should be revised to also evaluate the adequacy of an elder's social support network. What accounts for the apparent health risk of social isolation and how to best assess for an elder's social support networks are the topics of this chapter. Additional information on the assessment of social support is found in Chapter 26.

IMPORTANCE OF SOCIAL SUPPORT NETWORKS TO HEALTH

Theories for the Apparent Relationship of Social Support Network and Health

The most common explanation for the apparent link between health and social support networks is that strong social ties provide a buffering effect from stress, thereby reducing the vulnerability of an individual to stress related illnesses.[5-9] In practice, it is also noteworthy to remember that many practitioner–patient encounters are inherently stressful, increasing the relevance of this theory to assisting in desired clinical outcomes. This theory supposes that

Various theories have been proposed as to why social support networks may influence one's health status.

an elder with a nurturing social support network is more equipped to manage the stress normally associated with major health events as well as other stressful events common in old age. Perhaps the popular Beatles song that includes the refrain "I get by with a little help from my friends.... I'm going to try with a little help from my friends" captures the essence of this theory.

A related theory suggests that social isolation can have a direct physiologic effect increasing vulnerability to morbidity and mortality.[10] Details of this theory often include reference to how social ties may stimulate the immune system to better ward off illnesses. There is less hard evidence supporting this specific theory; however some very current research involving persons with imune disorders (e.g., cancer, AIDS, etc.) should further clarify the veracity of this theory.

Another common theory is that social networks provide essential support at times of illness, thereby facilitating adaptation and speeding recovery.[11, 12] Case examples have often illustrated these phenomena in past practice. It may be even more relevant today in the era of managed health care. Indeed, much of the current reliance on outpatient medical care requires the presence of a functional social support network to provide care to the elder that previously would have been delivered by nurses or nurses aides in a hospital. This theory would advise that those elders without an adequate social support network are at increased risk of complications and are likely to have a slower recovery period.

A fourth theory states that social support networks can encourage an elder to observe health promoting behaviors and quit bad practices.[10, 11, 13] This may be especially important when considering nutrition or exercise. Further, an elder's family or friends may facilitate a person's seeking timely medical attention for a specific health condition before it becomes a larger and more difficult to treat problem.

Summary of Research Findings on Social Support Networks

What is most surprising about the research findings regarding the connection between social support networks and health is that they were obtained despite a lack of clarity in defining social support networks and an inconsistency in measuring health. Indeed, the diversity of these studies adds extra significance to the convergence of their findings. Research shows that social support networks correlate with mortality rates,[2, 14–16] various morbidity indicators,[10, 17–22] and several different psychological well-being measures.[23–25] Similarly, measures of quality of life in old age including activity of daily living (ADL) measures or life satisfaction or morale measures consistently correlate with measures of an elder's social support network.[26] Social support networks also significantly correlate with various measures of health care use including all cause hospitalization rates.[3]

Where longitudinal studies have been conducted, it is possible to move beyond the cautionary associational statements and more boldly state that social support networks have a causal relationship to health. In fact, some social scientists have pointed out that the evidence now available regarding the relationship of social support networks to health is as strong as that which was available linking smoking to health at the time the U.S. Surgeon General issued the warning about the health consequences of smoking.[2,27] Conceivably, a similar admonition needs to be made regarding the health consequences of social isolation to health.

Current research has generally failed to examine the etiology of social isolation. Case examples from practice, however, suggest that there are important differences. For example, the widower who withdraws from social contact out of bereavement is likely to be quite different than the wife who, consumed with spousal caretaking responsibilities, is forced to withdraw from social interaction with her friends. An elder's own deteriorating physical health is another likely cause of isolation. Also, depression is another factor associated with isolation.[1,25] The literature would suggest that there are relatively few life-long isolates but some do exist.[28]

Even with this preliminary taxonomy of isolates drawn from practice, it is evident that more research must be done on this topic. The nature and etiology of these types of isolation suggest alternative strategies for intervening. For example, the widower might benefit from counseling whereas the over-burdened spousal caretaker might best benefit from a respite program. Clearly, a generic intervention attempting to address the needs of all types of isolates would be doomed for failure.

> Social isolation may have as much influence on health status as does cigarette smoking, drinking, or poor nutrition.

REFINING THE DEFINITION OF SOCIAL SUPPORT NETWORKS

Distinguishing Social Networks from Social Supports

Social networks and social supports are not identical.[29] Social networks refer to the structural aspects of social integration, whereas social supports consider functional aspects. Social networks are the web of social relationships that surround an elderly person and the characteristics of those social ties.[17] The functional nature of social support suggests specific dimensions such as emotional or instrumental support.[30] Social supports are those aspects of one's social network drawn upon at a time of need. Thus, an adequate social network precedes the existence of social support. Further, it is helpful to think of an elder's social supports as a subset of one's total social network. Not everyone within an elder's social network are equally adept at supplying social support, in general, and a particular kind of support (e.g., emotional versus instrumental), in particular.[31] Accordingly, an elder may have adequate support for some needs but may have insufficient for other life contingencies. A diversified and well-stocked reservoir of social networks increases the likelihood that the appropriate social support would be available to the elder for life's various emergencies.

Social supports are not the same as social networks.

Illustrations of Social Networks

Social networks consist of both quantitative and qualitative aspects.[4, 24, 32, 33] For example, knowing that an elder comes from a large family does not say much about how good the relationships are within the family. Besides size, another commonly used quantitative measure of social networks is frequency of contact. Knowing that a client is seen by a reliable family member or friend on a daily basis as opposed to infrequent social support should influence whether the health care provider sends a frail elder home from the hospital sooner or whether extra inpatient days may be required to minimize rehospitalization.

Qualitative measures of social networks include evaluation of the value of an elder's social network. For example, clarifying how many family members or friends the elder can "count on for help" or "speak to about private matters" is qualitatively different than merely noting how many family members or friends the elder has.

Illustrations of Social Supports

Similar to social networks, social supports can also be conceived along both quantitative and qualitative dimensions. Again, the health care provider could count how many people provide instrumental support to the elder as opposed to evaluating the quality and extent of that support. Another commonly used measure of quality of social supports evaluates its availability in times of acute crisis as opposed to being there for the long haul associated with caring for a chronic illness. Few people can shift their work schedules for these long-haul assignments whereas dependent care releases from one's work place are becoming increasingly available. A related dimension is the responsiveness of help at times of need. It may be possible to provide some sort of emotional support by long distance given modern communication technology. It is quite another thing to provide tangible instrumental support by long distance. In the modern work world in which children often measure their distance from elder parents in terms of time zones, it becomes essential for practitioners to consider such distance when evaluating the quality and likely durability of an elder's social support system.

The Distinctive Roles of Family and Friends

It is important to note that family and friends function quite differently in one's social support network. Friends, perhaps because they are more discretionary, are more highly correlated with positive mental health measures than are family social support network measures. At times of physical illness or infirmity, however, family members are much more likely to carry the burden than friends. Part of this distinction is that an elder's friendships tend to be contemporary in age with the elder whereas family social networks are likely to cross age cohorts. This age homogeneity of friends may increase understanding and trust relationships among friendships, whereas the great heterogeneity of ages among families may inhibit the building of relationships that are most predictive of positive mental health indicators. The fact that most of an elder's friends are equally old, however, tends to limit their ability to perform rigorous instrumental tasks at times of the elder's infirmity. Generally, the stronger social support networks are those that include strong bonds across age cohorts.

Family and friends generally provide different types of social support.

PRACTICE APPLICATIONS

Illustrations of Importance of Social Support Networks to Clinical Practice

Case Vignette: Mr. Smith, a retired federal employee, and his wife of more than 40 years seemed to be coping well on his relatively generous retirement pay and extensive health insurance plan. For more than 40 years, they lived together in a traditional blue-collar neighborhood in a house they had inherited from Mrs. Smith's parents. The Smith's two children both live more than 2000 miles away but regularly talk on the telephone. At least once a year, the children along with grandchildren visit the Smiths. From all external appearances, the Smiths are an octogenarian couple successfully aging. That misconception was shattered late one evening when Mrs. Smith tumbled down a flight of stairs breaking both wrists and cracking a vertebrae in her neck. The fall was partially caused beacuse Mrs. Smith did not want to turn on a light while she went to the bathroom for fear that the light would awaken Mr. Smith. Given Mrs. Smith's severe osteoporosis, her broken wrists required extensive treatment and many weeks of hospitalization.

During Mrs. Smith's prolonged hospitalization, Mr. Smith's own health problems became more evident. His wife had concealed his increasing frailty including the fact that he had incurred a number of falls around the house. These falls may have been associated with a drinking problem that Mr. Smith had developed. He drank partially to escape the loneliness brought on by his no longer being able to see friends from his former place of employment. He was never an outgoing person and seemed less so after his retirement. Thus, he never developed new friends to compensate for those he once had at work. When he retired from his job, he essentially also retired from his friendship network and, over time, developed a severe case of depression. His increasing problem with drinking alcohol was most likely a case of self-medication.

With the deception uncovered, the Smith's two children became more involved in monitoring their parent's situation. They also secured formal care management and home health care services to facilitate Mrs. Smith's recovery. The children also provided extensive periods of social support to both infirm parents during Mrs. Smith's rehabilitation. Once she regained much of her strength, the children backed off allowing Mrs. Smith to again resume much of the responsibility for caring for her husband. Children also empowered close friends and neighbors to regularly check on the older Smith couple and to call either of the children at the first sign of any difficulties.

The case of Mr. and Mrs. Smith illustrates why physicians, nurses, social workers, and other health care professionals all need to pay more heed to evaluating social support networks in community health settings. Mr. Smith's symptoms of depression and corresponding drinking problem could have probably been detected years before Mrs. Smith's tragic fall down the stairs. Indeed, had Mr. Smith's problems been detected earlier, many of the ensuing events may never have happened. Mrs. Smith would not have become so burdened with caring for her husband and covering his drinking problem. The final results demonstrated that both family and neighbor social support networks were willing to rally around the Smiths. For far too long, however, no one wanted to "interfere" with an elderly couple who perpetuated a myth of successful aging, when in fact they were an unnecessary accident waiting to happen.

Institutional settings also offer compelling cases for examining social support networks in clinical practice. There is strong evidence that most families do not abandon their elders when they move into a nursing home. Thus, health care providers should regularly ask the institutionalized elder about family visits. For those institutionalized elders with severe cognitive impairment, self-report regarding outside social support network contact may have to be gained through a proxy. Regardless of whether the elder has severe cognitive impairment or not, sudden declines in family visits or other social contact may be markers for increased vulnerability of the elderly person in institutional settings.

> The case of Mr. and Mrs. Smith illustrates the importance of social support networks to care management for a couple facing health problems in old age.

Screening for Isolation

Health promotion and wellness programs for elders should adopt screening for social isolation. Although truly isolated elders in the community may be relatively rare, perhaps as many as one in five elders is either clinically isolated or at high risk for such. Some of the assessment instruments described later in this chapter can be readily incorporated into health screening instruments.

Besides inclusion in health screening instruments, general assessment regimes should also be adapted to include at least a few items that might alert the health care provider of potential social isolation.[30] Increased sensitivity of providers to the importance of social support networks for well being in old age might help flag those elders in need of a more comprehensive assessment by a social worker or other practitioner.

Designing Interventions to Strengthen Social Support Networks

More than one type of intervention will be needed to address the diversity of social isolates and strengthen social support networks. Respite care programs would be one type of intervention. Some spouses become so burdened with caretaking responsibilities that they no longer see their own friends. Cognizant of the importance of friendship to mental health, it is clear that spousal and other over-burdened elder caretakers need a break. Some caretakers assume almost a martyr type dedication to their charges. Perhaps using the approach of providing respite so as to allow the caretaker to continue friendships might be another way to resolve this problem.

Interventions need to be tailored for the different types of social isolation.

Counseling programs would be most appropriate for those elders whose social support networks may be diminished because of the elder's own despondency. Ecological and social systems clinical paradigms are especially appropriate for this form of counseling. Many of these elders might also benefit from social activity programs. These programs provide a mechanism to help fabricate social support networks where they do not already exist. In the case of Mr. Smith, such activity programs at a much earlier stage of his loneliness may have actually prevented the eventual despair.

Among the most successful efforts to both strengthen existing and fabricate new social support networks are senior peer support and other self-help programs. In such programs, elders learn successful coping techniques for particular problems faced in aging as well as ways to maximize prevention of many problems. Further, because the elders are themselves the counselors, they are engaged in a social activity that brings increased social contact and self-esteem.

How about life-long isolates? First, few elders have been life-long isolates. Even in those who have coped in the past with relatively small social support networks, however, increased frailty diminishes the likelihood that these elders will continue to be able to cope. Thus, while there is still time, efforts should be made to help these elders both appreciate the importance of social support networks to their future well-being but also acquire improved social skills to strengthen what networks they have. There is no upper age limit after which it is not possible to change this aspect of a human being.

ASSESSING SOCIAL SUPPORT NETWORKS

Types of Social Support Network Measures

Although there have been some attempts to identify single-item indicators of social support networks, most of these indicators have proven faulty. Two of the most common examples include asking the elder whether he or she lives alone or not and asking whether they are married or not. Living alone was once thought to be a good proxy for social connectedness but has proven to be a better indicator of physical and mental functional capability. Indeed, only those with good functional skills can live alone. Also, many elders who live alone turn out to be quite socially active. Marital status has proven equally tricky as a proxy for social integration. The case of Mr. and Mrs. Smith illustrates the problems with both of these single-item indicators. On both counts, the Smith's problems would have continued undetected. Indeed, their marital status and living together while seemingly coping, created a social moat around their household that was only shattered with a medical crisis.

Better single-item indicators might include whether the elder has a confidant or not and whether they have someone they can call on for help in times of emergency. Actually identifying a name for such persons and follow-up inquiry with those persons might validate adequacy of support where there are reasons for doubt.

Another approach to measuring social support networks is to examine specific areas of an elder's network such as that of their family or that of their friends or neighbors. Additionally, some health care providers may wish to concentrate on selected facets of the support network such as instrumental help or emotional help. The area of social support networks selected might be determined by the focus of the agency sponsoring the health care provider. For example, those working in agencies sponsoring homemaker chore services are apt to focus on a narrow range of items that directly impact on appropriate treatment planning for those services.

Researchers, particularly, employ another approach to measurement. They often create composite social support network measures. These composite measures are generally more reliable than single-item indicators or indexes constructed from just a few items. These desirable properties, however, come at a cost for those who wish to use the same measurement tool in clinical settings. The composite social support network measures are generally too lengthy or unwieldy for clinical applications. Thus, there has been a push to develop more abbreviated measures.

One example of a relatively short composite measure is the Lubben Social Network Scale (LSNS).[29, 34] This 10-item scale was one of the earliest attempts to design a social support network measure specifically for use among an elderly population. The LSNS has been successfully employed in both research and clinical settings[3, 18, 28, 35] and its psychometric properties have been documented.[29]

Another commonly used social support network scale is the Medical Outcomes Study Social Support Scale (MOS-SSS). It was

TABLE 4-1. LUBBEN SOCIAL NETWORK SCALE-ABBREVIATED (LSNS-A)[a]

1. How many RELATIVES do you see or hear from at least once a month?
2. How many RELATIVES do you feel close to that you can call on them for help?
3. How many RELATIVES do you feel at ease with that you can talk about private matters?
4. How many FRIENDS/NEIGHBORS do you see or hear from at least once a month?
5. How many FRIENDS/NEIGHBORS do you feel close to that you can call on them for help?
6. How many FRIENDS/NEIGHBORS do you feel at ease with that you can talk about private matters?

Response options and scoring for all six LSNS-A items:

0 = none
1 = one
2 = two
3 = 3 or 4
4 = 5–8
5 = nine or more

[a]alpha = 0.77.

developed for the RAND Medical Outcomes Study[30] and is largely a measure emotional support. Because of a great deal of redundancy in items, however, many suggestions have been made to abbreviate the MOS-SSS.[29, 36] Its current length (20-items) makes it particularly cumbersome for clinical settings.

Abbreviated versions of both the LSNS and MOS-SSS are good candidates for a battery of assessment measures employed in clinical settings. We propose a 6-item abbreviated version of the LSNS and refer to it as the LSNS-A,* to distinguish it from the longer version of the LSNS that remains more appropriate for research settings. The six items selected are shown in Table 4-1. They assess two critical domains of social support networks: (1) family; and (2) friends and neighbors. These items can be combined to form a family subscale, a friends and neighbors subscale, as well as a composite scale (LSNS-A). All three measures (family, friends and neighbors, and LSNS-A) have a relatively good internal consistency for such short scales (alphas over 0.74).

An additional advantage of the three measures is that in a clinical setting, it can be useful to determine particular strengths or weaknesses in family ties separate from those of an elderly person's relationships with friends or neighbors. Thus, the subscales

*The LSNS-A has recently been re-named the LSNS-6.

can be used individually. The two subscales can also be combined to form a composite LSNS-A score that, in turn, could be used as a marker for possible social isolation and suggestive of particular types of clinical interventions.

Scores for the LSNS-A items is similar to that for the original LSNS. Each of the selected items is scored from 0 (low social support networks) to 5 (high social support networks). These scores reflect a modified logarithmic scale acknowledging that marginal benefit of unitary change in any one of these items diminishes after a certain level. In particular, zero is coded as 0, one as 1, two as 2. Three and four, however, are both evaluated as a 3 on the scale. Five through eight are evaluated as 4 whereas nine and above are scored as 5. This scaling remains the same as that which has proven effective in the original LSNS.

A 3-item abbreviated version of the MOS-SSS is also proposed. The following are selected MOS-SSS items that particularly differ from those that make up the LSNS-A. These three items show high internal consistency and are correlated with total MOS-SSS score. The three items are scored on a Likert-type response. Although the original MOS-SSS was scored on a 5-point scale, a 6-level response option (Never = 0; Seldom = 1; Sometimes = 2; Often = 3; Very Often = 4 and Always = 5) is recommended to facilitate comparison with the LSNS-A, which employs a 6-level response pattern. The SSS-A items are shown in Table 4-2.

Preliminary work has also been done to combine the six LSNS-A items with these three SSS-A items. The proposed nine-item social support network clinical screening instrument (SSN-CSI) has very good internal consistency (alpha = .84) and the anticipated three factor structure (emotional support, family, and friends/neighbors) (see Appendix #43). More work is needed to develop abbreviated social support network scales suitable for both research and clinical settings.

Abbreviated scales appropriate for both clinical practice and research are identified.

TABLE 4-2. ABBREVIATED RAND SOCIAL SUPPORT SCALE (SSS-A)

1. How often do you have someone to love?
2. How often does someone show love and affection to you?
3. How often do you have someone to share worries?

   Response options and scoring for all three SSSA items:

   0 = never
   1 = seldom
   2 = sometimes
   3 = often
   4 = very often
   5 = always

[a]alpha = 0.87.

Practical Applications of Abbreviated Versions of Scales

The suggested abbreviated scales, or combinations thereof, can readily be incorporated into an assessment battery allowing clinicians to gather social health information in a systematic manner. Thus, they can readily share this knowledge with other team members in quantifiable, measurable terms. Also, the systematic use of such scales facilitates more accurate description of aspects of social network that may require tailored intervention. Additionally, global scales that quantify an elder's social environment might also be useful for monitoring systemic changes over time. The use of such tools may also increase attention of the elder to his or her own social health. Elders might be encouraged by the nature of the inquiry contained in these scales to evaluate and identify (on their own) areas of weakness in social network or areas of strength or potential resources. Finally, the LSNS-A could be used as a screener for social isolation that might not be otherwise detected. Similarly, the MOS-SSS abbreviated scale would be sensitive to detecting deficiencies in emotional support that might not be otherwise detected in less tailored instruments. Together, these two abbreviated scales could facilitate better community care and prescription for such programs as respite, peer support, or group counseling programs.

There are practical benefits for including social support network measures in a clinical battery.

SOME IMPORTANT VARIATIONS IN SOCIAL SUPPORT NETWORKS

Gender Differences

The social support networks of elderly women and men differ.[19,37–39] Among the current cohort of elderly, men were much more likely to be employed throughout much of their lifetime than were women. Accordingly, men are more likely than women to have workplace based friendships that become increasingly difficult to maintain in old age. Alternatively, those women who did not leave the home and go to a formal place of employment more often developed social relationships in the neighborhoods where they may still reside. Further, the women may have developed stronger ties with children because childcare was more apt to be performed by mothers than fathers among the current cohort of elders. Thus, men more than women severed important social ties when they retired from work whereas earlier life investments in social relationship building with both family and neighbors are more apt to reap dividends for women than men.

Another important gender difference among the current cohort of elders is that these women tended to develop more nurturing social relationships whereas their male counterparts more often engaged in competitive social interaction. In old age, when competition becomes more problematic, the males may be at a greater disadvantage continuing their social relationships than the women. Perhaps in old age nurturing may be even more important to maintaining social ties than it was at a younger age. Some males, noting the relative advantages of nurturing patterns, actually adopt more nurturing patterns in their social relationships in later life than they did at an earlier age.

Cultural Variations

Besides gender differences in social support networks, cultural differences are also prevalent.[40] Frequently one thinks of ethnic and racial intergroup differences in this regard and there are some important differences in social support patterns. For example, many first generation Asian and Hispanic Americans stress lineal family relationships more than friendships whereas their counterparts who are second or later generation immigrants are more apt to trade such extensive social contact with offspring to be able to spend more time with peers (either siblings or friends). Data shown in Figure 4-1 suggest that all ethnic and racial groups will face increasing challenges in providing adequate parent support care.

Rural and urban differences are another form of cultural variation.[41] Some of these differences may be due to relative size of communities that in turn afford more opportunities to build stable social relationships. Also, there is thought to be a greater sense of social interdependence and obligation among rural communities

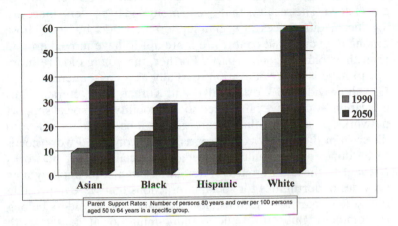

Parent Support Ratos: Number of persons 80 years and over per 100 persons aged 50 to 64 years in a specific group.

FIGURE 4-1   Parent support ratios by race and hispanic origin

than urban communities. Such stereotypes, however, are dangerous in a rapidly changing world that early in the century was noted by mass population movements away from rural areas and more recently, there is some indication of return migration from urban areas back into suburban and even rural areas.

Social support networks among gay and lesbian elders are topics for which there are very limited data.[42] Many gays and lesbians were socialized in an era when openness about one's homosexuality was dangerous. Indeed, they often had to develop very tight but limited social support network structures. Many continue to face significant social consequences of past discrimination from society in general and ostracization from their families in particular. Although little is known about this population, gay and lesbian elders might be especially at risk of social isolation as they age for some of the reasons mentioned.

There are some data on cross-national comparisons of social support networks providing a glimpse at future trends. China provides a unique case whereby the implementation of a "one child" policy to control birthrates will have a tremendous impact on future cohorts of elderly. Although not by deliberate social policy, many developed countries of the world, including the United States, are approaching similar consequences with fewer children expected to care for more elderly in the future. An increasing proportion of elders in the United States have no living children.[43] Indeed, the increasing lack of living or proximal offspring will become a driving force to foster alternative forms of social support networks for elders throughout the world.

Cohort Variations

The present generation of elders has experienced tremendous social change. The result is that even among today's elders, there are significant differences in social support networks by age. Those among the young-old cohort are more apt to have moved around than their old-old counterparts. Further, the young-old are more apt to have a better education, partially as a consequence of the GI Bill provided to World War II and Korean War veterans. This education would have influenced social mobility and social support networks. It is likely that future generations of elders will also differ from their older counterparts. Thus, continued work needs to be done to help build knowledge of social support networks relevant to these different cohorts. For example, technology now provides opportunities for social interactions that were impossible only a few years ago, such as electronic mail. Some elders belong to computer clubs for seniors maintaining social contact with friends they have never met in person. Some even have a home page on the Internet suggesting future ways of fabricating new network patterns.

SUMMARY

There is a growing recognition of the importance of social support networks to health. As gerontologists and geriatricians begin to identify the means to increase active life expectancy, rather than mere life expectancy, it is likely that an elder's social networks will be shown to be even more indispensable to health and successful aging.

Because social networks and social support are relatively distinct constructs, there is a need for separate measures of each. From applied research and clinical perspectives, there is growing pressure to develop short and efficient scales. Some elderly populations may not do well with long questionnaires. Time constraints in most clinical practice settings necessitate efficient and effective screening tools. Shorter scales require less time and energy for both the administrator and respondent. Thus, parsimonious and effective screening tools will be more acceptable to both elders as well as health care providers. This chapter presents two abbreviated scales of social support networks suitable as screening tools in a variety of health care settings.

REFERENCES

1. Kaplan GA, Seeman TE, Cohen RD, Knudsen LP, Guralnik J. Mortality among the elderly in the Alameda County study: behavioral and demographic risk factors. *Am J Public Health.* 1987;77:307–312.
2. House JS, Landis KR, Umberson D. Social relationships and health. *Science.* 1988;241,540–545.
3. Lubben JE, Weiler PG, Chi I. Health practices of the elderly poor. *Am J Public Health.* 1989;79,731–734.
4. Rook KS. Assessing the health-related dimensions of older adults' social relationships. In: Lawton MP, Teresi JA (eds). *Annual Review of Gerontology and Geriatrics.* New York: Springer Publishing Company; 1994;142–181.
5. Cassel J. The contribution of the social Environment to host resistance. *Am J Epidemio.* 1976;104:107–123.
6. Cobb S. Social support as a moderator of life stress. *Psychosom Med.* 1976;38:300–314.
7. Thoits PA. Conceptual, methodological, and theoretical problems in studying social support as a buffer against life stress. *J Health Soc Behav.* 1982;23:145–159.

8. Cutrona C, Russell D. Rose J. Social support and adaptation to stress by the elderly. *Psychol Aging.* 1986;1:47–54.

9. Krause N, Herzog AR, Baker E. Providing support to others and well-being in later life. *J Geronto B: Psychol Sci Soc Sci.* 1992;47:P300-P311.

10. Berkman LF. (1985). The relationship of social networks and social supports to morbidity and mortality. In: Cohen S, Syme SL. (eds). *Social Support and Health.* Orlando, FL: Academic Press; 1985: 241–262.

11. Cohen S, Syme SL. Issues in the study and application of social support. In: Cohen S, Syme SL (eds). *Social Support and Health.* New York: Academic Press; 1985:3–22.

12. Berkman LF. Social networks, support, and health: taking the next step forward. *Am J Epidemiol.* 1986; 123:559–562.

13. Crawford G. Support networks and health related changes in the elderly: theory-based nursing strategies. *Fam Commun Health.* 1987;10:39–48.

14. Berkman LF, Syme SL. Social networks, host resistance, and mortality: a nine year follow-up study of Alameda County residents. *A J Epidemiol.* 1979;109:186–204.

15. Blazer DG. Social support and mortality in an elderly community population. *Am J Epidemiol.* 1982;116:684–694.

16. Zuckerman DM, Kasl SV, Ostfeld AM. Psychosocial predictors of mortality among the elderly poor: the role of religion, well-being and social contacts. *Am J Epidemiol.* 1984;119:410–423.

17. Ell K. Social networks, social support, and health status: a review. *Soc Serv Rev.* 1984;58:133–149.

18. Mor-Barak ME, Miller LS. A longitudinal study of the causal relationship between social networks and health of the poor frail elderly. *J Appl Gerontol.* 1991;10(3):293–310.

19. Torres CC, McIntosh WA, Kubena KS. Social network and social background characteristics of elderly who live and eat alone. *J Aging Health.* 1992;4:564–578.

20. Mor-Barak ME. Major determinants of social networks in frail elderly community residents. *Home Health Care Serv Q.* 1997;16(1–2): 121–137.

21. Bosworth HB, Schaie KW. The relationship of social environment, social networks and health outcomes in the Seattle Longitudinal Study: two analytical approaches, *J Gerontol B Psychol Sci Soc Sci.* 1997;52(5):197–205.

22. Stuck AE, Walthert JM, Nikolaus T, et al. Risk factors for the functional status decline in community-living elderly people: a systematic literature review. *Soc Sci Med.* 1999;48:445–469.

23. Hurwicz ML, Berkanovic E. The stress process of rheumatoid arthritis. *J Rheumatol.* 1993;20:1836–1844.

24. Chappell NL. The role of family and friends in quality of life. In:Birren JE, Lubben JE, Rowe JC, Deutchman DE (eds). *The Concept and Measurement of Quality of Life in the Frail Elderly.* New York: Academic Press; 1991:171–190.

25. Dorfman RA, Lubben JE, Mayer-Oakes SA, et al. Screening for depression among the well-elderly. *Social Work.* 1995;40:295–304.

26. Seeman TS, Bruce ML, McAvay GJ. Social network characteristics and the onset of ADL disability: MacArthur studies of successful aging. *J Geronto B Soc Psychol Sci.* 1996;51B:S191–S200.

27. Bassuk SS, Glass TA, Berkman LF. Social disengagement and incident cognitive decline in community-dwelling elderly persons. *Ann Int Med.* 1999;131:165–173.

28. Rubinstein RL, Lubben JE, Mintzer JE. Social isolation and social support: an applied perspective. *J Appl Gerontol* 1994;13(1):58–72.

29. Lubben JE, Gironda M. Social support networks among older people in the United States. In: Litwin H (ed). *The Social Networks of Older People.* Westport, CT: Praeger; 1997:143–161.

30. Sherbourne CD, Stewart AL. The MOS Social Support Survey. *Soc Sci Med.* 1991;32: 705–714.

31. Berkman LF. Assessing the physical health effects of social networks and social support. *Ann Rev Public Health.* 1984;5:413–432.

32. Antonucci TC, Jackson JS. Social support, interpersonal efficacy, and health: a life course perspective. In: Carstensen LL, Edelstein BA (eds). *Handbook of Clinical Gerontology.* New York: Pergamon Press; 1987:291–311.

33. Wenger GC. Support networks and dementia. *Int J Geriatr Psychiatry.* 9:181–194.

34. Lubben JE. Assessing social networks among elderly populations. *Fam Commun Health.* 1988;11:42–52.

35. Luggen AS, Rini AG. Assessment of social networks and isolation in community-based elderly men and women. *Geriatr Nurs.* 1995;16:179–181.

36. Steiner A, Raube K, Stuck AE, et al. Measuring psychosocial aspects of well-being in older community residents: performance of four short scales. *Gerontologist.* 1996;36(1):54–62.

37. Barush AS, Peak T. Support groups for older men: building on strengths and facilitating relationships. In: Kosberg J, Kaye LW, (eds). *Elderly Men: Special Problems and Professional Challenges.* New York: Springer; 1997:262–278.

38. Adams RG. Older men's friendship patterns. In: Thompson, EH (ed). *Older Men's Lives.* Thousand Oaks, CA: Sage; 1994:159–177.

39. Matthews SH. Men's ties to siblings in old age. In: Thompson EH (ed). *Older Mens Lives.* Thousand Oaks, CA: Sage; 1994:178–195.

40. Lubben JE, Becerra RM. Social Support among black, Mexican and Chinese elderly. In: Gelfand DE, Barresi CM (eds). *Ethnic Dimensions of Aging.* New York: Springer Publishing Co.; 1987:130–144.

41. Coward RT, Dwyer JW. Health and well-being of rural elders. In: Ginsberg LH (ed). *Social Work in Rural Communities.* Alexandra, VA: Council on Social Work Education; 1993:164–182.

42. Dorfman R, Walters K, Burke P, et al. Old, sad and alone: the myth of the aging homosexual. *J Gerontol Social Work.* 1995;24:29–44.

43. Gironda MW, Lubben JE, Atchison KA. Social support networks of elders without children. *J Gerontol Social Work.* 1999;31:63–84.

ASSESSMENT IN REHABILITATION

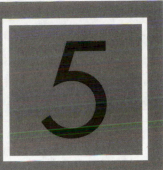

KENNETH BRUMMEL-SMITH

INTRODUCTION

Geriatrics, assessment, and rehabilitation are inextricably linked. Rehabilitation is the process whereby a person's abilities to perform daily activities are measured and a care plan is designed to enhance or recover any abilities that have been lost. Function is conceptualized as the product of physical, psychological, and social activities (Figure 5-1). Rehabilitation cannot begin without first assessing the person's skills in these areas. Disabling conditions much more commonly affect the older population than all others. Data from the Uniform Data System (UDS) for Medical Rehabilitation illustrate that the average age of patients in rehabilitation in the United States was 68 years. Strokes were the most frequently cited problem for which rehabilitation was provided (34% of all cases) and orthopedic conditions were second. In these cases, the average ages were 71 and 75 years, respectively.[1]

In the field of geriatrics, assessment is used for many purposes: to detect an individual's functional problems; to characterize a sample population's functional status; or to develop health care financing plans, to name a few. As a result, instruments that have been developed often measure performance in three levels, those

The Agency for Health Care Policy and Research (AHCPR) was renamed in December 1999.
This agency is now known as the Agency for Healthcare Research and Quality (AHRQ).

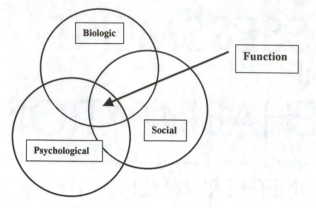

FIGURE 5-1 Conceptual model of function. Function is conceptualized as interplay between physical, psychological, and social components of a person's life.

Assessment in rehabilitation must be sensitive to small changes in performance. A change, for instance, from requiring maximal assistance to minimal assistance in dressing would not be detected using the Katz scale, but may allow the patient with a stroke to return home with a frail caregiver.

needing complete assistance, minimal assistance, or independent. Because rehabilitation involves close observation of the patient's performance over a period of time, measurement in assessment must be sensitive to detect small changes that characterize the process of recovery. Hence, in many rehabilitation programs the direct observation of the patient's performance by a skilled therapist has often supplanted the use of formal instruments of assessment. Because of the recent emphasis on outcome measures and the pressures of reimbursement, this tradition is shifting.

This chapter reviews the conceptual framework of assessment in rehabilitation, the use of assessment in rehabilitation prognostication and performance measurement, and the use of assessment in measuring outcomes. Attention is also directed to the use of disability-specific assessment instruments. The reader is encouraged to consult Chapters 3, 4, 10, 11, 15, 16, 19, 20, 21, 22, 23, and 26.

Impairment, Disability, and Handicap

There is little correlation between disease and function. Most traditional medical assessment systems have concentrated on characterizing diagnoses. This orientation is, however, inadequate when dealing with those in need of rehabilitation. To say that the patient has a "stroke with left hemiparesis" tells us nothing about the patient's capabilities to care for himself or herself, mobility status, or caregiving needs. A new classification system was needed to better describe the needs of the patient in functional terms.

TABLE 5-1.	DEFINITIONS OF IMPAIRMENT, DISABILITY, AND HANDICAP
Impairment	Any loss or abnormality of psychological, physiologic, or anatomic function. As such, this is usually experienced at the organ level.
Disability	Any restriction or lack (resulting from an impairment) of ability to perform an activity in the manner or within the range considered normal for a human being. These abilities are then experienced at the personal level.
Handicap	A disadvantage for a given individual, resulting from an impairment or disability, which limits or prevents fulfillment of a role that is normal for that individual. This effect represents the social consequences to the person of their disability or impairment.

Only recently has there been significant attention paid to the classification of disability and handicap. The World Health Organization, building on work by Nagi[2] and Wood,[3] has promulgated the use of the terms "impairment," "disability," and "handicap," (Table 5-1).[4] This change in viewpoint is at the heart of both the rehabilitation process and geriatrics. The focus of attention is shifted from the disease (causation) to its effect (disablement). Because of the rise in the aging population in our society and the associated increase in the number of persons with difficulties in daily activities, this paradigm shift is timely. The relationship of these terms is illustrated in Figure 5-2.

Assessment and measurement of impairments is a classic endeavor of medicine. Evaluation of cardiac size or rhythm, examination of the skin, or detection of pulmonary diseases are techniques familiar to health care providers. Yet assessment of a patient's functional abilities or social needs are domains often neglected in the traditional medical encounter. Even within the rehabilitation community there has been a tendency to view disability in primarily physical terms. As pointed out by Meyer, however, "Over time, the term has been broadened to include mental and emotional impairment, chronic illness, and aging as well."[5]

One of the most novel approaches to designing a new terminology of disablement was suggested by Duckworth, who proposed that a classification system should be adapted to those by whom it is to be used.[6] This proposal emphasizes a critical point in geriatric assessment: the definition of the functional deficit must incorporate the value system of the individual being assessed. Failure to pay attention to this factor may explain why some elderly patients are

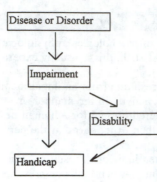

FIGURE 5-2   The relationship between disease and handicap. This diagram represents the relationships between diseases, impairments, disability, and handicap. Disease such as diabetes may cause impairments (e.g., retinal changes). That impairment affects the person's vision. With proper adaptive devices (prescription eyeglasses), however, the person with the disability can still function normally. If glasses are not available due to insurance limitations, the person is handicapped (a societal limitation). Some impairment may directly lead to handicap if there is no way to provide accommodation (e.g., an airline pilot who becomes blind).

Social support is one of the most critical determinants of whether older persons are offered rehabilitation and their outcomes.

labeled as "poorly motivated" when they chose not to participate in certain rehabilitation activities. The patient may simply not value the examiner's determination that the impairment found (poor balance after a stroke) is affecting her ability to walk safely (disability). Perhaps this is the reason older persons have significantly higher rates of disability and handicap. In fact, in a study of aging with a spinal cord injury, increased chronological age significantly increased measured disability, handicap, and costs of care regardless of degree of neurologic impairment.[7]

The importance of this model to geriatrics cannot be overstated, especially in the area of social functioning. The patient's social support situation is a major determinant of whether or not he or she is offered rehabilitation and on the outcome of that intervention. Many elderly patients are handicapped by society's view that their disabilities are expected for old age or that they would not be responsive to rehabilitation interventions. For instance, the life satisfaction of persons with spinal cord injury has been shown to be influenced by aspects of their social role performance, but not by their degree of impairment or disability.[8] Age exerts the largest single influence on individual expectations of roles and performance so it is appropriate that assessment strategies be used in geriatrics to identify, and ameliorate, any reductions in those areas (Figure 5-3).[9] As Wood and Badley observe, "The reality is that circumstances associated with aging aggravate disablement regardless of the underlying diagnoses."[10]

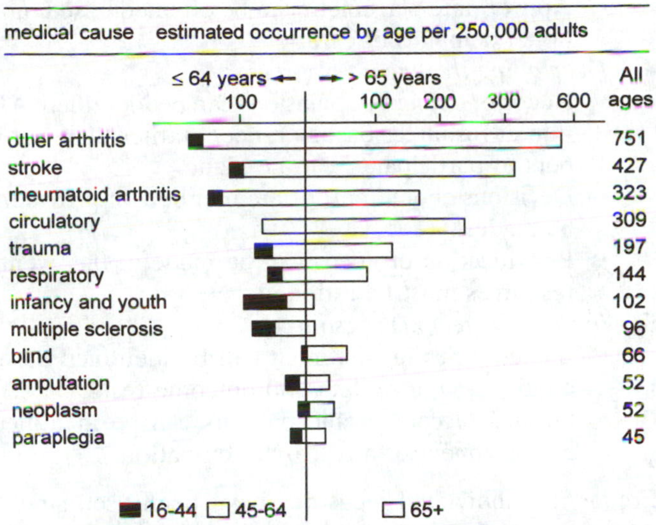

medical cause   estimated occurrence by age per 250,000 adults

FIGURE 5-3   Age distribution of the impairments. This figure illustrates how impairments are much more common in the older age groups. (Reproduced, with permission, from Granger CV, Gresham GE. Functional Assessment in Rehabilitation Medicine. Baltimore: Williams & Wilkins; 1984:35.)

The Goals of Functional Assessment in Geriatric Rehabilitation

The primary uses of functional assessment in rehabilitation have been elucidated by Granger[11] and include the following.

1. *Planning treatment:* A problem list that is comprehensive and inclusive of functional problems allows for appropriate targeting of interventions.
2. *Determining the effectiveness and efficiency of care:*
   - Measures of function before and after treatment can be compared.
   - Cost-benefit measurements can be applied using functional outcome data.
   - Utilization review for necessity of level of care can be conducted based on functional status measures.
3. *Maintaining continuity of care:*
   - Patients can be tracked through the system and over time.
   - Care management can be facilitated by allowing targeting of those with greater degrees of disablement or handicap to receive additional support.

- Appropriate placement can be effected based on functional demands of care.
4. *Developing treatment resources:*
   - Needs of defined populations can be identified. Allocation of resources based on need, rather than just numbers of participants, can be made.
   - Decisions about appropriate numbers of providers can be made.
   - Prioritization of needs can be made in the event that resources must be rationed.
5. *Improving treatment resources:*
   - Inadequacies in treatment can be identified based on quality assurance data and outcome results.
   - Groups of comparable patients can be identified for establishment of a research population.

Frequently, individual measures have been used simultaneously to satisfy a number of these roles. This presents certain methodological problems in that the measure may not have been developed to be used in that manner, studies of reliability and validity may have been conducted only in one of the areas and may not be applicable to another, or experience of using the measure in one area may be particularly limited.

Limits of Functional Assessment Tools in Rehabilitation

It is interesting that the use of assessment tools has been rather limited in both rehabilitation and geriatrics. Though tools for measurement of function have existed for decades, and are used extensively in research, many well-known programs either use no standardized tools or only a limited number. Findings are often recorded in narrative reports. Part of the reason for this phenomenon is that there is a long history in rehabilitation of individual providers conducting extensive, hands-on assessments of function by clinical examination. For instance, while an occupational therapist may have never used the Katz ADL scale, he or she would probably spend over an hour assessing ADL functions in a newly admitted stroke patient. That assessment would entail reports of functional abilities by both the patient and proxy, as well as detailed testing of functional performance in a variety of settings over a protracted period of time. Given that assessment, the patient's impairments and disabilities could be accurately catalogued and a care plan developed. Hence, many therapists believed that the use of a standardized tool was often superfluous, time-consuming, and sometimes simply inadequate to classify all the subtle deficits that could be detected. With closer observation of care by outside parties (third party payers, managed care organizations, etc.), that situation is rapidly changing.

A major problem in the use of assessment instruments in rehabilitation is the construction of the instrument itself. As representations of the reality of daily functioning, they must attempt to measure subtle changes in complicated human behaviors. Most of the scales have been ordinally based, presenting the assumption that there is a more or less equal difference between one performance level and another.[12] For simplicity in measurement, many scales utilize three levels of function: independent, those needing some assistance, and total dependence. Yet the experience of rehabilitation providers is far different than this simplistic analysis. Small, barely measurable changes in performance may mean a major gain in rehabilitation has occurred. For instance, the change from maximum assist in transfers to minimum assist can allow a person with a stroke to return home to a frail caregiver.

Furthermore, there often is an assumption that the reacquisition of physical skills is characterized by steady progress. Indeed, the patient's failure to progress according to this viewpoint often leads to refusals of reimbursement by third party payers. Yet, typically, progress in rehabilitation is one of "stops and starts" and the process is often variable in speed. Finally, as with any ordinal scale, even one with many levels of performance such as the Functional Independence Measure (FIM) (see Appendix #15), there is the possibility that greater clinical significance may be found between two levels that is not present between two other levels.[13]

Because of these concerns, researchers have developed methods to analyze the results of ordinal scales and use statistical techniques to transform them into interval measurements.[14] Rasch analysis is a statistical technique that allows for such a transformation.[15] Using this methodology, researchers were able to show that stair climbing, tub/shower transfers, and locomotion were the most difficult motor activities, and problem solving was the most difficult cognitive activity, on the FIM scoring system. Other researchers have used Rasch analysis to develop a scaling system that allows comparison between the findings from different functional scales.[16] Such analysis is still virtually unknown to the average rehabilitation provider but will probably play an increasing role in the evaluation of rehabilitation outcomes in the future.

ASSESSMENT OF REHABILITATION POTENTIAL

Health care providers caring for elders are often faced with the decision whether to request rehabilitation for a particular patient.

With the increase in use of home care and nursing home services, many physicians receive calls from nurses or allied health providers requesting approval for physical, occupational, or speech pathology services. How does the health care provider decide if the patient has the potential to benefit from rehabilitation?

Unfortunately, there has been little research in this area. While many studies can be found that purport to describe the ability to predict outcomes in rehabilitation, almost all of them have already accepted the patient into a rehabilitation program at the time that the patient is assessed for "potential." As most rehabilitation research is conducted in clinical situations for which reimbursement is a necessity, the mere fact that the patient was accepted means that someone must have felt there was some potential for a good outcome. This is, to some degree, a *post hoc* analysis and there are few studies that have measured the potential to respond to rehabilitation interventions before the patient is accepted into a rehabilitation program. What is really needed is an instrument that can be used to detect those patients who are most likely to benefit from a rehabilitation evaluation. Unfortunately, that does not exist at this time.

One study was conducted on acute stroke patients to evaluate the use of prognostic scoring in predicting rehabilitation outcomes. The Orpington Score, a modification of the Edinburgh Prognostic Score whereby mental status questions from the Mental Test Score of Hodkinson,[17] was used (see Appendix #35).[18] The Barthel Index was used as the "gold standard" (see Appendix #4). Assessments were first completed within 72 hours of admission to the acute hospital, then at 1, 2, and 4 weeks post-stroke. The mean age of the subjects was 81 years old and dementia was present in 23 percent of the patients. The outcomes are shown in Figure 5-4. The Orpington score at 1 week showed a significant correlation with the Barthel Index at discharge in the short staying patients but not in the longer admissions that still were able to return home. In the discussion, the authors point out that predicting rehabilitation success in minimally impaired persons is no dilemma. But predicting success in the largest group of patients, those with moderately severe deficits, who score between 3 and 5 on the Orpington scale, is much more difficult.

It will never be possible to design a single simple mathematical model which can predict outcome in every single stroke patient because of the heterogeneity of stroke and distortions introduced by other variables.

Several authors have developed statistical models for predicting outcomes.[19, 20, 21, 22] Most of these studies have used multivariate linear regression to base their predictions. It may well be that the variables that influence outcomes in rehabilitation however, are not linear. Recently, the use of simulated neural networks has been tested in that this new method of analysis is particularly well suited to nonlinear data. Grigsby and associates were able to accurately predict outcomes (86% accuracy compared to regression equation accuracy of 81%), length of stay (87% accuracy compared

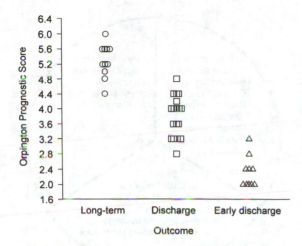

FIGURE 5-4 Orpington scores and rehabilitation outcomes. Patients with higher Orpington scores on admission had better outcomes with rehabilitation. (Reproduced, with permission, from Kalra L, Crome P. The role of prognostic scores in targeting stroke rehabilitation in elderly patients. *J Am Geriatr Soc.* 1993;41:396–400.)

to a regression equation accuracy of 35%), and costs (91% accuracy compared to 39%) using this system.[23] Perhaps in the future, rehabilitation providers will examine prospective patients with a hand-held computer to judge rehabilitation potential. Until such models exist in practice, we will be forced to use standard clinical judgements.

The health care provider is, therefore, left with a primarily clinical decision. In many ways, the evaluation of a patient's rehabilitation potential is a form of comprehensive geriatric assessment. There are, however, certain domains that are particularly important to predicting rehabilitation outcome (Figure 5-5). Assessment of functional status will not be addressed here as obviously the consideration for possible rehabilitation is prompted by the presence of functional deficits. Suffice it to say that the more severe and the longer duration of the functional deficit, the lower the chance of a "successful" rehabilitation outcome.

In the future, older persons with disability will be evaluated for rehabilitation potential using computer-based predictive models. Until that occurs, an evaluation based on the principles of comprehensive geriatric assessment is the best clinical method available.

Cognitive and Psychological Assessment

This area is arguably the most important in determining whether or not rehabilitation should be provided. Although much attention is paid by third party reimbursement systems to the physical disability, the patient's underlying cognitive status, psychological reactions

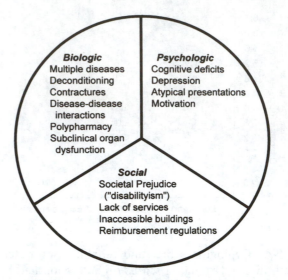

Biologic
Multiple diseases
Deconditioning
Contractures
Disease-disease
  interactions
Polypharmacy
Subclinical organ
  dysfunction

Psychologic
Cognitive deficits
Depression
Atypical presentations
Motivation

Social
Societal Prejudice
  ("disabilityism")
Lack of services
Inaccessible buildings
Reimbursement regulations

FIGURE 5-5 Factors to consider in assessing rehabilitation potential. Various conditions in the biologic, psychological, and social realms must be considered when deciding whether an elder can participate in rehabilitation. (Reproduced, with permission, from Brummel-Smith K. Introduction. In: Kemp B, Brummel-Smith K, Ramsdell JW (eds). *Geriatric Rehabilitation.* Austin, TX: Pro-Ed Press; 1990:12.)

to the disability, and motivation to learn new skills are factors that even more strongly affect rehabilitation outcomes. These areas should be assessed when evaluating the patient's potential to participate in rehabilitation.

The patient's cognitive status is the strongest factor affecting rehabilitation and cognitive deficits have been shown to limit success in traditional rehabilitation programs.[24] Assessment by interview and use of a standardized scale, such as the Folstein Mini-Mental Status Examination (MMSE) is warranted, though no clear cut points on the MMSE have been established for participation in a rehabilitation program. Certain components of the MMSE are particularly useful.[25] The ability to register and recall is a useful indicator of the patient's ability to learn new information. Attention also plays a critical role in learning, so poor scoring in this area is a negative prognostic sign. The inability to follow multistep commands often characterizes those patients who have difficulties in rehabilitation. Finally, if the patient shows evidence of visual neglect on the pentagram or clock drawing tests, he or she may have difficulty performing physical activities. Problems in these areas may occur as a result of delirium, which clearly limits involvement in rehabilitation. Another assessment for potential may be required after the delirium resolves. In summary, the key perfor-

To judge rehabilitation potential, examine certain key areas in the MMSE: attention, recall, ability to follow a three step command, and pentagram copying.

mance-based tests to administer when assessing cognitive ability to participate in rehabilitation are the ability to recall three objects after 2 minutes, follow a two-step command, maintain attention, and tests of visual-spatial skills.

Depression is also a critical factor in rehabilitation. It is a common sequel to newly acquired disabling conditions, and limits progress in new learning. Depression is extremely common following strokes, affecting as many as 70 percent of those with a left hemisphere lesion. Depressed patients often lack initiative and have poor attention, downplay their ability to accomplish demanding tasks, experience lethargy and a lack of energy, and have a hopeless outlook on the prospect of being able to regain independence. Fortunately, when detected, depression is usually responsive to treatment and the skills learned in rehabilitation often facilitate recovery as well. Unfortunately, depression is overlooked often by rehabilitation health care providers. The best method of assessment is a combination of the clinical interview and formal testing. Both may be limited by a person's aphasia and hindered by dysarthric speech. The Geriatric Depression Scale is a useful adjunct to the interview.

Motivation is probably the most difficult area to assess. Standardized instruments to assess motivation in a disabled geriatric population have not been developed. Patients who are depressed, delirious, or demented may appear unmotivated. Those who have experienced right hemisphere strokes are often seen as apathetic and lacking of motivation. The ageist attitude of society that says "you can't teach an old dog new tricks," promotes a feeling of hopelessness or impossibility when considering the potential of recovery from a serious disabling event. The patient may share those views as well.

Many rehabilitation providers have a mistaken notion about motivation. It is often stated in interdisciplinary team meetings a particular patient is not motivated because "he won't follow the directions I am giving." In other words, the patient is not doing what the health care provider thinks should be done. The real issue in motivation is whether the patient is doing what the patient thinks and believes should be done. Kemp[26] described a model for assessing depression that takes these issues into account. Motivation is seen as an interaction among four variables: (1) what the patient wants to accomplish in a rehabilitation program; (2) what beliefs the patient has about his or her abilities to recover or participate in such a process; (3) what rewards the patient expects to gain from this activity; and (4) the costs of participation. Costs are viewed broadly, not being limited to only financial ones, but also threats to personal safety, fears of loss of control, and others. If the wants, beliefs, and rewards outweigh the costs, from the patient's viewpoint, the person will appear motivated.

Social Assessment

Like the psychological area, the patient's social support system is critical to success in a rehabilitation program. Patients with much more severe difficulty in performing activities of daily living are more likely to go home if they have an adequate support than those who live alone and have less disability. Similarly, most assessments for rehabilitation potential are made preceding the offering of a service that must be reimbursed. Clearly, providers consider the patient's "potential" for participation in light of whether there is adequate coverage for that service. These facts provides a difficult ethical dilemma: should rehabilitation not be offered to patients with no support or insurance, even if they have physical and psychological factors that predict good outcomes?

Be careful not to let judgments about the quality of the patient's social support system exert too strong an effect on the decision to offer rehabilitation. This has ethical implications that are risky.

Fortunately, most patients have some support. The key questions in assessing potential are the quality and extent of support that is available, and the possibility that it can be modified. An extremely over-supportive family can be as detrimental as no support. Older persons with disability will take longer to perform activities. If family members become frustrated and assist the patient too quickly, the patient quickly learns that the "work" involved in rehabilitation is not necessary. Disablement also is a great stressor to families and it is common to see old family problems brought to the surface during a rehabilitation program.

When evaluating the patient's potential for participation in rehabilitation, assessment of social support should include observations of the family's interactions with the patient. Do they include the patient in discussions? Do they express an active interest in the patient's outcome? Do they have realistic expectations for recovery and future demands? Have they considered the impact of caregiving on themselves? It is also helpful to know if they have any experience in rehabilitation, how many persons comprise the system, and what are their future plans.

A final area within the social realm plays an important role in the decision to provide rehabilitation: finances. For most programs the decision to offer rehabilitation or the choice of site as to where the services will be rendered is heavily influenced by this consideration. Choices based solely on financial considerations are suspect on ethical grounds. Yet many patients opt to purchase insurance plans that state limits on the care provided at the outset. Perhaps these patients just did not expect to ever develop a disabling condition. A more troubling development is when frail older persons choose Medicare health maintenance organizations that limit access to rehabilitation in acute rehabilitation facilities. This limit on site of care is not usually presented in the marketing or benefits literature.

Physical Assessment

Although this is often the first area considered in traditional "medical rehabilitation," in geriatrics, the physical condition may play a lesser role than the psychological or social areas. Yet it is still vitally important, as the older person is much more likely to have multiple coexisting medical conditions that can affect the rehabilitation process. The cardiovascular, pulmonary, and neuromuscular systems are most likely to impact the patient's success in rehabilitation.

The evaluation of the patient's cardiovascular status is similar to a preoperative evaluation. Unfortunately, there have been no controlled studies that have developed predictive criteria for rehabilitation similar to the Goldman criteria for noncardiac surgery. A history of severe intermittent claudication, unstable angina, recent congestive heart failure, or uncontrolled hypertension are important to elicit, as rehabilitation is physically demanding and can lead to further destabilization. Echocardiography can also be helpful in estimating ejection fraction (EF). Clinical experience has shown those patients with an EF of less than 30 percent have difficulty participating in intensive rehabilitation programs. Those patients who have more serious cardiovascular conditions may still benefit from rehabilitation but are perhaps best served in sites where the demand can be lessened, such as in the skilled nursing facility.

Pulmonary diseases are common in elders and a history of having smoked is frequently found. Baseline evaluation includes a careful review of pulmonary symptoms predisability. A history of dyspnea on exertion may not be obtained, however, because the patient may have voluntarily restricted their activities. Pulmonary function testing is helpful and very low forced vital capacity or forced expiratory volumes can limit the patient's ability to participate in intensive rehabilitation programs. An arterial blood gas or pulse oximetry measurement can also be helpful, particularly if it is done while the patient attempts mild exercise such as using a upper extremity bicycle ergometer to determine if desaturation occurs during exercise. Hypoxia during exercise may be less limiting, however, than restrictive pulmonary deficits.

Neuromuscular assessment should include a careful evaluation of the patient's premorbid and present state of mobility, including sitting and standing balance, transfer ability, and gait, if possible. The presence of preexisting peripheral neuropathy is important to establish. Joint mobility and the presence of any significant arthritic involvement is likewise important. The view of the patient's condition should take into account the anticipated stresses that will be encountered once rehabilitation begins in earnest. For instance, a mild degree of hip osteoarthritis may be tolerable when the patient is using bipedal ambulation. Post-stroke, however, that same level of arthritic involvement on the unaffected side may limit the extra demands the patient will experience using a hemiplegic gait. Similarly, the development of hip or knee flexion contractures can significantly limit success in rehabilitation following an amputation.

In summary, the evaluation of rehabilitation potential is primarily a clinical decision. No one feature should categorically deny a patient from a trial of therapy. In an elder, the concept of "medical stability" is often elusive and a patient may actually have a better chance of achieving stability when their functional needs are met. When in doubt, the patient should be offered the chance to improve his or her functional capabilities.

ASSESSMENT OF PROGRESS AND OUTCOMES IN REHABILITATION

The measurement of function is the cornerstone in rehabilitation care. Such measurements establish a baseline from which it is hoped the patient will improve with therapy, allow for determination of improvements during therapy, and help to establish when the patient is ready to be discharged from rehabilitation or moved to a different level of care. They are also used to determine when a person is no longer in need of rehabilitation. Finally, aggregate results of measures of functional improvement may be used by programs to review the success of their interventions (as in quality review management programs), and are reviewed during accreditation evaluations, or may be used in determining reimbursement. In the future, health care plans or the Health Care Financing Administration (HCFA) may even publish outcomes of care to allow consumers to "compete on the basis of quality."

Yet this all-important area of measurement is plagued with many pitfalls. What functions should be measured in rehabilitation? Clearly, activities of daily living (ADL) and mobility are most frequently evaluated. Evaluation of cognition seems intuitively obvious, however, cognitive deficits have been shown to be frequently missed in rehabilitation programs. The same phenomenon has been encountered with depression, which also is often undetected. Instrumental activities of daily living (IADL) may be important to the person who goes home to live by himself or herself but many older men never shopped, cooked, or cleaned house.

The problems regarding validity and reliability of an instrument that were addressed in Chapter 2 clearly apply to measurements in rehabilitation. In fact, they are more difficult because the goals of rehabilitation are not just to establish where the patient is at a point in time but to sequentially measure where they go over a period of time. Measures that divide abilities into three levels of independent, needing assistance, or dependent are usually too gross to use during the process of rehabilitation. For instance, small changes in function can have important implications for caregiving needs yet not be measurable using a system of only three levels of function. Those instruments that use many levels of performance, however, are more difficult to administer and introduce the risk of inter-rater unreliability. There is also the problem in using global measures of function. Real change in one domain such as physical functioning may be obscured by changes in other areas (like social functioning).

Finally, there is the problem of what is the best source of data: the patient's own report, a therapist's professional assessment, or a directly observed, performance-based test (See Chapter 2). The patient's personal viewpoint is important because it reflects his or her values and perspective. But it may be quite different than other observer's opinions. A professional assessment is likely to be more standardized but can be affected by personal bias if the treating and evaluating health care provider are the same person. A performance-based test seems to be reliable, yet patients often have variable responses depending on the day they were tested, performance anxiety, or other factors. Furthermore, testing done in the controlled environment of the rehabilitation unit may not reflect the real performance the patient would exhibit in his or her own home.

The next section addresses the scales commonly used in rehabilitation. Many programs utilize the same instruments used in comprehensive assessment, such as the Katz ADL scale, the Lawton-Brody IADL scale, and the Mini-Mental Status Examination (see Appendix #s 24, 25, and 29). Because they have been covered in other chapters, they will not be reviewed here.

In selecting an assessment instrument to be used in rehabilitation, choose those that are able to measure changes over a relatively short period of time, can detect small changes in function, and are based on a variety of sources of information.

Early Instruments Used in Rehabilitation

One of the earliest forms of a global scale was the PULSES profile.[27] This acronym included the six categories of physical condition (P), self-care as expressed in the ability to use the upper extremities (U), mobility in terms of lower extremity function (L), sensory intactness and function (S), excretory function (E), and psychosocial status (S). Measurement was made on an ordinal scale with 1 being independent and 4 being totally dependent. A score of 6 would indicate full independence while a completely dependent person would score 24. Granger adapted the original scale in 1975 and found it to be reliable, valid, and sensitive to change; however, it lacks specific subscore detail in the ADL area to be truly useful.

The Kinney Self-Care Evaluation was introduced in 1965. It is basically an ADL scale but has been used extensively in rehabilitation in the United Kingdom. It uses a scoring system of 0 (completely dependent) to 4 (completely independent) in bed activities, transfers, locomotion, dressing, personal hygiene, and feeding. It has been shown to be very sensitive in documenting changes. It has been used to document rehabilitation outcomes and to quantify rehabilitation nursing workload.

A common criticism of these scales has been the assignment of relative equality to all functions. Common sense and clinical experience would indicate that not all physical functions are of equal value to the patient, and the absence of one of those functions does not have an equal impact on caregivers. Difficulty with bathing can be accommodated by caregivers on a once or twice weekly basis whereas impairments in feeding require assistance many times a day.

Perhaps the most widely used scale in rehabilitation in the past was the Barthel Index (Appendix #4). Developed by Barthel, a physical therapist, and Mahoney, a physiatrist, in Maryland in 1965, it was the first scale to attempt to assign different weights to different functions. Ten ADL variables were chosen, many specifically to reflect the kinds of problems seen in rehabilitation. Different relative weights were assigned according to the authors' clinical experience and judgement. Of particular interest to rehabilitation health care providers, they utilized the role that assistive devices play in determining independence. For instance, if the patient were unable to walk, but could "ambulate" with a wheelchair, he or she would score higher. The ability to put on a brace or prosthesis was added in a later iteration. Walking was assessed in terms of the patient's ability to go 50 yards, a distance that probably accurately reflects the capacity to be a household ambulator. Because of these features, the Barthel Index was widely used in both traditional rehabilitation and geriatric units.

Studies of its utility in stroke rehabilitation have revealed that those who score below 29 on admission to a rehabilitation unit are unlikely to return home or achieve significant independence in ADL. Those who score above 60 usually are discharged home and are basically independent. In spite of its utility and appropriateness to rehabilitation populations, the Barthel Index does have some limitations. Patients can be capable of performing an activity but not have the drive or initiative to do so. Some older patients may have both the cognitive capacity and drive but are so deconditioned that they cannot accomplish the task in a reasonable time frame. Finally, there is no inherent method for determining the component of the task that must be carried out by the caregiver. This consideration is extremely important to some elderly caregivers as they may have health problems themselves.

Early Comprehensive Scales

Because the scales mentioned previously are primarily focused on activities of daily living, global scales were developed that attempted to address the issues of cognition or social supports. Two scales were widely used in rehabilitation in the past and are still used by some programs. The Functional Life Scale (FLS) developed by Sarno[28] included scales for ADL, cognition, home activities (similar to IADL items), outside activities, and social interaction. It probably never achieved wide enough use to validate across all impairment groups.

The Long Range Evaluation System (LRES) combines the PULSES profile previously mentioned and an adapted Barthel Index, with the ESCROW profile.[29] The ESCROW is also an acronym, standing for environment (housing), social interactions and dependence, cluster of family members who may provide support, resources (financial), outlook (mental and psychological), and work or educational training. It includes diagnostic data that could be used for program management and assessment. It also includes a method for recording any adaptive equipment used.

Although it was an auspicious attempt to create a global measurement of function to be used in rehabilitation programs, it was extremely cumbersome. It required the use of many different measurement systems and, hence, much training to achieve inter-rater reliability. Many of the items are subjectively based and subject to bias. It did, however, set the stage for the development of the present state of the art in functional assessment in rehabilitation: the Functional Independence Measure (FIM).

Functional Independence Measure

The Functional Independence Measure is the most widely used functional status measurement system in rehabilitation today (see Appendix #15). It is an outgrowth of work by Granger and Hamilton conducted over the last 20 years as part of the Uniform Data System (UDS) of Medical Rehabilitation. A national task force convened by the American Academy of Physical Medicine and Rehabilitation and the American Congress of Rehabilitation developed it. Subsequently, Granger and others refined it at the State University of New York at Buffalo. It is now used by hundreds of rehabilitation facilities throughout the United States and in dozens of foreign countries. An important aspect of the FIM is that examiner must be trained and certified in its use before data can be accepted for inclusion in the Uniform Data System of Medical Rehabilitation. It, therefore, allows for nationwide comparison of rehabilitation interventions as well as an incredibly large data set

The Functional Independence Measure (FIM) is the most widely used assessment tool in rehabilitation today. It has now been used in tens of thousands of geriatric patients to measure progress and outcomes in rehabilitation.

for analysis. Its use in geriatric-specific settings has been more limited, however, data from the large data set reveals that in most of the rehabilitation categories studied (e.g., stroke, neurologic dysfunction, amputation, etc.), the majority of patients are over age 65 years.

The FIM has been extensively validated. Inter-rater reliability and stability of functional assessment has been tested,[30] it has been compared to the Barthel Index,[31] the use of seven levels of function has also been validated,[32] different institutions have compared scores to test agreement,[33] and it has been shown to closely correlate with patient self-ratings.[34] It has even been modified to be used in pediatric rehabilitation settings.[35] As of 1991, over 40,000 patients had been assessed using the FIM. The average age was 68 years and 42 percent of the patients were over 75 years old.[36] Because the FIM is used within 72 hours of admission and then at discharge, it is possible to measure total FIM score improvements related to length of stay. This ratio is called the "length of stay efficiency" and is used by programs and reimbursement agencies to measure their performance in rehabilitation.

The Functional Independence Measure is comprised of 18 items. Thirteen of the items are related to motor function and five are dedicated to cognitive function. An interesting aspect of the FIM is the use of percent of a particular activity that the participant is able to accomplish to measure levels of performance. Whereas the seven levels are basically the same for each function, during training, the examiner learns specific guidelines that are used to rate the performance of a particular function. An intensive study course is provided to train the examiners in the use of the FIM, including videotapes and case examples. Many providers use the FIM without being formally involved in the system.

Typically, different providers perform FIM measurements and then the results are discussed at team meetings. The FIM scores are used to decide on rehabilitation needs, measure progress, predict likely outcomes, and decide when a plateau has been reached. Occupational therapy usually measures the self-care items, nursing assesses sphincter control, and physical therapy the mobility and locomotion sections. Speech pathologists or psychologists may assess the areas of cognition. In actual practice, the measurements are often discussed and "negotiated" because, as a performance-based examination, different examiners may observe the patient performing at different levels. For instance, nursing input is crucial to all the measurements because of the extended time period of observation. In addition, patients are usually scored at the highest level that has been observed by a trained examiner. This is because one can always perform at a lower level than is expected but one cannot perform at a higher level than one is capable.

A very interesting aspect of the use of the FIM is one method for recording the results. By using a visual analog scale, a health care provider can quickly see a representation of the patient's performance and whether or not there have been improvements (Figure 5-6). Some programs make use of the graphic representation during team meetings, believing that the visual image is more useful than discussing "numbers."

Many investigators studied the performance of the FIM. In one study of over 25,000 patients, motor scores were a stronger predictor of length of stay than was cognitive function.[37] Admission motor function was the most powerful predictor for all impairment groups, which included stroke, arthritis, orthopedic problems, neurologic conditions, and others. Age was a significant predictor in the pulmonary, traumatic brain dysfunction, and nontraumatic brain dysfunction groups, but not in arthritis or cardiac groups. Admission cognitive function was also significant in that those patients with higher levels on function showed greater gains than those with lower cognitive function. Interestingly, older patients also had shorter lengths of stay. Whether this is because this group tended to show less improvement so were discharged earlier or actually improved faster than younger persons is unknown. Payer status did not correlate with length of stay but the authors do not report

The FIM can be scored in a team meeting. This allows for collaboration between various disciplines to arrive at the "truest" depiction of the patient's capabilities.

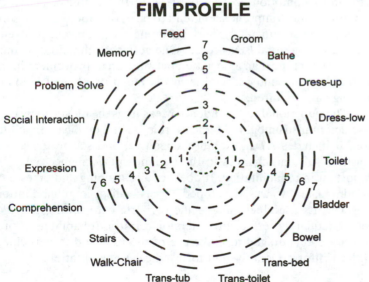

FIM PROFILE

FIGURE 5-6   The Functional Independence Measure (FIM) profile graph. Using the FIM profile graph, a line is drawn indicating the FIM score for each item at admission. Subsequent evaluations can then be indicated with additional lines, thereby depicting progress or lack thereof in each item.

the percentage of patients under a managed care plan, as the data was taken from records of admissions from 1987 to 1989.

Although the FIM addresses a number of difficulties that have been found with the use of other scales (such a floor and ceiling effects seen in the Barthel Index), it is not without its own problems. Perhaps the greatest problem is the need for training of examiners and the complexity of measurement. New users frequently must refer to the scoring booklet. Most find that with practice they can memorize the tool. It also takes some time to administer and collate the information. There have also been concerns about whether the intervals between the different levels reflect equal differences; for instance, is the difference between a 2 (maximal assistance) and a 3 (moderate assistance) the same as the difference between a 6 (uses a device) and a 7 (independent without a device)? If there is a difference, does it have clinical significance? Studies by a number of investigators have shown that even though there are conceptual differences, they do not appear to affect the ability of the instrument to measure performance or progress during rehabilitation.[38, 39]

Another aspect of the FIM to be aware of is that although all items are scored in the same manner, different activities have different levels of difficulty. For instance, of the motor items, eating and grooming are the easiest, and stair climbing, tub/shower transfers, and locomotion are the hardest. In the cognitive activities, expression and comprehension tend to be easier and problem solving is the most difficult.[40] These differences can present problems in the use of a "total FIM score." One geriatric rehabilitation unit, however, did report an association between an improvement in the total FIM score and a decrease in the mean number of hours of nursing care required.[41]

The Functional Independence Measure is the most widely used assessment instrument in Medicare-reimbursed medical rehabilitation. It includes ADL, mobility, cognitive, and social items. It is sensitive to small changes in the patient's performance, which is important in rehabilitation. It does require training and takes time to administer. It was developed by specialists in rehabilitation, however, its usefulness in specific geriatric care settings has not been adequately tested. Providers of geriatric rehabilitation programs are encouraged to make use of the FIM and to participate in the Uniform Data System for Medical Rehabilitation.

Health care providers should become familiar with the use of the FIM and evaluate whether their programs should participate in the Uniform Data System for Medical Rehabilitation.

ASSESSMENT METHODOLOGIES IN PROGRAM EVALUATION

Because improvement in functional status is the primary goal of rehabilitation, it is clear that the use of assessment information is critical to rehabilitation program evaluation. Traditionally, third party payers have used retrospective chart reviews of functional status on admission as compared to those measured near discharge as a means for determining appropriateness of care and payment. Rehabilitation health care providers sought to document any positive changes in functional status to ensure adequate reimbursement. Often, the areas of ADL function and mobility were "valued" more highly than psychological or social functioning. It is clear, however, that judgments regarding both quality and reimbursement for rehabilitation services will be tied to outcomes measured through functional assessment.

In the past, a major limitation in this process was the absence of quantifiable data. With the advent of the FIM, a validated, standardized system exists for measuring outcomes and assuring quality of care.[42] By participation in the Uniform Data System, data is collected on each patient's age, gender, living situation prior to admission, diagnosis leading to disability as well as the time since the onset, and functional status at admission and discharge. Other areas in the database include dates of admission and discharge (allowing for length of stay computation), admission source, and whether the rehabilitation stay was interrupted by an acute admission. As a result of having access to this information, many programs are now using FIM data for program evaluation. Because each item in the FIM can be used as a separate field in a statistical package, it is possible to perform a variety of analyses that compare outcomes in different areas of functioning, to such things as length of stay, diagnosis groups, age, or time to initiation of rehabilitation, to name a few.

Data from FIM assessments can also be used in reimbursement decisions. Freestanding and hospital-based rehabilitation units have been exempt from the Prospective Payment System, which is based on diagnosis related groups (DRGs). This exemption is because diagnoses are poor predictors of function and would not allow for rational reimbursement.[43] On the other hand, a study conducted by the Medical College of Wisconsin and the RAND Corporation demonstrated that functional status was strongly associated with rehabilitation length of stay and charges.[44] Work is now in progress to develop a prospective system for payment that is tied to functional status.

One such system uses a "change-in-functional status" model as a method for providing reimbursement. Using data from the MCW-RAND study, Harada and others developed a framework for rehabilitation utilization called the Rehabilitation Outcomes Model (ROM).[45] Under this model, the clinical outcome of rehabilitation is measured by a change in the functional status resulting from the intervention. It proposes a relationship between the demand for services (patient needs), the supply to meet that demand (provider characteristics), and such factors as the type of treatment provided, costs, and clinical outcomes. In order to test the model, functional status data from the MCW–RAND study were used. Such data were primarily based on the Katz scale so change was measured only at three levels (dependent, assist, or independent). Patients with spinal cord and brain injury showed the most improvement, while rehabilitation for back pain showed the least. Of interest to geriatricians is the finding that age was the only demographic variable found to be a significant predictor, the older the patient, the less the improvement. In general, those admitted with poorer functional status had greater levels of improvement. The presence of a communication deficit had a significant negative impact on improvement.

The study also addressed a question often raised by providers caring for persons who acquire a new disability: when is the best time to admit a patient to a rehabilitation program? Harada and associates found that those admitted after 29 days had significantly poorer outcomes. There was no difference for those admitted in less than 7, from 15 to 21 days, or from 2 to 28 days. Finally, the use of a catheter or development of a pressure ulcer was also associated with limitations in improvement. Like the RAND study, Harada and colleagues, concluded that better information might come from a more comprehensive functional status measurement system. With the advent of the FIM, such a system exists.

Using data from over 53,000 patients in 125 participating rehabilitation facilities, Stineman and colleagues developed the Functional Independence Measure version of the Function Related Groups (FIM-FRG).[46] Length of stay (LOS) was used as a proxy for resource utilization. The 14 UDS impairment group categories (stroke, brain dysfunction, amputation, etc.) were modified slightly to create 18 rehabilitation impairment categories (RIC). FRGs were then constructed for each RIC, based on clinical considerations using advice from a national advisory panel of experts. There were from one to five FRGs per RIC for a total of 53 (as compared to over 350 DRGs). Motor and cognitive subscales that incorporated information from the FIM data were then developed and used as variables in examining the outcomes in each RIC. Age was added as a variable only in the stroke RIC.

In the future, FIM scores will probably be used to determine prospective payment based upon Functional Related Groups.

When the analysis was completed, it appeared that it would be feasible to create a prospective payment system that is based upon functional status rather than diagnosis. For instance, for the stroke RIC patients with the most severe FRG (most severe motor disability score and younger than age 75 years) had the longest LOS. They also found that diagnosis alone only explained 13.8 percent of the variance in rehabilitation LOS.

This investigation is still under development and it is unlikely that a FIM-FRG system will be instituted soon. A system that is

TABLE 5-2. SKILLED NURSING FACILITY REHABILITATION UTILIZATION GROUPS (RUG)

Ultra high (RUC, B or A) = 720 min/wk
Very high (RVC, B or A) = 500 min/wk
High (RHC, B or A) = 325 min/wk
Medium (RMC, B or A) = 150 min/wk
Low (RLB or A) = 45 min/wk

Determination of prospective payment category. Within each, the total rehabilitation services from physical therapy, occupational therapy, and speech and language pathology must equal the related number of minutes of service provided. Determination of internal levels (i.e., levels A, B, or C) is made based on how many different rehabilitation therapies are involved and the "ADL score" (see Table 5-3).

Abbreviations: RUC, Rehabilitation Ultra-high, level C; RVC, Rehabilitation Very-high, level C; RHC, Rehabilitation High, level C; RMC, Rehabilitation Medium, level C; and RLB, Rehabilitation Low, level B.

based on actual functional status measurements, however, would seem to be far preferable to the present system, which provides financial incentives for facilities to admit preferentially the least disabled and, hence, least costly patients.[47] Older, disabled patients are often bypassed for needed services under the present reimbursement system.

Also with OBRA 1997, prospective payment for rehabilitation services in skilled nursing facilities has begun. Using resource utilization groups (RUG), rehabilitation interventions are reimbursed not in relationship to the disability or impairment being treated, but based on the amount of time therapy is provided or the number of days or providers involved in treatment. Five rehabilitation resource utilization groups are used. Three of the categories have three subcategories and the other two have only two sublevels (Table 5-2). Rehabilitation is triggered by the computation of an "ADL score" derived from Minimum Data Set (MDS 2.0) assessment that nurses complete after a resident has been admitted to a skilled nursing facility (Table 5-3). Most facilities started using

TABLE 5-3. SKILLED NURSING FACILITY PROSPECTIVE PAYMENT ADL SCORE	
Bed mobility, toilet use, and transfer	
Independent or supervision	1
Limited assist	3
Dependent:	
1–2 person assist	4
2+ person assist	5
Eating	
Independent or supervision	1
Limited assist	2
Dependent	3

RUGs in 1999 so little is known as to the effect on rehabilitation in this setting.

DISABILITY-SPECIFIC ASSESSMENTS IN REHABILITATION

Because geriatric rehabilitation encompasses a wide variety of medical conditions, it is useful to review some of the work regarding assessment in those conditions. This section addresses a number of the common conditions for which elders receive rehabilitative care.

Arthritis and Orthopedic Conditions

The measurement of function has long been an important component of the care of patients with arthritis. The American Rheumatism Association published the Classification of Functional Capacity in 1949.[48] Other instruments, including the Arthritis Impact Measurement Scales (AIMS),[49] the Stanford Health Assessment Questionnaire (HAQ),[50] and the Functional Status Index (FSI)[51] have been used in population-based studies of elders. They have not however, been used to a great degree in physicians' offices. Concerns about paperwork, having to keep a supply of "forms" on hand, and time constraints have probably limited their use more than a simple lack of interest or familiarity. Arthritis (with the subcategories of rheumatoid, osteoarthritic, and "other") is one of the major impairment group categories of the Uniform Data System for Medical Rehabilitation.

Clinical assessment of the patient with arthritis should address impairments (joint range of motion, extent and degree of active joint inflammation, muscle strength across affected joints), disabilities (changes in function in ADL, IADL, and mobility), and handicap (impact on social functioning, limits of access, etc.). Many elders in the community will have negligible effects on ADL but significant effects on IADL and mobility. Some of the factors measured using the Lawton-Brody IADL scale will miss common deficits seen in patients with arthritis, such as ability to open jars.

Two areas to be assessed clinically in these patients deserve special mention: endurance and pain. Patients with long-standing arthritis frequently become deconditioned and adjust their lifestyles accordingly. They may be able to accomplish a performance-based examination of ADL capability under testing circumstances, however, in their own homes, they may be so fatigued by the end of the day that they are essentially dependent. Diminution in endurance is difficult to detect, as there are no formal tests to use.

Traditional measures of ADL and mobility in arthritis may miss important clinical findings such as fatigability, pain, and endurance. These findings often predict functional performance in the patient's home.

Perhaps the simplest indication is the patient who admits to feeling fatigued while performing ADL.

Pain is a limiting factor in the performance of all functional activities. Arthritis patients must be taught to respect their pain threshold and reduce their activities when pain begins. There are numerous scales for assessing pain, however, the simplest is to have the patient rate their pain on a scale of 1 to 10. Rehabilitation is geared towards enhancing strength and flexibility, thereby decreasing pain (see Chapter 15).

Hip and other fractures are extremely common in old age and a frequent cause for referral to a rehabilitation program. Using data from the Uniform Data System, orthopedic conditions accounted for 31 percent of the caseload in rehabilitation in 1991, second only to stroke. This category also had the highest mean age (75). Over the last decade, there has been a remarkable improvement in the surgical techniques used and the use of anticoagulation and other measures to prevent complications. As a result, fracture type, treatment, and ability for immediate weight bearing have less association with outcomes than other factors. Preexisting medical conditions significantly affect outcomes following surgery. Mental status and the availability of a caregiver have also been shown to strongly predict outcomes.[52] Premorbid functional status has also been shown to correlate closely with outcomes.[53]

Stroke

As the most common diagnosis in rehabilitation, it is no wonder that much of the research in assessment in this field has been with stroke patients. A recent publication of the Agency for Health Care Policy and Research on post-stroke rehabilitation reviewed the current knowledge of assessment in this condition.[54] In the guidelines, there are a number of recommendations of instruments to be used in the rehabilitation of patients with stroke.

The Functional Independence Measure has provoked a flurry of research in stroke rehabilitation. For instance, using the FIM as a prognostic indicator, Oczkowski and Barreca were able to show that the absolute admission FIM score, not the change in score, was the best predictor of outcome disability and place of discharge.[55] Patients with admission FIM scores of 36 or less were never discharged home, while those with scores above 97 all went home. Subgroups of stroke patients with differing rehabilitation needs could also be identified. Older patients and those with poor postural control or bowel or bladder incontinence had poorer outcomes. A limitation of this study was the fact that the average time since stroke to initiation of rehabilitation was 52 days, much longer than

In one study, stroke patients admitted to a rehabilitation program with FIM scores below 36 were never discharged home.

the recommended maximum of 21 days. Similar outcomes have been found using the Barthel Index.[56] Another method for predicting outcomes, the classification tree approach, was used by Falconer and associates.[57] This approach correctly classified 88 percent of the sample using only four of the predictor variables: level of independence in toilet management, bladder management, and toilet transfer, and adequacy of financial resources.

There are a number of other instruments used in stroke rehabilitation. The Chedoke-McMaster Stroke Assessment (Chedoke Assessment) is a 2-part measure made up of a physical impairment inventory and a disability inventory.[58] The impairment inventory addresses six dimensions, including shoulder pain, postural control, the hand, arm, leg, and foot. Each is measured using a 7-point scale, each of which corresponds to the normal pattern of motor recovery following a stroke. The disability inventory tests 15 maneuvers, which are scaled using the FIM gradations (Table 5-4). It has performed well in tests for validity and reliability.[59] It has the advantage over other instruments in that it measures changes in disability, not just impairment, and the impairment inventory can be used by therapists to classify patients into homogeneous subgroups based on the stage of motor recovery. Its main disadvantages are that it has not had extensive use in different sites, requires

---

TABLE 5-4. CHEDOKE-McMASTER STROKE ASSESSMENT DISABILITY INVENTORY

Gross motor function index

1. Supine to side lying on strong side
2. Supine to side lying on weak side
3. Side lying to long sitting through strong side
4. Side lying to sitting on side of the bed through strong side
5. Side lying to sitting on side of the bed through weak side
6. Standing
7. Transfer to and from bed toward strong side
8. Transfer to and from bed toward weak side
9. Transfer up and down from floor and chair
10. Transfer up and down from floor and standing

Walking index

11. Walking indoors
12. Walking outdoors, over rough ground, ramps, and curbs
13. Walking outdoors several blocks
14. Stairs
15. Age- and gender-appropriate walking distance for 2 min

Scoring key: Same as Functional Independence Measure with 1 being total assist and 7 being complete independence.

training in both the instrument and knowledge of use of the FIM, and takes some time to complete. Such an instrument would be valuable in research studies that look at the effect of physical interventions to ensure patient comparability. Clinically, it would be useful to target the intervention more specifically to the motor deficit in question.

The Fugl-Meyer Assessment scale is widely used in Europe to measure motor function in stroke rehabilitation.[60] Like the Chedoke Assessment, it examines volitional movement within patterns of synergistic muscle movement commonly found after a stroke. It has been criticized because the item measuring sitting balance, an important function in stroke rehabilitation, has shown poor validity. Sitting balance is probably more validly quantified using the Chedoke Assessment. There is a simple, bedside clinical assessment of sitting balance, which clinicians may want to use (Table 5-5).[61] Simply measuring gait speed has been shown to correlate with other measures of disability after a stroke.[62] The patient is directed to walk 5 m at his or her usual pace, turn around and walk back 5 m. This distance was selected to allow for testing in the home setting. Formal gait analysis using an electrical recording system is usually not needed in stroke rehabilitation but can be utilized when there are questions regarding choice of an ankle or foot orthosis or the exact nature of the gait disturbance. Small, portable units, which fit in the patient's shoes, are now available and easy to use.[63]

Finally, the Sickness Impact Profile (SIP)[64] has been used in stroke rehabilitation, along with the Brief Symptom Inventory,[65] to predict burden of care.[66] A change in the FIM score was found

---

TABLE 5-5.   BEDSIDE TEST OF STATIC AND DYNAMIC SITTING BALANCE

Have patient sit on side of bed, feet on the floor, back unsupported, hands in lap.

If the patient can hold this position for 15 sec, nudge him or her anteriorly, posteriorly, and laterally using approximately 5 to 10 foot-pounds of force (a gentle nudge).

Important: Guard the patient from falling.

Scoring

4 = Normal

3 = Good: able to maintain static position without difficulty but requiring assistance in righting from the hemiplegic side

2 = Fair: able to maintain static position without difficulty but requiring assistance in all righting tasks

1 = Unable to maintain static balance

Consider using measures of patient and caregiver satisfaction as part of the rehabilitation assessment. Managed care is paying an increasing amount of attention to this area.

to be equivalent to an average of 2.19 minutes of help from another person per day while a change in one point on the SIP was found to be equivalent to an average of 3.32 minutes of help. Together with the Brief Symptom Inventory, the FIM and the SIP were found to be useful in predicting the patient's general life satisfaction. In another study, however, the SIP was not recommended for use in stroke rehabilitation because it was difficult to administer and was not sensitive to change with improvements in functional capability. The measurement of caregiver burden and life satisfaction has particular importance to rehabilitation providers because of the strong association between good outcomes and caregiver stress. As elderly patients become increasingly involved in rehabilitation under managed care, patient satisfaction is likely to play a larger role in quality assurance assessment.

Role of Assessment in Other Conditions

Functional assessment tools have been used in a number of other conditions, such as spinal cord injury,[67] traumatic brain injury,[68] multiple sclerosis,[69] and end-stage renal disease.[70] Most of these conditions affect a larger proportion of younger persons so the studies tend to have few elders represented. In most studies, advanced age does appear to limit functional outcomes but it is unclear to what degree this fact is due to age alone or to comorbid conditions. An interesting method for using the FIM data was developed by Cook and associates.[71] A graphic representation of admission and discharge scores was made allowing for visualization of rather dramatic changes in some patients (Figure 5-7).

SUMMARY

The use of assessment instruments and evaluations in rehabilitation is critical to providing high quality care. Assessment forms the basis by which impairments, disabilities, and handicaps are detected and a care plan is developed. Treatment outcomes are monitored through the use of repeated assessments over time. Decisions to continue or stop rehabilitation can be made on the basis of objective data rather than personal whim or subjective opinions. Programs can use assessment data to measure quality assurance indicators and for accreditation reviews. It is important for all who practice to have a basic understanding of the range of instruments available to be used in geriatric rehabilitation.

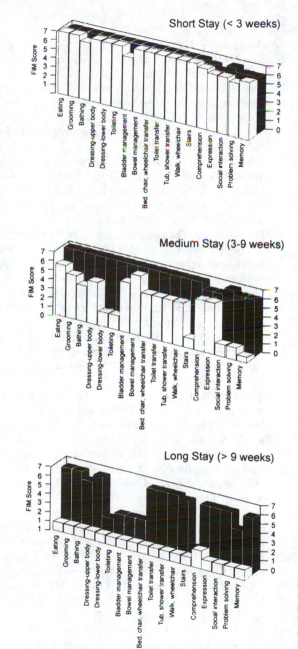

FIGURE 5-7   FIM profiles as an index of outcome. These three figures show how the Functional Independence Measure (FIM) admission and discharge scores can be used to indicate outcomes of care for different lengths of stay (c) patients in rehabilitation for brain injury. White bars are admission scores and shaded bars are discharge scores. **A.** Short stay (< 3 weeks). **B.** Medium stay (3–9 weeks). **C.** Long stay (> 9 weeks).

REFERENCES

1. Granger CV, Hamilton BB. The Uniform Data System for Medical Rehabilitation report of first admissions for 1991. *Am J Phys Med Rehabil.* 1993;72:33–38.
2. Nagi SZ. Some conceptual issues in disability and rehabilitation. In: Sussman MB. *Sociology and Rehabilitation.* Ohio State University Press; 1965:38.
3. Wood PHN, Bradley EM. Setting disablement in perspective. *Int Rehab Med.* 1978;1:32–37.
4. World Health Organization. *International Classification of Impairments, Disabilities, and Handicaps.* Geneva: WHO; 1980.
5. Meyer JK. Consequences and progression of disability. In: Sussman MB, ed. *Sociology and Rehabilitation.* Washington, DC: American Sociological Association; 1965:63.
6. Duckworth D. The need for a standard terminology and classification of disablement. In: Granger CV, Gresham GE, eds. *Functional Assessment in Rehabilitation Medicine.* Baltimore: Williams & Wilkins; 1984:chap 1.
7. Menter RR, Whiteneck GG, Charlifue SW, et al. Impairment, disability, handicap, and medical expenses of persons aging with a spinal cord injury. *Paraplegia.* 1991;29:613–619.
8. Fuhrer MJ, Rintala DH, Hart KA, Clearman R, Young ME. Relationship of life satisfaction to impairment, disability, and handicap among persons with spinal cord injury living in the community. *Arch Phys Med Rehabil.* 1992;73:552–557.
9. Wood PHN, Badley EM. Contribution of epidemiology to health care planning for people with disabilities. In: Granger CV, Gresham GE, eds. *Functional Assessment in Rehabilitation Medicine.* Baltimore: Williams & Wilkins; 1984:35.
10. Wood PHN, Badley EM. Contribution of epidemiology to health care planning for people with disabilities. In: Granger CV, Gresham GE, eds. *Functional Assessment in Rehabilitation Medicine.* Baltimore: Williams & Wilkins; 1984: p 35.
11. Granger CV. A conceptual model for functional assessment. In: Granger CV, Gresham GE, eds. *Functional Assessment in Rehabilitation Medicine.* Baltimore: Williams & Wilkins; 1984:19–21.
12. Bunch WH, Dvonch VM. The "value" of functional independence measure scores. *Am J Phys Med Rehabil.* 1994;73:40–43.
13. Granger CV, Hamilton BB, Linacre JM, Heinemann AW, Wright BD. Performance profiles of the Functional Independence Measure. *Am J Phys Med Rehabil.* 1993;72:84–89.
14. Heinemann AW, Linacre JM, Wright BD, Hamilton BB, Granger CV. Relationships between impairment and physical disability as measured by the Functional Independence Measure. *Arch Phys Med Rehabil.* 1993;74:566–573.
15. Wright BD, Masters G. Rating scale analysis. Rasch measurement. Chicago: MESA; 1982.
16. Fisher WP, Harvey RF, Taylor P, Kilgore KM, Kelly CK. Rehabits: a common language of functional assessment. *Arch Phys Med Rehabil.* 1995;76:113–122.

17. Quershi KN, Hodkinson HM. Evaluation of a ten-question mental test in the institutionalized elderly. *Age Ageing.* 1974;3:152–157.

18. Kalra L, Crome P. The role of prognostic scores in targeting stroke rehabilitation in elderly patients. *J Am Geriatr Soc.* 1993;41:396–400.

19. Osberg JS, DeJong G, Haley SM, et al. Predicting long term outcome among post-rehabilitation stroke patients. *Am J Phys Med Rehabil.* 1988;67:94–103.

20. Granger CV,Hamilton BB, Gresham GE, Kramer AA. The stroke rehabilitation outcome study: part II. Relative merits of the total Barthel Index score and a four-item subscore in predicting patient outcomes. *Arch Phys Med Rehabil.* 1989;70:100–103.

21. Magaziner J, Simonsick EM, Kashner TM, et al. Predictors of functional recovery one year following hospital discharge for hip fracture: a prospective study. *J Gerontol.* 1990;45:M101–107.

22. Stineman MG, Maislin G, Williams SV. Applying quantitative methods to the prediction of full functional recovery in adult rehabilitation patients. *Arch Phys Med Rehabil.* 1993;74:787–795.

23. Grigsby J, Kooken R, Hershberger J. Simulated neural networks to predict outcomes, costs, and length of stay among orthopedic rehabilitation patients. *Arch Phys Med Rehabil.* 1994;75:1077–1081.

24. Schuman JE, Beattie J, Steed DA. Geriatric patients with and without intellectual dysfunction: effectiveness of a standard rehabilitation program. *Arch Phys Med Rehabil.* 1981;62:612–618.

25. Mosqueda LA. Assessment of rehabilitation potential. *Clin Geriatr Med.* 1993;9:689–703.

26. Kemp B. Motivational dynamics in geriatric rehabilitation. In: Kemp B, Brummel-Smith K, Ramsdell JW, eds. *Geriatric Rehabilitation.* Austin, TX: Pro-Ed Press; 1990:297.

27. Moskowitz E, McCann CB. Classification of disability in the chronically ill and aging. *J Chronic Dis.* 1957;5:342–346.

28. Sarno JE, Sarno MT, Levita E. Functional life scale. *Arch Phys Med Rehabil.* 1973;54:214–220.

29. Granger CV, McNamara MA. Functional assessment utilization: The Long-Range Evaluation System (LRES). In: Granger CV, Gresham GE, eds. *Functional Assessment in Rehabilitation Medicine.* Baltimore: Williams & Wilkins, 1984.

30. Ottenbacher KJ, Mann WC, Granger CV, et al. Inter-rater reliability and stability of functional assessment in the community-based elderly. *Arch Phys Med Rehabil.* 1994;75:1297–1301.

31. Kidd D, Stewart G, Baldry J, et al. The functional Independence Measure: a comparative validity and reliability study. *Disabil Rehabil.* 1995;17:10–14.

32. Hamilton BB, Laughlin JA, Fiedler RC, Granger CV. Inter rater reliability of the 7-level functional Independence Measure (FIM). *Scand J Rehabil Med.* 1994;26:115–114.

33. Segal ME, Ditunno JF, Staas WE. Interinstitutional agreement of individual functional independence measure (FIM) items measured at two sites on one sample of SCI patients. *Paraplegia.* 1993:31:622–631.

34. Grey N, Kennedy P. The functional Independence Measure: a comparative study of clinician and self ratings. *Paraplegia.* 1993;31:457–461.

35. Msall ME, DiGaudio K, Duffy LC, et al. WeeFIM: normative sample of an instrument for tracking functional independence in children. *Clin Pediatr.* 1994; July 33(7), 431–438.

36. Granger CV, Hamilton BB. The Uniform Data System for Medical Rehabilitation report of first admissions for 1991. *Am J Phys Med Rehabil.* 1993;72:33–38.

37. Heinemann AW, Linacre JM, Wright BD, et al. Prediction of rehabilitation outcomes with disability measures. *Arch Phys Med Rehabil.* 1994;75:133–143.

38. Linacre JM, Heinemann AW, Wright BD, et al. The structure and stability of the Functional Independence Measure. *Arch Phys Med Rehabil.* 1994;75:127–132.

39. Heinemann AW, Linacre JM, Wright BD, et al. Relationships between impairment and physical disability as measured by the Functional Independence Measure. *Arch Phys Med Rehabil.* 1993;74: 566–573.

40. Granger CV, Hamilton BB, Linacre JM, et al. Performance profiles of the Functional Independence Measure. *Am J Phys Med Rehabil.* 1993;72:84–89.

41. Mason M, Bell J. Functional outcomes of rehabilitation in the frail elderly: a two-year retrospective review. *Perspectives.* 1994;18:7–9.

42. Dickson HG, Hodgkinson A, Kohler F. Inpatient quality assurance by local analysis of uniform data set data. *J Qual Clin Practice.* 1994; 14:145–148.

43. Batavia AI, DeJong G. Prospective payment for medical rehabilitation: the DHHS report to Congress. *Arch Phys Med Rehabil.* 1988: 69:377–342.

44. Hosek S, Kane R, Carney M, et al. *Charges and Outcomes for Rehabilitative Care. Implications for the Prospective Payment System.* (R-3424-HCFA) Santa Monica, CA: The RAND Corporation; 1986.

45. Harada N, Sofaer S, Kominski G. Functional status outcomes in rehabilitation: implications for prospective payment. *Med Care.* 1993; 31:345–357.

46. Stineman MG, Hamilton BB, Granger CV, et al. Four methods for characterizing disability in the formation of function related groups. *Arch Phys Med Rehabil.* 1994;75:1277–1283.

47. Stineman MG, Escarce JJ, Goin JE, et al. A case-mix classification system for medical rehabilitation. *Med Care.* 1994;32:366–379.

48. Steinbrocker O, Traeger CH, Botterman RC. Therapeutic criteria in rheumatoid arthritis. *JAMA.* 1949;140:659–662.

49. Meenam RF, Yelin EH, Nevitt M, et al. The impact of chronic disease: a sociomedical profile of rheumatoid arthritis. *Arthritis Rheum.* 1981;24:544–549.

50. Fries JF, Spitz R, Kraines RG. Measurement of patient outcomes in arthritis. *Arthritis Rheum.* 1980;23:137–145.

51. Jette AM. Functional status index: reliability of a chronic disease evaluation instrument. *Arch Phys Med Rehabil.* 1980;61:395–401.

52. van der Sluijs JA, Walenkamp GH. How predictable is rehabilitation

after hip fracture? A prospective study of 134 patients. *Acta Orthop Scand.* 1991;62:567–572.

53. Borquist L, Cedar L, Thorngren KG. Functional and social status 10 years after hip fracture. Prospective follow-up of 103 patients. *Acta Orthop Scand.* 1990;61:404–410.

54. Gresham GE, Duncan PW, Stason WB, et al. *Post-Stroke Rehabilitation.* Clinical Practice Guideline, No. 16. Rockville, MD: U.S. Department of Health and Human Services. Public Health Service, Agency for Health Care Policy and Research. AHCPR Publication No. 95-0662. May 1995.

55. Oczkowski WJ, Barreca S. The Functional Independence Measure: its use to identify rehabilitation needs in stroke survivors. *Arch Phys Med Rehabil.* 1993;74:1291–1294.

56. Loewen SC, Anderson BA. Predictors of stroke outcome using objective measurement scales. *Stroke.* 1990;21:78–81.

57. Falconer JA, Naughton BJ, Dunlop DD, et al. Predicting stroke inpatient rehabilitation outcome using a classification tree approach. *Arch Phys Med Rehabil.* 1994;75:619–625.

58. Gowland C, Torresin W, VanHullenaar S, Best L. Therapeutic exercise for stroke patients. In: Basmajian JV, Wolf SL, eds. *Therapeutic Exercise.* Baltimore, MD: Williams & Wilkins; 1990;207–229.

59. Gowland C, Stratford P, Ward M, et al. Measuring physical impairment and disability with the Chedoke-McMaster Stroke Assessment. *Stroke.* 1993;24:58–63.

60. Malouin F, Pichard L, Bonneau C, Durand A, Corriveau D. Evaluating motor recovery after stroke: comparison of the Fugl-Meyer Assessment and the motor assessment scale. *Arch Phys Med Rehabil.* 1994;75:1206–1212.

61. Sandin KJ, Smith BS. The measure of balance in sitting in stroke rehabilitation prognosis. *Stroke.* 1990;21:82–86.

62. Collen FM, Wade DT, Bradshaw CM. Mobility after stroke: reliability of measures of impairment and disability. *Int Disabil Studies.* 1990;12:6–9.

63. von Schroeder HP, Coutts RD, Lyden PD, Billings E, Nickel VL. Gait parameters following stroke: a practical assessment. *J Rehabil Res Dev.* 1995;32:25–31.

64. Bergner M, Bobbitt RA, Carter WB, Gilson BS. The sickness impact profile: development and final revision of a health status measure. *Med Care.* 1981;787–805.

65. Derogatis LR, Melisaratos N. The brief symptom inventory: an introductory report. *Psychol Med.* 1983;13:595–605.

66. Granger CV, Cotter AC, Hamilton BB, Fiedler RC. Functional assessment scales: a study of persons after stroke. *Arch Phys Med Rehabil.* 1993;74:133–138.

67. Menter RR, Whiteneck GG, Charlifue SW, et al. Impairment, disability, handicap, and medical expenses of persons aging with spinal cord injury. *Paraplegia.* 1991;29:613–619.

68. Granger CV, Divan N, Fiedler RC. Functional assessment scales: a study of persons after traumatic brain injury. *Am J Phys Med Rehabil.* 1995;74:107–113.

69. Granger CV, Cotter AC, Hamilton BB, Fiedler RC, Hens MM. Functional assessment scales: a study of persons with multiple sclerosis. *Arch Phys Med Rehabil.* 1990;71;870–875.

70. Cowen TD, Huang CH, Lebow J, DeVivo MJ, Hawkins LN. Functional outcomes after inpatient rehabilitation of patients with end-stage renal disease. *Arch Phys Med Rehabil.* 1995;76:355–359.

71. Cook L, Smith DS, Truman G.Using functional independence measures profiles as an index of outcome in the rehabilitation of brain-injured patients. *Arch Phys Med Rehabil.* 1994;75:390–393.

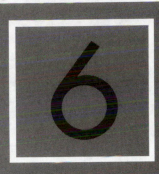

MULTIDIMENSIONAL ASSESSMENT IN THE COMMUNITY

DAVID B. REUBEN

The multiple complex health and social problems of older persons, particularly those above the age of 85 years, commonly lead to difficulties in accomplishing everyday activities. Multidimensional assessment allows health care professionals to identify these problems and develop preventive, treatment, and rehabilitation strategies designed to improve or maintain functional and health status. Multidimensional assessment extends beyond the traditional medical evaluation of an older person's health to include assessments of mental, functional, and social status. Other domains frequently included in the assessment are the patient's economic status, characteristics of the home environment, and a discussion of patient preferences regarding advanced directives.

Multidimensional assessment of elders can be conducted by individual practitioners or by a multidisciplinary team of health care providers (comprehensive geriatric assessment). This chapter describes practical methods for conducting multidimensional assessment by health care providers. The two approaches share common principles; however, the methods and resources required to implement the two differ substantially. To be successful, both approaches must be efficient and practical. Chapter 7 addresses the practical approaches to multidimensional assessment.

Fortunately, the majority of elders do not need an extensive multidimensional evaluation. Simple probes for the presence of common problems may suffice. More extensive evaluation, such as comprehensive geriatric assessment, should be reserved for those who are frail or at high risk for functional decline or nursing home placement.

GERIATRIC ASSESSMENT BY THE INDIVIDUAL PHYSICIAN

Structuring the Office Visit

Multidimensional assessment can be a slow, inefficient, and even disruptive process. If this assessment is to be readily incorporated into office practices, the assessment process must be streamlined. When properly organized, health care providers can conduct brief multidimensional assessments and render comprehensive care without spending an inordinate amount of time on the patient visit. Although every office setting is unique, some basic guidelines can be helpful.

First, health care providers need to discard the notion that each physician must personally gather every item of the patient's medical history. Much of this information can be obtained from old records, other professional or nonprofessional staff, or by self-report from patients or family members completing forms. Moreover, the amount of time the physician spends taking a medical history has been demonstrated to be inversely correlated with patient satisfaction.[1] In contrast, time spent conducting the physical examination, discussing treatment, and providing health education has been found to be positively correlated with patient satisfaction. A structured previsit questionnaire that gathers information on past medical history, medications, preventive measures, and functional status (including information on who helps when the patient is functionally dependent) can markedly reduce the time needed to conduct an initial assessment. If a patient is unable to complete the questionnaire, usually a family member or a caregiver can do so (see Appendix #38).

> A structured previsit questionnaire can markedly reduce the time needed to conduct an initial assessment.

Second, when case-finding for geriatric problems, trained office staff can administer screening instruments for many of the important dimensions. This approach enables the health care provider to spend only a short period of time reviewing the results of these screens and then decide which dimensions, if any, need greater evaluation.

Third, offices should take advantage of computer technology to improve record keeping. Although computerized medical record systems have not yet been widely implemented, templates generated on word processing programs can be used effectively. For example, a dictated previous note that has been saved in a word processing program and is available to the physician can be retrieved and updated to reflect the current office visit. In this manner, time spent keeping records is reduced, and records are kept current and legible. Essential components of each updated note include a problem list, preventive services, history, and current medication list.

Fourth, many elements of the treatment plan can be delegated to other health care providers. Follow-up telephone calls from office staff or health educators can reinforce instructions and improve adherence with recommended treatment. Each dimension should be systematically, if only briefly, evaluated to determine whether more in depth assessment is necessary.

Assessment Instruments

The use of assessment instruments can facilitate geriatric assessment. If used inappropriately, however, instruments can reduce efficiency and undermine the provider–patient relationship. Instruments cannot substitute for good clinical skills and judgment, including the skill of eliciting important items from the patient's history and physical examination. Information obtained from assessment instruments can, however, be used to focus on issues that are particularly germane to an individual patient. Instruments can also allow health care providers to dismiss certain dimensions as not needing further assessment.

To use assessment instruments in this manner, the principles of screening must be followed. To ensure that potential problems are not overlooked, assessment instruments should have high sensitivity even if specificity is low. If optimal test characteristics have not been determined, health care providers would be wise to use a low threshold to indicate the need for further evaluation.

If instruments are to improve the efficiency of the evaluation, nonprofessional personnel should administer them. For example, an office assistant might conduct a brief cognitive screen and, if abnormal, the physician would conduct a more extensive mental status evaluation. Several groups have demonstrated the feasibility and yield of utilizing office staff to administer case-finding and screening instruments that assess many of the dimensions described previously.[2, 3] This approach can dramatically improve the practitioner's efficiency and increase the number of new and treatable problems detected in patients. Using office-based staff to screen or case-find has cost implications. Office staff must be properly trained to administer these instruments and they can be quite time consuming. One published method takes approximately 22 minutes to administer and another takes an estimated 10 minutes to administer.[2, 3] This time must be taken from other office tasks and the cost of screening may be considerable.

What to Screen For and How to Do It

The individual health care provider's office-based multidimensional assessment for community-dwelling elders should include short screens for the domains of importance to elders. In addition to seeking common geriatric conditions, physicians should evaluate nonmedical issues that are of particular relevance to the health of elders (e.g., advanced directives, adequacy of social support, economic status, and environmental risks). These are briefly described in the following sections and longer assessments will also be mentioned. The reader is referred to other chapters in this book for the details of administering specific instruments for each dimension, as well as their test characteristics. The health care provider may choose to rely on less formal questions to probe into potential problems, however, and examples of open-ended questions will also be provided.

Physicians should evaluate nonmedical issues that are important to the health of elders.

MEDICAL ASSESSMENT

In addition to the standard medical history and physical examination, some specific conditions that are common among elders and have considerable impact on function should be searched for. These disorders include impairments of vision, hearing, and mobility, as well as the geriatric syndromes of malnutrition, urinary incontinence, and polypharmacy. In the course of the traditional medical evaluation, these problems may go unnoticed because elders fail to report them spontaneously. For example, they may not recognize that falls are indicative of treatable medical problems. They also may be embarrassed to mention problems with maintaining urinary continence. Finally, they may believe that these symptoms, such as hearing loss, are normal aspects of aging that cannot be helped.

Visual Impairment.
Although many older persons seek eye care from optometrists, opticians, and ophthalmologists, the high rates of vision disorders and impairment and the brevity of the screening process justify screening by primary care physicians. Each of the four major eye diseases (cataract, age-related macular degeneration, diabetic retinopathy, and glaucoma) increases in prevalence with age. Moreover, presbyopia is virtually universal and the vast majority of elders require eyeglasses. Among those over age 85 years, 20 percent have difficulty seeing even when wearing glasses.

Vision problems can increase the risk of injury due to falls and motor vehicle crashes and can also lead to impairment in physical and psychosocial function.

The standard method of screening for problems with visual acuity is Snellen's Eye Chart, which requires the patient to stand 20 feet from the chart and read letters, using corrective lenses. Patients fail the screen if they are unable to read all the letters on the 20/40 line. This simple screen can be performed by office staff at the time that vital signs are measured; thus, the physician can have the information to review at the time of the patient encounter.

Several interviewer and self-administered instruments to detect functional problems due to visual impairment have been developed, including the Activities of Daily Vision Scale and the VF-14.[4,5] These have primarily been used in research settings but may hold some promise as screening instruments in the future (see Appendix #s 1 and 46).

Hearing Impairment.

Hearing impairment is among the most common medical conditions reported by elders, affecting approximately one third of those 65 years of age or older. Hearing impairment is associated with reduced cognitive, emotional, social, and physical function in elders and the use of amplification devices has led to improvement in functional status and quality of life.

Screening for hearing loss can also be performed by office staff prior to the physician encounter using a Welch Allyn Audioscope™ (Welch Allyn, Inc., Skaneateles Falls, NY), a hand-held otoscope with a built-in audiometer. The audioscope can be set at a several different levels of intensity, but should be set at 40 dB to evaluate hearing in elders. A pretone at 60 dB is delivered and then four tones (500, 1000, 2000, and 4000 Hz) at 40 dB are delivered. Patients fail the screen if they are unable to hear either the 1000- or 2000-Hz frequency in both ears or are unable to hear both the 1000- and 2000-Hz frequencies in one ear.

An alternative is the whispered voice test, which is administered by whispering 3 to 6 random words (numbers, words, or letters) at a set distance (6, 8, 12, or 24 inches) from the person's ear and then asking him or her to repeat the words. The examiner should be behind the person to prevent speech reading and the opposite ear should be occluded during the examination. Failure to repeat 50 percent of the whispered words correctly indicates the need for audiology referral.

Similar to vision screening, a self-administered test of emotional and social problems associated with impaired hearing, the Hearing Handicap Inventory for the Elderly-Screening Version (HHIE-S), has been developed. Although this questionnaire (see Appendix #22) is brief and easy to administer, its accuracy when compared to audiometry is less than the audioscope.[6] More recently, a 6-item screen for hearing impairment based on questions from the National Health and Nutrition Examination Survey has been developed.[7] This simple screen is highly correlated with findings on pure-tone audiometry (see Chapter 10).

Malnutrition/Weight Loss.

Malnutrition is a global term that encompasses many different nutritional problems that are associated with diverse health consequences. The two most common nutritional disorders are obesity and energy undernutrition (including protein-energy undernutrition). Prevalence estimates of these disorders in community-based elders vary widely due to differences in defining malnutrition and the population studied. Both extremes of body weight place older people at risk for subsequent health problems.

The best brief assessment for nutritional status is weight expressed as body mass index [weight in $kg/(height\ in\ meters)^2$]. Particularly important is change in weight, especially recent weight loss. Accordingly, for established patients, weight should be measured every visit. Although guidelines have not been established for how frequently height should be measured, given the high rates of osteoporosis and some thinning of the intervertebral disks with aging, it is reasonable to measure height yearly. Patients who are new to the practice should be asked about weight loss or gain, which can be accomplished using a previsit questionnaire. One question for detecting weight loss asks. "Without trying to, have you lost or gained 10 pounds in the last six months?" Persons who answer yes to this question are at an increased risk of death over 4 years.

Several self-administered questionnaires have been developed, most notably the Nutrition Screening Initiative's 10-item checklist (see Appendix #33).[8] Although the validity of these instruments has been questioned, they are increasingly being used in community-based screening programs (see Chapter 12).

Urinary Incontinence.

Urinary incontinence is common, especially among community-dwelling elderly women, and is under-recognized for a variety of reasons. Women may be embarrassed to raise the issue, particularly if the health care provider is a male; they also may regard it as a normal aspect of aging that is best controlled with pads. Minor incontinence may have few medical consequences but may have substantial social ramifications. More severe incontinence may lead to skin breakdown and ulcers and is also associated with increased caregiver burden. In frail or demented elders, incontinence can be the precipitating factor that leads to institutionalization.

Incontinence can be screened for by asking two questions on a previsit questionnaire: (1) "In the last year, have you ever lost your urine and gotten wet?" and if the respondent answers yes to the first question, she or he is asked (2) "Have you lost urine at least six separate days?" Positive answers to both questions indicate a potential problem with urinary incontinence that needs further investigation by the clinician (see Chapter 22).[9]

Problems with Mobility and Balance.

Osteoarthritis is the most common chronic medical condition affecting elders. Particularly affected are the hips and knees. Neurologic conditions affecting sensory perception (e.g., neuropathies), motor function (e.g., stroke), and balance also frequently affect elders. Osteoporotic fractures of the hip almost exclusively affect elders. Each of these conditions individually or collectively can precipitate mobility problems. Impaired mobility can, in turn, lead to falls and/or further functional impairment.

A multidimensional assessment should assess both mobility problems and identify whether the patient has been falling. Mobility problems are best assessed by examination. Several methods have been advocated, including the Performance-Oriented Assessment of Mobility (see Appendix #36) instrument and the timed Get Up & Go Test (see Chapter 23).[10, 11] The former is a standardized instrument that measures gait and balance and the latter is a timed measure of the patient's ability to rise from a chair, walk 3 meters (10 feet), turn, walk back, and sit down again. Another method is the Berg Balance Test (see Chapter 23). This has proved valuable in research settings describing populations and predicting falls. A lower extremity battery has been developed that includes three items: a timed 8-foot walk, the time to perform 5 chair-rises, and a series of three balance maneuvers: side-by-side, semi-tandem, and full-tandem stances.[12] This test has demonstrated predictive validity for functional decline in community-based elders.

In clinical practice, there is no substitute for the observation of a patient's gait by the physician. It requires little time and provides an excellent evaluation of the patient's mobility. The physician must be trained to systematically observe gait and balance and this component of the examination should be routinely integrated into the office visit. The alert physician can perform a gait evaluation while the patient is entering or leaving the examining room. In clinical settings, the previously mentioned instruments may be the most valuable in helping physicians develop the observational skills needed to quickly evaluate this dimension. Brief assessment of a patient's resistance to a nudge and observation of a 360-degree turn can provide valuable insight to the patient's balance.

The presence of falls can be ascertained on a questionnaire by asking whether "During the past twelve months have you fallen all the way to the ground or fallen and hit something like a chair or stair?"[13] A yes answer is very sensitive but leads to many false positives and must be followed with subsequent questions by the health care provider (see Chapter 23).

Polypharmacy.   Most elders take at least one medication each day and many are prescribed several medications. As a result of increased medication use, elders are at increased risk for drug–drug interactions and adverse drug events. Inappropriate prescribing commonly occurs when patients see multiple providers or use multiple pharmacies.

A simple method of detecting potential problems with polypharmacy is to have each patient bring in all the medications (in their bottles or tubes) that he or she is currently taking to each visit. Office personnel can check these against a master medication list and discrepancies can be brought to the physician's attention at the time of the patient encounter. Using commercially available drug interaction programs, the patient's medication list can be investigated for possible interactions.

COGNITIVE ASSESSMENT

The incidence of dementia increases with age. The disorder is uncommon among those who are 65 to 74 years of age who are community-dwelling but rises substantially among those over age 85 years of age. Because of the progressive, relentless nature of the disorder and the low likelihood of finding completely or partially reversible causes (approximately 10 percent), screening for dementia has not been widely advocated. Several arguments support screening including new treatments for Alzheimer's disease that appear to be effective for some patients, the potential reversibility of the disorder of some cases, and the importance of providing prognostic information for patients and their families.

A variety of short screens are available, some of which can be administered by trained nonprofessional office staff. Patients and their families sometimes resent these questions and tasks, however, even when assessed by physicians. The most commonly used screen is the Mini-Mental State Examination, a 30-item interview-administered assessment of several dimensions of cognitive function.[14] (See Appendix #29) Shorter screens also have been validated including recall of 3 items at 1 minute, the clock drawing test (see Appendix #8), the serial sevens test (patients are asked to subtract seven from 100 five times) and the Time and Change Test.[15, 16] Normal results on these tests vastly reduce the probability of dementia, whereas abnormal results increase the odds of dementia.[15]

It must be recognized, however, that these tests rely on tasks that are not routine aspects of day life. Moreover, often they do not account for educational level, languages other than English, and cultural differences (see Chapters 3 and 21).

AFFECTIVE ASSESSMENT

Although the prevalence of major depression is low among community-dwelling elders (estimated at between 1 percent to 3 percent), symptoms of depression are much more common, affecting approximately 10 percent of the population. Depression tends to be under-recognized among patients and health care providers because of the similarity of depressive symptoms (e.g., fatigue, poor appetite, sleep disturbances) to those that accompany common medical illnesses. Among the current cohort of elders, there may also be some stigma associated with seeking help for mental health problems. Nevertheless, depressive symptoms and major depression are quite responsive to nonpharmacologic or medication therapy.

Patients can be asked about depression on a previsit questionnaire using the question "Do you often feel sad or depressed?"[17] A number of other brief self-administered screens are available, including the Mental Health Index from the Medical Outcomes Study SF-36 and the Geriatric Depression Scale, which has 15- and 30-item versions (see Appendix #40 and 16).[18]

ASSESSMENT OF FUNCTION

An assessment of function is a measure of the overall impact of diseases and disorders on the individual. It can be valuable as a stimulus to further diagnostic evaluation, to plan specific treatments, and to provide prognosis and plan for long-term care. Three levels of function are commonly evaluated in elders: basic activities of daily living (BADLs), instrumental or intermediate activities of daily living (IADLs), and advanced activities of daily living (AADLs).[19] BADLs assess the ability of the patient to complete basic self-care tasks (e.g., bathing, dressing, toileting, continence, feeding, and transferring). IADLs measure the patient's ability to live independently (e.g., shopping for groceries, driving or using public transportation, using the telephone, meal preparation, housework, repair work, laundry, taking medications, and handling finances). AADLs measure the patient's ability to fulfill societal, community, and family roles as well as participate in recreational or occupational tasks. Because AADLs are usually voluntary, they are more individualized than are BADLs and IADLs. These AADLs can be viewed as a person's "functional signature." (See Appendix #s 24 and 25).

The prevalence of functional impairment in the community varies by the level of the functional task and how impairment is defined. Although fewer than 10 percent of community-dwelling elders are dependent in BADLs, up to 80 percent are dependent in some AADLs, such as performing heavy housecleaning.

A variety of instruments, including those that measure function by direct observation, have been developed to assess functional status at each level. Questions that ask about specific BADL and IADL function can be incorporated into a previsit questionnaire. Some AADLs (e.g., exercise and leisure time physical activity) can be addressed in this manner, but global questions about how a person spends his or her days are often very revealing and can provide reference points that can be monitored at subsequent office visits.

ASSESSMENT OF SOCIAL SUPPORT

When elders become progressively frail, the need for social support becomes more important. The availability of assistance from family and friends is frequently the determining factor of whether a functionally dependent older person remains at home or is institutionalized. Even in healthy elders, it is often valuable to raise the question of who would be available to help if he or she becomes ill; early identification of problems with social support may prompt planning to develop resources should the necessity arise.

Formal brief screening instruments that are clinically useful in assessing social support are under development. Nevertheless, when assessing function, some idea of support can be gauged by asking who provides help for specific BADL and IADL functions and whether these persons are paid or voluntary help. The older patient's family structure can be assessed by a few questions on a previsit questionnaire. The quality of these relationships, however, must be assessed by the physician during the patient encounter (see Chapters 4 and 26).

ECONOMIC ASSESSMENT

Economic assessment also becomes more important in functionally impaired persons. These elders may qualify for state or local benefits depending on income or may need to plan to draw upon financial reserves in a strategic manner. It, therefore, is useful to know the specific threshold for assistance eligibility in the patient's individual state. The patient's income can be assessed on a previsit questionnaire and eligibility can usually be readily determined.

ENVIRONMENTAL ASSESSMENT

With progressive frailty, the home environment becomes a more critical determinant of the ability to live independently and safely.

Unsafe environments can increase the risk of falls and resulting fractures. Although physicians rarely personally conduct environmental assessments, patients and their families can be referred to the National Safety Council (800-621-7619; www.nsc.org) to obtain a booklet on home safety. When indicated (e.g., recurrent falls, visual impairment), community agencies such as visiting nurses can be enlisted to inspect homes for safety and can recommend the installation of adaptive devices (e.g., shower bars, raised toilet seats). Persons who are at risk for becoming dependent in IADLS should be evaluated for the geographic proximity of necessary services (e.g., grocery shopping, banking), their need for use of such services, and their ability to utilize these services in their current living situations. Unfortunately, simple brief screening instruments that assess the needs and match for these necessary services have yet to be developed. (See Chapter 8 and Appendix #23).

SPIRITUALITY

Spirituality, whether affiliated with a formal religious denomination or nonreligious intangible elements, has increasingly been recognized as an important influence on health. Recent data indicate that frequent attendance at religious services is associated with lower mortality rates. Formal instruments assessing spirituality have not been developed but asking elders whether religion or spirituality is important to them may provide insights that may facilitate their care. Especially in hospital settings, involvement of pastoral care can be valuable in supporting the patient and in framing medical decisions in the context of the patient's personal belief system.

ADVANCE DIRECTIVES

As part of a multidimensional assessment, patient's goals and preferences for care should be determined. In frail elders, these preferences are essential for determining a management plan. Specific advance directives are invaluable in guiding therapy if a patient is unable to speak for himself or herself at a future time. The durable power of attorney for healthy care, which asks the patient to designate a surrogate to make medical decisions if the patient loses decision-making capacity, is often less emotionally laden than specifying treatments that the patient may or may not want. Nevertheless, particularly in patients with early dementia, it is valuable to begin discussions about preferences for specific treatments while the patient still has the cognitive capacity to make these decisions.

Although it is often difficult to find the time to discuss advance directives in detail during the initial office visit, a previsit questionnaire can determine whether the patient already has such a directive and patients can be given information to read at home in preparation for subsequent discussions (see Chapter 25).

OFFICE-BASED COMPREHENSIVE GERIATRIC ASSESSMENT

Comprehensive geriatric assessment (CGA) is a process that provides more in-depth evaluations of the dimensions described previously and links these evaluations with specific services aimed to restore or maintain function and health. In CGA, the assessments are conducted by a team of health care providers rather than by one solitary physician. This process has been demonstrated to be effective in providing a variety of benefits when conducted in inpatient and rehabilitation unit settings. Theoretically, outpatient CGA should be able to confer the same benefits. Although the initial reports of outpatient CGA did not indicate that it was effective in this setting, more recent models have achieved health benefits in randomized clinical trials and controlled studies. These models included utilizing a geriatric nurse practitioner to provide periodic in-home assessments that were subsequently discussed with a multidisciplinary team, geriatric care management in multidisciplinary geriatrics clinics, and linking an adherence intervention to a single geriatrics consultation.[20–23]

Some health care systems have found outpatient CGA to be a valuable way of organizing services for frail elders. In the ambulatory setting, a different set of logistical and practical obstacles must be overcome for CGA to be successful. Scheduling difficulties, the labor intensity associated with CGA, and reimbursement issues are major barriers. For example, in fee-for-service settings, reimbursement of nonphysician team members for their services is often difficult. The low volume of patients that can be cared for by traditional CGA models compared to usual one-on-one provider patient care, makes this method of health care delivery expensive in all reimbursement systems. Finally, patient fatigue may be a major factor, particularly when CGA is structured as a sequential set of evaluations on the same day, often taking 3 to 4 hours, (see Chapter 7).

SUMMARY

Office-based assessment by a primary care provider is an effective way to categorize the needs of frail elders or those threatened with placement in a long-term care facility. To be efficient, physicians will need to share responsibilities for portions of the assessment with trained office staff members. For complicated cases, multidisciplinary assessment may be necessary.

REFERENCES

1. Robbins JA, Bertakis KD, Helms LJ, et al. The influence of physician practice behaviors on patient satisfaction. *Fam Med.* 1993;25:17–20.
2. Miller DK, Brunworth D, Brunworth DS, Hagan R, Morley JE. Efficiency of geriatric case-finding in a private practioner's office. *J Am Geriatr Soc.* 1995;43:533–537.
3. Moore AA, Siu AL. Screening for common problems in ambulatory elderly: clinical confirmation of a screening instrument. *Am J Med.* 1996;100:438.
4. Mangione CM, Phillips RS, Seddon JM, et al. Development of the "Activities of Daily Vision Scale": a measure of visual functional status. *Med Care.* 1992;30:1111–1126.
5. Steinberg EP, Tielsich JM, Schein OD, et al. The VF-14: an index of functional impairment in patients with cataract. *Arch Ophthalmol.* 1994;112:630.
6. McBride WS, Mulrow CD, Aguilar C, Tuley MR. Methods for screening for hearing loss in older adults. *Am J Med Sci.* 1994;307:40–42.
7. Reuben DB, Walsh K, Moore AA, Damesyn M, Greendale GA. Hearing loss in community-dwelling older persons: national prevalence data and identification using simple questions. *J Am Geriatr Soc.* 1998;46:1008.
8. White JV, Dwyer JT, Posner BM, Ham RJ, Lipschitz DA, Wellman NS. Nutrition Screening Initiative: development and implementation of the public awareness checklist and screening tools. *J Am Diet Assoc.* 1992;92:163.
9. Diokno AC, Brown MR, Brock BM, Herzog AR, Normolle DP. Clinical and cystometric characteristics of continent and incontinent noninstitutionalized elderly. *J Urol.* 1988;140:567–571.
10. Tinetti ME. Performance-oriented assessment of mobility problems in elderly patients. *J Am Geriatr Soc.* 1986;34:119–126.
11. Podsiadlo D, Richardson S. The timed "Up & Go": a test of basic functional mobility for frail elderly persons. *J Am Geriatr Soc.* 1991;39:142–148.
12. Guralnik JM, Simonsick EM, Ferrucci L, et al. A short physical performance battery assessing lower extremity function:association with self-reported disability and prediction of mortality and nursing home admission. *J Geron:Med Sci.* 1994;49:M85–M94.
13. Cummings SR, Nevitt MC, Kidd S. Forgetting falls: The limited accuracy of recall of falls in elderly. *J Am Geriatr Soc.* 1988;36:613–616.
14. Tombaugh TN, McIntyre NJ. The Mini-Mental State Examination: a comprehensive review. *J Am Geriatr Soc.* 1992;40:922–935.
15. Siu AL. Screening for dementia and investigating its causes. *Ann Intern Med.* 1991;115:122–132.

16. Froehlich TE, Robison JT, Inouye SK. Screening for dementia in the outpatient setting: the Time and Change test. *J Am Geriatr Soc.* 1998; 46:1506–1511.

17. Lachs MS, Feinstein AR, Cooney LM, et al. A simple procedure for general screening for functional disability in elderly patients. *Ann Intern Med.* 1990;112:699–706.

18. Sheikh JI, Yesavage, JA. Geriatric Depression Scale: recent evidence and development of a shorter version. *Clin Gerontol.* 1986;5:165.

19. Reuben DB, Wieland DL, Rubenstein LZ. Functional status assessment of older persons: concepts and implications. *Facts and Research in Gerontology.* 1993;7:731–240.

20. Stuck AE, Aronow HU, Steiner A, et al. A trial of annual in-home comprehensive geriatric assessments for elderly people living in the community. *N Eng J Med.* 1995;333:1184–1189.

21. Burns R, Nichols LO, Graney MJ, Cloar T. Impact of continued geriatric outpatient management on health outcomes of older veterans. *Arch Intern Med.* 1995;155:1313–1318.

22. Boult C, Boult L, Murphy C, Ebbitt B, Luptak M, Kane RL. A controlled trial of outpatient geriatric evaluation and management. *J Am Geriatr Sec.* 1994;42:465–470.

23. Reuben DB, Frank JC. Hirsch SH, McGuigan KA, Maly RC. A randomized clinical trial of outpatient comprehensive geriatric assessment coupled with an intervention to increase adherence to recommendations. *J Am Geriatr Soc.* 1999;47:269–276.

IMPLEMENTATION OF THE ASSESSMENT PROCESS IN THE AMBULATORY CLINIC

LAURA MOSQUEDA / KERRY BURNIGHT

Multidimensional assessment clinics are ideal for elders with complex medical, social, and psychological problems. The clinics employ a team of health care professionals, each with a special knowledge in geriatrics. Although the composition of the team varies among clinics, most teams have a geriatrician, nurse practitioner, and social worker. Teams may also include a pharmacist, psychologist, nutritionist, physical therapist, occupational therapist, psychiatrist, podiatrist, and dentist. During or following the assessment process, there is often an interdisciplinary team meeting to share and discuss observations. A conference is held at the completion of the assessments to develop a plan of action with the individual and family members.

It must be noted that in some assessment clinics the function is limited solely to assessment. Studies of such programs reveal that such assessments result in identification of more diagnosis and in the reduction of caregiver stress. They do not convincingly show an improved patient outcome. The clinics that tend to improve medical outcomes are those that provide follow-up care in addition to assessment.[2]

At the National Institute on Health Conference, *Geriatric Assessment Methods for Clinical Decision Making,* participants articulated five goals of multidimensional assessment: (1) improve diagnostic accuracy; (2) guide the selection of interventions to restore or preserve health; (3) recommend an optimal environment; (4) predict outcomes; and (5) monitor clinical change.[3] These goals highlight that fact that multidimensional assessment is not an end in itself, but instead, a "gateway to care."[4]

The 5 goals of multidimensional assessment:

- Improve diagnostic accuracy
- Guide the selection of interventions to restore or preserve health
- Recommend an optimal environment
- Predict outcomes
- Monitor clinical change

The chapter begins with a review of the characteristics of patients most likely to benefit from multidimensional assessment in an ambulatory setting. This is followed by a discussion of the composition of the assessment team. The next portion of the chapter is devoted to a review of the techniques used in conducting multidimensional assessment. Specifically, we review the components of the medical, functional, psychological, socioeconomic, and environmental assessment. Finally, there is a discussion of the special aspects of assessment in the ambulatory clinic.

INDICATIONS: IDENTIFYING APPROPRIATE PATIENTS TO ASSESS

The majority of people between the ages of 65 and 75 years would probably not benefit from a comprehensive assessment. As a person ages, however, the likelihood of developing multiple chronic illnesses and functional deficits rises dramatically. These are often accompanied by psychological problems such as depression or anxiety, which may further increase functional limitations. These changes also affect the social support system, which in turn can lead to greater use of institutional sources of care. The ultimate goal of comprehensive assessment is to enhance the patient's functional abilities so that he or she can live in the most satisfying and least restrictive environment.

Characteristics of Elders Most Likely to Benefit from Multidimensional Assessment in an Outpatient Setting:

> Has Complicated, Interacting Problems
> Is a possible candidate for SNF placement
> May be Demented
> Has Multiple subspecialists and No Primary Care Physician
> Exhibits "the Dwindles"

The Elder with Complicated, Interacting Problems

Elders who have complex, interacting medical, psychological, and social problems are appropriate to refer for assessment. It may be difficult, if not impossible, for the primary care physician to adequately assess a new patient who is an 84 year-old man with diabetes, congestive heart failure, atrial fibrillation, macular degeneration, and a right hemisphere stroke. The physician in an assessment program will have more time to spend with the patient and will have team members to rely on for many portions of the assessment. For example, screening by physical and occupational therapists may uncover the need for exercise and adaptive equipment. Recommendations for modifications of the home environment may be given. The social worker can assist in developing connections to agencies that provide in-home support to enable the elder to stay at home. Several team members can complete assessments and education of the caregivers. The assessment process provides time and multidisciplinary expertise that the elders with complicated problems need.

The Elder Who is a Possible Candidate for a Nursing Home

One of the most difficult and heart-wrenching decisions a family makes involves placing a loved one in a nursing home. When an elder has very poor physical function, yet has the cognitive ability to participate in the decision and is unwilling to go, the family is put in an even more difficult position. The doctor is often consulted when these decisions are being made.

Referral to a comprehensive assessment clinic is an excellent method for making sure all possible alternatives to placement have been explored. Perhaps a combination of medication adjustments, adaptive equipment, family training, and community programs (such as adult day care) will provide the individual and family with the knowledge and skills to keep the elder in his or her preferred environment. At times, the team may act as patient advocate, encouraging the family to let the cognitively intact elder take a chance and remain at home even though they may have concerns. The following case vignette demonstrates some of these points.

Case Vignette: A 79-year-old man has been living by himself following the death of his wife 6 years ago. He had an ischemic stroke in the right internal capsule, leaving him with a moderate left hemiplegia but no cognitive problems. Both he and his family worry about his safety in the bathroom and his ability to care for himself in the event of an incident such as a fall. His daughter, the primary caregiver, talked with her father about moving into an assisted living facility but he refuses. His primary care physician refers him for evaluation. Careful questioning about his medications reveals that he is taking over-the-counter sleeping pills (which he never told his private doctor). A physical therapist notes that he would ambulate safely with a brace on his left lower leg and that his store-bought cane is much too tall for him. An occupational therapist discusses equipment for his bathroom, such as a tub transfer bench and a long-handled shower hose that will make his bathing safer. The social worker tells him about a "life line" program that allows him to call a response team in an emergency situation with the push of a button that he wears around his neck. The team feels that involvement in a local adult day health care center would enable the patient to get needed rehabilitation and provide for socialization. After a discussion between the team and clients, he agrees to attend for two visits to see how he will like it. Because the patient and family are willing and able to follow through with the recommendations, he is able to remain in his own home.

Conversely, the assessment sometimes confirms the need for placement and gives the family permission and support for the decision. Whereas patients involved in traditional Medicare reimbursement may need a qualifying admission to an acute hospital before being eligible for skilled nursing reimbursement, those in health maintenance organization are not subject to this restriction. A preadmission comprehensive assessment is very valuable for identifying the needs of the patient and initiating restorative interventions in a timely manner.

The Elder With Dementia

The interdisciplinary nature of the comprehensive assessment clinic makes it a good resource for families of people with dementing illnesses. This is especially true if the diagnosis is unclear and/or there are significant behavioral problems accompanying the dementia. The geriatrician, neuropsychologist, psychiatrist, and neurologist (all of whom are usually available through the comprehensive clinic setting) may be needed when the patient's diagnosis and optimal treatment are unclear. Therapists with training in geriatrics will help family members to find strategies that make their lives easier while trying to help the patient and family formulate realistic goals. Families may need education to learn more about dementing illnesses, strategies that may be effective in addressing behavioral problems, and care planning options. For those with a more advanced dementia, the family will need training to help with activities of daily living such as toileting and dressing.

The team will investigate: (1) the etiology of the dementia; (2) whether there are any causes of excess disability (such as medications with anticholinergic side effects or previously undiagnosed illnesses such as hypothyroidism); (3) how best to assist the patient; and (4) how to assist the family. Thorough assessment ensures that treatable dementias are not missed, factors contributing to excess disability are found, and educational needs of patient and family are addressed (see Chapter 21).

The Importance of Functional Status:

Throughout the assessment process all team members place an emphasis on evaluating the patient's and family's functional status. This is a special and important aspect of geriatric assessment, as it takes us beyond traditional medical diagnoses and into quality of life issues.

Case Vignette: The family members of a woman with Alzheimer's disease are at their wits' end, because she is hallucinating, wandering at night, combative at times, and incontinent of urine. The assessment reveals multiple factors contributing to these problems, many of which are at least partially reversible. Sensory deficits (poor hearing and vision) contribute to her hallucinations. Multiple medications increase her level of confusion and make her agitated. Depression is diagnosed and is thought to be making her more irritable. A very stressed daugh-ter-in-law, who is the primary caregiver, thinks that the patient "could remember if she wants to." Finally, problems with visuospatial ability make it difficult for her to find the bath-room; this makes her appear incontinent when, in fact, her sphincter control is fine. When the appropriate interventions are instituted, the patient's symptoms subside and the duration of home care is extended. Many members of the team suggested different interventions: the physician, pharmacist, occupational therapist, psychologist, and social worker.

The Elder With Multiple Subspecialists and No Primary Care Physician

Some elders go directly to a subspecialist when they encounter a new medical problem. As managed care becomes more common among the elderly, this ability to bypass a primary care provider will be reduced. It is not uncommon, however, for an elder to be seeing a cardiologist for congestive heart failure, a neurologist for Parkinson's disease, an orthopedist for osteoarthritis, and a pulmonologist for reactive airway disease. The danger is that there is no one doctor with a holistic, global perspective of the patient. The subspecialists are less likely than the primary care physician to do complete medication reviews and think beyond the organ system for which their opinion was sought.

A comprehensive assessment clinic will examine all aspects of care, analyze medications, and take a holistic, functional approach. Medical care may then be consolidated under one primary care provider after an interdisciplinary assessment, when the treatment plan is initiated. The subspecialists will still be used for consultation, although perhaps on a less frequent basis. Advantages include: less potential for medication interactions, less travel for the elder, and the opportunity for the elder to establish health care provision with a provider who is clearly the coordinator or overseer of care.

The Elder With "the Dwindles"

Some elders, especially those over the age of 80 years, lose function for no apparent reason (the "dwindles"). The decline may have started with a relatively minor acute illness, such as an upper respi-ratory infection, or incident, such as a fall without apparent injury, from which the person never fully recovered. This is a very distressing situation for both the elder and family members, as they are witnessing a previously independent elder experience a relatively rapid decline. The reason can be quite difficult to identify, and can be due to a combination of many factors. A comprehensive assessment team is useful in these instances.

The health care provider often finds that the decline actually started at an earlier point than the patient and family recognized, and that the illness or incident was actually a marker for underlying problems. Common problems that are uncovered include: hearing loss, poor vision, malnutrition, depression, worsening heart disease, thyroid disease, and neurologic problems such as lacunar infarcts. Physical and occupational therapists are helpful in determining deficits in endurance and the presence of deconditioning. Programs to enhance strength, endurance, and balance have been shown to be effective in reversing these conditions. The social worker will have a particularly important role in identifying community resources, assessing and assisting the family, and gathering psychosocial information about the patient.

TEAMWORK

Given the considerable heterogeneity of patients appropriate for assessment, every patient does not necessarily require the involvement of every team member. Prior to, or during the initial appointment, the geriatrician, nurse practitioner, and/or social worker will often determine which other disciplines will be helpful to an individual elder.

Regardless of the composition of the team, training of the team is very important. Such training should serve several purposes:

1. Ensure that team members have an adequate understanding of the CGA process.
2. Raise the level of expertise of team members.
3. Develop standard approaches to problems that are commonly identified through CGA.
4. Define areas of responsibility of individual team members.
5. Learn to work effectively as a team.

Some teams hold retreats or in-service seminars when new members are added to the team.

During and following the assessment process, there often is an interdisciplinary team meeting. Communication among team members is critical. The team members have common goals, based on the elder's wishes, and reinforce each other's efforts while interacting with the individual and family. Team meetings are an opportunity to share information and observations and to develop a plan of care. Responsibility for carrying out the plan may also be decided during these meetings. Some teams use these meetings to review care protocols used during assessment.

One of the challenges in team meeting is allowing all members to present their information without spending an inordinate amount of time. It helps if there is an identified team leader (not necessarily the physician) who keeps the meeting moving forward and elicits the most relevant information from the team members. Relevance, however, needs to be defined in the context of the team. An experienced team works quickly but thoroughly, in part, because members know what information is useful to the others and what information is primarily useful to them.

At times, team members may not be able to meet together. Conference calls can be used in such circumstances. Other team members may ask a fellow health care provider to make their presentations. In some circumstances, the team may need to review written reports from absent members.

Record keeping offers another challenge. A vast amount of data is created through a comprehensive assessment. The team must record their findings to review at a later time and to compare future improvement or decline to measured baselines. A computerized data base, coupled with a team member trained in research methodology, enables systematic comparisons of such outcomes. Because such a wealth of assessment data is rarely useful to referring primary physicians, it is best to summarize the main findings and recommendations in a concise report that can be given to the patient and family, and sent to the referring physician or agency.

TECHNIQUES FOR CONDUCTING MULTIDIMENSIONAL ASSESSMENT

Medical Assessment

In a comprehensive assessment setting, the geriatrician has the luxury of more time to spend with a patient than does the physician in a typical office practice. This allows for a comprehensive history and physical examination. Particular attention is paid to nutritional status, ability to perform activities of daily living (ADLs) and instrumental activities of daily living (IADLs), alcohol use, fall risk, and change in cognition. Many of the answers received during the history can be verified or brought into question during the physical examination. For instance, the patient who states he has no problems getting in and out of bed, yet is unable to arise from the examination table may be exaggerating his abilities.

In addition to the usual review of systems, the history includes questions about falls and urinary incontinence. These are two common problems that the patient may experience, but may not discuss without prompting. It is also important to ask specific questions about alcohol intake. (The patient who reports "I have always had one martini in the evening, and I always will" may be now drinking his "one" martini from a 10-ounce glass).

A physician and/or pharmacist perform careful review of prescription and over-the-counter medications. Patients are asked to bring all medication to the clinic. The pharmacist can then make a variety of suggestions, including: (1) testing for drug levels; (2) discontinuation of potentially dangerous medications; (3) withdrawal of inappropriate medication; and (4) recommendations of appropriate substitutions.

The physical examination must be thorough, with an emphasis on geriatric problems. Special attention to the sensory examination is important. Some clinics utilize an optometrist to perform screening exams for acuity, glaucoma, and macular degeneration. Screening audiology is also performed in most comprehensive assessment clinics. Another important area to examine is the genitalia. Many older persons, even those cared for in primary care settings, have not had routine pelvic or external genitalia examinations. In addition to performing preventive screenings (such as Pap smears and prostate exams) as appropriate, this is an opportunity to look for evidence and etiology of urinary or fecal incontinence.

A screening test for cognitive impairment, such as the Folstein Mini-Mental State Exam is also performed.[5] (See Appendix #29) The health care provider must be alert to the fact that some patients who "pass" the screen may indeed be demented and vice versa. If cognitive impairment is found but the diagnosis is unclear, referral to a psychologist for neuropsychological testing is helpful. Functional assessment tools are also used during the physical examination (see Chapter 2).

Because there usually will not be an ongoing relationship with the patient, it may be prudent to order laboratory tests on the first visit unless recent results are available. This gives the health care provider an opportunity to review the results with the patient on the next visit or during the family conference. It also assures that conditions that may have been overlooked in the typical primary care setting will not be missed in the consultative setting of a comprehensive assessment clinic. In addition to the usual laboratory tests (chemistries and complete blood count), measurement of TSH, B_{12}, and nutritional indices are commonly performed. Electrocardiograms and other tests of cardiac function can be ordered if indicated.

In some comprehensive assessment clinics, a neurologist and psychiatrist participate in the team. Neurologic consultation is advised for patients with unusual presentations of dementing illness or other major neurologic problems. Psychiatry is particularly helpful in those patients presenting with unusual or complicated psychiatric disorders and those on complex psychopharmacologic regimens.

On completion of the medical evaluation, a comprehensive list of the diagnoses is generated. Such a list should emphasize those conditions that are: (1) treatable and being adequately addressed; (2) treatable, and in need of further attention; and (3) stable or untreatable and not needing further attention. A plan is then developed to attend to each of these categories.

Functional Assessment

Throughout the assessment process, all team members place an emphasis on evaluating the patient's and family's functional status. This is a special and important aspect of geriatric assessment, as it takes us beyond traditional medical diagnoses and into quality of life issues. Diagnoses are poor predictors of functional abilities and it is only through direct assessment that patient's functional needs can be determined. For example, one patient with the diagnoses of diabetes, stroke, hypertension, glaucoma, and depression may be functioning at a completely independent level, while another, with a only a diagnosis of osteoarthritis, may require a great deal of assistance with all of the basic activities of daily living. It is, therefore, helpful to maintain a separate functional problem list.

The functional examination focuses on daily activities such as mobility, toileting, dressing, grooming, and hygiene skills. The mobility component includes an assessment of gait, transfers, balance, and dynamic activities such as reaching up and bending over. Wheelchair skills are also assessed; some patients would be independent with wheelchair mobility if their chair was the appropriate size and proper training was provided. The mobility and transfer assessments are usually done by the physical therapist. The other activities of daily living are assessed by the occupational therapist. If therapists are not available in the clinic, the physician or nurse practitioner may perform basic screening. Standardized instruments such as the Katz ADL Scale or the Barthel Index are usually employed (see Appendix #s 24 and 4).[6,7]

Instrumental activities of daily living may also be assessed, depending upon the patient's needs, abilities, and living situation. As with the basic activities of daily living, screening instruments can be used to record the results of the assessment and decide if an intervention (such as referral to an occupational therapist) would be appropriate. The Lawton Brody IADL Scale is probably most frequently used.[8] (See Appendix #25). The social worker is

In Assessing the Elder with Dementia:

(1) What is the etiology of the dementia?;

(2) Are there any reversible factors aside from the primary cause of the dementia which are causing excess disability?;

(3) What can be done to assist the patient?;

(4) What can be done to assist the family?

often involved in this area of assessment because many of these activities relate to community integration. For example, a person who is quite independent with the basic ADLs may derive substantial benefit from a handicap parking permit, a pill organizer, and meals-on-wheels. Sometimes, these simple interventions make a major difference in quality of life and perceptions of independence.

The choice of tools used throughout the multidimensional assessment is guided by the preferences of the individual practitioners. Performance based tests, such as the Tinetti gait and balance examination (POMA) (see Appendix #36) or the Williams timed manual performance examination, are easily administered in the clinic setting.[9, 10] Team members are able to understand how the patient functions in the home environment utilizing specific assessments by occupational and physical therapists. For example, the occupational therapist may use a cart that carries a variety of household articles for testing the patient's ability to make a sandwich, operate a telephone, or manage a checkbook. The physical therapist may use a short segment of stairs in the clinic and have an assortment of walking aids available for immediate trials.

Psychological Assessment

Although there is a high prevalence of psychological disorders such as depression and anxiety among elders, they are often undiagnosed, and therefore, untreated. Psychologists and/or social workers with special training in geriatric syndromes assist with detection and treatment of these problems. The psychological assessment is an area where the benefits of interdisciplinary teamwork become obvious. The occupational therapist may report that the patient seems to be socially isolated and less functional than expected based on examination; the physician may notice weight loss and problems with concentration; both report these findings to the psychologist who is alerted to the possibility of depression and/or early cognitive impairment. The physician has already ordered screening tests that rule out medical causes for these problems. A psychologist with training in medical issues and geriatrics will help to distinguish if physical symptoms such as insomnia and lack of energy are related to the medical problems or due to depression.

Mental health professionals also evaluate cognitive status. Whereas cognitive tests, such as the Folstein Mini-Mental State Examination, can be helpful to the physician in screening for cognitive impairment, neuropsychological testing provides detailed information about specific areas of an individual's cognitive performance. For example, testing may reveal that an elder has difficulty with verbal memory but good ability with visual memory.

This information has practical, useful implications for the patient and his or her family. The testing can also be helpful for determining what type of dementing illness a person has when the history and physical examination do not lead to a clear answer. Finally, testing establishes a baseline against which later changes can be compared.

Socioeconomic Assessment

An understanding of the patient's socioeconomic situation is crucial to providing appropriate care. Insurance status has a great impact on medical, psychological, and social services available to the elder and his or her family. As the use of health maintenance organizations increases, it is important for elders to understand what benefits are offered by a particular health plan; however, there is a great deal of variability among insurance plans and determining what is available may be a daunting task for the untrained. A skilled social worker can assist the elder in evaluating health plan benefits and restrictions.

A social worker can also help identify available resources in the community. Few elders and their families are aware of existing resources such as senior housing, meals-on-wheels, and adult day care programs. Care management (sometimes still called case management or coordination) can also be arranged, which is especially important if the assessment team will not be responsible for continued management (see Chapter 26).

Environmental Assessment

Many assessment programs offer in-home evaluations prior to the first clinic visit. The advantages of interviewing an elder in his or her own home are described elsewhere (see Chapter 8). The home visit provides an excellent opportunity for reviewing medications. A good method for ensuring that all medicines are brought out for review is to follow the individual throughout the house while asking if there are any other places that pills are kept. This enables the interviewer to see several rooms of the house (as long as the person gives permission) and to make sure that all known medicines are located. This is also an ideal time to do a safety assessment of the home and to notice if there are stairs or other environmental barriers in or out of the home. The person doing the assessment should note if the neighborhood appears to be safe. Some elders limit their own activity outside the home because they are afraid to leave the house.

Information gathered during the home visit should be available to all members of the health care team prior to seeing the patient. This is helpful to the team members, who then have a significant amount of information about the patient before entering the examination room, and helpful to the patient/family, who do not have to repeat the same information many times as new team members enter the room.

SPECIAL ASPECTS OF ASSESSMENT IN THE AMBULATORY CLINIC

Patient "Flow" in the Clinic Setting

Patient Stress:

All attempts should be made to reduce the stress on the patient of seeing multiple providers and undergoing a variety of assessments.

Each comprehensive assessment clinic designs the flow of patients and health care providers in ways that fit in with its physical setting and number of providers. All attempts should be made to reduce the stress on the patient of seeing multiple providers and undergoing a variety of assessments. Often, patients remain in one examination room while the providers come and go. The team should ensure that different providers do not repeat tests that have been completed by one team member. Because some elders may have limited experience dealing with health care providers other than physicians and nurses, a short written description of the roles of each provider is helpful.

Family Members:

When patients look to their family members for answers, or when family members jump in too quickly, it helps to position the family behind (i.e. out of direct sight) of the patient.

Family Involvement

As family members are often present during the visit, it is important to obtain the patient's permission for their attendance before proceeding with the history. If permission is obtained, the health care provider should be careful not to address the family and ignore patient. When patients look to their family members for answers, or when family members jump in too quickly, it helps to position the family member behind (i.e., out of direct sight) of the patient.

Which family members, if any, are invited to the conference is ideally determined by the patient. Sometimes this is not possible if the patient has a significant cognitive impairment.

Many assessment clinics offer family conferences as part of their routine care. At the end of the assessment process, a family conference is a forum to exchange information with the patient and family at the same time. It is also an opportunity for the patient and family to ask questions and seek clarification.

Scheduling a family conference can be a difficult task. The team meeting is an ideal place to determine which team members need to be present at the family conference. It is rarely necessary for all members to be present. Some teams have regularly assigned times that conferences are scheduled; others have more flexibility and work with the family to find a time that is acceptable to all involved.

Prior to the conference, it is helpful for those health care providers, who will be attending to confer for a few minutes. This time is used to determine what information the team wants to communicate to the family and how they want to communicate it. It is also useful to identify who will take charge of the conference, making sure that the information is delivered in an understandable manner, the family and patient have had ample opportunity to ask questions and make comments, and that the meeting ends on time. Most family conferences can be held in 30 to 40 minutes.

Communicating With the Primary Care Physician

The method of communicating with the primary care physician depends on the setting in which the clinic is run. A comprehensive assessment clinic that is part of a larger system, such as occurs within some health maintenance organizations, may put its findings directly on the chart, which is then available to the patient's personal physician at the next visit. Clinics that are not affiliated with a larger program typically send a letter to the primary care doctor summarizing the findings and recommendations. In an attempt to increase adherence to recommendations, one assessment clinic telephoned the participant's primary care physician to convey the recommendations generated through the assessment.[2] This approach to consultations allows the primary care physician to provide his or her input on the recommendations. A letter describing the recommendation, a copy of the dictated consultation, and copies of full-text references specific to the patient's condition followed the telephone call. Some clinics offer ongoing follow-up for some aspects of care and others are purely for assessment. Clinics that provide several months of follow-up, thus helping assure that the plan is useful and practical, have much better outcomes than those which provide no follow-up (see Chapter 27).[2]

USING THE RESULTS OF THE ASSESSMENT

Interventions and Benefits

A 1993 meta-analysis of 28 controlled trials of five types of geriatric assessment models concluded that it is the programs that link evaluation with strong long-term management that are effective for improving survival and function in elders.[11] For those clinics that do not provide follow-up, it is up to the primary care provider, patient and family to decide which recommendations are practical.

Case Vignette: An 82-year-old woman with osteoarthritis, congestive heart failure, hypertension, and diabetes mellitus has curtailed her usual social activities. Her increasing withdrawal from her social network is linked to a moderate depression. Family members who live close by are involved and want to help, but work full time. Her primary care provider referred her to an assessment clinic because she has had a decline in her function for unknown reasons.

Assessment
A thorough history reveals she has been experiencing a great deal of fatigue and pain and occasional polyuria (which sometimes leads to embarrassing episodes of incontinence). Because she thought these were normal changes of aging, she never told her primary care physician. The geriatrician discovers that the congestive heart failure is not being optimally treated and that the arthritic pain in her left knee responds well to a local injection. Her hemoglobin A1c is significantly elevated, indicating that her blood sugar control has room for improvement. The pharmacist notes that her antihypertensive medication may be contributing to her depression and that she is not on adequate doses of acetaminophen for pain control. A physical therapist notes that she has become deconditioned, has weak hip extensors, and is at high risk of falling when standing up from a chair. Appropriate exercises, a single point cane, and a raised toilet seat are prescribed. The occupational therapist notes that the patient has weak grip strength secondary to osteoarthritis and informs the patient about simple assistive devices that make working in the kitchen and getting dressed easier. The psychologist interviews the patient and believes that if her function improves and she attends a few counseling sessions, her depression will also improve. The social worker gives her information about transportation services and local community programs for seniors. The nurse practitioner, who performed the home visit, has suggestions to make the home safer and shows the patient a variety of devices that are available for organizing medications. A summary of the findings and recommendations are given to the patient and her family during the family conference. A written summary is sent to the patient's primary care physician.

Results of Assessment

If the patient, her family, and her doctor choose to follow through with the recommendations, what are the potential benefits? Better control of the congestive heart failure and diabetes leads to a significant reduction in fatigue and polyuria. Medication changes and the new system for taking her medicines improve her pain control and lessen the depression. The adaptive equipment in combination with a simple exercise regimen improves her ability to perform ADLs in a safe manner. She is now able to arrange for her own transportation and knows what types of programs that meet her interests are available. Perhaps a fall, which often leads to a hip fracture, was averted.

Patient Adherence to Recommendations

Adherence can be improved by diligent follow through with the patient. In addition to receiving a written list of recommendations at the time of the assessment, clinics can mail a copy of the dictated assessment and a duplicate copy of the list of recommendations. Several weeks after receiving the team's recommendation, the elder can be telephoned by a health educator to review the recommendations, make sure that the elder understands the recommendations, and to assess his or her level of agreement with the recommendations.

CONCLUSION

In a study examining the type of recommendations made in a multidimensional assessment, researchers found that nearly one third of the recommendations concerned general medical problems, 26 percent prevention issues, 15 percent functional impairment/ falls, 12 percent urinary incontinence, and 8 percent depression. Patients were found to adhere to about two thirds of the recommendations.[12] In another study, patients adhered to 85 percent of physician implemented recommendations and 46 percent of self-care recommendations.[13]

It is clear that multidimensional assessment programs find new, treatable problems in medical and psychosocial realms and, when proper follow-up is provided, help the patient and family. The special training of the geriatric team members, in combination with the interdisciplinary nature of the team, provide a synergy that does not exist in the typical outpatient office setting. It allows for creative thinking and problem solving and informed decision making, which ultimately benefits the patient, the family, and the primary care provider.

REFERENCES

1. Boult C, Boult L, Morishita L, et al. Outpatient geriatric evaluation and management: models of geriatric practice. *J Am Geriatr Soc.* 1998;46:296–302.
2. Reuben DB, Frank JC, Hirsch SH, et al. A randomized clinical trial of outpatient comprehensive geriatric assessment coupled with an intervention to increase adherence to recommendations. *J Am Geriatr Soc.* 1999;47:269–276.
3. Solomon D. Chairman, Consensus Development Panel. National Institutes of Health Consensus Development Conference statement: geriatric assessment methods for clinical decision-making. *J Am Geriatr Soc.* 1988;36:342–347.
4. Kane RL. Using technology to enhance assessment. *Generations.* 1997;11:55–58.
5. Folstein MF, Folstein SE, McHugh PR. Mini-mental state: a practical method for grading the cognitive state of patients for the clinician. *J Psychiatr Res.* 1975;12:189–198.
6. Katz S, Ford AB, Moskowitz RW, et al. Studies of illness in the aged. The index of ADL: a standardized measure of biological and psychological function. *JAMA.* 1963;185:914–919.
7. Mahoney FI, Barthel DW. Functional evaluation: The Barthel Index. *Md State Med J.* 1965;14:61–65.
8. Lawton MP, Brody EM. Assessment of older people: self maintaining and instrumental activities of daily living. *Gerontologist.* 1969;9: 179–186.
9. Tinetti ME. Performance-oriented assessment of mobility problems in elderly patients. *J Am Geriatr Soc.* 1986;34:119–126.
10. Williams ME. Timed manual performance in a community elderly population. *J Am Geriatr Soc.* 1990;38:1120–1126.
11. Stuck AE, Siu AL, Wieland GD, et al. Comprehensive geriatric assessment: a meta-analysis of controlled trials. *Lancet.* 1993;342: 1032–1036.
12. Reuben DB, Maly RC, Hirsch SH, et al. Physician implementation of and patient adherence to recommendations from comprehensive geriatric assessment. *Am J Med.* 1996;100:444–451.
13. Shah, PN, Maly RC, Frank, JC, et al. Managing geriatric syndromes: what geriatric assessment teams recommend, what primary care physicians implement, what patients adhere to. *J Am Geriatr Soc.* 1997; 45:413–420.

IN-HOME ASSESSMENT

CHAPTER 8

PETER A. BOLING / LINDA J. ABBEY

The goal of in-home assessment is to provide the information needed to optimize the individual's health and functional status and, when possible and desirable, to support continued living in the home. The assessment requires a broad perspective, careful preparation, and sensitivity to the unique opportunities afforded by evaluation in the home setting. This chapter explains the rationale for in-home assessment, identifies populations warranting special attention, and offers a conceptual framework for comprehensive and focused interventions.

Individuals with severe functional limitation and immobility comprise about 1 percent to 3 percent of community-dwelling elders, or between 400,000 and 1.3 million persons nationwide, depending on varying definitions of functional limitation.[1, 2] These figures have been established by large population-based surveys, and even though there is debate about exact numbers, it appears that two to three elders live in the community with severe functional limitations for every severely impaired elder living in a long-term care facility. Yet, the frequency of physician in-home visits is far lower than the frequency of contact for either ambulatory elders in poor health (who see physicians 10 to 12 times a year), or residents in nursing homes (who are seen at least 6 times or more annually). Considering the cost of ambulance transportation, the burden on both the patient and the caregiver, and the value of the information that is gained, regular in-home assessment is becoming increasingly important. This importance is magnified in light of

Though more frail elders live at home than in nursing homes, few are afforded the opportunity of having their physician visit them in their most desired living arrangement.

203

expectations that the number of frail, immobile elders will more than double over the next 20 years.[3]

BENEFITS OF THE IN-HOME ASSESSMENT

Improved Clinical Relevance

Home assessment provides information about the person's ability to function within the most clinically relevant setting. In the office, the patient may have difficulty walking across the room, yet have furniture arranged at home so that holding on permits safe ambulation. Likewise, patients may have difficulty rising from a chair in the office but may have their own favorite chairs at home arranged with cushions or pillows so that they are able to rise from a higher starting level. Home assessment can, therefore, show a higher level of functioning than office evaluation because of such adaptations. At the same time, some homes contain hazards that would never be recognized without home assessment. Classic examples are loose rugs, long phone cords, or poor lighting that may predispose a person to fall. In some cases, the hazards create a very high risk, such as a loose ventilation grate in the hallway floor directly between the bedroom and bathroom, or a kerosene heater in a room where oxygen is used. Formal studies have shown that even after a thorough clinic-based assessment, home-based assessment reveals new information. One study revealed 1.7 new problems per patient and many problems were serious.[4] Other recent data indicate that initial home assessment, followed by quarterly reassessment by geriatric nurse practitioners, can improve functional status and reduce nursing home use in a community-dwelling population of people aged 75 years and above.[5] In addition, reassessment continued to reveal new data in years 2 and 3 of the 3-year study.[6]

> In-home assessment almost always reveals new information, unknown to even the most comprehensive office-based care team.

Improved Caregiver Evaluation

Home assessment provides a unique opportunity to observe the individual–caregiver interaction and environmental factors in caregiving such as adequacy of space, cleanliness, personal care arrangements, and hazards (Table 8-1). Direct observation of caregiving skills, such as dressing changes or positioning and transferring, allows the health care provider to offer suggestions and provide education. Incipient burnout is more readily detected (Table 8-2). Although caregiver assessment can be performed in the office or hospital, one meets only a few caregivers and may inaccurately

Table 8-1. CAREGIVER EVALUATION
Who is available to help the person?
Who has the primary responsibility?
Schedule of caregiving?
Motivation and knowledge of care plan?
Expectations regarding prognosis and goals of treatment?
Other demands on time and energy (other than caregiving)?
Long-standing family conflicts?

gauge their capabilities. It is common to underrate caregiver capabilities in these artificial settings, especially when the elder has extensive needs. Direct observation also provides a more accurate assessment of caregiver skills and attitudes in many cases. Also, by visiting the home over time, there is a greater chance of meeting all the various supporting people.

There is no better way to assess caregiver skills than by direct observation.

Improved Decisions Regarding Care Setting

Home assessment is especially helpful when evaluating an elder for possible institutional care. Important considerations are caregiver abilities and burdens; environmental safety and adequacy; possible benefits of institutional care such as increased socialization as contrasted with isolation at home; autonomy; the person's cultural milieu; evidence of neglect or abuse; and needs for specialized or complex medical care. Sometimes, the home setting can be modified to forestall institutional admission. The issues are always inter-

Table 8-2. SIGNS OF POTENTIAL CAREGIVER BURNOUT
Increased frequency of calls to clinicians about stable chronic health problems.
Desire of caregiver to discuss his or her problems rather than the elder's needs.
Elder withdrawal or reluctance to talk about the caregiver or home situation.
Caregiver impatience in dealing with the individual.
Frequent caregiver comments that more help is needed.
Change in cleanliness or safety of the person's personal environment.
Signs of neglect or physical abuse.
Decline in nutritional status not in keeping with medical conditions.
Dependent patient left alone for prolonged periods (hours).
Failure to comply with reasonable treatment plans after being reviewed with caregiver.

woven, but knowing the social context and caregiver resources well helps greatly when guiding these difficult decisions.

WHO SHOULD BE ASSESSED AT HOME

At present, there are no standard guidelines for identifying people who need in-home assessment, or for determining the frequency and intensity of the assessment. Informed recommendations follow. Suggested candidates are shown in Table 8-3.

Post-Hospital Patients

Home health agency referrals often follow hospital discharge, a time when home care needs are often recognized. Elders who need only a focused in-home assessment, however, can be more difficult to recognize than other home care candidates, such as those needing home care for terminal illness, or those with profound, permanent immobility and several active medical problems who will need ongoing interdisciplinary medical care at home. People with wound care needs are often noticed, as are those needing help with new devices such as gastrostomy tubes, Foley catheters, tracheostomies, or intravenous lines. The post-hospital home assessment needs of

Table 8-3. INDICATIONS FOR FOCUSED, CONSULTATIVE, OR BRIEF HOME ASSESSMENT

Ambulatory person recovering from acute problems: stroke, orthopedic surgery, pneumonia, congestive heart failure, or myocardial infarction.

Planning rehabilitative or restorative therapy.

Unexplained nonresponse to therapy such as recurrent admissions for asthma, uncontrolled diabetes, hypertension, or congestive heart failure.

Preventive care for elders at high risk for accidental injury, such as ones prone to falls, ones with osteoporosis, or ones with early, stable dementia.

Immobile person with complicated social situation in need of family meeting involving many members or members who are inaccessible.

Socially isolated people or ones who need to change residences for their own protection or the protection of others (e.g., dementia or having severe chronic mental illness).

Fact-finding related to weight loss, failure to thrive, or unexplained new cognitive or affective problem.

inpatients who are less technology-dependent are too often over-looked, even though it is known that many hospitalized elders have delayed functional recovery.[7] It is equally important to consider the person with short-term home care needs, such as one who may be temporarily homebound, or one who can seek medical care outside the home but may yet benefit from in-home assessment. The provider must consider assessing people with new activities of daily living (ADL) limitations at discharge, those with an environmentally driven condition such as asthma, patients with recurrent admissions or admission for medication-related problems, or those who cannot recall their medication regimens.

Ambulatory Patients

The place where a patient with home assessment needs is most easily overlooked is the outpatient setting, yet these assessments can have a beneficial impact.[8] Although a patient may not have suffered an acute event like a stroke, the office patient who recently started to fall repeatedly, whose incontinence is worsening, or whose osteoarthritis is now causing new, or significantly worsening instrumental activities of daily living (IADL) or ADL deficits may be appropriate for focused in-home assessment. Inconsistent or refractory response to treatment for such conditions as diabetes, hypertension, congestive heart failure, or anticoagulation, may also indicate hidden problems that might only be discovered by in-home assessment.

Another target group of outpatients are those who remain perplexing after office-based evaluation. The patient who presents with "failure to thrive" manifested as unexplained weight loss, depression, or confusion is an ideal candidate for in-home evaluation. When in doubt about the explanation, a brief home assessment may be cost-effective, especially when it can be timed prior to expensive diagnostic testing. Finally, cases in which social issues seem to play a significant role in the patient's complaints may be appropriate for in-home assessment. In-home evaluators have better access to the key observations, while favorably redefining the relationship between the individual, family, and provider.

The home assessment needs of chronically homebound elders may be easier to recognize, but these individuals also drop from view in a busy office practice because they often have great difficulty in traveling to the office, and because skilled home nursing, which can serve as the physician's "eyes and ears," cannot be maintained indefinitely under current federal regulations. These people get "lost in the cracks," unless there is a system for tracking them and arranging for in-home assessments at reasonable intervals.

An ideal candidate for a home visit is the patient whose problems remain perplexing even after an office-based evaluation.

Elders Who Live in Supported Housing

As the continuum of care becomes an increasingly real concept, people will more often be found in transition between settings. Moving from nursing home or adult (domiciliary) home back to independent or assisted independent living is another context where early home assessment can sometimes be very useful. Too often, the responsibility for determining the safety of the transition from institution is left to the family, and too often, the assessment of needs is based primarily on information gathered while the individual is still in the facility.

FREQUENCY AND INTENSITY OF ASSESSMENT

Specific assessment goals vary from one person to the next and from visit to visit according to the severity and the chronicity or acuity of illness. In contrast to urgent care situations where the approach is similar to emergency room geriatric assessment, ad hoc or consultative home visits to more stable people have a different flavor. In a longitudinal practice, a combination of acute and chronic problem visits are typical. Again, a complete annual review differs from a follow-up visit.

Elders usually need an initial complete assessment that addresses all dimensions of well-being: pathophysiology, function, psychology, social situation, spirituality, economic status, and environment. In every case, the depth of investigation along each dimension should vary with the situation. Comprehensive assessment, when required, is best done in collaboration with several disciplines and takes substantial time and effort. Here, a detailed assessment is undertaken for all of the previously listed domains. Periodic, regular reassessment of some intensity is also appropriate in any people with ongoing functional deficits. The nursing home model, where clinical practice has been better studied than home care, seems a reasonable source of guidelines for the frequency and intensity of assessment, as homebound and nursing home people have many similarities.[9] In the nursing home, after a complete admission assessment that varies in its intensity, residents have a focused reassessment monthly for 3 months, and are then evaluated every 2 months from then forward. A complete review of each case is planned once each year.

Comprehensive assessment is not always needed. Research suggests that this process is valuable for only a small, select subset of patients. In one successful program, only 8.5 percent of hospitalized

A home visit can be designed to conduct a comprehensive review of a single problem, for instance, terminal care needs, rather than the traditional complete assessment of all domains.

patients were included.[10] Even within this selected group, certain characteristics predicted better or worse outcomes; for example, patients with serious heart disease had worse outcomes.[11] Focused, goal-directed assessment is more cost-effective and appropriate for elders who do not need comprehensive assessment. Examples are described as follows:

- If one is called to the home of a demented, alcoholic elder to assess decisional capacity for an anticipated guardianship hearing, the focus may be on mental capacity, conditions expected to affect mental capacity, and the safety of the home situation.
- When a person's health problems are not complex and the prognosis is favorable, assessment may focus on preventive care.
- When an elder is terminally ill, key goals include evaluating comfort, pain control, and preferences regarding aggressive medical care.

The approach to home-based assessment is also influenced by the home itself. One needs to consider a person who has difficulty transferring from bed to chair, and contrast the home situation with an office or hospital. If the transfer at home is made from an antique four-poster bed, 3 feet off the floor, using a nearby dresser and night stand for help, the absence of helpers in the event of a fall may affect the transfer assessment. In an office based on an institutional setting, providers determine environment-specific functional capability. The results can be different at home. In fact, the focus at home may change entirely and center on measures to improve care in the bed, or on altering the environment by changing the bed.

ELEMENTS OF THE IN-HOME ASSESSMENT

Elders with complex, chronic, or long-term home care needs require a relatively comprehensive assessment. This includes a complete health evaluation because the individual typically has significant medical and/or psychiatric illnesses that cause him or her to be homebound. Physical and cognitive functioning in the home environment should also be evaluated in each case, as should the caregiver support system. This type of multidimensional assessment takes time and may require more than one visit. Several short visits can lessen patient fatigue. If multiple visits are needed, target the most active problems first.

Health History

The health history of homebound people is similar to that of other frail elders. Anticipate numerous coexisting chief complaints and interactive problems where treatment of one may worsen another. Emphasis should be placed on those illnesses that contribute to loss of functional independence and those that require active medical intervention. Traditional preventive medicine issues, such as hyper-cholesterolemia for example, may still be important, but are usually less immediately relevant. Likewise, remote inactive problems, such as a laminectomy 20 years ago, are relatively less important. The same is often true of information about most familial diseases, particularly in elders. Detailed knowledge of major prior surgeries, especially abdominal and thoracic procedures, is important, as is information about recent advanced or invasive diagnostic testing, such as reports from coronary angiography or echocardiograms and CT or magnetic resonance scans. For example, if a person has lower abdominal pain at home, knowing about a prior appendec-tomy is important. If the complaint is chest pain, the specifics of prior cardiac evaluations are important. Accessing these data is often less easily accomplished quickly during future home visits for acute problems, so time spent gathering the information at the start of care is time well spent.

A detailed, thorough medication review and history of adverse medication reactions is mandatory. Look not only in the medication cabinet, but also at bedside tables, kitchen cabinets, and on tables next to the lounge chair.

A detailed, thorough medication review and history of adverse medication reactions is mandatory. This also allows the clinician to address practical problems of scheduling doses. Time should be taken during this part of the history to educate individuals and caregivers about medications that may be hazardous or less effective in elders such as long-acting benzodiazepines. All medication bottles should be examined. There may be medications prescribed by multiple providers, unreported but important nonprescription drugs such as nonsteroidal anti-inflammatory medications, and sometimes, situations where patients are taking two or more simultaneous doses of the same medication from bottles labeled with two different names. One dangerous example is "digoxin" and "Lanoxin." For the medication review, one might again apply guidelines that are used for frail, nursing home residents, particularly for those receiving four or more medications. Every medication should have an associated diagnosis. Regular attempts should be made to reduce the number of prescriptions, including prn medications and over-the-counter medications. Medications used for behavior control, such as sedatives and opiates, should be used for clearly defined purposes and should be limited when possible. Inquiries about alcohol and illicit drug use should specifically be included in the history and direct observation in the home can sometimes add insight. For example, a liquor bottle beside the comfortable chair or empty beer cans in the wastebasket may prompt more detailed questions about alcohol intake, especially when alcohol use is denied.

In reviewing the medications, those who visit the home have a unique opportunity. Items to be looked for include outdated prescriptions, bottles that are difficult to open or which have been spilled, pill boxes that are improperly filled or incompletely utilized; and accessibility to the elder of prn medications such as those for pain or constipation, that are not physically accessible to the patient. Explore how medications are organized and who dispenses them. Check to see that medications are not left in full sunlight, on the top of the refrigerator, above a radiator, or where a child could inadvertently take them.

Functional History

Functional assessment is also essential in every case. Ask about and note the responses for each basic ADL item; awareness of specific functional deficits is more helpful in daily clinical practice than aggregate scores on formal functional assessment scales. It is important to know which ADL function is affected; inability to transfer from bed to chair indicates a greater degree of dependency than inability to dress, and incontinence may be poorly tolerated while help with feeding is acceptable to the caregiver. The baseline functional assessment also sets the stage for future reassessments. No matter how well or ill the patient seems, or how capable or frail the caregiver seems, do not make assumptions. Ask specifically about each ADL: who does it, how is it done, and what assistance (human or devices) is required (Table 8-4). Remember that caregivers can create artificial "deficits" by performing functions for elders rather than waiting for them to perform the functions themselves. The detailed functional history also defines the accuracy of the person's or caregiver's perception that will then be directly tested

Table 8-4.   IN-HOME ASSISTIVE DEVICES
Raised toilet seat
Shower chair and hand-held shower attachments
Beside commode
Walker or 4-prong cane
Phone within reach; programming for emergency numbers; large size numbers on dial; signal lights or amplifiers for incoming calls to those who are hard-of-hearing
Personal emergency response system

by the examination. Discrepancies are a "red flag" for the reliability of future reports.

Social Supports

Many people can stay in their homes only because of support from formal and/or informal caregivers. In general, it should be determined which caregivers are primarily responsible for various tasks and with which caregivers home health professionals should communicate. Assumptions in this area should not be made. Specifics of caregiver support systems are very important when making future decisions "at a distance" in response to telephone calls. Recording information about caregivers prominently in the chart along with key telephone numbers is helpful. Also, lists of agencies and other support services along with the telephone numbers and the services that they provide is useful. This information is usually more reliable when gathered in the home than in the office or hospital. For example, simply knowing that the elder has a home health aide does not always mean that this aide is highly capable and committed. Knowing of preexisting family conflicts that may affect the individual's medical care and exploring recent losses, which are common in elders is of value.

Financial Status

A brief of key financial issues such as adequacy of funds for medications, feedings, or medical supplies, plus insurance coverage for services by Medicaid, Medicare Parts A and B, and private insurance or coinsurance should be done. Involvement in Medicare managed care must also be noted. Complete evaluation of the financial situation usually requires a team effort and problems in this area benefit from social work participation. Table 8-5 lists indications for social work referral.

Table 8-5. INDICATIONS FOR SOCIAL WORK REFERRAL
Caregiver death, sudden catastrophic illness or absence of caregiver
Loss of home: eviction, fire
Financial situations that affect compliance
Exploring options and planning alternate living situation
Guiding families through Medicaid applications and health-related personal finance issues
Leading or participating in family meetings
Impending caregiver burnout

Home Medical Equipment

An increasingly sophisticated and expensive array of medical equipment is available for home care. It is important at a minimum to obtain and maintain a current inventory of the equipment that is being used, who provided it, whether it is a rental or purchase item, and whether it is adequate for the person's needs. Also make note of any items that are no longer needed. One strategy is to include a section on home medical equipment in the evaluation form. If a significant problem is identified related to assistive devices, including an occupational therapist or physical therapist in the assessment process can be appropriate.

Physical Examination

The physical examination of a homebound elder involves the same principles as examination in any other setting. Certain aspects of the examination at home deserve specific comment. Basic equipment should be available as outlined in Table 8-6. Specifically, one should seek causes for functional decline, and remember the often "atypical" presentation of common geriatric problems such as thyroid disease, depression, and urinary tract infection.

Table 8-6. DIAGNOSTIC EQUIPMENT FOR THE HOME VISIT

Basic equipment
  Battery-powered ophthalmoscope/otoscope with cerumen scoop
  Portable sphygmomanometer (with several size cuffs)
  Stethoscope
  Reflex hammer
  Tuning fork
  Tongue blade
  Hand-held vision card
  Digital thermometer with single-use covers
  Portable scale (optional)
Advanced equipment
  Syringes and other tools for gathering biologic specimens (blood, urine, feces)
  Portable devices for on-site diagnostic testing (chemistry, hematology, coagulation)
  Electrocardiogram machine
  Pulse oximeter
  X-ray machine
  Portable computer
  Advanced communication devices

One should look for common problems with special senses, particularly hearing and vision, by direct, simple testing. Seeing if the elder can hear and understand a whisper and asking him or her to read large print or a hand-held card should be done. The eyes and ears should be examined and simple equipment should be available to remove the impacted cerumen. Poor oral and dental hygiene is a common problem for homebound people because going to the dentist is logistically difficult and often is expensive. Oral health problems can, in turn, lead to serious nutritional deficits. If it can be measured, body weight is the most useful physical parameter to follow for nutrition, but this is often difficult at home. If so, secondary parameters such as triceps skin fold thickness or mid-arm circumference can be used, noting problems with accuracy in older patients due to normal loss of subcutaneous fat and increased skin elasticity. Biochemical measures may ultimately become the main standard for objective assessment of nutritional status.

Because of the high incidence of stroke, diabetic neuropathy, Parkinson's disease, and dementia in homebound elders, always obtain a good baseline neurologic examination: motor strength, cranial nerve function, peripheral sensation, deep tendon reflexes, coordination, gait, balance, and mental status. If and when new problems surface, the baseline examination becomes vitally important. Even healthy elders can also have some findings that would be pathologic in younger populations such as mildly decreased vibration sense, miotic pupils, and hypoactive deep tendon reflexes.

If severe functional impairment exists, such as when people are confined to bed or chair, examine the skin carefully for signs of pressure injury. Examining the lower torso usually requires turning the person. This effort should always be made, even though it may be difficult. Finally, the feet should be checked for toenail problems or foot ulcers. Unlike many other specialty services, home visits by podiatrists are usually easy to arrange.

Cognition

Cognitive examination deserves special mention because dementia is common in homebound elders, who are typically older than the general population. Many people with cognitive deficits can function well in their own familiar environments and, thereby, create an appearance of normalcy. Formal mental status testing is required to reliably detect dementia and assess its severity. Some elements within instruments such as the Folstein Mini-Mental State Examination have limited usefulness in a frail elder because they depend on ability to see and copy figures or pick up paper from the floor. Awareness of current events or the exact date may also be limited by lack of interest or exposure. In the authors' experience, the following specific elements over time may, therefore, be more useful than following aggregate scores. Orientation to self and place, general orientation to time, short-term memory (recall of three words), and verbal skills are robust, reliable reflections of important, useful cognitive functions. Relevant tests of memory for the homebound elder might include knowing the names and telephone numbers of people that he or she can call for help when needed. Tailor questions to the situation, but include basic safety issues in every assessment. For example, one should routinely ask what the person would do in the case of fire.

Affective Status

The person's affective status also deserves special mention, particularly because assessment of affect may be more difficult when cognition is impaired. Neglect, social isolation, depression, and anxiety are prevalent. Chronic mental illnesses, such as psychoses or bipolar disorders, should also be considered. Routine use of formal instruments is unnecessarily cumbersome but a brief depression inventory can detect the need for more extensive evaluation. Tools such as the Geriatric Depression Scale[12] are useful, although even then there are problems with interpretation of such scales when there is extensive medical illness or dementia. (See Appendix #16).

Functional Status

Direct observation of the person's function confirms information given by the patient or caregiver during the history, and may uncover discrepancies. Formal quantitative tests of observed function, such as the Barthel Index (see Appendix #4), can be used but may be of less practical value than simply watching a few selected activities. Focus first on those activities with which there is reported difficulty and start with ones that you think will be most challenging. For example, ask the person who claims to be ambulatory to walk into another room. If this proves difficult, test the ability to get out of bed or rise from a chair. Record these as baseline data. Some recorded assessment of all major ADLs is essential. An IADL checklist is also helpful.

Screening, Preventive Care, and Diagnostic Testing

In home care, the screening emphasis shifts away from typical ambulatory care issues like cancer, hypertension, and hypercholesterolemia, unless the homebound patient is relatively young and has a long life expectancy (> 10 years). In general, screening should target high-yield areas where intervention is likely to be beneficial. Particularly relevant in home care are risk of falls, immobility, malnutrition, polypharmacy, hearing and visual deficits, incontinence, depression, and impaired cognition.

Home safety assessment is complex. Hazards that would not be permitted in institutions are common in homes. One must evaluate both the severity of risk and the practicality of correcting the problem. For example, a loose rug on a slick kitchen floor is an obvious and simply corrected hazard. Similarly, a loose railing on a steep staircase should be fixed, if the person uses the stairs. On the other hand, a person who cannot use the stairs safely may need to stay on the second floor near the bathroom. A practical approach is to seek out common hazards (Table 8-7) and then discuss the risks with the elder and/or caregivers. Sometimes, home evaluators can direct families to sources of help in making repairs. The home evaluator should also explore the person's ability to react in an emergency.

Immunization status should be determined. Vaccines against influenza and pneumococcal pneumonia should be given to all unvaccinated elders unless there are clear contraindications. The pneumococcal vaccine should probably be repeated every 5 to 7 years and influenza vaccine should be given annually. Tetanus immunization is also appropriate every 10 years, particularly for patients who are ambulatory.

Cancer screening strategies should be consistent with life expectancy. For example, in the Medical College of Virginia Hospital (MCV) House Calls program, the average life expectancy is 15

Table 8-7. HOME ASSESSMENT SAFETY CHECK LIST

Living area	Bathroom/kitchen
_____ Clutter	_____ Shelves beyond easy reach
_____ Loose carpets	_____ Burners/oven left on
_____ Poor lighting	_____ No grab bars in tub/shower
_____ Loose/no handrails	_____ Hot water over 120°F
_____ Poor repair of steps	_____ Spoiled food in refrigerator
_____ Insects	_____ Perishables left out of refrigerator
_____ Other	_____ Plumbing in poor repair

General

_____ Environmental temperature	_____ Slippery slippers/socks
_____ Poor ventilation	_____ Unlocked first floor windows
_____ Absence of smoke detectors	_____ Outside door left unlocked
_____ Cigarette burns visible	_____ Pets underfoot
_____ Bed/chair too high for easy transfers	_____ Other

months and early detection of cancer is unlikely to add much benefit. The subset of elders who have longer life expectancies can benefit from selected cancer screening. Although it is difficult to accurately predict life expectancy, the examiner can take account of the severity of the person's illnesses and the "trajectory" of the individual's life to make a reasonable appraisal of whether long-term survival is likely. This said, for women, a breast examination should be a routine part of the assessment because it is comparatively easy to perform. Mammography is logistically more difficult and should be used more selectively. The examiner should consider whether a mass would be treated if it were found, which in turn depends on comorbid disease states and patient preference. The digital rectal examination is more helpful in detecting impaction than rectal or prostate cancer in patients who are bedfast. Pelvic examinations are difficult to perform at home and are usually not warranted for screening in homebound women unless they are young and relatively healthy, such as women aged 20 to 65 years who are homebound because of slowly progressive neurologic diseases like multiple sclerosis or cerebral palsy. Use of prostate specific antigen (PSA) levels or testing the stool for occult blood, again, depends on overall prognosis. Prior to ordering a test, one should consider what treatment would be recommended if cancer were found. If aggressive measures would not be chosen, screening should usually not be done.

> Screening for cancer may benefit some home care patients but the decision should be weighed against the life expectancy of the patient.

Diagnostic laboratory studies should also be done as appropriate for a homebound elder. Because both nursing home and home care individuals often develop acute illnesses, take multiple medications, and have frequent declines in health, baseline laboratory data are useful. Published guidelines for use in nursing homes can be useful here.[9] Initial assessment should include review of basic hematology and chemistry panels that would detect anemia, renal dysfunction, diabetes, and hepatic or nutritional disease. Thyroid dysfunction is common and can be assessed by using the thyroid stimulating hormone (TSH) level. Health care providers should have a low threshold for ordering this test once but it does not need to be frequently repeated. Demented people without a previous work-up should have laboratory tests including at least serum chemistry, hematology, thyroid function, and a B_{12} level.

On-site, portable diagnostic laboratory capabilities are rapidly evolving and bear mention. Devices are already commercially available that deliver reliable results on basic chemistry and hematology parameters from capillary blood. Oximeters fit easily in a coat pocket. Portable x-ray, electrocardiogram, and ultrasound are also available for home use. Although these tools will initially be employed only by people engaged full-time in serving medically ill and often unstable home care populations, the coming era of mobile medical care will likely include this component of home assessment as a standard feature for a wider array of health care providers. Advanced equipment is, therefore, also listed in Table 8-6. A home visit bag can also include equipment used for treatment.

Consideration of Care Preferences

Finally, statements of care preferences and advance directives for medical care are always important in geriatric care, but emergencies requiring their use are particularly common in the home care population. At the MCV House Calls program, despite having mobile care at home, elders average 3 urgent transports per program year, and about 25 percent of them die each year. Information about care preferences should be part of the standard assessment and database and resolving these questions is something the home care provider should pursue. The 1991 Cruzan decision by the U.S. Supreme Court places added emphasis on the importance of written advance directives that will protect the patient from later undergoing invasive procedures that they do not want. Visiting the home allows health care providers to evaluate the family and caregivers, identify conflicts that may exist, and emphasize the individual's right to make his or her own decision while still capable of decision making. Protocols vary by state for documenting these choices (see Chapters 24 and 25).

PERSONAL CONDUCT AND PRECAUTIONS

Unlike the hospital, nursing home, or office, the health care provider is a "guest" in the person's home.

As a guest in the home, the health care provider must leave social biases behind and set standards based on health care goals: is the patient adequately nourished, is the skin intact, is the patient content? Some homes appear suboptimal for socioeconomic reasons yet provide an acceptable setting for care when elder and family preferences, and available alternatives (e.g., domiciliary facilities or nursing homes), are considered.

The home environment is unpredictable. Each home is unique. Providing health care in the home requires flexibility of attitude and approach. The elder and caregivers are in control of the home setting, which is a private world and is much different from other care settings. Respect for autonomy is required. The health care provider must be creative. The environment varies widely from home to home; rural farm to urban senior apartment; prosperous suburban development to decaying inner-city neighborhood; central air conditioning or almost no air movement in the summer heat; brand new home or old place; cluttered or clean. A successful home visitor will make best use of the resources afforded by the situation.

The home visitor usually travels alone while institutionalized residents are frequently under the observation of multiple health care providers who provide diverse perspectives and can detect problems that an isolated observer might miss. The home care provider, therefore, must be especially observant. When health care providers are concentrated in one location, complex care plans can more easily be implemented. Interaction of team members is also logistically easier. Conversely, in the home, information-sharing strategies play a key role. Telephones, fax machines, and other electronic media, as well as occasional team meetings of the various health care providers, can be indispensable to coordinated care.

The health care provider who makes home visits should also assess his or her own personal safety. Danger to providers can limit home assessment. Real danger is relatively rare, even in an urban setting, but there are instances when home care providers have been injured or killed while working. Appropriate precautions should be taken. Know the area in which you travel. Be alert. Carry a cellular telephone if possible. In some areas, keep a lower profile, such as not wearing a white coat, travel early in the day, and travel in pairs when necessary. In the event that a high-risk situation develops, notify authorities such as Adult Protective Services if there is a question of patient safety, and also notify other home care providers involved in the case so that they can be aware of the risk.

Home care visitors must be careful not to become overly involved in the social situation. Complex social situations may be impossible for the evaluator to resolve and can also create an undesirable dependency. This is a greater risk during continuous home care than when providing consultations, possibly because of the closer relationship among the health care provider, elder, and family. Caution should be taken about providing informal medical advice to family and other caregivers with whom you have no professional relationship. Focus should always be on the elder.

FOLLOW-UP, REFERRAL, AND TEAM COMMUNICATIONS

Strategies to benefit the person and caregivers are the foremost consideration in performing an in-home assessment. The information obtained must then be shaped into a care plan that best meets the needs of the individual and caregiver, taking into account health care needs, prognosis, and the therapeutic efficacy of current and

Good communication is the key to good home care. All parties—health care providers, caregivers, family, and the elder—must be able to express their needs and discuss options.

proposed interventions. Communications are the vital link when implementing the care plan, as numerous health care providers can be involved and each is operating from a base site that is remote from the person, the caregiver(s), and the home. Assessment forms tend to be lengthy; communication is best done by telephone contact, periodic team meetings, or by sharing clinical information in a form that is useful to both parties and easy to read. If the assessment form is such a document, it can be shared by facsimile, electronic mail, or regular mail. In general, these communication strategies should be developed locally by teams, until the industry provides systematic approaches (see Chapter 27).

Elder and Caregiver Communications

An essential domain of every in-home assessment is the evaluation of caregiver competence and commitment, as well as the potential for burnout. Before the assessment is completed, it is also critically important to solicit the caregivers' views of the situation and their input in planning care, rather than issuing unilateral recommendations or developing plans that cannot be easily implemented. In some cases, there may be value in an early referral to a social worker. Such referrals should be discussed with the elder and caregiver to explain the rationale and benefits of the referral (see Table 8-5).

Assuming that the caregiver is able to meet the elder's needs, effective communication with the caregiver about the plan is essential. Practical suggestions by experienced home care providers can help the family cope. Impractical or ill-considered suggestions will undermine trust and reduce the likelihood of compliance.

In general, language used should be easily understood by both the elder and caregiver, and feedback should be sought to ascertain the family's level of understanding and acceptance. Equally important is assigning priorities when giving multiple recommendations, so that a logical sequence of actions will occur even if all of the recommendations cannot be implemented immediately. Starting by expressing an understanding of the stress and burden experienced by the family is often a good first step (see Table 8-2; see Chapter 26).

Sometimes, it is advisable to suggest rearranging the home environment. For example, care might be improved by having an individual move downstairs to a back room near a bathroom. Putting special knobs on the stove or a latch high on the back door may prevent misadventures by a confused or disoriented patient. Repairing a loose board outside the upstairs bathroom door or installing tub rails in the shower may prevent falls. Such changes and modifications may entail some cost and effort for the caregiver. If the changes solve problems acknowledged by the caregiver, they are usually accepted willingly. Sometimes, it is necessary to help the caregiver find community resources, like a church group, for larger projects like building a wheelchair ramp. Conversely, corrections for hazards that are not evident to the caregiver must be introduced gently and judiciously. Recommendations must be expressed in practical terms, including options to reduce work and cost.

Effective communication is also the dominant theme when relating to other home care providers. Too often, home care plans go astray because of communication lapses. For example, communication among nurse practitioners, physicians, social workers, and elders within a single practice group engenders different challenges than communication with team members who are part of another organization, such as the home health agencies who also serve many of the individuals. Regularly scheduled interdisciplinary team rounds are also useful for keeping multiple providers current and for sharing the variety of opinions about each case after an initial assessment or reassessment (see Chapter 27).

Documenting the Assessment

As home care becomes increasingly more sophisticated, use of standardized formats and computerized data storage has become increasingly prevalent, including not only initial evaluations, but also reassessments and continuing care records. Payer requirements are another important consideration. For example, Medicare now requires use of the data-set, The Outcomes and Assessment Information Set (OASIS-B) for home health agencies. OASIS-B is an 89-item inventory of the individual's physiologic, social, and functional status that was developed through extensive health services research to be used by home health agencies for assessment and quality improvement in home care. The full text of OASIS, version B-1 and other related information is available through **www.HCFA.gov/medicare/hsqb/oasis/hhoview/htm**; and a listing of the categorical areas covered by the instrument is shown in Table 8-8. Health care providers are also seeing formalized guidelines from Medicare, other payers, and oversight bodies, so that the content of clinical records both substantiates the validity of bills and to demonstrate the level of quality. At MCV House Calls, an initial assessment tool that covers all the key elements and satisfies the standards of the Joint Commission for Health Care Organiza-

Table 8-8. CATEGORICAL AREAS OF OASIS B-1
Demographics and patient history
Living arrangements
Supportive assistance
Sensory status
Integumentary status
Respiratory status
Elimination status
Neuro/emotional/behavioral status
ADL/IADLs
Medications
Equipment management
Emergent care

Abbreviations: ADLs, activities of daily living; IADLs, instrumental activities of daily living.

tions (JCAHO) was developed (pboling@hsc.vcu.edu). Unlike many standard physician charts, this record should reflect the needs of frail elders, include specific reference to all the elements described previously, and should specifically list as problems "geriatric" issues such as falls, incontinence, and weakened social supports. Most importantly, a well-organized record is easier for providers to read and use. Standardized data recording will ultimately facilitate sharing data among providers who are based in several different locations, plus sharing data with acute care providers in hospitals and emergency rooms. Electronic data transmission will further enhance communication.

SUMMARY

In-home assessment provides more accurate information about the elder's condition and needs because it is information that is gained in his or her usual environment. Functional status, social support systems, and environmental hazards or needs are among the most important items on which the home-based assessment focuses. A systematic or structured approach is valuable and should incorporate those aspects of assessment that are specific to the home setting. The health care provider's approach must be respectful and take into account the limited resources that may be available. With careful attention to these specific aspects of practice in the home, the health care provider has a unique opportunity to assess elders with severe functional impairment and to develop care plans that will improve quality of life, satisfaction with care, and health outcomes.

REFERENCES

1. Stone RI, Murtaugh CM. The elderly population with chronic functional disability: implications for home care eligibility. *Gerontologist.* 1990;30:491–496.

2. Weissert WG. Estimating the long-term care population: prevalence rate and selected characteristics. *Health Care Financing Rev.* 1985; 6(4):83–91.

3. Boling PA. Present and projected demands. In: *The Physician's Role in Home Health Care.* New York: Springer Publishing Company; 1997;193–213.

4. Ramsdell JW, Swart JA, Jackson E, Renvall M. The yield of a home visit in the assessment of geriatric patients. *J Am Geriatr Soc.* 1989; 37(1):17–24.

5. Stuck AE, Aronow HU, Steiner A, et al. A trial of in-home comprehensive geriatric assessments for elderly people living in the community. *New Engl J Med.* 1995;333(18):1184–1189.

6. Alessi CA, Stuck AE, Aronow HU, et al. The process of care in preventive in-home comprehensive geriatric assessment. *J Am Geriatr Soc.* 1997;45(9):1044.

7. Hirsch CH, Sommers L, Olsen A, Mullen L, Winograd CH. The natural history of functional mobility in hospitalized older patients. *J Am Geriatr Soc.* 1990;38:1296–1303.

8. Fabacher D, Josephson K, Pietruszka F, Linderborn K, Morely JE, Rubernstein LZ. An in-home preventive assessment program for independent older adults: a randomized controlled trial. *J Am Geriatr Soc.* 1994;42(6):630–638.

9. Ouslander JG, Osterweil D. Physician evaluation and management of nursing home residents. *Ann Intern Med.* 1994;121:584–592.

10. Rubenstein LZ, Josephson K, Weiland D, English PA, Sayre JA, Kane RL. The effectiveness of a geriatric evaluation unit: a randomized controlled trial. *N Engl J Med.* 1984;311(26):1664–1770.

11. Rubenstein LZ, Weiland D, Josephson KK, Rosbrook B, Sayre J, Kane RL. Improved survival for frail elderly inpatients on a geriatric evaluation unit: who benefits? *J Clin Epidemiol.* 1988;41(5):441–449.

12. Yesavage J, Brink TL. Development and validation of a Geriatric Depression Scale. Preliminary report. *J Psych Res.* 1983;17:37–49.

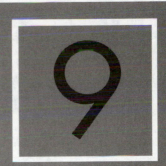

COMPREHENSIVE ASSESSMENT IN AN INSTITUTIONAL SETTING

MAGGIE DONIUS

The purpose of this chapter is to describe comprehensive assessment in the long-term care setting at admission and further assessment using the Minimum Data Set (MDS). Although it is a multidisciplinary process, this chapter focuses on the nurse as the focal evaluator. More extensive review of the physician's role can be found elsewhere.[1]

GOALS OF ASSESSMENT IN THE LONG-TERM CARE SETTING

Assessment in a long-term care facility serves many purposes including the following.

1. Establishing and documenting a baseline status at the time of admission so that change can be monitored over time.
2. Obtaining information about status prior to admission.
3. Discovering medical, functional, social, and psychological problems.
4. Obtaining information that can facilitate or make safer what an individual desires or is likely to do.
5. Placement/setting for services needed or recommending the optimal environment for care.

The Agency for Health Care Policy and Research (AHCPR) was renamed in December 1999.
This agency is now known as the Agency for Healthcare Research and Quality (AHRQ).

6. Detecting discharge issues if discharge to another setting is being considered or planned.
7. Developing an individualized plan of care that, to the degree possible, will facilitate an environment in which elders can live their lives as they direct or would have lived if they had stayed in their own homes.

If a change in status is detected, the assessment directs an appropriate intervention.

THE MANDATED COMPREHENSIVE ASSESSMENT TOOL

In the 1980s, Congress directed the Health Care Financing Administration (HCFA) to study how to improve nursing home regulation. HCFA contracted with the Institute of Medicine to conduct a study of existing regulations and to recommend changes that would enhance nursing homes' ability to ensure satisfactory care for their residents. As part of its response to the Institute of Medicine report, Congress passed the Omnibus Reconciliation Act 1987, which mandated a national resident assessment system that included a uniform set of items and definitions for assessing all residents in nursing homes in the country.

In a contract with HCFA, Brown University, the Hebrew Rehabilitation Center for Aged, University of Michigan, and the Research Triangle Institute developed the Minimum Data Set (MDS). The MDS is made up of items necessary for a comprehensive assessment of residents in nursing homes. The original MDS has been modified, MDS 2.0, in response to comments and suggestions by the nursing home industry, health care providers, advocacy groups, surveyors, and others.

The RN coordinator is responsible for completion of the MDS with input from interdisciplinary staff members.

The full MDS assessment form contains a core set of screening, clinical, and functional status items with definitions and coding instructions for each. It includes demographic, identification, and background information as well as 16 specific categories, B through Q, requesting specific information relevant to each category. The assessment periods are specified during which time involved persons observe the resident for the specified behavior and indicators. These assessments are then entered as numbers or checks as indicated on the form.

When the MDS has been completed, certain item responses identify or trigger one of 18 Resident Assessment Protocols (RAPs). RAPs include issues common to the nursing home population including: delirium, cognitive loss and dementia, visual function, communication, activities of daily living (ADL) functional rehabilitation potential, urinary incontinence and indwelling catheter, psychosocial well-being, mood state, behavioral symptoms, activities, falls, nutritional status, feeding tubes, dehydration and fluid maintenance, dental care, pressure ulcers, psychotropic drug use, and physical restraints. The RAPs have four parts: (1) general information about how the condition affects the nursing home population; (2) a list of the MDS items that trigger that particular RAP; (3) guidelines that provide information about issues to consider and gather more data about; and (4) a RAP key that lists the items that trigger and a summary of the guidelines including the MDS item number that might be helpful in the assessment process. The RAPs guide the interdisciplinary team through further assessment. The team, in conjunction with the wishes of the resident, and family if appropriate, will then decide if and how care will be planned for this clinical problem.

For example, if the RAP for pressure ulcers is triggered and the resident is in the dying process and requests minimal disruption by staff members and comfort care only, the care plan will be much different than for a resident where healing is a desired and realistic goal. The RAP summary sheet (Figure 9-1) is a quick way for the primary health care provider, who often spends less time with the resident than other members of the care team, to become aware of the issues that have been identified by the MDS.

Instructions for completing the MDS are not included here as the *Long Term Care Facility Resident Assessment User's Manual*, which fills a 2-inch 3-ring notebook, is readily available at any facility required to complete the instrument. The manual is a public document published by HCFA and can be copied freely or can be purchased through various long-term care associations. This information can also be obtained via the Internet at **www.hcfa.gov/ medicare/hsqb/mds2.0/default.htm.**

The MDS provides the framework for a comprehensive assessment and results in a plan of care. The MDS is completed for residents admitted for a non-Medicare stay within 14 days of admission, yearly, and when a significant permanent change in resident status occurs. In addition, an abbreviated MDS is completed quarterly. The plan of care is updated as indicated at each review.

At the present time, the MDS is completed more frequently for those who qualify for Medicare Part A reimbursement (postacute care—also often referred to as transitional, skilled, subacute or short stays). As part of the Prospective Payment System (PPS), the MDS must be completed on day 5, 14, 30, 60, 90, and when there is a significant change. A 2- to 5-day grace period applies in specified situations. If the person is rehospitalized, the completion cycle begins all over again. The plan of care is to be modified as

SECTION V. RESIDENT ASSESSMENT PROTOCOL SUMMARY

Resident's Name:	Medical Record No.:

1. Check if RAP is triggered.
2. For each triggered RAP, use the RAP guidelines to identify areas needing further assessment. Document relevant assessment information regarding the resident's status.
   - Describe:
     — Nature of the condition (may include presence or lack of objective data and subjective complaints).
     — Complications and risk factors that affect your decision to proceed to care planning.
     — Factors that must be considered in developing individualized care plan interventions.
     — Need for referrals/further evaluation by appropriate health professionals.
   - Documentation should support your decision-making regarding whether to proceed with a care plan for a triggered RAP and the type(s) of care plan interventions that are appropriate for a particular resident.
   - Documentation may appear anywhere in the clinical record (e.g., progress notes, consults, flowsheets, etc.).
3. Indicate under the Location of RAP Assessment Documentation column where information related to the RAP assessment can be found.
4. For each triggered RAP, indicate whether a new care plan, care plan revision, or continuation of current care plan is necessary to address the problem(s) identified in your assessment. The Care Planning Decision column must be completed within 7 days of completing the RAI (MDS and RAPs).

A. RAP PROBLEM AREA	(a) Check if triggered	Location and Date of RAP Assessment Documentation	(b) Care Planning Decision—check if addressed in care plan
1. DELIRIUM			
2. COGNITIVE LOSS			
3. VISUAL FUNCTION			
4. COMMUNICATION			
5. ADL FUNCTIONAL/ REHABILITATION POTENTIAL			
6. URINARY INCONTINENCE AND INDWELLING CATHETER			
7. PSYCHOSOCIAL WELL-BEING			
8. MOOD STATE			
9. BEHAVIORAL SYMPTOMS			
10. ACTIVITIES			
11. FALLS			
12. NUTRITIONAL STATUS			
13. FEEDING TUBES			
14. DEHYDRATION/FLUID MAINTENANCE			
15. DENTAL CARE			
16. PRESSURE ULCERS			
17. PSYCHOTROPIC DRUG USE			
18. PHYSICAL RESTRAINTS			

B.

1. Signature of RN Coordinator for RAP Assessment Process
2. Month Day Year
3. Signature of Person Completing Care Planning Decision
4. Month Day Year

FIGURE 9-1   Resident Assessment Protocol Summary form. (Courtesy of Briggs Corporation, Des Moines, Iowa).

TABLE 9-1. MDS SECTIONS WITH PARTICULAR RELEVANCE TO THE PRIMARY CARE PROVIDER			
MDS	SECTION	ITEMS	INFORMATION
AC	Customary, routine	g, k	Tobacco and alcohol use
A	Identification and background	9, 10	Responsibility Legal guardian Advance directives
F	Psychosocial well-being	2	Unsettled relationships Losses of close friends or family members
I	Disease diagnoses	1	Disease impacting current functional, cognitive, and mood status
J	Health condition	1, 2	Problems presenting in last 7 days such as weight change, dehydration, vertigo, shortness of breath, vomiting, etc.
Q	Discharge potential	1, 2	Preferences, support system

indicated at each review. Selected items determine the level of reimbursement the facility will receive.

Sections With Particular Relevance to the Primary Care Provider

If the primary care provider knew the patient prior to admission, MDS information known by the provider can be added or communicated to staff members who can enter the information. Sections which the primary care provider may have specific knowledge of or interest in are shown in Table 9–1.

The RAP assessment documentation note addresses each RAP triggered by the MDS with the rationale for the plan that may be helpful to the primary care provider, especially if the patient is new to the provider.

ASSESSMENT: LONG-TERM ADMISSION VERSUS SHORT-TERM ADMISSION

Elders entering a long-term care facility come for a long-term (permanent) stay or a short term (transitional) stay. The assessment needs of these two groups are different because their goals are different.

Long-Term Admissions

The following case scenario describes a nursing home resident admitted for a long-term stay.

> *Case Vignette: Mr. Jones has been cared for in his home by his wife of 51 years. He is suffering from dementia, has become somewhat resistant to care, has insulin-treated diabetes, is frequently up at night, and is incontinent. Mrs. Jones had a "small" stroke and the doctor doubts her ability to continue to care for her husband. Mrs. Jones and her children agree and Mr. Jones is being admitted to a facility nearby so Mrs. Jones can visit frequently.*
>
> *Mr. Jones is a person who is classically thought of as a long-term care resident. When a person is dependent and there is no caregiver or the caregiver is unable to provide needed care, long term or permanent placement is needed. Some long-stay placements turn out to be temporary if there is improvement in the status of the resident and/or the caregiving situation. The initial intent, however, is for a long stay and improvement occurs slowly, if at all.*

As an example, in the case of Mr. Jones, the MDS will likely trigger the cognitive loss and dementia and urinary incontinence RAPs among others. The cognitive loss and dementia RAP will direct the health care providers to consider depression among other things. Use of the Geriatric Depression Scale (GDS) or other tools mentioned in Chapter 19 to assess depression will be helpful in working through this RAP.

The goal in a long-stay situation is to create a living environment that will support people as they wish. This can simulate, to the extent possible, what their lives would have been like had they been able to stay in their own homes and/or introduce new options that might be enjoyable, monitor health status, and provide or assist with personal care as indicated. The MDS and RAPs provide the framework for the assessment and resulting care plan that has the capability to do this.

Short-Term Admissions

A growing number of individuals are admitted to long-term care facilities for a short stay just after hospitalization. These stays may qualify for Medicare Part A or private insurance reimbursement. The majority of short stays in a long-term care facility occur due to early discharge from the acute care setting after a major change in health or physical status such as a hip fracture or cerebrovascular accident (CVA).

> *Case Vignette: Mrs. White is admitted to the facility 4 days after hip surgery. She was living independently in her home of 53 years when she tripped and fell on an uneven sidewalk leading to her back door. After surgery, she is unable to walk because of pain and is unable to care for herself at home. Mrs. White's daughter will return from vacation in 1 week. Mrs. White feels that she will be ready to return home at that time with the support of her daughter.*

Hospitalized patients who are unable to return home at discharge enter a care facility on their way home. The goal for people admitted for a short stay is to leave. These people often make it known that they are not interested in the activity and other offerings of the facility because they "won't be staying." The goal in these situations is to assist the individual in obtaining a level of function that allows discharge to the desired setting as soon as possible. Managed care organizations are increasingly involved with this population and an efficient stay is their goal as well. Short stays involve matching what the person is able to do with what a spouse, caregiver, or setting is willing to provide. A complete return to their previous level of function and further recuperation and rehabilitation occurs in his or her home or a less intensive, less expensive level of care with the support of home health or out-patient treatment.

SPECIAL PROBLEMS IN THIS SETTING

The original HCFA MDS was not designed for the person who is admitted for a transitional or short stay. In fact, the term "resident" does not fit either. Many people admitted to what are often referred to as skilled or Medicare units or facilities better fit the "patient" description. Prior to reimbursement changes which encourage shorter hospital stays (Prospective Payment System), however, these patients, would still be in the hospital. The acuity of this group will continue to rise as managed care organizations use long-term care facilities as hospital step-down units.

Discharge Planning

People admitted for a short stay rarely benefit from the completion of the present MDS because its focus is not on discharge. The only area of the MDS directly addressing discharge is section Q (discharge potential and overall status). Item 1 asks if the resident or support person indicates a preference for discharge and if discharge is expected to be within 90 days. This does not trigger a RAP. Other MDS items that can be helpful for discharge include B4 (cognitive skills for daily decision making), C4 & 6 (making self understood and ability to understand others), G1-9 (physical functioning and structural problems), M1 (skin ulcers), O3 (injections), and P1 (special treatments, procedures and programs). Although the injection item simply asks number per week, for those planning discharge to another setting or lower level of care, a home health referral and/or caregiver teaching may be needed if the individual is unable to prepare a syringe and self-inject. For discharge, one must know not only how much assistance a person needs but also what family members, caregivers, or a care setting is willing and able to provide.

Significant time on short-stay units is spent on assessment and monitoring unstable health conditions, which is not included in the MDS. Changes in condition and treatment are so frequent that the care plan or the approach needs modification more often than the required MDS assessment cycles. The MDS lags behind or follows rather than leads the plan of care. When caregiver issues are paramount, the MDS may have little to do with the care plan.

When the condition of the person has changed, which is common, the MDS is to be revised. The discharge is fast approaching or has already occurred and staff have spent a tremendous amount of time on the MDS, which may not benefit the person and will not effect the outcome/discharge in anyway. Much of what happens during a short stay is not included in the MDS, so as a reimbursement tool, it also falls short. The staff members are generally highly involved in assessments and clinical decisions related to the details of discharge. Will home health be able to manage and monitor Mrs. King's wound? Can Mrs. Rose draw up her insulin, can she give it, will she remember to give it? Will Mr. Tomkins be safe at home alone while his wife does shopping and errands? Is an emergency response system appropriate?

The MDS is much more useful for the long- or permanent-stay resident, for whom it was designed. The long-stay resident is often in a more stable condition or changes more slowly and stays long enough to benefit from the outcome of the assessment tool and process.

The MDS-Post Acute Care

The MDS-Post Acute Care (PAC), which has been designed for the short-stay population referred to as "patients" on the form, is currently being field tested and will be much more useful. Items relevant to discharge have been added, many responses have been expanded providing more detail, and most assessment periods have been shortened to 3 days unless otherwise specified. Training was expanded to patient and family training in the procedures/services section. Comparative (now versus before the precipitating event) functional status information is requested and instrumental activities of daily living (IADLs), medical complexities, functional prognosis, and resources for discharge sections were added.

Admission Assessment

This section describes the admission assessment for the person admitted to a long-term care facility. This initial assessment, however, with some exceptions, is applicable in other community-based settings as well. This assessment gets at the immediate care needs, which enables staff members to provide care and a safe environment during the time recuperation or further assessment is being done. The suggested assessment strategies in this admission assessment assist in the completion of certain MDS items as well as complement the assessment suggestions in many of the RAPs. The assessment strategies and tools outlined in other chapters in this book are also helpful in implementing triggered RAPs.

The admission assessment described is modeled after the functional screening exam developed by Lachs and associates and influenced by the MDS.[2] This framework fits the long-term care setting because it is functionally related to a medical or health problem that results in admission. When the medical or health problem is stabilized, if these functions can be restored or a caregiver instructed, the person can be discharged. If these functions cannot be restored or a caregiver instructed, a care setting that can provide or assist with these functions can be located and a permanent stay planned. Most elders care more about their functional ability and their ability to care for themselves than their various diseases, so attending to functional needs is generally a more helpful approach.

WHAT TO DO WITH THE INFORMATION OBTAINED

Assessment information must be documented and recorded in the plan of care so that all staff members can participate. The plan includes staff members providing assistance that compensates for self-care deficits as well as monitoring and managing health and medical problems. The plan of care should be developed in consultation with the patient/resident or family/significant other, if the elder is unable to participate. An interim plan can be developed based on the assessment and modified later if the family or significant other is not present at the time of admission. Mutual goals and expectations should be determined at this time. When family is involved in a discharge plan, they should be included all along the way as appropriate.

HOW TO ASSESS AT ADMISSION

Information that accompanies the patient/resident should be reviewed prior to the admission assessment. Limited information may be available for people admitted from home so more time will be needed for their initial assessment. People admitted from hospitals are generally sent with reports of a history and physical examination and operative reports, nursing assessment, home medications, a list of medications given in the hospital, laboratory work, x-ray reports, and physicians orders at transfer. Review of the orders alerts the health care providers to contraindicated activities, such as no weight-bearing, which will alter the assessment. Certain portions of the assessment may need to be omitted or deferred depending on the medical problems or diagnosis. In many situations, it is appropriate for physical, occupational, and/or speech therapists to complete portions of the initial assessment. If therapy is ordered, their assessment should be used.

The health care provider should begin the assessment with a welcome, introducing himself or herself, making sure that the patient/resident is comfortable, and then explaining what will be done. When the person is suffering from a cognitive impairment or dementing illness, explanations should be short and concrete. The assessment needs to focus on objective rather than subjective information and some information will need to be obtained from family members or significant others.

Vital Signs

The temperature of an elder is frequently lower than the accepted normal. This has implications for the "definition" of fever.

Obtain vital signs, temperature, pulse and heart rate, respiration, and blood pressure. The vital signs obtained at admission may not be a reflection of the person's normal ones. They may be having medical problems at admission, and admission to a long-term care setting is generally an anxious time. It is not uncommon for people admitted from the hospital to be angry at finding themselves out of the hospital before they are ready to go home.

Hearing Ability

To assess hearing, whisper a question such as "what is your name" near each ear standing behind or to the side of the person so your lips can not be seen. If the person wears hearing aids, they should be used for the test.

It is important to identify hearing difficulty since it can easily be mistaken for cognitive impairment.

If the person is unable to respond to the question or responds differently with each ear, check for a build up of wax. Hearing will likely improve after wax impaction removal. Wax impactions are not uncommon, especially in those who wear hearing aids, because each time the aid is placed, wax can be further packed into the ear. Repeat the question in front of the person with your lips visible to see if you can be understood with the additional cue of lip movement. If the person is unable or has difficulty responding to the question, ask if they have noticed a change in their hearing. Family can be consulted if needed. The best way to facilitate verbal communication should be noted on the care plan.

If the person describes a quick or abrupt change in his or her hearing, intervention from the health care provider is needed as soon as possible for investigation. If the loss or change has been gradual, and he or she has not had this evaluated, further assessment from the primary health care provider may be helpful. The primary care provider can then determine if referral to an audiologist is appropriate (see Chapter 10).

Hearing assessment in the MDS, section C (communication/hearing patterns), item 1 asks that one of four descriptive responses be chosen based on the observations and interview of the assessor, other staff members, and family during the past 7 days. Hearing difficulty triggers the communication RAP, which guides staff members to further assessment issues and to consider corrective communication interventions.

Communication Ability

If the person is unable to comprehend verbal information, explore other modes of communication such as writing, communication boards, and gestures as appropriate. Family or significant others can often supply information in this regard. The best method of facilitating communication should be noted on the care plan. Referral to a speech-language pathologist may be appropriate and generally requires an order from the primary care provider. If the person is already receiving such services, the speech pathologist may be the most appropriate person to provide assessment data and input for this section of the MDS.

MDS section C (communication/hearing patterns) items 2

through 7 collect additional communication information. Difficulties in these items will trigger the RAPs on communication, cognitive loss and dementia, and/or psychotropic drug use if antipsychotic, antianxiety, and/or antidepressant drugs have been given in the previous 7 days. This drug information is collected in section O (medications) item 4.

Skin Test and Immunizations

Two-step PPD skin testing is recommended for TB screening. Influenza, pneumonia, and tetanus vaccinations can be safely readministered.

Most states require PPD skin testing in long-term care facilities. One needs to ask the resident if he or she has previously tested positive, as readministration may not be warranted in this case. PPD skin testing requires a physician's order. A chest x-ray should be ordered if indicated. Flu shots, pneumovax, and tetanus should be asked about and offered, when appropriate, if they have not already received them.

Visual Ability

Vision is assessed with a vision screening card held 14 to 16 inches away from the eyes. If the person wears glasses, he or she should wear them for the test. Vision screening cards include the directional E for those who do not recognize letters. Other available material such as a newspaper, telephone book, or greeting card, can be used instead. For those unable to follow instructions or communicate, watch to see if their eyes follow moving objects. When vision difficulty is found, it should be noted on the care plan and appropriate environmental modifications should be made.

Difficulty reading a vision screening card or other material at the 20/40 level, indicates need for referral and further evaluation. When appropriate, the primary care provider may want to perform a fundoscopic examination for possible macular degeneration, cataracts, glaucoma, and diabetic retinopathy. The need for referral to low vision services can be determined (see Chapter 11).

The MDS guides that vision assessment, section D (vision patterns) item 1, be based on interview of the resident and staff members as well as observation of the resident's visual ability. The resident is to read aloud headlines and gradually down to the smallest print. The assessor selects one of four descriptive responses. The variation for those who cannot follow instructions or communicate verbally is described in the user's manual. Difficulties trigger the visual function RAP, which guides staff to consider treatable conditions to prevent permanent blindness and quality of life enhancement with visual appliances.

Physical Functioning

ARMS/HANDS

The following activities test movements that are required for hair combing, washing, brushing teeth, eating, dressing, getting items from upper shelves and so forth. The person should be asked:

1. Place the palm of the right then the left hand on the back of the head.
2. Pick up a small object placed within reach, such as a pen or spoon, using each hand.
3. Put both arms up over the head.
4. Put both hands together behind the waist.
5. Bend over while sitting in a chair and touch each foot with the opposite hand.

If the individual is unable to perform these activities and the reason is not readily apparent, further evaluation by the primary health care provider and/or physical or occupational therapy intervention may be appropriate, if not already ordered. The person admitted with right hemiplegia may not be able to use the left side because of an old CVA or orthopedic problem. In no case should one assume level of functioning without proper assessment.

MOBILITY

Asking those who are able to respond if they have trouble with slips, trips, stairs, or have fallen getting around their home, is helpful in revealing a history of falls. "Fallers" tend to fall again, so this is helpful information to have at admission. Asking about falls, MDS section J. (health conditions) item 4 (accidents), just prior to the required completion (day 5 or 14 of stay) may be too late. If a hip fracture has been repaired, but the cause of the fall not investigated, the person may fall again. A blood pressure measure should be obtained when appropriate to detect orthostatic blood pressure changes. This may be particularly appropriate in the case of a history of falls, anticholinergic medications, complaints of light headedness, dizziness, etc. The primary health care provider will want to evaluate the elder who falls if this has not already been done so that correctable conditions can be dealt with (see Chapter 23 for information on falls).

If the elder has fallen in the previous 30 to 180 days, the RAPs for falls and psychotropic drug use are triggered. If a hip fracture occurred in the previous 180 days, the psychotropic drug use RAP will trigger if psychotropic drugs have been given in the past 7 days.

The Morse Fall Scale[3] is a brief 6-item tool that assesses risk level and is useful in directing fall prevention interventions as

To do the Get Up and Go assessment observe the person doing the following:

1. Going from supine to sitting
2. Standing from the bed
3. Walking to the bathroom or transferring to a bedside commode
4. Toileting, including clothing management, etc.
5. Standing from the toilet or bedside commode
6. Turning in a 360-degree circle
7. Walking or transferring back to the bed
8. Sitting to supine

Restraints are associated with increased injury.

Siderails are considered physical restraints when they prevent an able resident from leaving the bed.

well. This tool includes a question about history of falling (see Appendix #31).

To assess mobility, ask the individual to perform the Get Up and Go Test (see Chapter 23). Ideally, this observation is done when the individual has to use the toilet. This evaluation is a variation of the Get Up and Go described by Mathias and colleagues,[4] with turning around and a toileting observation added. Many falls occur during attempts to get to the toilet in time. Observing toileting is critical because nearly all people want to avoid incontinence. The decreased warning time many elders experience makes waiting for assistance difficult. Staff members need to know if a person can safely toilet. If not, an alternate plan needs to be implemented. This is especially true if the elder is suffering from a cognitive impairment and may attempt to toilet even if he or she is physically unable.

If the individual is able to do the Get Up and Go Test safely, it is unlikely that side rails and physical restraints need consideration. The goal is generally to maximize abilities; therefore, use of side rails and physical restraints, given their potentially negative consequences, is inappropriate when people are physically able. If the individual is not ambulatory and uses a wheelchair, the test is done using the wheelchair. Use of physical therapy staff members can be helpful when implementing the RAP on falls.

The Physical Performance and Mobility Examination[5] is similar, but is a more structured, 3-level scored tool (see Appendix #36). It was developed as a practical performance measure of physical functioning and mobility for hospitalized and frail elders. The tool takes 10 minutes, on average, to administer after brief training. The person must be ambulatory, and toileting is not included.

MDS section G (physical functioning and structural problems) asks for information during the last 7 days about how much the resident does on his or her own and how much assistance staff members must provide related to ADLs. If the person is receiving physical and or occupational therapy, the involved therapist/s can participate in the completion of this section of the MDS. The RAPs for ADL-rehabilitation, pressure ulcer, and psychotropic drug use, if psychotropic drugs have been given in the previous 7 days, are triggered by certain responses. The ADL-functional rehabilitation RAP guides staff members in establishing specific, realistic, and positive goals considering both the risks and benefits of independence.

The use of side rails, often considered a benign or routine practice, should be an issue that receives significant attention. Side rails can result in feelings of being caged or trapped and can contribute to trauma and death. Side rails are one of many things that can erode autonomy in an institutional setting. When a person is unable or does not wish to leave the bed unassisted, rails serve no purpose. Side rails can facilitate independent turning and repositioning, or restrict mobility and make individuals totally dependent on staff members. Half rather than full rails may be appropriate. When rails restrict freedom of movement in those who desire it, they can be a hazard. There are no data to indicate that side rails increase safety, but there are data that rails increase the risk of injury if someone crawls over them. Therefore, side rail use must be evaluated, individualized, and noted on the care plan.

The Side Rail Decision Tree (Figure 9-2) is an example of how this decision can be made. Choice about side rail use is one way that health care providers can address the issue of autonomy as well as safety.[6] When any manual method, or physical or mechanical device, material, or equipment attached or adjacent to the body is used that the elder cannot easily remove, and which restricts his

> The Side Rail Decision Tree can simplify documentation by marking directly on the tool and including it in the record.

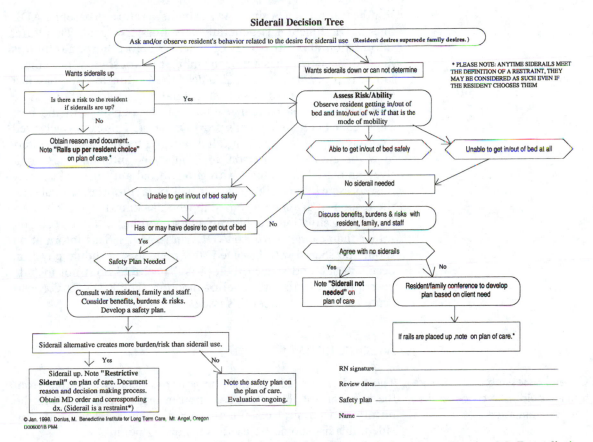

FIGURE 9-2   Siderail Decision Tree. (Reproduced, with permission, from Donius M. Benedictine Institute for Long Term Care, Mt. Angel, Oregon.)

or her freedom of movement or normal access to the body, a physician's order is required because it meets the definition of a physical restraint.

The primary health care provider should be alert to atypical presentation of illness, which could present as impaired physical functioning including falls, and deal with any unstable chronic and/or acute illness that could be effecting function. An in-depth neurologic examination may be needed as well.

MDS section G (physical functioning and structural problems) item 6 and section P (special treatments and procedures) item 4, collect information about side rail and restraint use. Certain responses to item P4 trigger the RAPs on falls, physical restraints, and/or pressure ulcers.

Self-Care Abilities

For the transitional or short-stay patients, a return to baseline ADL and IADL function is generally the long-term goal. Therefore, information about the level of function before hospitalization is needed. If a person has not been ambulatory for some years, ambulation is probably not a goal unless the reason for this has just been corrected. Preadmission functional status information can be obtained from the patient/resident, or the person with the best knowledge of the individual's previous status. This can be achieved by using a questionnaire, or, alternatively, facility staff can interview the appropriate person and collect the information. Cognitively impaired individuals with good verbal and social skills may misrepresent their abilities, so, it will be appropriate to validate the responses given with someone who has knowledge of the person's living situation. People can, but sometimes will not or do not, rather than cannot perform ADLs and IADLs. This information should be shared with involved staff members including physical, occupational, and speech therapists. The MDS does not include descriptions of previous level of function. The MDS-PAC (post-acute care) does address this issue.

Medications

Careful assessment of medications should take place at the time of admission.

The medication regime must be assessed. Elders admitted from the hospital usually have medication information included in the history and physical examination or nursing assessment. If provided, this list should be used as a starting point.

Section U assists nursing home staff members to identify potential problems related to polypharmacy, drug reactions, and interactions. One counts the number of tablets, capsules, suppositories, or liquid administered in the last 7 days, including prn medications. To record required information, current physician orders and a current medication administration record of the last 7 days are needed. The National Drug Code (NDC) is used to code the drugs. (Information on NDC can be found in the *Physicians' Desk Reference.*) This section can be completed by the pharmacist or other nursing home personnel who must certify its accuracy with their signatures in Section R.2. Coding instructions and more information are available. An *Official Replica Edition of the Long Term Care Facility Resident Assessment Instrument (RAI) User's Manual,* April, 1999, can be obtained from Eliot Press, 508-655-8123.

A stay in a long-term care facility is an ideal time for the primary care provider to examine the medication regimen and eliminate unnecessary medications because the individual can be monitored during changes. A medication review by a pharmacist is required and the primary provider should attend to the outcome of this review.

MDS section O (medications) is limited to number, new medication, injections and if antipsychotic, antianxiety, antidepressant, hypnotic and/or diuretic medications have been given in the previous 7 days. These drugs, excluding hypnotics, will trigger the falls, dehydration/fluid maintenance, and/or psychotropic drug use RAPs.

Mental Functioning

While it is tempting to assess cognitive function early in the process, being a sensitive matter, it should be deferred to a later time when rapport has been established with the resident. All should have a screening mental status examination to obtain baseline data. Because people may be unfamiliar with this type of testing or fear failure, the mental status examination should be prefaced with an explanation that it is a routine part of the admission process for everyone. There may be fear of permanent institutionalization if memory problems are detected. Some of the anxiety commonly related to mental status examination may be alleviated by explaining that memory is commonly affected by illness so memory testing information is often helpful in determining if an acute illness is present.

The 10-question Short Portable Mental Status Questionnaire[7] (SPMSQ) (See Appendix #41) or a similar examination that is a quick test of orientation, recent and long-term memory, and serial calculation should be administered. The answers to the questions asked need to be available for verification. It is helpful to use a test that can be administered quickly, and repeatedly for comparison. If there were errors, the more comprehensive 30-question Mini Mental State Examination[8] (MMSE) (see Appendix #29) should be administered at a later time. When changes in mental function are detected, an in-depth assessment by the primary care provider or mental health professional may be needed.

For short-term memory testing, the person should be asked to repeat and remember three items, for example *book*, *watch*, and *table*. Engage in other conversation for 5 minutes then ask the person to repeat the three items. A Cognitive Performance Scale (CPS) made up of 5 items from the MDS (comatose status, short-term memory, ability to make decisions, making self understood, and eating performance) is described by Morris and Associates (see Appendix #9).[9] This scale corresponded closely with scores generated by the MMSE and the Test for Severe Impairment. Appendix F of the MDS User's Manual contains the scoring rules. A disadvantage of the CPS is that it is only familiar to those providers who have intimate knowledge of the MDS. The decision-making item may be difficult to score at admission and the eating observation is to be based on a 7-day observation period so the CPS cannot be scored at admission.

Explain the operation of the call light. Observe the individual turning it on. Those who are physically unable to turn on the call light and have the cognitive ability to do so will need an alternate means of calling. Those who have demonstrated poor short-term memory may not remember instructions for call light use. After the explanation, instruct them to signal for you after you leave the room. Leave the room and see if the instructions are followed. Often it is apparent that those suffering from cognitive impairment are unable to use the call light. This should be noted on the plan of care so that staff are alerted to the fact that the person will not call, they must check.

A brief screening method for depression may utilize a question such as, "Do you often feel sad or depressed?"[10] A "yes" response will trigger administration of a more comprehensive screening tool such as the Geriatric Depression Scale or a similar tool (see Chapter 19). If he or she scores in the depressed range, additional assessment and intervention from the primary care provider and/or a mental health provider is indicated. For those unable to participate in question/answer dialogue because of dementia, the 19-item Cornell Scale[11] is heavily reliant (see Appendix #13) on observations by caregivers. Either of these tools will be helpful in working through the mood state RAP.

Depression specific information is included in section E (mood and behavior patterns) item 1 of the MDS. Responses are to be based on observations over the previous 30 days. Specific responses will trigger the RAPs on psychosocial well-being, mood state, and/

or psychotropic drug use if use is indicated in Section O (medications, item 4).

Elimination

A catheter is often present when a patient/resident is admitted from the hospital. Review the information sent from the hospital to see if there were urinary retention problems. Unless indicated otherwise, the catheter should be removed and the person monitored. The RAP on urinary incontinence and indwelling catheter describes this process.

To assess continence ask "Some people lose urine or stool before they get to the toilet. Is that something that happens to you?" Leaving the word incontinence out of the question eliminates the dilemma of the many definitions of that term. If the answer is "yes", further assessment is indicated.

The RAP on urinary incontinence and indwelling catheter describes the assessment process. The primary care provider will need to order such things as urinalysis and catheterization for postvoid residual (PVR). Certain aspects of the evaluation may need to be performed by the primary provider such as a pelvic or prostate examination. Need for referral to a urologist should also be determined. Chapters 17 and 22 contain information about urinary incontinence and bowel disorders that may be helpful in implementing this RAP. Ask about usual urinary and bowel patterns and routines so that both can be facilitated and maintained during their stay.

It is unrealistic to expect cognitively impaired individuals to use the call light and wait for help when they have to go to the bathroom. A plan, such as offering toileting on a schedule, is needed. If they are likely and able to crawl over a side rail, environmental modifications, such as a low bed, are needed as in this case side rails are hazards, not safety devices.

Information gathered from the Get Up and Go Test should be utilized to develop a plan that will facilitate safe and, when possible, independent toileting. This could include no side rails with a clear path to the bathroom, a bedside commode, a urinal (male or female), or scheduled toileting, which should be noted on the care plan. Individuals who can independently manage elimination in some way will have more discharge options.

Section H of the MDS collects information about continence of bowel and bladder over the previous 14 days. Certain responses will trigger the RAPs on urinary incontinence and indwelling catheter, pressure ulcer, and/or psychotropic drug use in section O, item 4.

Nutrition and Hydration

If a feeding tube is present, this should be noted. The tube may or may not be permanent. This issue will be sorted out during the stay and depend on the patient/resident status. Speech therapy and a dietitian are usually involved. Presence of a feeding tube noted in MDS section K (oral/nutritional status) item 5, will trigger the feeding tube and dehydration/fluid maintenance RAPs. The primary health care provider will need to write orders depending on the tube type and if x-ray verification is needed after replacement and appropriate change interval if the tube is long term.

To assess nutritional status, obtain height and weight and ask about unintentional weight loss. Height, commonly used in the calculation of body mass index (BMI), is difficult to measure in elders who are unable to stand (see Chapter 12).

The knee height measurement using a knee height caliper is an alternate method of measuring height. This requires someone trained to do the measurement and calculation as well as the caliper used in obtaining the measurement. Another method of measuring height is arm-span, which has been shown to be a reliable and practical estimate of height. The measurement is done using a flexible tape measure with arms held out in line with the shoulders. Support at the elbows may be needed. When only one arm can be outstretched, the measurement taken from the center of the sternal notch to the fingertip is doubled.[12]

Unintentional weight loss should trigger an evaluation by a dietitian and a primary health care provider. The evaluation should include examination of the oral cavity, chewing, swallowing and observation of food intake.

MDS section K collects information related to oral and nutritional status. RAPs that may be triggered include nutritional status, feeding tubes, dehydration/fluid maintenance, dental care, and psychotropic drug use if use is indicated in section O, item 4. The dietitian may be the most appropriate person to provide or contribute information for this section of the MDS.

If evidence of malnutrition or indicators of high risk are needed to justify intervention by a dietitian, the 18-question Mini Nutritional Assessment,[13] which takes 10 to 20 minutes to complete can be used (see Appendix #30). Calculation of the BMI (weight in kilograms/height in meters^2) and measurement of mid-arm and calf circumference complete this tool. Accurate knowledge of previous intake patterns needs to be ascertained several days after admission.

Ability to assess hydration is somewhat limited. Decreased skin elasticity, medication use, and mouth breathing are unreliable parameters in this population. Objective findings such as postural blood pressure changes, decreased urinary output, and laboratory data are more reliable and should be monitored on an ongoing basis when dehydration is suspected. For those at risk for dehydration, the care plan should include hydration strategies.

Although there is no hydration section on the MDS, items that will trigger the dehydration/fluid maintenance status RAP include section J (health conditions) items 1a, c, d, h, j; section I (disease diagnosis) item 2j or 3; section K (oral nutritional status) item 5a or b, and section O (medications) item 4e.

Pressure Ulcer Risk

The prevalence of pressure ulcers in skilled care and nursing home-type facilities may be as high as 23 percent. Since pressure ulcers are the cause of significant pain and suffering, and are expensive to treat, prevention is a high priority. Individuals who are unable to reposition themselves and are chair or bed bound should be evaluated. Risk for pressure ulcer development can be assessed using the Braden Scale (see Appendix #6).[14] This assessment may be repeated at a later time. There are 6 items graded on a 1 to 3 or 4 scale. The lower the score, the higher the risk. Interventions should be implemented as indicated and noted on the care plan. Those who do not score at risk can be spared sleep disruption by routine turning during the night if other health conditions allow (see Chapter 13).

Skin condition, section M on the MDS, collects information on various skin problems including pressure ulcers and foot problems. Items in this section may trigger the nutrition and/or pressure ulcer RAPs.

Proper positioning and/or pressure reducing/relieving devices can decrease discomfort, and prevent pressure ulcers.

Physical Discomfort

In spite of the estimated prevalence of pain in people over age 60 years to be twice as high as in younger people, there is little research on efficient assessment of pain in elders. Few, if any, tools have been validated with elders. Many elders have difficulty communicating about their pain. Hearing, vision, and cognitive impairments further complicate assessment. Although it is not clear which tools works best for older people, it is clear that providers need to ask about pain. Failure to complain about pain does not mean that pain is not present. Cultural and social background, coping styles, anxiety, and depression, among other things, affects how a person expresses pain, so reliance on observation of what we may consider pain behaviors can be problematic[15] (see Chapter 15).

Standard pain assessments include onset and temporal pattern, description, location, intensity and severity, precipitating and relieving factors, previous treatment, and its effect on physical and social functioning. The Initial Pain Assessment tool by McCaffrey and Beebe is an example.[16] Most important is the person's perception of whether or not the pain is under control.[17] If the person reports inadequate pain control, additional assessment using tools described as follows and further intervention is indicated.

There are tools to assess various aspects of pain including intensity and severity tools, many of which include vertical or horizontal lines, some with corresponding numbers and/or words such as the Visual Analog Scale (see Appendix #45), the 0–10 Numeric Pain Distress Scale, and the Simple Descriptive Pain Distress Scale. Some tools include a body chart on which the location of pain can be marked and described with symbols. The Pain Affect Faces Scale, representing levels of discomfort with facial expressions, can be helpful for those with language or cognitive deficits. These tools can be found in the AHCPR Clinical Practice Guidelines on Management of Cancer Pain (#9) and Acute Pain Management (#1). The Clinical Practice Guidelines from the American Geriatrics Society on the management of chronic pain in elders contains assessment tools and recommendations specific to elders.[18] The pain thermometer, which has a vertical orientation and word descriptions, has also been suggested.[19] For noncommunicative people with advanced Alzheimer's disease, a very difficult population to assess, a 9-item Discomfort Scale has been developed.[20]

All efforts must be made to provide comfort and freedom from pain, which is essential to quality of life. Physical and occupational therapists, if involved, may be able to provide important information about pain. The primary care provider should be responsive to requests and suggestions from the patient/resident and staff members regarding pain relief measures that require a physician's order.

Two MDS items deal with pain. Section J (health conditions), item 2 asks about frequency and intensity of, and item 3 about pain site. There is no RAP for pain.

Sleep and Night Issues

Sleep can be especially difficult in a facility setting. To facilitate sleep, ask about daytime naps and nighttime rituals. These should be maintained to the extent possible as this will prevent the need for sleeping medications. Asking about nighttime elimination allows appropriate preparation related to the environment, equipment, or staff response. Daytime alertness is a good indicator of adequate sleep. Those who have difficulty staying awake during the day may need additional assessment and or intervention. See Chapter 16 for additional information.

There is no MDS section specific to sleep. Section AC (customary/routine) asks about staying up after 9 PM, naps of at least 1 hour during the day, and if he or she wakens at night to urinate. There is no RAP for sleep. Section E (mood and behavior patterns) item 1j & k, sleep cycle issues, asks about unpleasant mood in the morning and insomnia and change in usual sleep pattern. If it is indicated that any of these occurred 5 days per week or more in the last 30 days, the mood state RAP will trigger. Section N (activity pursuit patterns) items 1 and/or 2 may trigger the activity RAP. Section O (medications) collects the number of days a resident has received a hypnotic medication in the previous week. This item does not trigger a RAP.

Psychosocial Resources

Social support is very important and often crucial for discharge. To briefly assess social support, ask the person "Who would or do you contact if you need to talk or for help in case of illness or an emergency?" If the person is not able to identify a support person or if the support person lives far away, additional support may be needed. A discharge plan may need to be modified. Some may have an extensive social support network and have many people to contact, which increases their resources for discharge if needed. See Chapter 4 for more information on this topic.

Some idea about psychosocial resources can be obtained from section AC (customary/routine), as this section asks about daily contact with relatives or close friends, church attendance, finds strength in faith, and group activities. Section F (psychosocial well-being) item 2 asks about unsettled relationships. Certain responses to items a–d will trigger the psychosocial well-being RAP.

Sexuality

The MDS does not include a section on sexuality. There are MDS items tangential to the issue (for example, the past roles item 3 in section F), but not specific to it. Admission to a long-term care facility can significantly change intimate relationships and how the person interacts with a partner. Aspects of sexuality to consider include intimacy, touch, affection, body image, sexual identity, and intercourse. Asking the patients/residents or their partners, if they have partners, if they shared a bed/bedroom, if hugging and touching was common, if they are still sexually active, and what staff members can do to help maintain those aspects of their relationship, sends a message that these activities are important and can continue in the facility. Explanations about where or how privacy can be maintained in nonprivate rooms can occur during this conversation. It is an unfortunate reality that we may not be able to live with our partner, but the relationship can be maintained.

Economic Resources

The social service worker is often the staff member who inquires about financial issues. Finances often influence options and access to services at discharge. Asking the person if they are troubled by financial concerns related to their stay or discharge is helpful in starting the referral process when indicated.

MDS section A (identification and background information) item 7 asks for current payment sources for the nursing home stay but does not include concern regarding finances.

Home or Discharge Environment

When the goal is discharge, basic information about the discharge location is needed. This includes but is not limited to the presence of stairs, grab bars, wheelchair accessibility, and so forth. See Chapters 6, 7, and 8 for more information on assessment in the community and home. If the individual requires a caregiver at discharge, caregiver instruction should be started as soon as it is possible.

Physical Examination

Doing the physical examination at the end of the assessment allows rapport building. The examination includes the standard head to toe observations and auscultation to detect any problems that need monitoring or intervention. Observations can validate or reveal inconsistencies in other parts of the assessment that will need further evaluation or referral during the stay.

Examination of certain parts of the body such as teeth, mouth (section L), and skin condition (section M) is necessary.

Integrating Assessment Findings with Care Plans

Each area of the initial assessment results in a specific plan of care that should be documented in a way that makes it easy for all staff members to be aware of and follow the plan. The plan should be continually updated and modified during the stay to reflect the current needs. Additional referrals such as to optometry, audiology, podiatry and dentistry should be made when indicated to maximize function when this is consistent with goals.

During discharge planning, appropriate residential modifications that may be needed at the discharge location, caregiver training and medication instruction should be implemented. Referral to a home health agency should be made when appropriate and, for continuity, the plan of care should accompany the individual to his or her new location.

For long-stay residents, the emphasis of the plan of care is to create an environment that is supportive to the residents and their families. Completing the MDS and triggered RAPs will assist in

Behavioral Symptoms Risks | Month, Day, Year | **IMMEDIATE PLAN OF CARE** | **BEVERLY HEALTHCARE**

Problem	Interventions	Resp	Family/Responsible Party Involvement
Behavioral Symptoms Risks related to: ☐ Wandering [E4aA=1, 2, 3](1,2,4,9) ☐ Verbally abusive [E4bA=1,2,3](3,4,5,6,7,8,11) ☐ Physically Abusive [E4cA=1, 2, 3](3,4,5,6,8,11) ☐ Socially Inappropriate [E4dA=1, 2, 3] (3,4,5,6,7,8,10,11) ☐ Resists Care [E4eA=1, 2, 3] (3,4,6,8,10) *(The italicized numbers in the Problem Column designate the boxes to be considered in the Intervention Column. Place a ✔ in all boxes that apply)* Plan of Care Completed By _____ (Signature) Plan of Care Reviewed with Resident ☐	☐ 1.Evaluate need for wandering management program ☐ 2.Wandering Management Program initiated: ☐ 3.Reinforce positive behaviors as they occur ☐ 4.Maintain consistent daily routine ☐ 5.Separate from others when demonstrating socially inappropriate behaviors by _____ ☐ 6.Initiate monitoring program to identify situation/ condition which triggers inappropriate behavior ☐ 7.During episodes of verbally abusive behavior redirect by _____ ☐ 8.Schedule care/treatments around _____ which, if interrupted, causes resident to demonstrate socially inappropriate behavior ☐ 9.Use Personal alarm system ☐ 10.Encourage customary sleep pattern of going to at _____ and waking up at _____ ☐ 11.During episodes of socially inappropriate behavior, redirect by _____ ☐ Other:		**WHAT CAN YOU DO TO HELP:** Tell us what may be causing the problem. Bring in personal possessions. Include the resident in decision making. Tell us how the person coped with stress Encourage activities which minimize inappropriate behaviors Inform us if this is new behavior What activities worked at home to decrease inappropriate behaviors Provide us with accurate contact phone numbers for family members/responsible parties Other: Discussed with family/responsible party on ___/___/___. _____ Name of Family Member/Responsible Party Staff Signature_____

Goal: Resident safety and management of behaviors which may present risk of injury to self or others.

Patient Name _____ | Room # ____ | Attending Physician ____

Clinical Services 4/5/99
BE 556

FIGURE 9-3 Example of care plan implementation of behavioral MDS items. (Courtesy of Mary Tellis-Nayak, RN.)

this process. For the short-stay patient, the emphasis of the plan of care is on discharge. When finalized and implemented, the new MDS-PAC will be more helpful. Ending the assessment with a thank you and offering any assistance that may be desired or enhances comfort sets the stage for a positive outcome.

After completion of the MDS, individual items or combinations of items will identify or trigger specific resident assessment protocols (RAPs). Triggered RAPs will be reviewed, further assessment done as indicated, and suggestions for the care planning process will be considered by the care team. Figure 9-3 is an example of care plan implementation of behavioral MDS items. Utilizing the assessment strategies described in this and other chapters of this book in assessment and implementation of the RAPs will result in a more systematic and positive outcome. A care conference is held including appropriate staff members, resident, and family or significant others, and the findings of the assessment are shared and the care plan is further refined. This process is repeated at specified intervals.

REFERENCES

1. Ouslander JG, Osterweil D, Morley J. *Medical Care in the Nursing Home,* 2nd ed. New York: McGraw-Hill; 1997.
2. Lachs MS, Feinstein AR, Cooney LM, et al. A simple procedure for general screening for functional disability in elderly patients. *Ann Intern Med.* 1990;112:699–706.
3. Morse JM, Morse RM, Tylko SJ. Development of a scale to identify the fall-prone patient. *Can J Aging.* 1989;8:366–377.
4. Mathias S, Nayak U, Isaacs B. Balance in elderly patients: the Get-up and Go Test. *Arch Phys Med Rehabil.* 1986; 67:387–389.
5. Winograd CH, Lemsky CM, Nevitt MC, et al. Development of a physical performance and mobility examination. *J Am Geriatr Soc.* 1994;42:743–749.
6. Donius M, Rader J. Use of side rails: rethinking a standard of practice. *J Gerontol Nurs.* 1994;20(11):23–27.
7. Pfeiffer E. A short portable mental status questionnaire for the assessment of organic brain deficit in elderly patients. *J Am Geriatr Soc.* 1975;23:433–441.
8. Folstein MF, Folstein SE, McHugh PR. Mini-mental state: a practical method for grading the cognitive state of patients for the clinician. *J Psychiatr Res.* 1975;12:189–198.
9. Morris JN, Fries BE, Mehr DR, et al. MDS cognitive performance scale. *J Gerontol.*: Medical Sciences 1994;49(4):M174–M182.
10. Mahoney J, Drinka TJ, Abler R, et al. Screening for depression: single question versus GDS. *J Am Geriatr Soc.* 1994;42:1006–1008.
11. Alexopoulos GS, Abrams RC, Young RC, Shomian CA. Cornell scale for depression in dementia. *Biol Psychiatry.* 1988;23:271–284.

12. Kwok T, Whitelaw MN. The use of arm-span in nutritional assessment of the elderly. *J Am Geriatr Soc.* 1991;39:492–496.

13. Guigoz Y, Vellas B, Garry PJ. Mini nutritional assessment: a practical assessment tool for grading the nutritional state of elderly patients. *Facts Res Gerontol.* 1994;2(suppl):15–59.

14. Braden BJ, Bergstrom N. Clinical utility of the Braden scale for predicting pressure sore risk. *Decubitus.* 1989;2:44–51.

15. Closs SJ, Phil M. Pain in elderly patients: a neglected phenomenon? *J Adv Nurs.* 1994;19:1072–1081.

16. McCaffery M, Pasero C. *Pain: Clinical Manual* (2nd ed.). St Louis: Mosby; 1999.

17. Walker JM, Akinsanya JA, Davis BD, Marcer D. The nursing management of elderly patients with pain in the community: study and recommendations. *J Adv Nurs* 1990;15:1154–1161.

18. AGS Panel on Chronic Pain in Older Persons. The management of chronic pain in older persons. *J Am Geriatr Soc.* 1998;46:635–651.

19. Herr KA, Mobily PR. Comparison of selected pain assessment tools for use with the elderly. *Appl Nurs Res.* 1993;6:39–46.

20. Hurley AC, Volicer BJ, Hanrahan PA, Houde S, Volicer L. Assessment of discomfort in advanced Alzheimer patients. *Res Nurs Health.* 1992;15:369–377.

ASSESSMENT AND TREATMENT OF HEARING LOSS AMONG ELDERS

DONALD E. MORGAN

Hearing loss of sufficient magnitude to influence the ability to hear and understand conversational speech is the third most common chronic problem in elders affecting approximately 30 percent of community-dwelling elders over age 65 years, and affecting 70 percent to 80 percent of residents of nursing facilities.[1,2] When the etiology of hearing loss in the person is limited to the process of aging (presbycusis), the characteristics of the hearing loss are predictable, the effects are reasonably constant across individuals, and the treatment strategies are common for most patients.

The impact of significant hearing loss is most apparent as it affects the ability to communicate efficiently. People with new onset hearing loss are typically frustrated and often confused by the absence of clarity in the perceived speech of others. People engaged in conversation with the hearing impaired individual often question the attentiveness of the listener and, sometimes, assume that the listener is evidencing problems more appropriately associated with dementia or senility. The general ignorance of the impact of hearing loss associated with aging compounds the confusion of both the individual with hearing loss and the person seeking to communicate with that individual. Understanding the common problems encountered by aging individuals with hearing loss requires knowledge of the means by which we assess magnitude and configuration of hearing loss and the effects of hearing loss on communication.

ASSESSMENT OF HEARING LOSS

Assessment Setting

The assessment of hearing loss in an elder may be dictated, to some degree, by the setting in which the person resides. For individuals who live independently and have no ambulatory restrictions, the assessment is likely to be conducted in an outpatient facility equipped with state-of-the-art instruments and equipment, enabling the most complete and accurate assessment. When the individual's physical and/or psychosocial conditions limit him or her to long-term care facilities, the conditions under which the assessment must be conducted can be restrictive.

Ideally, physical examination would be conducted in an examination room enabling microscopic or hand-held otoscopic (illuminated and magnified) examination of the external ear and tympanic membrane. In addition, measurement of hearing loss (tuning fork and/or electronic testing) would be conducted in an acoustically controlled environment. Both the physical examination and the measurement of hearing loss can be conducted at bedside when the circumstances dictate. When the decision is made to sacrifice the ideal examination and test condition, the examiner must be knowledgeable of the limitations inherent in the decision to conduct the procedure under less than ideal conditions. Specifically, room lighting and physical access to the patient will affect the physical examination; room noise will affect the measurement of hearing. Typically, the more naive and inexperienced the examiner, the less knowledgeable he or she will be regarding the impact of the setting on the results obtained; the more knowledgeable the examiner, the greater the understanding of the effects of the setting on the results obtained. Therefore, when patients are to be assessed under less than ideal conditions, "experts" should be consulted to evaluate the quality of the results and to advise regarding interpretation of the results.

Physical Examination

Assessment of hearing loss should begin with otoscopic examination of the outer ear and tympanic membrane. Cerumen accumulation in the external auditory canal is a common source of hearing loss in elders, and can be visualized with successful otoscopy. Significant accumulation of cerumen (any amount sufficient to preclude visualization of the tympanic membrane) should be removed before formal hearing assessment is scheduled. In the event cerumen is not removed before hearing assessment is conducted, any air conduction hearing loss measured is subject to influence of the cerumen on the magnitude of hearing loss measured, and will affect the ability to conduct immittance measures and obtain earmold impressions.

If otoscopy reveals a patent external auditory canal, the examination will reveal evidence of external auditory canal conditions that can affect hearing. Any external ear canal pathology can affect hearing sensitivity and must be considered as a potential contributing source for any hearing loss evidenced by the patient. Successful visualization of the tympanic membrane can also reveal evidence of middle ear pathology. Middle ear effusion (when evident upon visualization of the tympanic membrane) will affect hearing sensitivity. Most other middle ear conditions, and all inner ear conditions affecting hearing sensitivity, will not be evident on otoscopic examination of the ear.

Therefore, careful otoscopic examination of the external ear and tympanic membrane is essential in the assessment of hearing loss, but the absence of visual evidence of a source for any hearing loss of which the person complains does not rule out the possibility of either a middle ear or an inner ear site of lesion affecting hearing sensitivity. Finally, it can be erroneous to assume that cerumen (or any other space-occupying condition of the external ear) may be the sole source for hearing loss evidenced by a patient, and that removal of the external ear occlusion will return hearing sensitivity to normal. Removal of space-occupying occlusions from the external ear canal will typically provide physical relief to the patient, and commonly will provide an increase in hearing sensitivity, which he or she may express as "normal hearing." In the absence of formal hearing assesment, however, it is not possible to determine if hearing sensitivity is normal following successful removal of cerumen (or other foreign substance).

Measurement of Hearing Loss

There are two major reasons for conducting measures of hearing loss: first, to provide information leading to determination of the anatomic site of auditory lesion and; second, to assess the receptive communication capabilities of the patient. Tuning fork tests and some informal procedures can enable an initial impression by the examiner of the need for formal audiologic assessment. Furthermore, hand-held devices for screening for hearing loss can be useful additions to the office or bedside assessment of persons presenting with a complaint of hearing loss.

Tuning Fork Tests of Hearing

Upon completion of a physical examination of the external ear and tympanic membrane, an initial question is whether or not the patient deviates in sensitivity from normal-hearing individuals. Prior to the development of the clinical audiometer, assessment of hearing was typically conducted with tuning fork tests. Tuning forks continue to be an integral part of the initial assessment of patients presenting with hearing loss, particularly at the bedside or in the office. A 512 Hz tuning fork is most appropriate for an initial screening.

Each tuning fork emits a pure tone of a particular frequency depending on the physical characteristics (mass and inertia) of the fork. An experienced practitioner can activate the fork by striking it a "standard" blow. By comparing the length of time the patient can hear the slowly damping intensity of the fork relative to that of the practitioner (assuming the practitioner has normal hearing), it is possible to determine the relative magnitude of hearing loss the patient has at a particular frequency. Because of the problem in reliably striking a "standard" blow and the inability to control noise levels in most clinical examination settings, tuning forks are more commonly used in a qualitative manner to assess type of hearing loss. A calibrated audiometer is the procedure of choice in determining more precisely the magnitude and configuration of hearing loss evidenced by a patient. Certain tuning fork tests, however, provide substantive subjective information regarding the integrity of the auditory system.

SCHWABACH TEST

The Schwabach Test provides a tuning fork estimate of hearing loss. The vibrating fork is held at the entrance to the external auditory canal (not touching the pinna) for air conduction measures or the hilt of the vibrating fork is held against the mastoid process for bone conduction measures. The Schwabach Test result for the patient is considered "shortened" or "prolonged" relative to the hearing of the examiner. Experienced examiners are able to obtain rough estimates of magnitude of hearing loss by determining the degree (time) to which the Schwabach is shortened.

RINNÉ TEST

The Rinné Test compares the patient's response to air conduction and bone conduction sensitivity. For those with normal hearing, and for people with sensorineural hearing loss, the tuning fork is heard longer by air conduction than by bone conduction. This result reveals the advantage provided by the air conduction signal in the normal middle ear system. Under conditions when the patient hears bone conduction longer than air conduction, however, a conductive (middle ear) hearing loss is suggested. This result ensues when the air conduction route of transmission is no longer the more efficient route to the cochlea.

WEBER TEST

The Weber Test assesses the ear to which the auditory image is referred when the tuning fork is placed at the center of the forehead and the patient is instructed to indicate in which ear the signal is heard. When both ears are normal or symmetrically abnormal, the auditory image will be localized to the center of the head. If there is a unilateral middle-ear (conductive) loss, the sound will lateralize to the ear with the conductive loss. If there is a unilateral sensorineural loss, the sound will lateralize to the ear with the better sensorineural sensitivity.

Tuning fork tests provide the examiner with an initial impression of the probability of hearing loss and of the possible site of the auditory lesion affecting hearing sensitivity. Tuning forks seldom provide definitive information regarding the magnitude and configuration of hearing loss, and provide no information regarding the effect of any hearing loss on the ability to understand speech for communicative purposes. Other assessment techniques that can be applied during an office or bedside evaluation include hand-held hearing screening devices and self-assessment questionnaires.

Hearing Screening Devices

Figure 10-1 is an example of a commercially available device that enables otoscopic examination of the external ear and screening for hearing loss at several discrete frequencies and intensities. The otoscope (which enables magnified visualization of the external canal) is equipped with a rechargeable, battery-operated, pure tone generator. With the speculum of the scope securely placed in the external auditory canal, pure tones can be presented at one of three presentation levels (20, 25, or 40 dB) to determine if the patient is able to hear and respond to the presentation of the sound. Pure tones at octave frequencies between 500 and 4000 Hz can be presented.

The results of such a screening procedure can provide information regarding asymmetries between ears, differences in hearing as a function of frequency, and initial information regarding the probable magnitude of hearing loss as a function of frequency (e.g., less than or more than a 40 dB hearing loss). More importantly,

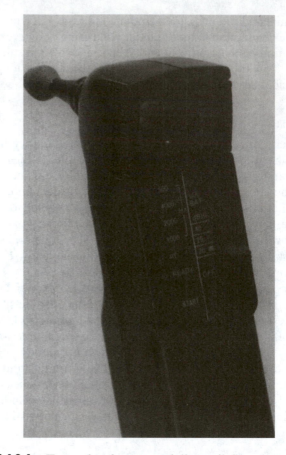

FIGURE 10-1   Example of commercially available otoscope/hearing screening device. The hand held, battery-operated unit enables otoscopic examination of the external ear canal and tympanic membrane and provides pure tones at octave frequencies from 500–4000 Hz at preset intensity levels (20, 25, or 40 dB HL).

the screening procedure can provide information regarding the probable value of formal audiologic evaluation.

Self-Assessment Questionnaires

Another tool in the identification of people with significant hearing loss can be standardized self-assessment questionnaires. Hearing difficulty has been variously described in the clinical literature. Typically, two terms are used to define auditory dysfunction: *hearing impairment* and *hearing handicap*.[3, 4] *Hearing impairment* has emerged as the term used to identify the condition of abnormal hearing, typically defined as the magnitude by which an individual's hearing loss exceeds "normal." The term does not directly address the effects of the hearing loss on the person's ability to function in life experiences. *Hearing handicap* has evolved to refer directly to the effect of the hearing impairment on the person's everyday situation. The term refers specifically to the disadvantage imposed by the hearing loss of the patient on that person's ability to communicate effectively in the activities of daily living. *Hearing impairment* can be determined by using hearing testing procedures; *hearing handicap* is determined using standardized questionnaires that assess the degree to which any particular hearing loss limits the fulfillment of a communication role that is normal for that individual. Hearing impairment is quantifiable solely on the basis of information from the audiologic evaluation. Hearing handicap requires assessment of the perception of the individual, and is quantifiable only following an analysis of the perceived experiences of the person.

In response to the inadequacy of formal hearing tests in predicting handicap, several instruments have been developed to directly assess the degree to which an individual patient perceives a handicap in communication. These instruments do not depend on the results of hearing tests, and can be applied by health care providers interested in determining whether or not a problem with hearing is perceived by a particular person (or family member). The hearing handicap instruments vary in focus, but typically include questions regarding the person's ability to perform activities of daily living without awareness of "difficulty" hearing. The Hearing Handicap Scale[5] was among the earliest instruments, focusing on speech communication and environmental sounds. The Hearing Performance Inventory[6] has more than 150 items and assesses speech understanding, social situations, and personal and occupational issues. Some instruments have been developed specifically to assess performance with hearing aids (e.g., the Hearing Aid Performance Inventory).[7] An example of one tool that has enjoyed widespread investigation and application is the Hearing Handicap Inventory for the Elderly (HHIE) (see Appendix #22).[8] This 25-item self-administered questionnaire assesses the self-perceived emotional and social consequences of hearing loss. The HHIE was standardized on adults over 60 years of age and, therefore, is particularly applicable for use with elders.

Scores indicating the experience of "handicap" secondary to hearing loss can be used as a mechanism for identifying the patient in need of formal assessment of hearing loss and in need of rehabilitative measures. The instrument also can be used to evaluate whether the hearing loss measured during formal hearing testing is perceived by the individual to have an effect on activities of daily

Hearing impairment is a term used to identify the condition of abnormal hearing. *Hearing handicap* refers directly to the effect of hearing impairment on an individual's everyday situation.

living. Additionally, some inventories can be used to differentially assess performance with and without hearing aids. Health care providers may consider use of self-assessment inventories as an additional means by which to identify people with hearing loss. Any such instruments considered for use by a health care provider need to be evaluated for reliability and sensitivity before application in the clinical setting.

Observational Assessments

Finally, informal impressions regarding the possible presence of hearing loss can be obtained by observing the person's response to simple commands and/or the person's apparent ability to follow a conversation during an office or bedside consultation. To be more specific, the health care provider can have the person repeat a list of words (without use of visual cues, i.e., "lipreading") to informally assess whether the individual is having difficulty understanding speech because of impaired hearing, or if cognitive function may be involved in the inability to communicate. Consultation with an audiologist would enable development of lists of words or phrases that could be used for such informal assessments of speech recognition.

Suggested words for informal assessment of speech understanding

Easy words	Difficult words
Airplane	Coke
Baseball	Folk
Cowboy	Hits
Hotdog	Peak
Railroad	Sick

When it is apparent to the health care provider that formal assessment of hearing is indicated, an audiologic evaluation should be conducted. That evaluation, conducted by an audiologist, will include not only measures of pure tone hearing sensitivity, but also measures of speech recognition perhaps both in quiet and with various types of competing noise or speech. The evaluation provides definitive information regarding the magnitude and configuration of hearing loss in each ear, and formal assessment of the ability of the listener to hear and understand speech at various intensity levels. The assessment provides the information from which diagnostic decisions regarding etiology of the hearing loss can be made, and from which rehabilitative decisions regarding the possible need for hearing aids can be made.

Audiologic Evaluation

Pure Tone Audiometry

Hearing loss is quantified audiometrically by plotting the threshold sensitivity responses from the individual under test against a "norm" (0 dB HL) for the general population. Any deviation from 0 dB across the frequency range 250 to 8000 Hz represents the

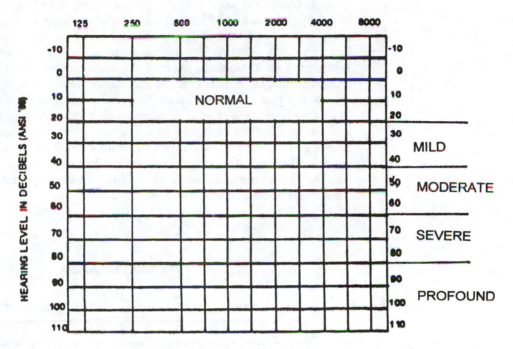

FIGURE 10-2   Standard audiogram on which hearing loss (in dB HL) is plotted as a function of frequency (in Hz). Normal hearing range (0–20 dB HL) and designations of magnitude of hearing loss are also noted.

magnitude of hearing loss at a particular frequency. Figure 10-2 is an example of the standard audiogram form on which pure tone hearing test results will be summarized. Frequency (250 to 8000 Hz) is plotted on the abscissa: hearing loss (in dB) is plotted on the ordinate. Figure 10-2 also includes descriptive terms by which the magnitude of hearing loss is often characterized. Specifically, for adults, *normal* hearing sensitivity includes any deviation from 0 dB to no greater than 20 dB. *Mild* hearing loss includes hearing sensitivity between 20 and 40 dB HL. Hearing loss in the 40 to 60 dB range would be described as a *moderate* loss; a *severe* loss is between 60 and 80 dB HL. *Profound* hearing loss exceeds 80 dB HL. Because hearing loss is assessed at each frequency, it is common to observe differences in hearing sensitivity as a function of frequency (as is developed more fully in subsequent sections of this chapter).

Tests are conducted to determine threshold sensitivity by air conduction and bone conduction. The difference in air and bone conduction sensitivity reveals whether the hearing loss is *conductive* in origin (outer ear and/or middle ear pathology) or *sensorineural* in origin (inner ear and central auditory pathways). Figure 10-3 presents three examples of pure tone test results for octave frequencies from 250 to 8000 Hz (0 = air conduction; = bone conduction). When the loss is conductive (panel A), bone conduction is more sensitive than air conduction. In the sensorineural hearing loss (panel B), there is equal deviation from normal hearing sensitivity (0 dB) for both air and bone conduction. It is possible to observe a *mixed* hearing loss (panel C) in which the patient presents with both a conductive and sensorineural component. In such a case, bone conduction sensitivity would show a deviation from normal hearing (0 dB); air conduction sensitivity would reveal an even greater deviation from 0 dB.

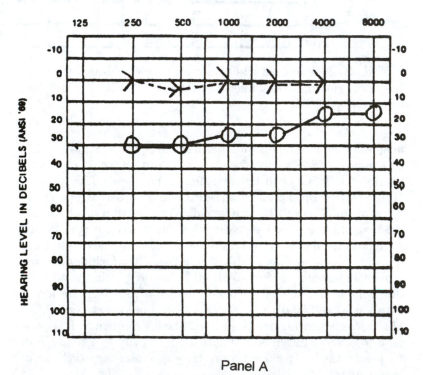

Panel A

FIGURE 10-3   Panel A is a conductive hearing loss (note the difference between air and bone conduction sensitivity);

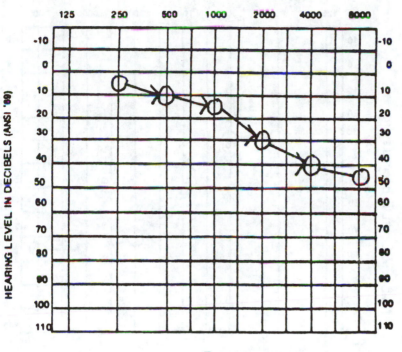

Panel B

FIGURE 10-3   Panel B is a configuration of sensorineural hearing loss (note that air and bone conduction symbols are interweaving).

Speech Audiometry

Reduced speech recognition is among the most common problems encountered by persons with hearing loss. Speech audiometry is used to assess the receptive communication ability of the patient and to predict the site of auditory lesion. Two speech tests are performed in a standard auditory battery: a measurement of the sensitivity for speech, referred to as the Speech Recognition Threshold (SRT), and a measurement of the recognition (discrimination) ability at suprathreshold levels, sometimes referred to as the Speech Discrimination Score (SDS).

Speech Recognition Threshold (SRT).   Traditionally, the SRT is measured using spondee words: two-syllable words in which equal stress is placed on each syllable (e.g., hotdog, baseball, cow-

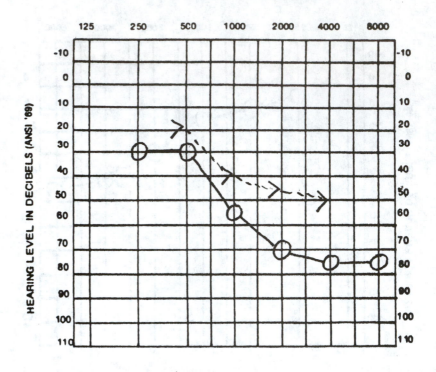

Panel C

FIGURE 10-3   Panel C is a mixed loss which has both a conductive and sensorineural component.

boy, sidewalk). The SRT is reported as the dB hearing level below which the patient cannot successfully recognize 50 percent of the two-syllable words. It is expected that the SRT will be approximately equal to the average hearing loss for pure tones in the mid-frequency region (500 to 2000 Hz), regardless of the type of hearing loss (conductive or sensorineural). As such the SRT has little differential diagnostic significance but is used to provide a descriptive measure of magnitude of hearing loss for speech.

Speech Discrimination Score (SDS).   The measurement of speech recognition at suprathreshold levels is conducted using standardized lists of words or sentences. The standardized materials have been chosen to meet specific criteria that enable comparison with "everyday speech." The materials available for use include monosyllabic word lists, nonsense syllables, and sentence materials.

The results are reported in percent-correct scores at specified supra-threshold levels.[9]

People with conductive hearing loss typically obtain high (> 80 percent) percent-correct scores on these suprathreshold speech recognition measures. Individuals with sensorineural hearing loss will evidence decreased "discrimination," depending on the magnitude and configuration of the sensorineural hearing loss and the site of the auditory lesion (cochlear versus retrocochlear). To explain, recognition of isolated speech segments is unaffected by conductive hearing loss (when materials are presented at amplitude levels sufficiently above threshold to be readily audible) because the encoding mechanisms of the cochlea and central pathways are normal. Therefore, when the threshold sensitivity loss is surpassed by the amplitude of the speech signal, the ability to understand the speech segment is excellent.

When the conductive mechanism is normal and cochlear or retrocochlear structures are affected by lesions of the auditory system, however, the ability to understand consonantal elements of speech is affected. Typically, the more central the site of the auditory lesion, the greater the effect of the lesion on the ability to understand speech at suprathreshold levels.

Objective Measures of Auditory System Function

In addition to the *subjective* measures of hearing described previously, there are *objective* measures by which auditory system function can be assessed. When individuals are unwilling or incapable of cooperating in the performance of subjective tests of hearing, or when information specific to the function of certain aspects of the auditory system is needed, one or more of the objective measures can be employed to predict the probable site of an auditory lesion, and possibly to gain indirect information regarding magnitude of hearing loss. The conduct and interpretation of these tests require referral to an audiologist.

IMMITTANCE STUDIES

Among the most significant advances in the differential diagnosis of middle ear impairments, and the procedure which provides definitive information regarding the integrity of the acoustic reflex arc, is acoustic immittance studies. *Tympanometry* provides indirect evidence of the mechanical integrity of middle ear structures when ear canal air pressure changes are introduced. Pathologic conditions including middle ear effusion, ossicular chain fixation, or ossicular chain discontinuity, are differentially identifiable from the tympanogram.[10] *Acoustic reflex* measures provide indirect evidence of the integrity of the stapedius muscle contraction in response to acoustic stimulation. Results from the tests of the acoustic reflex provide information regarding cranial nerve VIII (sensory), low brainstem (cranial nerve VII nucleus), and cranial nerve VII (motor) integrity.[11]

AUDITORY BRAINSTEM EVOKED RESPONSE (ABR) MEASURES

The ABR is one of several clinically useful evoked auditory potentials. The ABR is indicated to determine presence or absence of hearing loss (in cases where the person is incapable of cooperating for standard hearing tests) or in cases in which a low brainstem, space-occupying lesion is suspected. The procedure is most commonly employed for differential diagnostic purposes, and is not typically required in the audiologic evaluation of elders.

OTO-ACOUSTIC EMISSION (OAE) MEASURES

Auditory physiologists have identified the emission of acoustic energy in the external canal of participants following stimulation of normal cochlear structures.[12] Following the early reports, evidence has accumulated confirming that such acoustic energy leakage is a biochemical property of the healthy, functioning cochlea. Several methods are available for evoking and recording the oto-acoustic emission (OAE). Each procedure enables the presentation of an acoustic stimulus to the ear, and the monitoring of energy in the ear canal. The OAE has been determined to be a product of the outer hair cells of the cochlea. As such, the procedure is an objective measure of the integrity of the auditory system through the level of the outer hair cells of the cochlea. Normal OAEs are expected among individuals of all ages when hearing sensitivity is better than 35 dB HL. Hearing loss of cochlear origin that exceeds 35 dB HL will result in no identifiable evoked OAE.[13] Because many elders have hearing loss exceeding 35 dB HL, the OAE is not commonly employed in the evaluation of such patients. As with the ABR, however, when differential diagnostic questions are being resolved, the OAE can contribute additional objective evidence of auditory system function.

MANIFESTATIONS OF PRESBYCUSIS

Pure Tone Audiometric Patterns

Presbycusis typically presents as a sensorineural hearing loss, bilaterally symmetrical, with better hearing sensitivity in the low frequency region relative to the high frequency region. Audiometrically, the characteristic pattern is exemplified in panel B of Figure 10-3. Among persons with presbycusis, the absolute magnitude of hearing loss is not predictable but varies across individuals; however, regardless of differences across individuals in absolute magnitude of hearing loss, the general configuration of a "sloping" (low frequency to high frequency) pattern is typically preserved.

Hearing loss of presbycusic origin may be evidenced as early as the fifth decade of life, but more commonly does not emerge until the sixth decade of life. Onset is typically gradual with no sudden changes in hearing sensitivity. The changes in pure tone sensitivity typically are evident first in the high frequency (> 2000 Hz) region. As the hearing loss progresses, and invades the lower frequency (500 to 2000 Hz) regions, effects on understanding speech become more evident. Specifically, when hearing loss invades the frequency region lower than 3000 Hz, the ability to understand conversational speech will decrease. As the magnitude of hearing loss increases throughout the frequency range 300 to 3000 Hz, the ability to recognize the presence of speech will decrease and the ability to understand speech will also decrease. The pure tone audiogram provides the most definitive information by which to identify the individual who is likely to have significant difficulty understanding conversational speech due to peripheral hearing loss secondary to aging.

Hearing Loss and the Understanding of Speech

The complaints of individuals with presbycusis are predictable. Most individuals report that they can "hear" speech but cannot "understand" speech. For individuals with normal hearing sensitivity, such statements have no experiential counterpart. Specifically, for the normal hearing individual, there is no difference between "hearing" and "understanding" the speech signal. Said differently, any message loud enough to be "heard" will be "understood." An understanding of how one might "hear" but not "understand" a speech signal requires an appreciation for some of the acoustic properties of speech and how those acoustic properties interact with sensorineural hearing loss to affect "understanding."

Figure 10-4 (panel A) provides a schematic representation of the average energy available in a long-term speech sample. If one calculates the spectral (frequency and intensity) characteristics of any long sample of speech, the amplitude of the energy represented in the sample will vary as a function of frequency. The variance across individual speakers, however, will not vary greatly from the

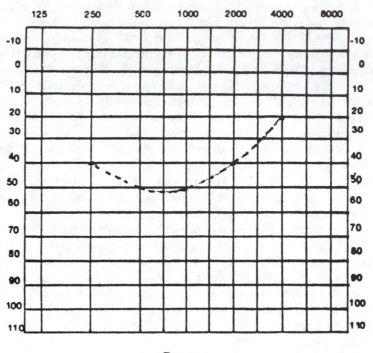

Panel A

FIGURE 10-4   Schematic representation of the long-term average spectrum of soft conversational speech (Panel A).

"average long-term spectrum of speech." Therefore, the schematized representation of speech in Panel A Figure 10-4 provides a reasonably accurate representation of the frequency-and-intensity information any listener's auditory system must encode in order for the listener to accurately understand the segmental elements of the speech signal. To explain, the spectrum of speech includes both high intensity, low frequency energy (predominantly coming from vowels: a, e, i, o, and u), and low intensity, high frequency energy (predominantly coming from the voiceless consonants in our language: s, sh, f, th, k, t, p, and h).

Panel B in Figure 10-4 reveals how the characteristics of a presbycusic hearing loss interact with the energy of speech to affect the clarity ("understanding") of the speech signal. In this example, threshold sensitivity in the frequency region up to 1000 Hz is sensitive enough that the individual is able to hear all the low frequency components of the speech signal. The threshold sensitivity loss for frequencies at 2000 Hz and higher, however, is greater than the

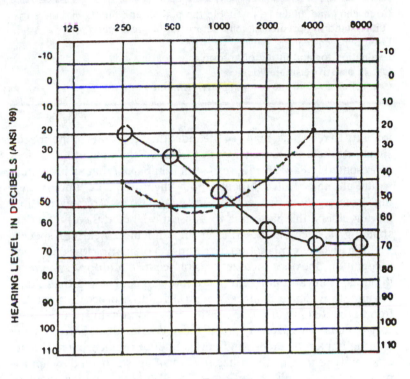

Panel B

FIGURE 10-4   Panel B includes the spectrum of speech with a sensorineural hearing loss superimposed.

amplitude of the energy available in the speech signal. All of the speech signals in the frequency range 1200 to 4000 Hz will be inaudible to the listener. For the listener with the hearing loss represented in this example, soft, conversational speech would have an indistinct, muffled quality, with little to no clarity differentiating the high frequency consonant elements of the message. Consequently, the listener would "hear" the speech (because of the audible low frequency energy), but the listener would not "understand" the speech (because of the inaudible high frequency energy).

The impact of this interaction between the spectral characteristics of conversational speech and the threshold sensitivity loss is the underlying source for the hearing impaired listener's perception that speech is "heard" but not "understood." One should consider the difficulty presented by hearing the vowel sounds of speech, but not hearing approximately one third of all consonant sounds. The result is an awareness of the presence of a speech signal, but an

TABLE 10-1.   MANAGEMENT STRATEGIES FOR ELDERS WITH PRESBYCUSIS
Counseling and guidance to enable the patient and family members to understand the predictable characteristics of presbycusis
Use of speech-reading skills
Evaluation for and fitting of appropriate hearing aids
Use of assistive listening devices
Control of noise in the listening environment

inability to recognize many of the individual elements of the speech signal. As hearing loss increases to exceed the magnitude of loss represented in Panel B Figure 10-4, it is apparent that an individual would ultimately have difficulty both "hearing" and "understanding" conversational speech. In virtually all cases of hearing loss among elders, the pattern is to first experience difficulty "understanding" speech before experiencing difficulty "hearing" speech.

Finally, this explanation of the impact of hearing loss on speech recognition does not include possible central auditory system influences. Clinical reports are unanimous in concluding that elders commonly evidence changes in central auditory processing in addition to the loss in pure tone sensitivity. Additionally, central auditory deficits can adversely affect the self-assessed handicap of the hearing-impaired person, and may influence the hearing aid wearer's ability to maximally utilize the advantages provided by appropriately-fitted amplification devices.[14] Therefore, management of the person with presbycusis requires a thorough understanding of the information provided in the audiologic assessment, as well as the complex interactions between peripheral and central auditory mechanisms, and the potential ways in which these factors interplay with the physical, cognitive, and social limitations sometimes accompanying the aging process.

People evidencing classic presbycusis, with no concomitant, transient medical condition affecting the auditory system (e.g., cerumen impaction, otitis media) typically require some or all of the management strategies listed in Table 10-1. These are discussed more fully in the following paragraphs.

MANAGEMENT OF PRESBYCUSIS

Counseling of Individual and Family

People with presbycusis typically do not seek help for hearing loss during the early stages of onset. They often attribute the problems they are encountering to poor speech habits of speakers. Family members often mistake hearing loss for "senility" because the family members observe that the elder seems to "hear everything," but only "understands" familiar speech. The family typically has no appreciation for the impact of even mild hearing loss on the ability to understand speech. Consequently, family members may not question the possibility of hearing loss until the magnitude and configuration of hearing loss affects the patient's ability to "hear" normal conversational speech. When the hearing loss has been explained to family members, it is no less important that they understand the limitations inherent in successful use of hearing aids (if worn by the individual). That counseling should include the audiologist, who is in the best position to understand the unique interrelationships among the factors of hearing loss, speech recognition, any unique limitations of the patient, and performance with the hearing aid.

Counseling of the individual and family members toward an understanding of the reality of the hearing loss, and the impact such a loss has on the understanding of speech, enhances understanding of the elder and often leads to heightened communication even without the benefit of other rehabilitative strategies. For those individuals in whom there is a complex interaction including peripheral hearing loss, disordered central auditory processing, and cognition, the counseling of family members will be critical to the maintenance of the highest possible quality of life for the person. In such cases, the use of hearing aids or assistive listening devices will be limited relative to the degree to which the amplification device, in isolation, can enhance the return of the individual to effective interpersonal communication. Under such circumstances, the counseling by the audiologist with family members or other care providers is crucial to an understanding of the complexity of the hearing handicap under which the individual must perform.

Individuals with presbycusis typically do not seek help for hearing loss during the early stages of onset, and the family typically has no appreciation for the impact of even mild hearing loss on the ability to understand speech.

Speech Reading Skills

Because presbycusis involves depopulation of hair cells and neural fibers required in the encoding of acoustic information, even when the person is fitted with appropriate hearing aids, the ability to communicate efficiently cannot be expected to approximate that of the normal listener. The decrease in available encoding units results in less redundancy in the auditory information available to the central auditory system for processing. Therefore, elders often are helped by learning speech reading skills. Aural rehabilitation sessions and formal speech-reading classes are available at many community speech and hearing centers as well as many graduate training institutions. Such sessions enhance the natural use of visual cues as an aid to understanding conversational speech.

Many elders express an aversion to the use of "lipreading," and assume the skills are too difficult to master. Most elders with adequate visual acuity, however, can make use of visual cues to enhance their use of auditory information, with or without the aid of amplification.

Hearing Aids

Developments in the hearing aid industry have resulted in the availability of prosthetic devices that can be tailored to the individual hearing loss characteristics of a particular person. It is no longer the case that hearing aids "do not work for individuals with sensorineural hearing loss." In fact, the majority of hearing aids manufactured today are designed to accommodate the unique needs of the individual with sensorineural hearing loss.

The purpose of an appropriately fitted amplification system is to make audible the frequency components of conversational speech (via electronic amplification), and secondly, to make important environmental sounds audible. The goal is to ensure that the information of conversational speech is audible throughout the frequency range ~ 300 to 4000 Hz. The frequency-specific amplification is coupled with output-limiting features designed together to make soft speech audible and to prevent loud speech from being intolerable.

Electronic and acoustic features of the hearing aid and/or the earmold are designed to enhance listening in the presence of background noise; but no hearing aid currently available is capable of completely canceling out the negative impact of background noise on the understanding of speech under hearing aided conditions. It should be kept in mind that listening in noise for the person with hearing loss is an extremely difficult task (even with appropriately fitted hearing aids). Therefore, the expectations of elders, family members, and other care providers must be tempered to include the realistic expectation that listening in noise will continue to pose problems even for the person well fitted with hearing aids.

Hearing aids are available in a wide range of styles, models, and strategies. The two primary models commonly used are illustrated in Figure 10-5 and include behind-the-ear devices and in-the-ear devices. The differences between the two primary models include cost, overall size, and cosmetic factors. Additionally, the behind-the-ear instruments separate the hearing aid from the earmold with clear tubing (not shown); whereas, the in-the-ear devices contain all components of the hearing aid within the chassis of the instrument, which is typically custom molded from an impression

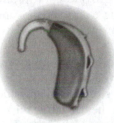

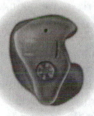

A. Behind-the-ear   B. Full shell

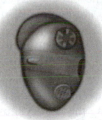

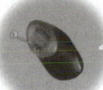

C. Canal   D. Completely-in-canal

FIGURE 10-5   Examples of common types of hearing aids. A = behind-the-ear device in which the hearing aid chassis is separated from the earmold (earmold not shown). B, C, D = in-the-ear devices in which the components of the hearing aid are housed in the chassis custom-molded to fit the ear (full shell); C represents a "canal" instrument, which fits within the ear canal of the wearer but with a smaller portion seated in the inferior part of the concha; and D, which represents a "completely-in-canal" (CIC) device that fits entirely into the canal and has a small string puller used to remove the aid.

of the user's ear. Costs for hearing aids vary dramatically based on the complexity of the amplification circuit and the overall size of the housing. It is not necessarily the case that a higher priced instrument provides either a more sophisticated circuitry or a more satisfied user. Hearing aids receiving the widest interest currently are so-called "digital" or "digitally programmable" hearing aids. These instruments are typically more versatile with respect to the acoustic features that can be manipulated in the device. The fundamental characteristics of frequency response, gain, and output limiting, however, must still be chosen to fit the unique needs of the individual wearer. For many individuals with hearing loss, conventional amplification systems equipped to provide appropriate frequency response, gain, and output limiting characteristics may be as satisfying to the wearer, at a lower overall cost, as the more expensive, completely digital devices.

For the person with presbycusis, the decision regarding the management strategies that will be employed is complex. The decision includes the multidimensional factors of: the magnitude and configuration of the bilateral sensorineural hearing loss; the degree to which the person is limited in manual dexterity; the demands on the person for social and/or vocational communication; the overall, independent functional capabilities of the patient; and the motivation of the person to use hearing aids.

For example, an individual may present with hearing loss sufficient to warrant use of hearing aids. If the person has severely limited use of the hands and fingers, it may not be possible for the person to manipulate the instrument into the ears for successful usage. In such a case, successful use of the hearing aids requires that there be a caregiver who can be responsible for inserting and manipulating the hearing aids. As another example, a person may present with only mild hearing loss, insufficient to warrant use of hearing aids for most people. If, upon taking the history, however, it is revealed that the individual has high demands on communication due to an active social, volunteer, or vocational life, such a person may be an excellent candidate for hearing aids. The decision whether to include hearing aids in the rehabilitative management of the person needs to be made by the audiologist following thorough audiologic evaluation and consideration of the factors influencing the successful use of the hearing aids in each particular person's case. The decision to fit hearing aids is far more complex than can be made on the basis of magnitude of hearing loss alone.

Hearing aids have been shown to positively affect not only the person's ability to communicate, but also to improve the quality of life overall.

Hearing aids that have been appropriately chosen and fitted have been shown to positively affect not only the person's ability to communicate, but also to improve the quality of life overall. Specifically, hearing aids successfully reduce the social, emotional, and communication dysfunctions reported by elders[15] and lead to enhanced self-concept.[16] It has also been shown that interference with psychosocial well-being can be minimized if rehabilitation services, including hearing aids, are provided to elders.[17,18]

The success of hearing aid use among elders will be affected by factors specifically related to the degree of independent living evidenced by the hearing aid wearer. For example, it has been shown that hearing aid use is not as successful among nursing home residents as among elders living independently.[19] Furthermore, there are predictable problems with hearing aid use, which require either the attention of the wearer or surveillance by an alert care provider. The problems include factors summarized in the following sections.

FEEDBACK

Acoustic feedback is the annoying, high-pitched "squeal" that is audible to anyone in the immediate vicinity of the hearing aid wearer, and sometimes audible to the wearer (depending on magnitude of hearing loss). The feedback occurs when the acoustic energy of the amplified signal "escapes" from any acoustic leak beyond the receiver of the hearing aid, and reenters the microphone of the hearing aid. Feedback is often associated with a poor-fitting earmold in the ear of the wearer, but also can be due to intentional venting in the hearing aid, to cracked or split tubing, and occasionally, to more complex acoustic coupling factors associated with the fit of the hearing aid in the ear.

Troubleshooting the source of feedback in the individual case can be difficult, but can be enhanced by removing the hearing aid from the ear of the wearer, covering the tip where sound enters the ear, with the instrument in the "on" position. If feedback is eliminated under that condition, the likelihood is that the problem lies in the fit of the hearing aid and earmold in the ear of the wearer. The instrument should be fitted to the ear of the wearer, being careful to completely "seat" the hearing aid and earmold in the ear and turn the hearing aid to "on." If feedback is eliminated with careful seating of the hearing aid and earmold, it is likely that the wearer is not accurately seating the instrument in the ear (thus leading to an acoustic leak around the earmold). When feedback is not eliminated even after careful seating of the device, be sure there is no open vent through which acoustic energy can be escaping back to the microphone. If feedback is not eliminated even after careful seating of the device in the ear and closure of the vent, it is possible that a remake of the earmold impression can be required to eliminate feedback. Consult the dispensing audiologist to resolve the problem of persistent feedback before deciding a remake of the earmold is required.

CERUMEN BLOCKED EARMOLDS

The hearing aid must be checked periodically to assure that cerumen does not accumulate in the tip and block sound from being transmitted to the ear. When cerumen is identified in the earmold tip, it must be removed. For in-the-ear instruments, the tip must be dry-cleaned with the specific "pick" provided by the hearing aid manufacturer. Do not use any small sharp device other than the tool provided by the hearing aid manufacturer, as it may be possible to damage the receiver and other parts of the hearing aid by invading too deeply into the chassis using an unauthorized cleaning device.

The only exception to dry-cleaning cerumen from the tip occurs if the hearing aid is behind the ear and, therefore, coupled to the earmold by clear tubing. Under these conditions, the earmold tip can be dry-cleaned, or can be separated from the hearing aid at the tubing and cleaned with warm water and cleaning solution. The dispensing audiologist should be consulted before cleaning the earmold with water and cleaning solution. Any water contact with the electronic components of the hearing aid can be damaging to the instrument.

BATTERY CARE

Hearing aids require batteries to power the device. Each hearing aid has a specified battery "number" with which it is designed to function. Batteries have a positive (+) and a negative (−) pole, which must be appropriately oriented in the battery compartment of the hearing aid. If the battery polarity is reversed, the hearing aid will not amplify. Under normal usage batteries provide 75 to 225 hours of hearing aid use depending on the model of hearing aid. A "dead" battery should be removed and replaced immediately to prevent corrosion of the battery in the compartment. When any hearing aid is not in use (removed from the ear during sleeping or for any other reason), the power switch should be turned off and the battery compartment disengaged to be assured that there is no drainage of battery power during periods of nonuse.

If a hearing aid is not functioning in the "on" position and there is no cerumen or debris occluding the earmold, the most likely problem is a dead or polarity-reversed battery. The first step is to correct the battery polarity and turn the instrument to "on." If the aid is still not receiving power, the battery should be replaced and checked again. If there is still no power, the instrument must be evaluated by the dispensing audiologist for possible repair.

RIGHT AND LEFT EAR HEARING AIDS

A hearing aid will have been chosen for a particular ear (or for each ear individually) for any hearing aid wearer. It is practical to put an identifying mark on the hearing aid (or earmold) to indicate which ear it fits. In fact, many hearing aids are "color-coded" by the manufacturer. The industry protocol is to indicate the right ear with a red marking and the left ear with a blue marking.

Assistive Listening Devices

Individuals with hearing loss often express difficulty hearing and understanding speech under specific conditions. Listening to television with other family members can pose problems in the determination of the loudness level at which all members of the family can be satisfied. Additionally, attendance at concerts, theater performances, church or synagogue gatherings, and other public meetings, often pose a unique problem for the hearing impaired individual even when successfully fitted with conventional hearing aids. Use of telephones by the hearing impaired may be difficult. Finally, individuals with hearing loss often experience difficulty recognizing doorbells, alarm clocks, and other uniquely auditory alerting signals. When people with hearing loss are successfully fitted with hearing aids but continue to encounter difficulties with these and other experiences of daily living, or when a hearing aid cannot be provided for an individual, a variety of assistive listening devices are available.

PERSONAL LISTENING SYSTEMS

Personal listening systems can provide the hearing impaired person with enhanced communication when a hearing aid is not used. Such devices are hard-wired systems that include a microphone (sometimes separated from the amplification unit and sometimes housed within the amplification box), an amplifier, and headphones, which deliver the amplified signal to the ears of the wearer. The units provide control over the amount of amplification, and some are equipped with equalizer circuits that provide minor additional control over the relative amplification in discrete frequency bands. The devices are not designed uniquely for the individual wearer and, therefore, can be used in settings where hearing impaired individuals might commonly be seen, but where some individuals may not have been fitted with hearing aids. For example, geriatricians or other health care providers commonly dealing with elders could have a personal listening device available so that communication with patients with significant hearing loss could be enhanced during office or bedside evaluations. The cost of such devices is commonly less than 10 percent of the cost of a conventional hearing aid. Such an assistive device enhances communication between patient and practitioner and can also provide an initial impression regarding the potential the person may have for conventional hearing aid use.

TELEVISION ACCESS SYSTEMS

For television viewing in the home, devices are available that enable the hearing impaired person to control the volume of sound received differentially from that heard from the standard speaker system of the television set. Such systems typically include a hard-wired interface with the audio output of the television, provide independent control of volume, and can be connected to the headphones by hard-wire or using infrared or an FM-loop system. Any of these systems enables the hearing impaired person to enjoy the same programming as the rest of the individuals in the room, but with independent control of the loudness. Additionally, since the device is directly interfaced with the audio output of the television, the distracting noises in the room and distortion from the loud-speaker system are minimized.

Closed-captioning, as an additional visual cue, is an option available with most current television sets, and is available as a programming option on many commercial and public television programs. Access to the closed-captioning option requires a deciphering interface either external to, or housed within, the television set.

LARGE GROUP SYSTEMS

Many concert halls and some churches and synagogues are equipped with infrared and other wireless amplification systems that enhance the auditory signal available to the hearing impaired in the audience. Some devices require a receiving headset, and some systems can be used in association with the wearer's hearing aid. Such systems are designed to equalize the fidelity of the auditory signal available to the person in the audience, regardless of seat location relative to the sound source.

TELEPHONE AIDS

Telephone usage can be particularly disturbing for the individual with hearing impairment since telephone technology is designed for use by normal-hearing individuals. Portable and permanent amplification can be obtained for use with standard telephone equipment. In addition, some hearing aids are equipped with a telephone switch, enabling the use of the hearing aid to amplify the signal from the earpiece of the telephone. It should be noted, however, that not all telephone manufacturers use compatible circuitry for use with standard hearing aid circuitry. In any community, audiologists, otolaryngologists, and some hearing aid dispensers will have information regarding the compatibility of local telephone equipment with hearing aid telephone circuits.

ALERTING DEVICES

Hearing impaired individuals often can be assisted by use of devices that translate common household auditory signals into visual or tactile signals. For example, doorbells, alarm clocks, fire alarms, and telephone rings can be interfaced with equipment that provides visual (light) and/or tactile (vibratory) signals to alert the hearing impaired individual. Many such devices are available from mail-order catalogs. The range of assistive devices available in any geo-graphical area should be well known by local audiologists, otolaryn-gologists, and hearing aid dispensers.

Factors Affecting Use of Electronic Devices

A very common problem encountered by hearing impaired elders is aggressive marketing of the sale of hearing aids (and other assistive devices) without adequate assessment of the capability of the person to use the device unassisted. It is possible that an elder may have the magnitude and configuration of hearing loss to require use of hearing aids, but may not have the manual dexterity or mental capacity to put the hearing aid(s) into the ear and adjust the devices for use. Responsible individuals providing hearing aids to elders will ensure that the person (or an available caregiver) is able to use the device before fitting and selling the instrument. When the history and audiologic evaluation of an elder reveals significant hearing loss, assessment of the capability to understand the function of the hearing aid, and assessment of the manual dexterity of the individual, must precede the decision to fit and sell the device to the individual. Conventional hearing aids may not be the most efficient and practical rehabilitative strategy for every elderly hearing impaired individual.

> A common problem encountered by hearing impaired elders is aggressive marketing of hearing aids without adequate assessment of the capability of the person to use the device unassisted.

The communicative needs of the elder with sensorineural hearing loss can be met with adequate assessment and appropriate management. In fact, the quality of life for an elder with hearing loss can be maintained or even enhanced by the appropriate choice of hearing aids and other assistive devices when there are no medical or surgical treatments available. All assistive devices (including hearing aids), however, require that the person (or a caregiver) be able to manipulate the device to ensure its proper use.

Noise and Noise Control

The single most universally negative experience of the hearing impaired is the confounding influence of noise in the listening environment. In this context, "noise" refers to any sound not contributing to the audibility of the primary auditory signal to which the listener is attending. For example, the quiet banter of several individuals in friendly conversation will be "noise" to a hearing impaired person trying to engage in conversation with another individual in the same vicinity. Similarly, sounds common to specific environments (plate/utensil noises in a restaurant or children's

The single, most universally negative experience of the hearing impaired is the confounding influence of noise in the listening environment.

voices on a playground) can be experienced as particularly distracting "noise" to the hearing impaired listener. Clinical reports reveal that persons with even mild sensorineural hearing loss, and elders in general (with or without hearing loss), require a more advantageous signal-to-noise ratio to achieve the same performance criteria as young individuals with no hearing loss.[20] That is, elders experience increased "masking" of speech by "noise." Hearing aids do not typically improve significantly the listener's ability to tolerate background noise. Consequently, many hearing aid wearers find use of hearing aids particularly limited in noisy environments.

Unfortunately, many institutional-care environments have relatively high noise levels. Room acoustics often include high levels of reverberation, due to the use of hard wall and floor coverings for ease of cleaning. These acoustic conditions often exacerbate the already difficult time the hearing impaired experience understanding speech. Measures taken to decrease or diffuse the noise levels in group meeting rooms, cafeterias, or examining room areas will decrease the fatigue and irritability of occupants, and will enhance the ability to communicate for the hearing impaired.

COMMUNICATION STRATEGIES

Previous sections included the common characteristics associated with hearing loss in elders. The configuration of hearing loss in this group is relatively predictable, although, as reviewed, the absolute magnitude of hearing loss can vary among individuals. The common features of bilateral symmetry, sloping configuration, and difficulty understanding speech, however, suggest that strategies for effectively communicating with these patients might also be predictable. Indeed, there are common strategies which, when followed, will enhance communication between a speaker and the hearing impaired individual. The strategies require attention by the speaker to three features of the communication process: the environment, the speech, and the process required of the listener.

The Communication Environment

Competing noise will make conversations very difficult for the hearing impaired; when possible, choose an environment which is quiet. Good lighting on the face of the speaker will enhance the hearing impaired listener's use of facial expressions and lip and mouth movement. The health care provider should position himself or herself so, that he or she is at eye level with the listener and the face is fully visible to the listener. The best distance when speaking to hearing impaired elders is typically three to six feet.

The Speaker

The health care provider should speak clearly and distinctly and not exaggerate lip and mouth movement in an effort to aid the person's ability to understand; and speak at a normal rate because slowing the rate of speech typically distorts clarity. He or she should avoid chewing, eating, or covering the mouth with the hand when speaking. Rapid changes in the topic of conversation may be difficult for the hearing impaired; if possible, the person should be cued that the topic of conversation is changing.

The Process Required of the Listener

Some sounds of speech are naturally louder and more visible than others; this makes certain sounds and words easier to understand than others. Because hearing loss among elders typically affects the higher frequencies, they will often confuse the high-pitched sounds: s, sh, f, th, k, t, p, h. Because the hearing impaired often must process a message that has only been partially intelligible, they may take longer to respond. The person should be given sufficient time to respond before assuming that they have not understood the message. When the listener appears not to understand, the statement is rephrased in another short, simple sentence.

SUMMARY

The focus of this chapter has been on those characteristics of hearing loss in elders which are common across individuals. Much of the scientific and clinical literature related to this subject focuses on the complexity of the auditory profile presented by this population. Specifically, the literature is clear in revealing that auditory sensitivity, as reflected in the pure tone audiogram, seldom is predictive of the level of difficulty an individual will evidence when confronted with signals as complex as speech, especially speech in the presence of competing noise.

The literature suggests that the process of aging results in the degeneration of encoding mechanisms throughout the peripheral and central auditory system. The pure tone audiogram summarizes only one simple measure of auditory system function. Therefore, it is common to encounter people with the same magnitude and configuration of pure tone hearing loss, each of whom evidences a wide difference in speech recognition ability. The most common explanation for the differences is that aging is characterized by wide variance in the effects of the degenerative changes on the function of the central auditory system. As the depopulation of hair cells at the peripheral level is increasingly associated with a depopulation of neural elements in the central auditory system, there will be a resultant increasing difficulty accurately recognizing the subtle complexities of speech. When speech recognition is further complicated by the presence of a competing signal, the person may be overwhelmed by the complexity of the task. The explanation of the difficulty understanding speech encountered by an elder does not include any contribution of failure in cognition or invoke other sequelae of aging. The aging auditory system continues to challenge investigators regarding the etiology and rehabilitation of hearing loss. Bergman reminded those working to understand the complexity of hearing loss among elders of an important fact: "as we age we are increasingly more unlike each other than when we were young adults."[21]

ACKNOWLEDGEMENT

The editors acknowledge the assistance and editorial comments of Leonard Reid, PhD.

REFERENCES

1. National Center for Health Statistics (NCHS). Current estimates from the National Health Interview Survey: United States, 1987. *Vital and Health Statistics.* Series 10, Public Health Service. Washington, DC: U.S. Government Printing Office; 1987.
2. Schow R, Nerbonne M. Hearing levels among elderly nursing home residents. *J Speech Hear Res.* 1980;45:124–132.
3. American Academy of Otolaryngology committee on hearing and equilibrium and the American Council of Otolaryngology committee on the medical aspects of noise. Guide for the evaluation of hearing handicap. *JAMA.* 1979;241:2055–2059.
4. American Speech and Hearing Association (ASHA) Executive Board. On the definition of hearing handicap. *ASHA.* 1981;23:293–297.
5. High W, Fairbanks G, Glorig A. Scale for self-assessment of hearing handicap. *J Speech Hear Dis.* 1964;29:215–230.
6. Giolas T, Owens E, Lamb S, Schubert E. Hearing performance inventory. *J Speech Hear Dis.* 1979;44:169–195.
7. Walden B, Demorest M, Hepler E. Self-report approach to assessing benefit derived from amplification. *J Speech Hear Res.* 1984;27:49–56.

8. Ventry I, Weinstein B. The hearing handicap inventory for the elderly: a new tool. *Ear and Hear.* 1982;83:128–134.

9. Gordon-Salant S. Basic hearing evaluation. In: Mueller H, Geoffrey V, eds. *Communication Disorders in Aging.* Washington, DC: Gallaudet University Press; 1987:301–333.

10. Hall J, Chandler D. Tympanometry in clinical audiology. In: Katz J, ed. *Handbook of Clinical Audiology.* 4th ed. Baltimore: Williams & Wilkins; 1994:283–299.

11. Northern J, Abbott-Gabbard S. The acoustic reflex. In: Katz J, ed. *Handbook of Clinical Audiology.* 4th ed. Baltimore: Williams & Wilkins; 1994:300–316.

12. Kemp D. Stimulated acoustic emissions from within the human auditory system. *J Acoust Soc Am.* 1978;64:1386–1391.

13. Stover L, Norton S. The effects of aging on otoacoustic emissions. *J Acoust Soc Am.* 1993;94:2670–2681.

14. Chmiel R, Jerger J. Hearing aid use, central auditory disorder, and hearing handicap in elderly persons. *J Am Acad Audiol.* 1996;7:190–202.

15. Mulrow C, Aguilar C, Endicott J, et al. Quality of life changes and hearing impairment: a randomized trial. *Ann Intern Med.* 1990;113:188–194.

16. Harless B, McConnel F. Effects of hearing aid use on self-concept in older persons. *J Speech Hear Dis.* 1982;47:305–309.

17. Weinstein B. Hearing aids at my age: why bother? *ASHA.* 1991;33:38–40.

18. Firman J, Holmes C. The consequences of untreated hearing loss in older persons. *Innovations in Aging.* 1999;1:21–25.

19. Schow R. Success of hearing aid fitting in nursing homes. *Ear and Hear.* 1982;3:173–177.

20. Dubno J, Dirks D, Morgan D. Effects of age and mild hearing loss on speech recognition in noise. *J Acoust Soc Amer.* 1984;76:87–96.

21. Bergman M. *Aging and the Perception of Speech.* Baltimore: University Park Press; 1980.

VISION

CAROL M. MANGIONE

Vision problems are one of the most common treatable causes of disability associated with aging. This chapter briefly reviews the prevalence of common eye conditions which are age-related and the current disease-specific screening recommendations. It then addresses some newly developed vision-targeted measures as potential screening tools, and summarizes the increasing number of self-report measures for the assessment of visual functioning.

PREVALENCE OF COMMON EYE CONDITIONS ASSOCIATED WITH AGING AND CURRENT DISEASE-SPECIFIC SCREENING RECOMMENDATIONS

Thirteen percent of Americans ages 65 and older have some form of visual impairment and 8 percent have an inability to read newsprint or blindness in both eyes.[1] Among persons ages 65 to 74 years, a visual acuity of 20/50 or less was measured in 11 percent of those who wear glasses and 26 percent of those who do not.[2] Up to 25 percent of older adults may be using an incorrect lens

The Agency for Health Care Policy and Research (AHCPR) was renamed in December 1999.
This agency is now known as the Agency for Healthcare Research and Quality (AHRQ).

prescription.[3] The prevalence of vision problems reaches nearly 50 percent in adults over 75 years. A population-based prevalence study of nursing home residents in Baltimore demonstrated that 17 percent of all residents had bilateral blindness, defined as a corrected visual acuity of 20/200 or worse.[4] In this study, among those 90 years or older, 28.6 percent had bilateral blindness.

It is essential to screen for vision problems because elders may view deterioration of their vision as a normal aspect of aging, and may not be aware that most causes of visual impairment are treatable. This is partially because most eye diseases associated with aging lead to gradual declines in visual function that may not create obvious symptoms. Additionally, the normal aging eye can create symptoms due to senile miosis, increased intraocular light scatter from increased opacity of the lens and vitreous, and presbyopia, or decreased amplitude of accommodation of the lens.[5] The challenge for visual screening tests is to differentiate between the changes associated with normal aging and treatable eye diseases in the older eye. Early detection and treatment of visual impairment is essential, because if left untreated, eye diseases can lead to increased risk for functional decline, social isolation, falls, hip fractures, and accidents.[6-14] For these reasons, a comprehensive geriatric assessment should include an evaluation of visual function.[15-16]

Age-Related Cataracts

The most common cause of visual loss associated with aging are bilateral cataracts. Cataracts occur in 18 percent of people aged 65 to 74 years and 46 percent of those over age 75 years.[17] Cataracts are the leading cause of reversible blindness and the second leading cause of overall blindness in the United States. For this reason, cataract extraction is the most frequently performed surgical intervention in the Medicare population with approximately 1.2 million cases a year, accounting for more than 8 million office visits per year.[18] It has been reported, however, that among urban nursing home residents, unoperated cataract is the leading cause of blindness.[4] In the Baltimore Eye Survey, 27 percent of all blindness among African-Americans was from unoperated cataract.[19] These investigations indicate that although cataract extraction is the most frequently performed surgery among Medicare beneficiaries, there is evidence of underuse of this highly effective procedure among older persons with less access to preventive or screening eye examinations.

Cataracts can usually be detected with direct ophthalmoscopy. Not every cataract affects vision and a person's ability to pursue activities that require vision. Published guidelines for the management of age-related cataracts indicate that surgical removal and replacement with an intraocular lens should only be considered if the cataracts are creating limitations in visual functioning.[20-22] For this reason, assessment of age-related cataracts should incorporate short patient surveys that assess visual functioning and symptoms as part of the screening ophthalmologic examination.

Primary Open-Angle Glaucoma

Glaucoma is the second leading cause of blindness in the United States.[23] Primary open-angle glaucoma accounts for 90 percent of glaucoma in the United States, and it usually progresses in the absence of symptoms until irreversible field loss has occurred.[24] Increased age is a risk factor for glaucoma. Population-based prevalence studies suggest that 4 to 9 percent of older persons have glaucoma.[25-26] Data from the Baltimore Eye Survey indicate that the prevalence and the number of persons who develop blindness from glaucoma is much higher among older African-Americans.[19] In addition to age and race, those elders with a first-degree relative with glaucoma or a personal history of coronary artery disease, hypertension, or diabetes mellitus, are at increased risk for developing this condition.[27]

Tonometry, or measurement, of intraocular pressure alone, or in combination with direct visual examination of the fundus, have unacceptably high false negative and false positive rates to be used as screening tests by noneye care specialists.[28] The diagnosis of glaucoma depends on the presence of optic nerve excavation, or cupping, and evidence of visual field defects. The use of stereoscopic equipment and field testing increases the accuracy of diagnosis, therefore, periodic referral to a vision care provider, with training in fundoscopic examination and interpretation of visual field defects, is the optimal screening strategy for the detection of this condition.

Age-Related Macular Degeneration

Age-related macular degeneration (ARMD) is the leading cause of blindness among Caucasians in the United States. This condition is present in 3 percent to 9 percent of persons older than 80 years.[19,29-31] Although less treatable than cataract or glaucoma, early laser treatment is effective at slowing progression of ARMD for some patients. In general, although patients with ARMD lose central acuity, peripheral vision is preserved. Therefore, with appropriate referral to low vision rehabilitation services, many elders with ARMD can learn to use their peripheral vision to improve their ability to pursue instrumental activities of daily living (IADL) independently.

A dilated fundoscopic examination in combination with measured visual acuity are used to diagnose ARMD. As with the detection of glaucoma, periodic referral to a vision care provider with training in fundoscopic examination is the optimal screening strategy for the detection of ARMD.

Diabetic Retinopathy

The prevalence of diabetic retinopathy is correlated with the duration of diabetes mellitus. Therefore, the prevalence has increased as people with adult-onset diabetes live longer. The Early Treatment of Diabetic Retinopathy Study (ETDRS) determined that laser treatment is beneficial in certain patients with early diabetic retinopathy and macular edema before perceptible vision loss has occurred. Appropriate use of laser photocoagulation can reduce the risk of severe visual loss by 50 percent.[32] Therefore, it is critical that a screening strategy for diabetic retinopathy detect this condition during the asymptomatic phase. For this reason, annual referral for a dilated fundoscopic examination is the recommended screening strategy for elders with known diabetes mellitus.[33]

Uncorrected Refractive Error

Recent community- and nursing home-based prevalence studies have identified uncorrected refractive error as one of the leading causes of reversible visual impairment among elders. Among people aged 65 to 74 years, a visual acuity of 20/50 or less was measured in 11 percent of those who wear glasses and 26 percent of those who do not.[34] Previous investigations indicate that up to 25 percent of elders may be using an incorrect lens prescription.[35] It is difficult to estimate the precise prevalence of uncorrected refractive error, but a study of nursing home residents in Baltimore indicated that 20 percent of the cohort had functional blindness from uncorrected refractive error and an additional 37 percent had visual impairment secondary to uncorrected refractive error.[4] Deterioration of refractive correction with aging may be due to change in the axis of astigmatism and or decreased amplitude of accommodation of the lens (presbyopia) with aging.[5] In addition, early cataract can change the curvature of the lens and the refractive correction.

Because decline in visual function from uncorrected refractive error is easily detected with standardized measurement of visual acuity, periodic examination with an eye chart is currently the best screening strategy. The eye charts developed for use in the Early Treatment Diabetic Retinopathy Study (ETDRS) have greater reliability than the more common assessment tools such as the Snellen Eye Chart.[36] Measurement of visual acuity while wearing current correction with ETDRS charts can be integrated into an annual geriatric assessment. All people with a decline of greater than 10 characters or two lines from their previous best corrected visual acuity, and all those without known eye disease whose visual acuity while wearing current correction is worse than 20/40, should be referred for a refraction and a comprehensive ophthalmic examination by a vision care provider. The sensitivity and specificity of questionnaires designed to assess visual function for the detection of uncorrected refractive error have not been described and should not be considered an acceptable alternative to an eye chart evaluation.

VISION-TARGETED MEASURES AS POTENTIAL SCREENING TOOLS

Vision-targeted measures can be classified by the degree and type of patient participation required to complete the assessment.[37] The first group of measures are the physical measures, such as lens or retinal photographs. These require cooperation but little participation from the participant. Thus, one strength of physical measures is the limited opportunity for participants to introduce bias into data collection. As potential screening tools, physical measures are attractive for the detection of presymptomatic stages of eye diseases. This characteristic is particularly useful for conditions such as diabetic retinopathy where presymptomatic detection and treatment can prevent blindness. Most physical measures are not feasible screening tools because they require costly equipment, time, and training for the reliable assessment of visual structures and interpretation of physical data. Also, it is likely that physical measures would have an unacceptable high false positive rate due to the lack of information about the clinical or functional implications of abnormal findings on these tests. For example, many of the retinal photographic abnormalities associated with the diagnosis of age-related macular degeneration are also observed to a lesser degree in the normal aging eye.[38]

The second group of assessment tools are the performance-based measures such as eye chart measurement of visual acuity and automated perimetry to assess visual fields. These measures are principally used in clinical practice, and therefore, abnormal findings on these tests are frequently used as diagnostic criteria for many eye diseases.[36] The comprehensive eye examination consists of a battery of performance-based tests and, currently, these measures are widely recognized as the most valuable for screening purposes. All performance-based measures are effort-dependent and require a cooperative and cognitively intact participant. Therefore, their usefulness as screening tools among nursing home residents and other elders with impairments in cognitive and physical capacity may be limited. Additionally, an accurate assessment with these measures requires training and standardization of procedures. Because most performance-based measures require special lighting and test conditions, these measures may not be feasible for in-home screening assessments. Sources of random error and systematic bias in performance-based measures include the participant, the equipment, and the operator who conducts and interprets the test.

The third group of measures are self-reports of visual functioning.[39-43] The majority of these self-assessments are questionnaires that estimate the elder's perception of visual disability or limitations in the performance of visual activities. The advantages of self-report measures are that they do not require special equipment and they can easily be integrated into settings other than eye care practices such as a person's home, other community-based locations, or primary care offices. It is likely, however, that self-report measures will only be useful for the detection of treatable eye diseases that cause symptoms such as age-related cataracts or uncorrected refractive error. For diseases where detection and treatment is considered most effective during the presymptomatic phase, such as glaucoma, diabetic retinopathy, and some types of ARMD, it is unlikely that surveys will be useful for the detection of these conditions in their most treatable phase. Therefore, it is likely that even the most carefully designed self-report measure as a stand-alone assessment tool will have a high false positive rate and more importantly, an unacceptably high false negative rate for the detection of glaucoma, diabetic retinopathy, and ARMD to be useful as a screening tool.

Since only those people with cataracts who report limitations in visual functioning are in need of further evaluation, self-report surveys are promising as tools for the detection of elders with visually significant cataracts who may wish to consider cataract surgery. Additionally, although there have not been published descriptions of the diagnostic accuracy of questionnaires for the detection of uncorrected refractive error, self-report measures can be useful for this purpose. Because of the high prevalence of visually significant cataracts and uncorrected refractive error, a comprehensive screening strategy directed at visual impairment should incorporate a brief questionnaire that assesses visual function in addition

Since only those people with cataracts who report limitations in visual functioning are in need of further evaluation, self-report surveys are promising as tools for the detection of elders with visually significant cataracts who may wish to consider cataract surgery.

to a mandatory periodic referral for a comprehensive, dilated eye examination for the detection of presymptomatic glaucoma, diabetic retinopathy, and age-related macular degeneration.

All questionnaires are dependent on cooperative and cognitively able participants, and are limited by respondent bias. Because normal aging of ocular structures can cause visual symptoms, self-report measures can be especially susceptible to a high false positive rate. Questionnaire data are also limited by potential confounding from other chronic medical conditions. Finally, because of limitations in feasible length and investigator's bias about the areas of greatest importance for questionnaires as screening tools, self-report measures may omit aspects of visual functioning that are associated with the onset and early detection of eye diseases.

SUMMARY OF PUBLISHED SELF-REPORT MEASURES FOR THE ASSESSMENT OF VISUAL FUNCTIONING

There are a number of questionnaires designed for the assessment of visual functioning. None of the published self-report measures in the medical literature was designed for use as screening tools or diagnostic tests. Most of these measures were specifically constructed to evaluate the effectiveness of cataract extraction. One of the earliest of these measures is the Visual Function Index developed by Bernth-Petersen.[44] The Visual Function Index evaluates 11 vision-specific tasks that most of the subsequent scales in the literature and currently under development include such as reading, distance vision, and watching television. Additionally, this survey includes items that address mobility limitations due to visual loss. During 1992 as part of a study of outcomes after cataract extraction, Mangione and associates developed a survey entitled the Activities of Daily Vision Scale[40] (see Appendix #1). This questionnaire allows the participants to rate their difficulty with 20 common visual activities that were identified during open-ended interviews with elders with bilateral cataracts. A newer vision-targeted survey in the literature is the VF-14[42] (see Appendix #46). The VF-14 was also developed for use in a national study of outcomes after cataract extraction and intraocular lens implantation. This measure consists of 14 items that assess many of the visual activities included in the Visual Function Index and the Activities of Daily Vision Scale. The VF-14 has the advantage of being shorter, yet it has high reliability (Cronbach's $\alpha = 0.85$). To the author's knowledge, none of these surveys designed to assess people with age-related cataracts has been tested as a screening tool among community or nursing home-dwelling elders.

The Visual Activity Questionnaire developed by Sloane and coworkers,[41] is one of two published visual functioning questionnaires that was not specifically designed for the evaluation of people with cataracts. This questionnaire has strong face validity because the goal of the item selection strategy was to target areas of visual functioning that have been previously identified to be affected by the normal aging process. Because of this orientation, the Visual Activity Questionnaire may have a high false positive rate if used as a screening tool for the detection of eye diseases among elders. This survey consists of 33 items and also has high internal consistency (Cronbach's $\alpha > 0.82$ for all subscales).[41]

To address the absence of a vision-targeted questionnaire with known psychometric properties that could be used for eye diseases other than cataract, the National Eye Institute sponsored a research program to develop such a questionnaire. The questionnaire covers the areas of functioning and well-being identified as important by people with one of five major eye diseases. This National Eye Institute sponsored questionnaire is the first measure of visual functioning to derive items from a formal, multicondition focus group process. Items were derived from a content analysis of the transcripts from 25 focus groups that consisted of 8 to 10 patients with the same chronic eye condition. The conditions represented in the focus groups include age-related cataract, age-related macular degeneration, glaucoma, diabetic retinopathy, and cytomegalovirus retinitis.[45] The 51-item version of this measure, called the NEIVFQ-51, has excellent reliability and validity when used among elders with age-related cataracts, macular degeneration, diabetic retinopathy, or glaucoma.[43] Currently, development of a 25-item version of this measure is underway. Whether this measure will function well as a screening test for the detection of eye diseases or uncorrected refractive error among elders is not known.

INTEGRATION OF MEASURES OF VISUAL FUNCTIONING AND DISABILITY INTO ROUTINE CARE

The published surveys designed to assess visual functioning are all short, and easily administered by interview. Because the majority of the surveys designed to assess visual function were created for those with known eye diseases and some visual impairment, most of these measures have only been used in an interview format. Therefore, little is known about the reliability and validity of these questionnaires when they are self-administered. Clearly, due to cost considerations, questionnaires that can be reliably self-administered have greater potential for integration into routine clinical care or community-based screening programs than measures that require a trained interviewer.

SUMMARY

Whether patient reported descriptions of visual functioning are valuable for the detection of treatable eye conditions in the absence of information from the ophthalmologic examination is not known. Because of the high prevalence of treatable eye conditions that are associated with aging, however, it is clear that persons who report difficulty with visual functioning or other visual complaints should be referred to an appropriately trained vision care provider for a dilated comprehensive ophthalmologic examination. Additionally, because of the high prevalence of asymptomatic chronic eye conditions in this age group, the asymptomatic elder also needs a dilated comprehensive eye examination on at least a biannual basis.[46] Augmentation of the comprehensive ophthalmologic examination with standardized assessments of visual functioning has a clear advantage for the evaluation of cataracts, and may also be useful when evaluating how well pharmacologic treatment for glaucoma is tolerated.[47] Additionally, for people with age-related macular degeneration and end-stage glaucoma or diabetic retinopathy, patient-reported descriptions of visual functioning will identify unmet need for low vision services and need for training in the use of visual aids.

The majority of the published questionnaires that assess visual functioning were designed for those with cataracts and may not adequately capture visual disability from other common eye conditions such as uncorrected refractive error, age-related macular degeneration, or glaucoma. Because of the absence of published data that describe the diagnostic test characteristics of these questionnaires for the detection of chronic and potentially treatable eye conditions, it is not possible to know which of these surveys holds the most promise for being a useful diagnostic tool in nursing home or nonmedical community-based settings. Further research is needed that will assess the sensitivity and specificity of self-report measures as visual screening tools before they can be widely used in nursing homes or community-based settings. Because it is not known how often a questionnaire-based screening strategy, either alone or in combination with an eye chart evaluation, will miss potentially treatable ophthalmologic conditions, currently, the most prudent approach for screening is a regularly scheduled dilated ophthalmologic examination.

REFERENCES

1. Nelson KA. Visual impairment among elderly Americans: statistics in transition. *J Vis Impair Blind.* 1987;81:331–334.
2. National Center for Health Statistics. Refractive status and mobility defects of persons 4–74 years, United States, 1971–1972. *Vital and Health Statistics,* series 11, no. 206. Washington, DC: National Center for Health Statistics, 1978:89–93. Publication no. DHEW (PHS) 78-1654.
3. Stults BM. Preventive health care for the elderly. *West J Med.* 1984; 141:832–845.
4. Tielsch JM, Javitt JC, Coleman A, et al. The prevalence of blindness and visual impairment among nursing home residents in Baltimore. *N Engl J Med.* 1995;332:1205–1209.
5. Owsley C, Sloane M. Vision and aging. *Handbook Neuropsychol.* 1990(4):229–249.
6. Marx MS, Werner P, Cohen-Mansfield J, Feldman R. The relationship between low vision and performance of activities of daily living in nursing home residents. *J Am Geriatr Soc.* 1994;40:1018–1020.
7. Scott IU, Schein OD, West S, Bandeen-Roche K, Enger C, Folstein MF. Functional status and quality of life measurement among ophthalmic patients. *Arch Ophthalmol.* 1994;112:329–335.
8. Carabellese C, Appolonio I, Rozzini R, et al. Sensory impairment and quality of life in a community elderly population. *J Am Geriatr Soc.* 1993;41:401–407.
9. Tinetti ME, Speechley M, Ginter SF. Risk factors for falls among elderly persons living in the community. *N Engl J Med.* 1988;319: 1701–1707.
10. Glynn RJ, Seddon JM, Krug JH et al. Falls in elderly patients with glaucoma. *Arch Ophthalmol.* 1991;109:205–210.
11. Cummings SR, Nevitt MC, Browner WS, et al. Risk factors for hip fractures in white women. *N Engl J Med.* 1995;332:767–773.
12. Ensrud CE, Nevitt MC, Yunis C, et al. Correlates of impaired function in older women. *J Am Geriatr Soc.* 1994;42:481–489.
13. Nevitt MC, Cummings SR, Kidd S, et al. Risk factors for recurrent nonsyncopal falls. A prospective study. *JAMA.* 1989;261:2663–2668.
14. Kelsey JL, Browner WS, Seeley DG, et al. Risk factors for fractures if the distal forearm and proximal humerus. *Am J Epidemiol.* 1992; 135:477–489.
15. Bulpitt CJ, Benos CG, Nicholl AE. Should medical screening of the elderly population be promoted? *Gerontology.* 1990;36:230–245.
16. Beers MH, Fink A, Beck J. Screening recommendations for the elderly. *Am J Public Health.* 1991;81:1131–1140.
17. Kahn HA, Liebowitz HM, Ganley JP, et al. The Framingham Eye Study: outline and major prevalence findings. *Am J Epidemiol.* 1977;106:17–32.
18. Steinberg EP, Javitt JC, Sharkey PD, et al. The content and cost of cataract surgery. *Arch Ophthalmol.* 1993;111:1041–1049.
19. Sommer A, Tielsch JM, Katz J, et al. Racial differences in the cause-specific prevalence of blindness in East Baltimore. *N Engl J Med.* 1991;325:1412–1417.

20. Cincotti A. Evaluation of indications of cataract surgery. *Ophthalmic Surg.* 1979;10:25.

21. Cataract Management Guideline Panel. *Management of Cataract in Adults: Clinical Practice Guideline: Quick Reference Guide for Clinicians,* Number 4. Rockville, MD: U.S. Department of Health and Human Services, Agency for Health Care Policy and Research; February 1993. AHCPR publication 93-0543.

22. *Cataract Surgery: Patient-Reported Data on Appropriateness and Outcomes.* United States General Accounting Office April 1993;3.

23. National Center for Health Statistics. Prevalence of selected chronic conditions, United States, 1979–81. *Vital and Health Statistics,* series 10, no. 155. Washington, DC: Government Printing Office, 1986. Publication no. DHHS (PHS) 86-1583.

24. National Institutes of Health. Vision research—a national plan: 1983–1987. *Report of the Glaucoma Panel,* vol. 2, part 4. Bethesda, MD: Department of Health and Human Services, 1984. Publication no. DHHS (NIH) 84-2474.

25. Klein BEK, Klein R, Sponsel WE, et al. Prevalence of glaucoma, the Beaver Dam Eye Study. *Ophthalmology.* 1992;99:1499–1504.

26. Tielsch JM, Sommer A, Katz J, Royall RM, Quigley HA, Javitt J. Racial variations in the prevalence of primary open-angle glaucoma, the Baltimore Eye Survey. *JAMA.* 1991;266:369–374.

27. Trobe JD. *The Physician's Guide to Eye Care.* American Academy of Ophthalmology, San Francisco, CA; 1993:137–139.

28. Quigley HA, West SK, Munoz B, Mmbaga BBO, Glovinsky Y. Examination methods for glaucoma prevalence surveys. *Arch Ophthalmol.* 1993;111:1409–1415.

29. Klein R, Rowland ML, Harris MI. Racial/ethnic differences in age-related maculopathy. Third National Health Interview Survey. *Ophthalmology.* 1995;102:371–381.

30. Klein R, Wang Q, Klein BEK, Moss SE, Meuer SM. The relationship of age-related maculopathy, cataract, and glaucoma to visual acuity. *Invest Ophthalmol Vis Sci.* 1995;36:182–191.

31. Macular Photocoagulation Study Group. Laser photocoagulation of subfoveal neovascular lesions of age-related macular degeneration. *Arch Ophthalmol.* 1993;111:1200–1209.

32. Early photocoagulation for diabetic retinopathy. ETDRS report number 9. Early Treatment Diabetic Retinopathy Study Research Group. *Ophthalmology.* 1991;98:766–785.

33. American Academy of Ophthalmology, San Francisco, CA: *Diabetic Retinopathy Preferred Practice Patterns.* 1998.

34. National Center for Health Statistics. Refractive status and motility defects of persons 4–74 years, United States, 1971–1972. *Vital and Health Statistics,* series 11, no. 206. Washington, DC: National Center for Health Statistics, 1978:89–93. Publication no. DHEW (PHS) 78-1654.

35. Stults BM. Preventive health care for the elderly. *West J Med.* 1984;141:832–845.

36. Ferris FL, Kassoff A, Bresnick GH, Bailey I. New visual acuity charts for clinical research. *Am J Ophthal.* 1982;94:91–96.

37. Mangione CM, Lee PP, Hays RD. Measurement of visual functioning and health-related quality of life in eye disease and cataract surgery. In: Spilker B, ed. *Quality of Life and Pharmacoeconomics in Clinical Trials.* 2nd ed. New York: Raven Press. 1995;108:1045–1051.

38. Sarks SH, Sarks JP. Age-related macular degeneration: atrophic form. In: Schachat AP, Murphy RP, Patz AP, eds. *Retina.* Vol 2. St Louis, MO: CV Mosby; 1989:152–155.

39. Bernth-Petersen P. Visual functioning in cataract patients—methods for measuring and results. *Acta Ophthalmol.* (Copenh) 1981;59: 198–205.

40. Mangione CM, Phillips RS, Seddon JM, et al. Development of the "Activities of Daily Vision Scale": a measure of visual functional status. *Med Care.* 1992;30:1111–1126.

41. Sloane ME, Ball K, Owsley C, et al. The visual activities questionnaire: developing an instrument for assessing problems in everyday visual tasks. *Tech Dig Noninvas Assess Vis Sys.* 1992;1:26–29.

42. Steinberg EP, Tielsch JM, Schein OD, et al. The VF-14 an index of functional impairment in patients with cataract. *Arch Ophthalmol.* 1994;112:630–638.

43. Mangione CM, Lee PP, Pitts J, et al. Psychometric properties of the National Eye Institute Visual Function Questionnaire (NEI-VFQ). *Arch Ophthalmol.* 1998;116;1496–1504.

44. Bernth-Petersen P. Cataract surgery outcome assessments and epidemiologic aspects. *Acta Ophthalmol.* (Copenh) 1985;63:s174.

45. Mangione CM, Lee PP, Berry SH, et al. Identifying the content area for the 51 item National Eye Institute Visual Function Questionnaire. *Arch Ophthalmol.* 1998;116:227–233.

46. Trobe JD. The Physician's Guide to Eye Care. American Academy of Ophthalmology, San Francisco, CA. 1993:1–13.

47. Lee BL, Gutierrez P, Gordon M, et al. The Glaucoma Symptom Scale: a brief index of glaucoma specific symptoms. *Arch Ophthalmol.* 1998;116:861–866.

C H A P T E R

12

NUTRITIONAL ASSESSMENT

DAVID B. REUBEN

Nutritional assessment falls into two general categories, screening or case-finding for malnutrition and more extensive evaluation of nutritional status. This chapter focuses on screening, case-finding, and the use of commonly available assessment instruments and tests needed to guide most clinical decisions. Although more sophisticated high technology assessments of nutritional status are available, they require equipment that is not available to most clinicians and are primarily used for research purposes.

WHY ASSESS NUTRITION? THE BURDEN OF SUFFERING

When considering the impact of malnutrition on the health of elders, both the prevalence of specific nutritional disorders and the nature and severity of the associated adverse health consequences must be considered. From a public health perspective, the combination of prevalence and health consequences has been termed the "burden of suffering."

Malnutrition among elders is a particularly complex issue because three populations must be considered: community-dwelling, hospitalized, and nursing home elders. Although there is considerable overlap among these three populations, the burden of acute and chronic disease differs among the three groups. In addition, the prevalence and types of disorders vary substantially depending on the definition employed and the population considered. It is

297

useful to consider community-dwelling elders treated in ambulatory settings, hospitalized elders, and elders living in nursing homes separately. For each, the prevalence of specific nutritional disorders and the health consequences are described briefly. The approach to malnutrition is further complicated by the broad range of conditions that this term encompasses, ranging from undernutrition (e.g., protein energy undernutrition) to nutritional excesses (e.g., obesity, hypervitaminosis). This chapter focuses specifically on energy undernutrition, as well as on obesity; thus, vitamin, mineral, and micronutrients are not considered further.

Energy undernutrition states include adult marasmus (energy undernutrition), in which normal serum proteins are maintained, and adult kwashiorkor (protein energy undernutrition). Protein energy undernutrition is defined by the presence of clinical (physical signs such as wasting, low body mass index) *and* biochemical (albumin or other protein) evidence of insufficient intake. Obesity has been defined variably by different organizations. Traditionally, thresholds for overweight have been body mass index (BMI) exceeding 27.8 for men and 27.3 for women. Recently, however, the threshold has been revised such that BMI of 25–29.9 is considered overweight and BMI of 30 or higher is considered obese.

Community-Based Population

Among community-dwelling elders, if energy undernutrition is defined as having a body weight of less than 45.4 kg (100 lb), slightly more than 3 percent of those age 60 years or older may be affected.[1] If it is defined by caloric or nutrient intake, 37 percent to 40 percent of elderly community-dwelling men and women (those age 65 and over) report energy intakes less than two thirds of the recommended daily allowance (RDA).[2] Although other surveys have suggested that 30 percent of community-dwelling elders have energy intakes below the RDA, the same surveys indicate that protein intake has generally been above the RDA. It should be noted, however, that recommended dietary allowances should not used as a criterion standard for assessing individual nutritional adequacy; rather, they are a population standard. Moreover, RDAs do not acknowledge different nutrient requirements for persons over 65 years of age compared to younger persons. Adipose mass and body weight are subnormal in fewer than 5 percent of community-dwelling elders.[3]

Body weight and weight loss have been identified as important nutritional measures. Although some studies have identified low body mass as a predictor of increased risk of mortality, a history of weight loss from middle to old age may be more important than actual low body weight *per se*. An analysis of data from the Established Populations for Epidemiologic Studies of the Elderly (EPESE) noted that after exclusion of participants who lost more than 10 percent of their weight after age 50 years and adjustment for health status, the higher risk of death associated with low weight was eliminated.[4]

Objectively determined weight change has prognostic significance. In one sample of elders admitted to a geriatric rehabilitation unit, weight loss (derived from medical records) predicted whether complications would develop on the unit and 1-year mortality.[5, 6] A VA study defined 4 percent weight loss over 1 year as having the best test characteristics (sensitivity and specificity) in predicting subsequent mortality during a 2-year follow-up period; 28 percent of those with involuntary weight loss died compared to 11 percent of those without weight loss.[7] In that study, the annual incidence of involuntary weight loss of 4 percent or more was 13.1 percent.

Serum albumin also has predictive validity for 3, 5, and 9 to 10 year mortality in community-dwelling older persons.[8–10] In the EPESE study, older men with albumin levels of 35 g/L had an adjusted relative risk of 5.3 for all-cause mortality within 1 year compared to those with levels greater than 43 g/L; for women the relative risk was 4.9. Moreover, this risk was greatly increased in persons with mobility disorders or disability in activities of daily living, or both.[9] Among community-dwelling elders, the combination of low serum albumin and low serum cholesterol predicts even greater risk of subsequent functional decline or mortality.[11]

The prevalence of overweight increases with age between the ages of 22 to 55 years, but then stabilizes in women and declines in men. The percentage of overweight (BMI 25–29.9) people in the 65 to 74 year old age range remains substantial, however, at about 44% in men and about 34% in women. Older African Americans, Latinas, and poor women have higher rates of overweight.

Data on the risks associated with obesity in elders are less consistent than for those for undernutrition. A substantial body of evidence links overweight to hypertension, hypercholesterolemia, heart disease, insulin resistance and diabetes, cholelithiasis, respiratory impairment, gout, and arthritis. The relation between obesity and occurrence rates of specific diseases or overall mortality in persons over 65, however, has received limited study. There is some evidence that the obesity-associated relative risk of disease occurrence is less in older than in younger persons. Moreover, several cohort studies have demonstrated that high BMI does not predict mortality, and that it may even be protective against early death in older persons.[12–14] Other studies indicate that obesity is related to the development of functional impairment.[15, 16] In addi-

> Low serum albumin is a simple sign of potential malnutrition.

> Unexplained weight loss is a greater risk than mild to moderate obesity.

tion, overweight is newly emerging as a protective factor for hip fracture (independent of its relation to bone density); thus, perhaps unique to elders, benefits versus risks of weight reduction should be analyzed.

Hospitalized Older Persons

In hospitalized patients, the prevalence of malnutrition is considerably higher than that in community-based samples; prevalence estimates usually range from 35 percent to 65 percent. A Department of Veterans Affairs (DVA) case series defined malnutrition as meeting two of the following four measures: (1) weight/height percent < 90 percent of normal; (2) mid-arm muscle circumference < 90 percent of normal; (3) albumin < 3.5 g/dL; and (4) transferrin < 200 mg/dL. Of patients 65 years of age or older 61 percent met this criterion compared to 28 percent of those younger than 65 years.[17] Sixty-four percent of those who met this criterion for malnutrition had infections during their illness (compared to 26 percent of those who were not malnourished) and 28 percent died (compared to 4 percent who were not malnourished). A Norwegian case series identified 55 percent of medical inpatients aged 70 years or older who were admitted to a medical ward as having weight/height ratios less than 90 percent of the expected values.[18]

Among hospitalized elders, the health consequences of malnutrition can be profound. Several markers of malnutrition in hospitalized elders, including low body mass index, low serum albumin, and hospital-acquired hypocholesterolemia, have been associated with adverse outcomes. Low serum albumin in hospitalized elders (measured at various times during the hospitalization) predicts a higher rate of in-hospital complications, longer hospital stays, more frequent readmissions, in-hospital mortality, and increased mortality at 90 days and 1 year.[19] When considering mortality, the lower the albumin level, the higher the risk of death. Serum prealbumin has also been studied as a prognostic factor among hospitalized elders. In a study of hip fracture, patients who had complications did not show improvement in prealbumin (or albumin) during their hospitalization, whereas those without complications did.[20] Among nursing home residents who were hospitalized, severe hypoprealbuminemia predicted extended hospitalization, but not mortality.[21]

Data from hospitalized elders also support the prognostic importance of a drop in serum cholesterol levels during the hospitalization. In a case-control study, elders whose cholesterol fell from 160 mg/dL or higher, to 120 mg/dL or lower during hospitalization had more infectious and noninfectious complications. Length of stay was nearly 3 times as long; and mortality was higher in the

Acute hospitalization can lead to the development of malnutrition.

acquired hypocholesterolemia group, though not significantly.[22] In that study, approximately 10 percent of elders who were hospitalized experienced a drop in cholesterol of that magnitude.

Institutionalized Elders

A summary of 14 surveys of nutritional status conducted among the chronically institutionalized elders concluded that only 5 percent to 18 percent of residents had energy intakes below the RDA but up to 30 percent consumed less than 0.8 g protein/kg body weight per day and 15 percent to 60 percent had substandard mid-arm muscle circumference, serum albumin, or both.[3] In a study conducted in one Canadian nursing home, a rating system based on 7 anthropometric measurements identified severe undernutrition in 18 percent of residents, moderate undernutrition in 27 percent, and mild/moderate overnutrition in 18 percent.[23] Data from 26 DVA nursing homes indicated that 12 percent of residents had body weight less than 80 percent of standard and 28 percent had albumin levels less than 3.5 g/dL.[24]

Serum cholesterol has also been identified as a possible nutritional measure among nursing home residents. In a study at a DVA nursing home, a variety of demographic and nutrition-related variables were used to predict 1-year mortality, in multivariate analysis, only serum cholesterol and hematocrit remained significant. The authors reported a "mortality risk index" using the equation: 0.1 (cholesterol) + (hematocrit) < 60 with specificity of 85 percent and sensitivity of 90 percent.[3]

EFFECTIVENESS OF CURRENTLY AVAILABLE NUTRITIONAL ASSESSMENT INSTRUMENTS

In addition to considering the burden of suffering, the value of nutritional assessment (particularly when considering screening) is contingent on its potential effectiveness. To be effective, the nutrition assessment must be accurate, and those identified as having nutritional problems should benefit from intervention. Screening tests and assessments that detect problems for which there is no effective treatment are of little or no benefit.

The remainder of this chapter focuses on nutritional assessments that can be conducted by the primary care provider in a variety of settings. These assessments include short questionnaires (either self-administered or interviewer-administered), anthropometric measures, subjective assessments by health care providers, short measures of food intake (both whole diet and nutrient-specific), specific biochemical tests, and multimethod techniques.

Nutritional Risk Factors

The most important risk factors for poor dietary quality include low income, social isolation, level of stress, poor appetite, visual impairment, and medical illness. The assessment of food security (defined as stable, sustainable access in socially acceptable ways to enough food of sufficient quality to lead a healthy life) is emerging as a central concern in nutritional assessment and surveillance. Indicators to assess hunger or food insufficiency have been developed and validated. Currently, however, most food sufficiency information is limited to that collected by consumer advocacy groups, which tends to be anecdotal and qualitative.

An assessment kit (Table 12-1), designed in the United Kingdom for use by social workers to detect nutritional neediness among the homebound, utilizes ten risk factors: fewer than eight main meals a week; less than one half pint of milk per day; little or no fruit and vegetable intake; wastage of food even if supplied; long periods of the day without food; depression or loneliness; unexpected weight change or loss; shopping difficulties; low income; and indications of disabilities (including alcoholism).[25]

Other risk factors include chronic diseases that can affect appetite and interfere with the ability to chew, digest, or absorb food. Chronic diseases can also affect nutrition through medication–nutrient interactions.

Formal instruments to assess risk factors for nutritional disorders have yet to be developed. In their absence, health care providers may wish to probe for the answers to the questions in Table 12-2.

TABLE 12-1. DETECTION OF NUTRITIONAL NEEDS
Fewer than eight main meals a week
Less than one-half pint of milk per day
Little or no fruit and vegetable intake
Wastage of food
Long periods of the day without food
Depression or loneliness
Unexpected weight change or loss
Shopping difficulties
Low income
Indications of disabilities

TABLE 12-2. RISK FACTOR QUESTIONS
Does economic status pose a barrier?
Is food of sufficiently high nutritional quality available?
Are there dental problems that prohibit ingesting foods?
Do medical illnesses interfere with the digestion or absorption of foods or cause additional nutritional requirements?
Do limitations in functional capacity interfere?
Do food preferences or cultural beliefs interfere?
Does the individual have a good appetite?
Does the individual have high levels of stress or depressive symptoms?

Nutritional Intake Measures

There are four major methods for measuring dietary intake of energy and nutrients. These are diet recall, diet record, diet history, and food frequency questionnaires.[19]

DIET RECALL

A diet recall is performed by asking participants to recollect the foods that they have ingested during a given time frame, usually 24 hours; therefore, it measures current dietary intake. Memory-related measurement error can occur. Respondent burden is modest; most individuals require about 20 minutes to complete a 24-hour or previous-day diet recall. Data entry can be time-consuming, however, and, in general, best results are obtained when nutritionists perform this task. For the purpose of estimating mean nutrient intake for a group, the 24-hour recall appears to perform as well as actual food weighing or longer periods of diary recording.

Intra-individual (day-to-day and other time-related) variation in diet, however, makes a single 24-hour recall inappropriate for estimation of an individual's customary intake. The number of 24-hour recalls or records required to approximate the average value derived from all the recalls or records varies greatly depending on the dietary component measured.

FOOD RECORDS

Food records are more burdensome for subjects than diet recalls. During a specified time frame, participants record all the food they eat; the amounts can be estimated or weighed by the subjects. Respondent burden is high, and although the recording should be done contemporaneously, many participants complete the record at the end of the day, leading to potential memory-related error.

Similar to diet recall, data entry requires expertise and is fairly time consuming. Individual food records suffer the same shortcomings as individual 24-hour recalls, due to the instability of daily diet.

DIET HISTORY

Diet histories are performed by interviewers and consist of open-ended questions that attempt to ascertain the participant's usual intake of food. They require at least an hour to complete and highly trained personnel to administer. Advantages include the ability to assist the participant in considering seasonal variations in food, and to account for ethnic foods not generally included on standard survey instruments. Diet histories are impractical as screening tools.

FOOD FREQUENCY QUESTIONNAIRES

Food frequency questionnaires (FFQ) attempt to estimate the customary dietary intake over a specified period of time (e.g., 1 year). Participants report on their usual frequency and portion size of various foods from a predetermined list. FFQs that measure the complete diet can include more than 100 items and take up to an hour to complete. Limited FFQs, intended to measure the usual intake of certain nutrients, such as calcium, vitamin A, and vitamin E, have also been developed. These are much shorter (average food item list is roughly 20) and thus, less time consuming. Food frequency questionnaires are useful to estimate nutrient intakes among groups of persons and to rank subjects in relation to nutrient intakes but not for screening of individual participants.

Self-Report Brief Screening Instruments

NUTRITION SCREENING INITIATIVE

The American Academy of Family Physicians, the American Dietetic Association, and the National Council on Aging, Inc. have developed a tiered approach to nutrition screening, the Nutrition Screening Initiative (NSI) checklist. The first tier consists of a checklists for older Americans and/or their caregivers to complete. Those who are identified at risk of poor nutritional status based on the checklist are eligible for level I screening, which is designed for any setting in which older Americans come into contact with professionals in the health care and social service system. Included at this level screen are height and weight (and calculated body mass index) as well as questions about 10 pound weight gain or loss within 6 months, eating habits, living environment, and functional status. Level II screening is designed to obtain more diagnostic information in clinical settings. Included are anthropometric measurements (body mass index, mid-arm circumference, mid-arm muscle circumference, and triceps skin fold); laboratory data (serum albumin and cholesterol); and information on therapeutic drug use, clinical problems that might affect eating, eating habits, living environment, functional status, and cognitive and affective status.

Based on review by the NSIs technical review committee, a checklist score of 6 was selected for identifying elders at high nutritional risk. An estimated 24 percent of all Medicare beneficiaries would fall into this high-risk group. In a validation study, those at high risk were more likely to have been hospitalized overnight during the past year. Using the cut-point of 6 to predict inadequate nutrient intake (3 or more nutrients below 75 percent of RDA) on a single 24-hour recall, the sensitivity, specificity, and positive predictive value of the NSI checklist was 36 percent, 85 percent, and 38 percent; using the same cut-point, the comparable test-characteristics to predict perceived fair or poor health status were 46 percent, 85 percent, and 56 percent (see Appendix #33).[26]

Other studies have evaluated the cross-sectional and longitudinal predictive validity of NSI checklist items. A cross-sectional study of rural elders found that only a few of the NSI checklist items were independently associated with functional status limitation or average monthly charges for medical care.[27] A longitudinal study found that several individual items predicted 8-to-12 year mortality, but the summary score for the entire instrument had a considerably lower predictive value than the individual items.[28]

Anthropometric Measures

Anthropometric measures have long been used in assessing nutritional status and reference values derived from elderly white persons have been published. Anthropometric measures can be used in two ways to assess nutritional status, either monitoring change in a measure for an individual or comparing a person's value to reference normal (or malnourished) values. The most widely used anthropometric indices are height, weight, and the derived body mass index (BMI) (kg/m^2). Because of narrowing of intervertebral disk spaces and osteoporotic vertebral fractures, measured height may not be accurate for calculation of BMI in elders and in some situations, they may be unable to stand to have height measured. In these cases, total arm length and armspan have been used as proxies.

Measures such as midarm circumference and skin folds have long been used in research and in some clinical settings to identify elders with malnutrition. Because triceps skin fold thickness spans a wide range among normal individuals, sequential changes in the same individual can be more valuable than one-time measurements.[29] Measurement error increases, however, with size of skin fold, and inter- and intra-observer variation may be large.[30] Moreover, these anthropometric measurements suffer from poorer reliability in elders compared to younger participants, even among experienced researchers. This is due, in part, to the difficulties in accurately locating anatomic landmarks and age-related changes in skin elasticity.[31] For example, a triceps skin fold measurement taken at the level of the midarm can vary by as much as 150 percent from a measurement taken only 1 to 2 centimeters above or below this point.[31] With aging, a smaller proportion of total body fat is subcutaneous; therefore, skin fold thickness is less likely to indicate total body fat in older compared to younger persons.

Biochemical and Laboratory Measures

PROTEIN STATUS

The most commonly used biochemical indicators of protein status are serum proteins that are synthesized in the liver. As measures of nutritional status, serum proteins vary in their degree of specificity for malnutrition across care settings. For example, changes in serum protein among hospitalized older persons can be more reflective of inflammation and the acute phase reaction than of malnutrition *per se*, whereas such changes *may* be more likely to indicate protein-energy malnutrition in community-dwelling elders. In addition, nursing home residents can have chronic inflammation, which complicates the diagnosis and management of malnutrition. Nevertheless, changes in these traditional indicators frequently have prognostic and clinical meaning and are, therefore, considered in this chapter.

Serum albumin is the best studied serum protein. As mentioned previously, it has been shown to have prognostic value for subsequent mortality and morbidity but, it has several limitations. A relatively large extravascular pool provides a buffer in the acute states of deprivation; thus, albumin is a better indicator of chronic protein status and generally does not fall unless undernutrition is moderately severe and prolonged, or accompanied by trauma, sepsis, or significant infection. The latter events alone (without protein deprivation) also cause a fall in serum albumin, leading some to suggest that low serum albumin levels in acute care settings should be regarded more as a negative acute-phase reactant than a direct measure of protein status. Because serum albumin does not fall quickly in protein deprivation, it can be quite a useful indicator for chronic moderate to severe undernutrition. A recent study identified risk factors for hypoalbuminemia among community-dwelling elders included the following: age 65 years or greater, being on welfare, having a condition interfering with eating, vomiting 3 or more days per month, previous surgery for a gastrointestinal tumor, heart failure, recurring cough attacks, feeling tired or worn-out, poor teeth condition, little or no exercise, low salt diet, and current smoking.[32]

Proteins with shorter half-lives and smaller body pools, such as retinol-binding protein and thyroxine-binding prealbumin may be better suited to monitor nutritional status during acute illness and convalescence. Prealbumin has been highly correlated with serum albumin and has also been shown to predict in-hospital mortality[33] and its half-life of 48 hours allows it to be a sensitive measure of early response to treatment.

SERUM CHOLESTEROL

Recently, low or falling serum cholesterol has been explored as a nutritional marker. Some cases of hypocholesterolemia, however, may not be nutritionally mediated. Recent reports support the hypotheses that on-going inflammation and proinflammatory cytokines, particularly IL-6, may be responsible for acquired hypocholesterolemia.[34]

Multimethod Techniques

Several instruments have used patient-report, anthropometrics, health care provider subjective assessment, laboratory values, and skin tests in combination to assess nutritional status. A frequently employed approach is to analyze data obtained by administering large batteries of questions, anthropometric measures, dietary intake measures, and laboratory values and then examining bivariate associations and multivariable models for determining test characteristics. Most often, these studies have been conducted in selected subpopulations of hospitalized persons.

SUBJECTIVE GLOBAL ASSESSMENT

The Subjective Global Assessment (SGA) relies on items from the patient history, physical examination findings, and the health care provider's overall judgment of a person's global nutritional status.[35] Historical items include: (1) weight loss within the previous 6 months and whether there has been any recent change (within the previous 2 weeks); (2) dietary intake relative to usual intake, with classifications of duration and degree of deviations; (3) presence of persistent (greater than 2 weeks) gastrointestinal symptoms;

(4) functional capacity, with duration and degree of incapacity classified; and (5) an assessment of the metabolic demand of the patient's primary diagnosis. Five components of the physical examination (loss of subcutaneous fat, muscle wasting, ankle edema, sacral edema, and ascites) are subjectively graded from 0 (normal) to 3+ (severe). Finally, the overall SGA ranking (normal, mildly malnourished, significantly malnourished) is determined, again subjectively, with instructions for raters to place most of their judgment on weight loss, poor dietary intake, loss of subcutaneous tissue, and muscle wasting (Table 12-3). The instrument has been administered by research nurses, nurse practitioners, and physicians who had substantial training in use of the instrument. Interrater reliability has been high, but appears to be higher when examining younger compared to older patients.[35, 36] Overall SGA rankings are most highly correlated with subjective estimates of loss of subcutaneous fat and muscle wasting.

Reports describing the validity of SGA have focused primarily on selected populations (e.g., younger persons who are admitted to surgical wards for major gastrointestinal surgery, dialysis patients). In these studies, SGA has demonstrated construct validity and was predictive of surgical complications.[37, 38] Despite showing some promise, several aspects of SGA limit its potential use as a screening method for elders. First, it requires a trained health care provider to administer. Second, its administration requires that patients undress and be turned, resulting in administration times that are likely to be too long for mass screening even in hospitalized patients, unless incorporated into an admission history and physical examination. Finally, the test's performance may differ substantially in populations with lower disease prevalence, such as community-dwelling elders. Nevertheless, SGA may prove valuable as a secondary assessment by a health care provider and may prove valuable in monitoring elders. The instrument's sensitivity to changes, however, has yet to be determined.

TABLE 12-3.   COMPONENTS OF SUBJECTIVE GLOBAL ASSESSMENT

Weight loss within the previous 6 months and change within previous 2 weeks
Dietary intake relative to usual, with classifications of duration and degree of deviations
Presence of persistent (> 2 weeks) gastrointestinal symptoms
Functional capacity, with duration and degree of incapacity classified
Assessment of the metabolic demand of the patient's primary diagnosis
Physical examination findings of malnutrition
An overall subjective ranking of nutritional status

MINI-NUTRITIONAL ASSESSMENT

The Mini-Nutritional Assessment (MNA) is an 18-item instrument requiring 20 minutes to complete. It incorporates several anthropometric measures, dietary intake questions, and health and functional status questions (see Appendix #30). The developers used discriminant analysis techniques applied to several cross-sectional samples to establish cut-points for being "at risk" of malnutrition and being undernourished. The instrument has been validated against clinical judgment of nutritional status, dietary intake, and biochemical measures.[39] Predictive validity for weight loss, the occurrence of acute disease, and need of assistance has been demonstrated in a Danish study.[40]

PROGNOSTIC NUTRITIONAL INDEX

The Prognostic Nutritional Index (PNI) was derived using stepwise regression and discriminant analysis methods from a set of 161 patients who had nutritional assessment on admission prior to major elective general surgery. PNI is reported as the risk (0–100, with 100 being highest risk) of developing a complication based on an equation that includes albumin, triceps skinfold, serum transferrin, and cutaneous delayed hypersensitivity to mumps, streptokinase-streptodornase, or *Candida*. PNI scores have been trichotomized into high risk, intermediate risk, and low risk. Thirty-three percent of high risk patients died during the hospitalization compared to 3 percent who were at low risk.[41] Sepsis, major sepsis, and all complications were similarly significantly increased in those at high risk. Using a cut-point of 50 or more, sensitivity of the PNI was 86 percent and specificity was 69 percent for in-hospital mortality; using a cut-point of more than 40 the values are 93 percent and 44 percent, respectively.

HOSPITAL PROGNOSTIC INDEX

The Hospital Prognostic Index (HPI) was derived from medical and surgical hospitalzed persons (mean age 59) who received consultations for metabolic and nutritional support. Discriminant function equations were generated to predict subsequent sepsis and in hospital mortality. Cancer diagnosis and serum transferrin level were predictive of subsequent sepsis (sensitivity of the equation was 65 percent and specificity was 61 percent). Serum albumin level, cutaneous delayed hypersensitivity response, concurrent sepsis, and cancer were predictive of in-hospital mortality (sensitivity 74 percent, specificity 66 percent).[43]

OTHER METHODS USED IN ASSESSING HOSPITALIZED PATIENTS

Several other methods have been used to gauge nutritional status among hospitalized patients but are used less frequently.[38] These have predictive validity for complications during the hospitalization, though are less are less valuable once diseases and measures of disease severity were also considered.

The Nutritional Risk Index uses serum albumin and the ratio of actual to usual weight according to the following equation.

Nutritional Risk Index = $(1.489 \times$ serum albumin, g/L$) + 41.7 \times$ (present weight/usual weight ≥ 6 months prior to admission)

A score of more than 100 indicates no malnutrition, 97.5–100 indicates mild malnutrition, 83.5 to 97.4 indicates moderate malnutrition, and less than 83.5 indicates severe malnutrition.

The Maastricht Index uses serum albumin, prealbumin, blood lymphocyte count, and percentage of ideal body weight according to the following equation.

Maastricht Index = $20.68 - (0.24 \times$ albumin, g/L$) - (19.21 \times$ prealbumin, g/L$) - (1.86 \times$ lymphocytes, 10^6/L$) - (0.04 \times$ ideal weight).

Those with an Index score greater than 0 are considered malnourished.

IMPLEMENTING NUTRITIONAL ASSESSMENT INTO PRACTICE SETTINGS

Formal studies demonstrating the value of routine nutritional assessment in office, hospital, and nursing home settings have not been conducted. Furthermore, despite the availability and current usage of nutritional screening instruments and methods in ambulatory, hospital, and nursing home populations of elders, there is little evidence to support nutritional screening. Accordingly, the decision of when to conduct nutritional assessment must follow clinical judgment rather than established guidelines.

Community-Based Practice

At the time of the initial visit, patients should be asked about involuntary weight loss. Patients should be weighed at this and all subsequent visits. It is also reasonable to measure height yearly so that changes in body mass index can be determined. Self-administered screens like the Nutrition Screening Initiative checklist can be administered in waiting rooms or mailed to patients to complete prior to the visit. These instruments can provide additional insight into potential nutritional problems but their limitations must be recognized. Currently used dietary assessment methods do not appear to be promising as office assessments because of daily intra-individual variations, respondent burden, and training needed for interviewers. Brief food frequency questionnaires that can be entered into personal computers may eventually be clinically valuable. Among biochemical measures, low levels of serum albumin and cholesterol can identify severe chronic undernutrition but the yield may be quite low. Hence, their use should be guided by clinical indications rather than as a routine assessment.

Hospital Settings

Hospitalizations in elders are sentinel events that frequently change the course of their health. Frequently, the acute events precipitating hospital admissions and complications that prolong hospital stays are overwhelming, even for elders with adequate nutritional status prior to hospitalization. Thus, in hospital settings, more acute measures of nutritional status, such as serum proteins and cholesterol, may hold more promise as assessment methods than self-reports of previous dietary habits. For patients undergoing elective surgery, Subjective Global Assessment can provide a good idea of preoperative nutritional status. For those who are already malnourished or are at risk of malnutrition because of thin body habitus, poor dietary intake while hospitalized, or low serum albumin, monitoring of dietary intake and shorter half-life proteins (e.g., serum prealbumin) can be valuable in assessing response to treatment such as nutritional supplements or enteral or parenteral feedings.

Institutional Settings

The nursing home population is different from community-dwelling and hospitalized elders for a number of reasons. First, the locus of control of dietary intake is no longer solely with the individual but shifts to a partnership with the institution, which provides meals and assistance with feeding, if necessary. Second, the potential health outcomes of malnutrition are more difficult to define and operationalize. For example, the decision of whether or not to hospitalize a nursing home resident may depend more on the services that can be provided at that institution, and the resident's and family's wishes for level of aggressiveness of care, than on the type or severity of the acute illness. Finally, for this population, the ability to intervene and improve health outcomes will be more difficult because of disease processes (e.g., dementia) that are already in motion, and frequently were the factors that precipitated institutionalization. The Minimum Data Set has items that assess oral problems, height and weight, weight loss of 5 percent within the last 30 and 180 days, dietary behavior and intake, and a rating of oral and dental status.[44] Based on responses to these items, resident assessment protocols (RAPs) may be triggered leading to more comprehensive assessment and treatment. Measurement of cholesterol and albumin is appropriate for those whom the MDS questions raise suspicion of undernutrition.

SUMMARY

This chapter provides ample assessment instruments that are all in the early stages of development and use. So far, there is no evidence that interventions triggered by them lead to better outcomes. Therefore, the author has reserved recommendations for use of instruments to the discretion of the reader. The instruments that appear in the Appendix were selected by the editors.

REFERENCES

1. Manson A, Shea S. Malnutrition in elderly ambulatory medical patients. *Am J Public Health.* 1991;81:1195–1197.
2. Ryan AS, Craig LD, Finn SC. Nutrient intakes and dietary patterns of older Americans: a national study. *J Gerontol A Biol Sci: Med Sci.* 1992;47:M145–M150.
3. Rudman D, Feller AG. Protein-calorie undernutrition in the nursing home. *J Am Geriatr Soc.* 1989;37:173–183.
4. Losconczy KG, Harris TB, Cornoni-Huntley J, et al. Does weight loss from middle age to old age explain the inverse weight mortality relation in old age? *Am J Epidemiol.* 1995;141:312–321.
5. Sullivan DH, Patch GA, Walls RC, Lipschitz DA. Impact of nutrition status on morbidity and mortality in a select population of geriatric rehabilitation patients. *Am J Clin Nutr.* 1990;51:749–758.
6. Sullivan DH, Walls RC, Lipschitz DA. Protein-energy undernutrition and the risk of mortality within 1 year of hospital dischrge in a select population of geriatric rehabilitation patients. *Am J Clin Nutr.* 1991;53:599–605.
7. Wallace JI, Schwartz RS, La Croix AZ, Uhlmann RF, Pearlman RA. Involuntary weight loss in older outpatients: incidence and clinical significance. *J Am Geriatr Soc.* 1995;43:329–337.
8. Klonoff-Cohen H, Barrett-Connor EL, Edelstein SL. Albumin levels as a predictor of mortality in the healthy elderly. *J Clin Epidemiol.* 1992;45:207–212.

9. Corti M-C, Guralnik JM, Salive ME, Sorkin JD. Serum albumin level and physical disability as predictors of mortality in older persons. *JAMA*. 1994;272:1036–1042.

10. Sahyoun NR, Jacques PF, Dallal G, Russell RM. Use of albumin as a predictor of mortality in community-dwelling and institutionalized elderly populations. *J Clin Epidemiol*. 1996;49:981–988.

11. Reuben DB, Ix JH, Greendale GA, Seeman TE. The predictive value of combined hypoalbuminemia and hypocholesterolemia in high functioning community-dwelling older persons: MacArthur studies of successful aging. *J Am Geriatr Soc*. 1999;47:402–406.

12. Diehr P, Bild DE, Harris TB, et al. Body mass index and mortality in nonsmoking older adults: the Cardiovascular Health Study. *Am J Public Health*. 1998;88:623–629.

13. Stevens J, Cai J, Pamuk ER, Williamson DF, Thun MJ, Wood JL. The effect of age on the association between body-mass index and mortality. *N Engl J Med*. 1998;338:1–7.

14. Fried LP, Kronmal RA, Newman AB, et al. Risk factors for 5-year mortality in older adults. *JAMA*. 1998;279:585–592.

15. Galanos AN, Pieper CF, Cornoni-Huntley JC, Bales CW, Fillenbaum GG. Nutrition and function: is there a relationship between body mass index and the functional capabilities of community-dwelling elderly? *J Am Geriatr Soc*. 1994;42:368–373.

16. Vita AJ, Terry RB, Hubert HB, Fries JF. Aging, health risks, and cumulative disability. *N Engl J Med*. 1998;338:1035–1041.

17. Bienia R, Ratcliff S, Barbour GL, Kummer M. Malnutrition in the hospitalized geriatric patient. *J Am Geriatr Soc*. 1982;30:433–436.

18. Mowe M, Bohmer T. The prevalence of undiagnosed protein-calorie undernutrition in a population of hospitalized elderly patients. *J Am Geriatr Soc*. 1991;39:1089–1092.

19. Reuben DB, Greendale GA, Harrison GG. Nutrition screening in older persons. *J Am Geriatr Soc*. 1995;43:415–425.

20. Patterson BM, Cornell CN, Carbone B, Levine B, Chapman D. Protein depletion and metabolic stress in elderly patients who have a fracture of the hip. *J Bone Joint Surg*. 1992;74-A:251–260.

21. Ferguson RP, O'Connor P, Crabtree B, et al. Serum albumin and prealbumin as predictors of clinical outcomes of hospitalized elderly nursing home residents. *J Am Geriatr Soc*. 1993;41:545–549.

22. Noel MA, Smith TK, Ettinger WH. Characteristics and outcomes of hospitalized older patients who develop hypocholesterolemia. *J Am Geriatr Soc*. 1991;39:455–461.

23. Keller, HH. Malnutrition in institutionalized elderly: how and why? *J Am Geriatr Soc*. 1993;41:1212–1218.

24. Abbasi AA, Rudman D. Observations on the prevalence of protein-calories undernutrition in VA nursing homes. *J Am Geriatr Soc*. 1993;41:117–121.

25. Davies L. Nutrition and the elderly: identifying those at risk. *Proc Nutr Soc*. 1984;43:295–302.

26. Posner BM, Jette AM, Smith KW, Miller DR. Nutrition and health risks in the elderly: the nutrition screening initiative. *Am J Public Health*. 1993;83(7):973–978.

27. Jensen GL, Kita K, Fish J, Heydt D, Frey C. Nutrition risk screening characteristics of rural older persons: relation to functional limitations and health care charges. *Am J Clin Nutr.* 1997;66:819–828.

28. Sahyoun NR, Jacques PF, Dallal GE, Russell RM. Nutrition Screening Initiative checklist may be a better awareness/educational tool than a screening one. *J Am Diet Assoc.* 1997;97:760–764.

29. Shenkin A, Cederblad G, Elia M, Isaksson B. Laboratory assessment of protein-energy status. *Clin Chim Acta.* 1996;253:S5–S59.

30. Fuller NJ, Jebb SA, Goldberg GR, et al. Inter-observer variability in the measurement of body composition. *Eur J Clin Nutr.* 1991; 45:43–49.

31. Sullivan DH, Patch GA, Baden AL, Lipschitz DA. An approach to assessing the reliability of anthropometrics in elderly patients. *J Am Geriatr Soc.* 1989;37:607–613.

32. Reuben DB, Moore AA, Damesyn M, Keeler E, Harrison GG, Greendale G. Correlates of hypoalbuminemia in community-dwelling older persons. *Am J Clin Nutr.* 1997;66:38–45.

33. Fulop T, Herrmann F, Rapin CH. Prognostic role of serum albumin and prealbumin levels in elderly patients at admission to a geriatric hospital. *Arch Gerontol Geriatr.* 1991;12:31–39.

34. Ettinger WH, Harris T, Verdery RB, Tracy R, Kouba E. Evidence for inflammation as a cause of hypocholesterolemia in older people. *J Am Geriatr Soc.* 1995;43:264–266.

35. Detsky AS, McLaughlin JR, Baker JP, et al. What is subjective global assessment of nutritional status? *JPEN.* 1987;11:8–13.

36. Anna-Christina E, Unosson M, Larsson J, Ganowiak W, Jurulf P. Interrater variability and validity in subjective nutritional assessment of elderly patients. *Scan J Caring Sci.* 1996;10:163–168.

37. Jeejeebhoy KN, Detsky AS, Baker JP. Assessment of nutritional status. *J Paren Ent Nutr.* 1990;14:193S–196S.

38. Naber THJ, Schermer T, de Bree A, et al. Prevalence of malnutrition in nonsurgical hospitalized patients and its association with disease complications. *Am J Clin Nutr.* 1997;66:1232–1239.

39. Guigoz Y, Velas BJ, Garry PJ. The Mini Nutritional Assessment (MNA): a practical assessment tool for grading the nutritional state of elderly patients. *Facts and Research in Gerontology 1994* (suppl. 2). New York, NY: Springer Publishing Co; 1994:

40. Beck AM, Ovesen LF. The predictive capacity of the Mini Nutritional Assessment method. *Ugeskr Laeger* 1997;159:6377–6381.

41. Buzby GP, Mullen JL, Matthews DC, Hobbs CL, Rosato EF. Prognostic nutritional index in gastrointestinal surgery. *Am J Surg.* 1980;139:160–67.

42. Dempsey DT, Mullen JL. Prognostic value of nutritional indices. *J Paren Ent Nutr.* 1987;11:109S–114S.

43. Harvey KB, Moldwer LL, Bistrian BR, Blackburn GL. Biological measures for the formulation of a hospital prognostic index. *Am J Clin Nutr.* 1981;34:2013–2022.

44. Morris JN, Hawes C, Murphy K, et al. *Resident Assessment Instrument Training Manual and Resource Guide.* Natick MA: Eliot Press; 1991.

PRESSURE ULCERS

BARBARA BATES-JENSEN

Pressure ulcers are areas of local tissue trauma usually developing where soft tissues are compressed between bony prominences and external surfaces for prolonged periods. The mechanical injury to the skin and tissues causes hypoxia and ischemia, leading to tissue necrosis. The chronic recalcitrant nature of pressure ulcers is a frustration for health care providers because of the time and resources that are often invested in the management of these wounds. Pressure ulcers are a pervasive and resource-draining problem for all health care settings. In acute care, the incidence has been reported as high as 29.5 percent, with prevalence ranging from 10.1 percent to 29.5 percent.[1-3] Long-term care facilities have higher rates of pressure sore development, with prevalence reported at 23 percent and incidence at 1 year of facility residency of 13.2 percent, rising to 21.6 percent during the second year in the facility.[4-6] Community home health incidence has ranged from 16.5 percent to 20 percent with prevalence in one community home health setting at 29 percent.[7-8]

Pressure ulcers are costly. The estimated mean hospital charge for a patient admitted with a primary diagnosis of pressure ulcer was $21,675, with estimated physician charges of $2,900 per case for 1992.[9] Estimated charges for secondary diagnosis of pressure ulcer using hip fracture as the primary diagnosis were $10,986, with associated physician charges of $1,200 per case.[9] Total annual estimated national health care expenditure is $1.3 billion.[9] The cost of treatment increases as the severity of the wound increases. Direct cost estimates for healing one pressure ulcer range from $7,000 to

$25,000, depending on the severity of the wound. Not all pressure ulcers heal and many heal slowly causing a continual drain on resources. The significance of the problem in terms of number of patients afflicted and actual dollars spent is evident.

There is interest in pressure ulcer management at the regulatory level with pressure ulcers used as an indicator of the quality of care delivered in all health care settings. There is business interest in pressure ulcer treatment and prevention. Pressure ulcers and other chronic wounds are big business with the wound care products industry competing with over 2400 different wound care products on the market in the United States. There is growth in bioengineering and technological development of bioengineered tissues and use of technology for healing. Manufacturers of support surfaces and devices abound and there is rapid growth in the number of wound healing centers throughout the country.

Pressure ulcers are associated with loss of function and a fourfold risk of death. There is a cost for care givers too. Depression, social isolation, and frustration are often caregiver complaints. The cost of care, regulatory and business interest in the clinical condition, and the human toll associated with the wounds underscore the impact of pressure ulcers on health care. The goal is always to prevent pressure ulcer development and if unsuccessful, to intervene in the early stages of tissue trauma. This chapter reviews risk assessment for targeting prevention strategies to those at risk of developing pressure ulcers, and assessment of individuals with pressure ulcers.

ASSESSMENT OF RISK

Factors associated with pressure ulcer development can be thought of as those that affect the pressure force over the bony prominence and those that affect the tolerance of the tissues to pressure. The primary risk factors affecting pressure over the bony prominence are conditions that lead to immobility, inactivity, and loss of sensory perception.

Immobility, inactivity, and decreased sensory perception all affect the duration and intensity of the pressure over the bony prominence. Normal capillary pressure ranges from 12 to 32 mm Hg. High intensity pressure between the bony prominence and the external surface over a short period of time can induce tissue necrosis. Lower pressures for longer periods of time without relief can also produce tissue necrosis. High pressures can be tolerated for short periods of time if intermittent relief is offered to provide for tissue reperfusion. Pressure causes tissue ischemia, with resultant cellular damage by occluding capillary flow, allowing build up

Color Plate 1
Pressure Ulcer Stages.

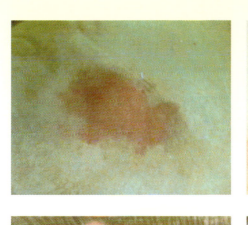
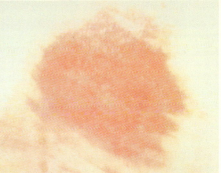

A. clinical demonstration
of Stage I pressure
damage.

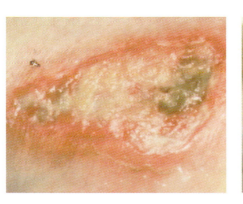
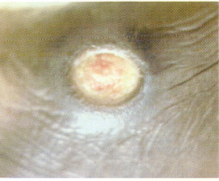

B. Stage II damage to
the epidermis and
dermal tissue layers.
Photographs present
clinical presentation of
Stage II pressure ulcers.

C. Stage III pressure
ulcers.

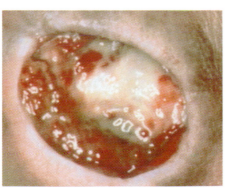
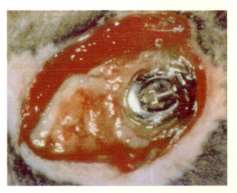

D. Stage IV pressure
ulcers with damage to
underlying tissues
including muscle, joint,
and bone. The bone may
be seen in Picture 1 and
the steel prosthetic hip
device may be seen in
Picture 2.

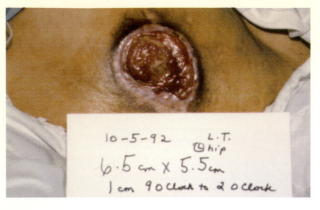

Color Plate 2
This photograph illustrates the rolled, thickened and hyperpigmented color of the wound edge in chronic pressure ulcers.
Reprinted with permission copyright
© Barbara M. Bates-Jensen

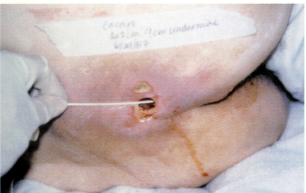

Color Plate 3
Extensive undermining in a pressure ulcer. There is 9 cm of undermining present towards the rectal area of the patient.
Reprinted with permission copyright
© Barbara M. Bates-Jensen

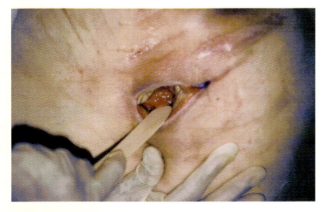

Color Plate 4
Tunneling in a pressure ulcer. The tongue blade points to the opening of the tunneled area of the wound.
Reprinted with permission copyright
© Barbara M. Bates-Jensen

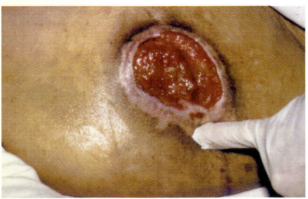

Color Plate 5
Photo of pressure ulcer with 75–100% of the wound filled with bright red, beefy granulation tissue. Note that where the finger is pointing, the granulation tissue has filled the wound to even with the wound edge and the process of epithelialization is evident.
Reprinted with permission copyright
© Barbara M. Bates-Jensen

of metabolic waste products, and cellular hypoxia. Deeper tissues are commonly affected initially with the skin often being the last tissue layer to demonstrate ischemic injury. Because of the nature of the damage, bony prominences are more prone to pressure induced necrosis.

Most pressure ulcers develop over the sacrum, ischial tuberosities, greater trochanters, heels and lateral malleoli, with the sacralcoccyxgeal area the most common site as noted in Figure 13-1. One study showed that ulcers on the greater trochanter are more severe in depth of trauma.[10] Reports indicate as many as 75 percent of pressure ulcers occur in the hip and sacral area.[11]

The risk factors that can affect tissue tolerance to pressure can be grouped into extrinsic and intrinsic factors. Extrinsic factors include moisture, friction, and shearing forces. Intrinsic factors include nutritional status, age, temperature, and psychological factors.

Moisture alters the resiliency of the epidermis to external forces. As such, it is not surprising that urinary and fecal incontinence are common risk factors associated with pressure ulcer development, with fecal incontinence more significant in pressure ulceration than urinary incontinence.[6, 12, 13] Both shearing force and friction increase in the presence of mild to moderate moisture. Friction acts on the tissue tolerance to pressure by abrading and damaging the epidermal and upper dermal layers of the skin. Additionally, friction acts with gravity to cause shear. Shear is caused

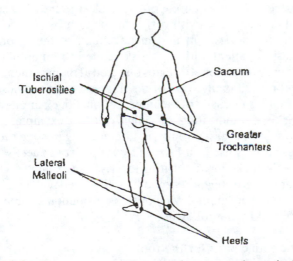

FIGURE 13-1   Pressure sore. The sacralcoccyxgeal area is the most common site for pressure sores. (Reproduced, with permission, from Ouslander JG, Osterweil D, Morley J. *Medical Care in the Nursing Home,* 2nd ed. New York: McGraw-Hill; 1997:205.)

by the interplay of gravity and friction. Shear is a parallel force that acts to stretch and twist tissues and blood vessels at the bony tissue interface. Shear is responsible for the large undermined areas associated with pressure ulcers involving deep tissue trauma.

There is some disagreement on the major intrinsic risk factors affecting tissue tolerance to pressure, and various investigators offer different lists of major risk factors. Most investigators, however, identify nutritional status as playing a role in pressure ulcer development[12, 14, 15] Hypoalbuminemia, weight loss, cachexia, and malnutrition are all commonly identified as risk factors predisposing patients to pressure ulcer development. Altered mental status and certain surgical and chronic medical conditions (hip fractures, spinal cord injury, multiple sclerosis, diabetes mellitus, peripheral vascular disease, metastatic cancer, and contractures) have also been cited extensively as risk factors for pressure ulcer development.[12–14, 16–22] Others have examined psychological factors that may affect risk for pressure ulcer development and the impact of stress on pressure ulcer development.[23]

In order for health care providers to intervene cost effectively, a method of screening for risk factors is necessary. There are several risk assessment instruments available. Screening tools assist in prevention by distinguishing those persons who are at risk for pressure ulcer development from those who are not. The only purpose for identifying patients at risk for pressure ulcer development is to allow for appropriate use of resources for prevention. The use of a risk assessment tool allows for targeting of interventions to specific risk factors. For example, pressure ulcer prevention strategies for a patient identified with a risk factor of urinary incontinence would include assessment and management of the incontinence. In contrast, a patient with high risk related to immobility would benefit from prevention strategies targeted at management of tissue loads and repositioning. Use of a risk assessment tool also allows for determining intensity of the intervention. For example, a patient with a risk score indicating very high risk (for example, a Braden Scale score of 10 or less) would require more aggressive prevention strategies such as use of a low air loss support surface, whereas a patient with a risk score indicating low risk (an example is a Braden Scale score of 18 or higher) would be well served with less intensive interventions. Selection of which risk assessment instrument to use is determined by the following.

- Scientific basis for the tool
- Reliability of the tool for the intended raters
- Predictive validity of the tool for the intended population
- Sensitivity and specificity of the instrument for the intended health care setting
- Ease of use and time required to complete

This approach of selecting the aggressiveness of interventions according to risk assessment scores, was suggested at the 1999 National Pressure Ulcer Advisory Panel.

The most common risk assessment tools are Braden's Scale for Predicting Pressure Sore Risk (see Appendix #6) and Norton's Scale (see Appendix #32).[20, 24] Table 13-1 presents common characteristics of each scale for comparison.

The Braden scale was developed in 1987 and is composed of 6 subscales that conceptually reflect degrees of sensory perception, moisture, activity, nutrition, friction and shear, and mobility.[24, 25] All subscales are rated from 1 to 4, except for friction and shear, which is rated on 1 to 3. The subscales can be summed for a total score, with a range from 4 to 23. The cut-off score for hospitalized adults is considered to be 16, with scores of 16 and below indicating at risk status. In older patients, some have found cut off scores of 17 or 18 better predictors of risk status. The Braden scale has been tested in acute care and long-term care settings with several levels of nurse raters and demonstrates high inter-rater reliability with registered nurses.[25, 26] Validity has been established by expert opinion and predictive validity has been studied in several acute care and long-term care settings with good sensitivity and specificity demonstrated.[26, 27] Sensitivity and specificity vary with assessment times and with health care settings.

The Norton Tool is the oldest risk assessment instrument, developed in 1961, and consists of five subscales: physical condition, mental state, activity, mobility, and incontinence.[20] Each parameter is rated on a scale of 1 to 4, with the sum of the ratings for all five parameters yielding a total score ranging from 5 to 20. Lower scores indicate increased risk. A score of 14 indicates "onset of risk," and scores 12 and below indicate high risk for pressure ulcer formation. There are limited reliability data on the tool and some problems with content validity because of the lack of a nutrition parameter.

Risk assessment is most meaningful when performed by a health care provider with some knowledge of the individual.

TABLE 13-1. COMMON CHARACTERISTICS OF RISK ASSESSMENT INSTRUMENTS: THE BRADEN SCALE AND THE NORTON SCALE

RISK FACTORS	BRADEN SCALE	NORTON SCALE
Nutrition	X	—
Moisture or incontinence	X	X
Friction and shear	X	—
Mobility	X	X
Activity	X	X
Sensory perception	X	—
Mental state	—	X
Physical condition	—	X

Tools such as the Braden Scale or the Norton Scale are recommended for risk assessment.

The tool is easy to use and has been studied in many settings with a variety of health care providers.[28]

The Agency for Health Care Policy and Research recommended use of either the Norton Scale or the Braden Scale for risk assessment as both have been tested.[21] The Braden Scale recently has been automated and is a portion of the Wound and Skin Intelligence System (WSIS) software program.[29]

The WSIS is a comprehensive software program for wound management. The WSIS incorporates risk assessment with the Braden Scale, prevention guidelines and interventions, wound assessment, and general treatment guidelines. The WSIS allows for graphic reports at a variety of levels including individual patient level, unit or floor level, and organizational or facility level. The reports can be used to benchmark progress in prevention (and treatment) with other facilities using the same system. The Braden Scale has also been tested with preventive protocols derived from individual patient scores on the tool.[30] The Braden score itself is predictive of the use of prevention strategies (turning and repositioning and support surface use), with higher and lower scores most predictive of risk.[27, 31]

Regardless of the instrument chosen to evaluate risk status, the clinical relevance is three-fold. First, assessment for risk status must occur at frequent intervals. Assessment should be monitored at admission to the facility, at predetermined intervals, and whenever a significant change occurs in the patient's general health and status. There are suggested parameters for assessment intervals based on health care setting.[27] Suggested risk assessment intervals include the following.

- Acute care setting, critical care units
  On admission
  Then every day
- Acute care setting, general medical surgical units
  On admission
  Then every other day OR
  On a routine schedule (such as Monday, Wednesday, Friday)
- Long-term care setting
  On admission (as soon as possible during the initial 24-hour period)
  Every week for 4 weeks (suggested as most vulnerable time period for development of a pressure ulcer)
  Then on a routine schedule (such as quarterly)
- Home health care setting
  On admission
  Then every week

The second clinical implication is the targeting of specific prevention strategies to identified risk factors. This allows for individualization of the prevention protocol and improvement in outcomes. The final clinical implication is for those patients in whom prevention is not successful. For patients with an actual pressure ulcer, the continued monitoring of risk status can prevent further tissue trauma at the wound site and can prevent development of additional wound sites. Assessment of the patient with a pressure ulcer requires attention to three areas: diagnosis of severity of tissue trauma, differential diagnosis of wound etiology, and baseline and monitoring of wound status.

At a minimum, risk assessment should be performed on admission and at routine intervals for the specific health care setting (e.g., daily in critical care, weekly in home care and medical surgical units, and quarterly in long term care facilities)

ASSESSMENT OF WOUND SEVERITY

Assessment of wound severity refers to the use of a classification system for diagnosing the severity of tissue trauma by determining the tissue layers involved in the wound. There are multiple classification systems of which the Pressure Ulcer Staging System is one example. Classification systems such as staging pressure ulcers facilitate communication among health care providers regarding the wound severity and the tissue layers involved in the injury.

Pressure Ulcer Staging

Pressure ulcers are commonly classified according to grading or staging systems based on the depth of tissue destruction. Historically, one problem in assessment was the lack of a universal staging system for classifying the severity of pressure ulcers. The National Pressure Ulcer Advisory Panel (NPUAP) and the Agency for Health Care Policy and Research (AHCPR) recommend use of a universal four-stage classification system to describe depth of tissue damage. Staging systems only measure one characteristic of the wound and should not be viewed as a complete assessment independent of other indicators. Staging systems are best used as a diagnostic tool for indicating wound severity. Table 13-2 presents the pressure ulcer staging criteria according to the National Pressure Ulcer Advisory Panel and the Agency for Health Care Policy and Research. Figure 13-2 (see color plate 1) provides graphic illustration of the four stages of pressure ulcers.

Staging classification systems do not assess for criteria in the healing process and hinder tracking of progress because of the inability of the staging system to demonstrate change over time. The staging system does not allow for pressure ulcer development on a dynamic continuum, there is no room for movement within and between stages. Many health care providers attempt to use

TABLE 13-2. PRESSURE ULCER STAGING CRITERIA	
PRESSURE ULCER STAGE	DEFINITION
Stage I	A stage I pressure ulcer is an observable pressure-related alteration of intact skin whose indicators as compared to the adjacent or opposite area on the body may include changes in one or more of the following: Skin temperature (warmth or coolness) Tissue consistency (firm or boggy feel) Sensation (pain, itching) The ulcer appears as a defined area of persistent redness in lightly pigmented skin, whereas in darker skin tones, the ulcer may appear with persistent red, blue, or purple hues.
Stage II	Partial-thickness skin loss involving epidermis or dermis, or both. The ulcer is superficial and presents clinically as an abrasion, blister, or shallow crater.
Stage III	Full-thickness skin loss involving damage or necrosis of subcutaneous tissue, which may extend down to but not through underlying fascia. The ulcer presents clinically as a deep crater with or without undermining of adjacent tissue.
Stage IV	Full-thickness skin loss with extensive destruction, tissue necrosis, or damage to muscle bone or supporting structures (such as tendon, joint capsule).

Source: National Pressure Ulcer Advisory Panel, 1998.

the staging system as such a continuum, despite the difficulties associated with back-staging or down staging. The best use of the staging system is as a diagnostic tool. It presents a probable level of tissue injury and as such, has implications for the future course of the patient with a pressure ulcer.

There are problems associated with pressure ulcer staging. Accurate, meaningful communication is difficult, as health care providers may not have the experience necessary to recognize the various tissue layers that identify the stage or grade. In addition, they may interpret definitions of each stage differently. Staging requires practice and a certain amount of skill that develops with time spent examining wounds.

Additional problems regarding the validity of the staging system relate to the stage II lesion, characteristics of the Stage I lesion, and use of the system on wounds of various etiology. There is one theory of pressure ulcer development that purports pressure ulcer trauma starts at the bony tissue interface and works outward to

TABLE 13-3. DISADVANTAGES OF STAGING FOR USE AS A SINGLE OUTCOME MEASURE
It requires past experience and education in tissue layer identification
Different staging systems still abound
Reliability is an issue
Validity of the system as a whole may be questioned
It is a static tool and does not measure change
It is only one characteristic of the wound
It does not account for wound recovery

the top layer of the skin. With this model in mind, stage II lesions do not fit the model. Stage II lesions are usually caused by friction or shearing of the tissues causing superficial, partial thickness damage to the epidermis. Another theory of pressure ulcer development supports damage from the epidermis extending in, towards the bony surface. Stage II lesions start at the epidermis and work inward to deeper layers providing support for the latter theory. The reality may be that pressure ulcers form in multiple manners and present with a variety of clinical manifestations.

The validity problems associated with stage I lesions relate to the various presentations of this stage of tissue destruction. Some stage I lesions indicate severe deep tissue damage, with the surface of the skin the last tissue layer to indicate ischemic injury. Other stage I lesions indicate only superficial insult where damage is somewhat reversible and not indicative of underlying tissue death. Finally, wounds caused by factors other than pressure (for example, vascular, neurotrophic, traumatic, and moisture) are often classified using the same staging system, which further confuses the issue.

In summary, use of the staging system has the advantage of determining tissue layers involved in the wound and wound stage is acknowledged by payers for reimbursement of therapies. The disadvantages of staging as a single indicator of pressure ulcer status are listed in Table 13-3 and include the need for experience in tissue layer identification, reliability and validity issues and inability to measure change or account for wound recovery. These problems are not easily overcome and make staging of pressure ulcers an ineffective assessment when used alone.

ASSESSMENT OF WOUND ETIOLOGY

Diagnosis of wound etiology is essential for development of an effective treatment plan. Differential diagnosis requires general knowledge of the presentation of chronic wounds of various etiolo-

TABLE 13-4. CHARACTERISTICS OF WOUNDS BY ETIOLOGY

WOUND PRESENTATION	PRESSURE ULCERS	VENOUS DISEASE ULCERS	ARTERIAL AND ISCHEMIC ULCERS	DIABETIC NEUROPATHIC ULCERS	PERINEAL DERMATITIS
Patient history	Immobility, inactivity, decreased sensory perception (e.g., cerebral vascular accident, spinal cord injury, or diabetes), malnutrition, incontinence, altered mental status, orthopedic procedures, prolonged bedrest, and critical illness	Previous deep vein thrombosis and varicosities, obesity, phlebitis, traumatic injury to site, congestive heart failure, orthopedic procedures, and previous vascular ulcers	Diabetes, cerebral vascular accident, smoking, intermittent claudication, vascular procedures, hypertension, hyperlipidemia, arteriosclerosis and atherosclerosis, and traumatic injury to site	Diabetes, Hansen's disease	Urinary or fecal incontinence
Location	Bony prominences, most commonly sacral and coccyxgeal area, greater trochanters, ischial tuberosities, and heels	Medial and lateral aspect of lower leg and ankle, superior to malleolus	Toe tips and/or web spaces, phalangeal heads around lateral malleolus, areas exposed to repeated trauma or pressure	Plantar aspect of foot, metatarsal heads, heels	Buttocks including sacral and coccyxgeal area and perineal area; ulcers are multiple, appearing over the entire buttocks and sacral and coccyxgeal areas (not confined to the bony prominence)
Wound color	Variable, if significant necrosis, will have surrounding erythema, if ulcer chronic, will have hemosiderin staining at edges (appears as hyperpigmentation or purple color to wound margins)	Red and ruddy wound base	Extremity is pale on elevation and shows dependent rubor; ulcer bed may be pale in color	Normal skin color, ulcer color variable	Buttocks will have diffuse erythema with uneven borders, extending beyond bony prominence of sacrum or coccyx; ulcers are usually pink
Surrounding skin	Usually normal unless continuing pressure injury, then blanchable and nonblanchable erythema may be present	Erythema, brown staining (hemosiderin deposits)	Shiny, taut, thin, evidence of tissue and skin atrophy with hair loss on lower extremities.	May have callus formation (hyperkeratosis), fissures and cracks in skin	Denuded and erosions evident (particularly with fecal incontinence) flaking and scaling may also be present
Depth	Variable	Partial thickness or full thickness but usually shallow	Deep	Variable	Partial thickness and shallow
Wound margins	Usually regular and well-defined, in early stages will be irregular, ill-defined and diffuse	Irregular	Even and regular, a "punched out" appearance	Well-defined undermining may be present	Irregular and diffuse
Exudate	Variable	Moderate to heavy (dependent on amount of edema present in extremities)	Minimal	Variable	Minimal, depending on severity of skin denudation
Edema	Variable; in later stages, pitting or nonpitting and induration possible	Pitting or nonpitting, induration, cellulitis possible	Variable, depends on severity of arterial impairment	Cellulitis, erythema, and induration common	Usually not present

TABLE 13-4. CHARACTERISTICS OF WOUNDS BY ETIOLOGY (*Continued*)					
WOUND PRESENTATION	PRESSURE ULCERS	VENOUS DISEASE ULCERS	ARTERIAL AND ISCHEMIC ULCERS	DIABETIC NEUROPATHIC ULCERS	PERINEAL DERMATITIS
Skin temperature	Normal; in early stages, increased warmth to touch, in later stages, cool to touch.	Normal and warm to touch	Decreased, cool to touch	Normal, warm to touch	Normal, warm to touch
Granulation tissue	Usually present and red color in proliferative phase of healing	In partial thickness ulcers, evidence of epithelialization will be present; in full thickness ulcers granulation tissue is present and red	If present, pale pink in color	Frequently present	Partial thickness ulcers, no granulation tissue will be present, but evidence of epithelialization should be present
Infection	Not usually present, signs of inflammation will be present when necrotic tissue is present	Usually not present	Frequently present	Frequently present	Concomitant yeast infection may be present
Necrosis	Present when ulcer presents with more severe tissue insult, or when ulcer is chronic and long standing; can be yellow slough or eschar type	Usually not present; if present typically yellow slough and fibrin	Eschar, gangrene may be present	Variable, gangrene uncommon	Not typically present
Pain	Unknown, may be minimal or procedural in nature	Usually mild, but may be more severe or procedural in nature	Intermittent claudication, rest pain, positional (relieved with dependent position), nocturnal pain; ulcer may be very painful.	Painless, diminished sensitivity to touch, insensate foot	Moderate to severe depending on level of denudation and erosion of the skin
Peripheral perfusion	Peripheral pulses present and palpable (unless concomitant PVD)	Peripheral pulses present and palpable (unless edema hinders palpation); capillary refill: normal, less than 3 seconds	Peripheral pulses absent or diminished; capillary refill: delayed, more than 3 seconds; ankle/brachial index: less than 0.8	Peripheral pulses present and palpable; capillary refill: normal, less than 3 seconds; reflexes: diminished; altered gait, orthopedic deformities common	NA

gies. Differential diagnosis of pressure ulcers involves determining the etiology of the wound and intervening appropriately. Pressure ulcers on lower extremities must be differentiated from venous ulcers, arterial and ischemic ulcers, and neuropathic ulcers. Ulcers on the sacral and coccyxgeal area must be distinguished from perineal dermatitis. Table 13-4 presents typical presentations of various chronic wound types.

ASSESSMENT OF WOUND STATUS

Pressure ulcer assessment is the base for maintaining and evaluating the therapeutic plan of care. Initial assessment, and follow up assessments at regular intervals to monitor progress or deterioration of the ulcer, are necessary to determine effectiveness of the treatment plan. Indices for pressure ulcer assessment should provide data for multiple purposes.

1. Examining the severity of the lesion
2. Evaluating and monitoring changes in the lesion over time
3. Prescribing and evaluating appropriate treatment
4. Predicting outcomes or prognoses

The assessment data enables health care providers to communicate clearly about a patient's pressure ulcer, provide for continuity in the plan of care, and allow evaluation of treatment modalities. Assessment of wound status should be performed weekly and whenever a significant change is noted in the wound. Assessment should not be confused with monitoring the wound at each dressing change. Monitoring the wound can be performed by less skilled caregivers, however, assessment should be performed on a routine basis by health care providers.

Measurement

Early studies noted that the first obvious measurable aspect of pressure ulcer healing is wound size. Today, assessment of size of the ulcer remains a focal point for measurement of healing and for predicting healing outcomes. How size is best determined is an area of intensive study and debate. Size can be measured using two-dimensional or three-dimensional techniques. Techniques involve linear measurements of area, wound tracings, photography, planimetry, molds, and instillations. Other methods of determining size include: stereophotogrammetry; use of photographs and planimetry; acetate tracings of wounds subjected to planimetry, weighing, or counting blocks on graph paper, and use of casts or molds of the wound bed. Methods range from clinically friendly and familiar to complex and complicated. The most common method of determining size in clinical practice is area measurements. Table 13-5 lists suggestions for improving such measurements.

Methods of determining area measurements can involve manual two-dimensional or three-dimensional measurements. The usual method of obtaining area measurements involves measuring the length and width (and/or depth) of the wound in centimeters and recording area measurement on a flow sheet for tracking pur-

TABLE 13-5. SUGGESTIONS FOR IMPROVING MEASUREMENT RESULTS
Take measurements in a consistent manner; always measure the longest and widest aspect of the wound.
Calculate the surface area estimate from the length and width to allow tracking of a single number improving ability to monitor for changes over time.
Use caution in concluding minute changes in size are evidence of healing (more likely evidence of the unreliable nature of the measure).
Assess for overall gross changes in size as the indicator of wound healing.

poses. Consistent documentation of area measurements allows determination of whether the ulcer has decreased in size over a period of time.

The following three suggestions can improve the results obtained. Take measurements in a consistent manner; always measure the longest and widest aspect of the wound to increase the reliability of the results. Calculating the surface area estimates from the length and width allows for tracking of a single number, which can improve the ability to monitor for changes in size over time. Use caution in concluding that minute changes in size are evidence of healing (more likely evidence of the unreliable nature of the measure) and instead, assess for overall gross changes in size as the indicator of wound healing.

There are problems with area measurement reliability and used alone, area measurements may not indicate the rate of wound healing. The patient that is evaluated initially with a necrotic pressure ulcer and then debrided of the nonviable tissue presents a common problem with using size as the only indicator of wound healing. When an ulcer is debrided, the size increases, yet, the wound is generally improved. Wounds with irregular shapes and depth present additional problems with linear measurements of size. Irregularly shaped wounds pose the question of where, along an uneven wound edge, to place the measuring device to obtain the measurement reading. Some health care providers have difficulty recognizing the wound edge. This can impact the validity of size measurements as well. Ulcers with depth may make two-dimensional measurements meaningless and three-dimensional measurements are difficult.

Depth may be measured linearly as part of the determination of size by inserting a cotton-tipped applicator into the wound, marking the level of the skin, and measuring the applicator to the mark in centimeters. The difficulty in measuring depth with linear measurements relates to the imprecise nature of the measure.

Where to insert the cotton-tipped applicator on the uneven wound base topography is problematic and raises questions about the reliability and validity of the measure. Depth measurements can be more meaningful by use of the same reference points for each measurement, such as the deepest aspect or the 12 o'clock position of the wound.

Size is an important indicator for pressure ulcer assessment. As wounds heal, wound surface area must decrease. Rate of change in wound size has demonstrated predictive ability in several studies. Van Rijswijk examined patient and healing characteristics related to full-thickness pressure ulcers in 119 participants (48 had full-thickness pressure ulcers) in a variety of health care settings.[32] One of the objectives of the study was to determine if there was a specific time that distinguished wounds that healed from those that did not heal. Healing was measured with surface area tracings and wounds were followed for 15 months. The mean reduction in wound area was significantly different at 2 weeks (45 percent for healed, > 3 percent for nonhealed) and at 4 weeks (77 percent reduction for healed and 18 percent reduction for nonhealed) for the wounds that healed versus nonhealed. This suggests that reduction in surface area at 2 weeks and at 4 weeks may be a predictor to eventual wound healing.

In a secondary analysis of the same study data, Van Rijswijk and Polansky examined predictors of time to healing deep stage III and IV pressure sores. Time to healing analysis methods were used to evaluate healing time in stage III and IV sores as a function of patient and wound characteristics at baseline and after 2 weeks of therapy. Results demonstrated that patients whose ulcers reduced at least 39 percent in size after 2 weeks healed more quickly than those who did not have at least a 39 percent reduction in area (median time to healing 53 days versus 70 days).[33]

Bates-Jensen, in unpublished data, studied a sample of 143 participants with 51 partial-thickness and 92 full-thickness pressure ulcers to examine potential wound characteristics as predictors of healing. Results of the study indicated that time to 50 percent healing could be predicted by 1-week change in surface area ($p = .0001$). Assessment of wound size at weekly intervals can be a relatively easy method of predicting wounds that will progress to timely healing versus those that will not. It is only one characteristic of the wound, however, and should not be the only index to status of the ulcer. Size does not necessarily assist with development of a treatment plan and is not always helpful in evaluation of treatment effectiveness. A comprehensive assessment of multiple wound characteristics provides the best basis for evaluation of wound status, determination of treatment options, and outcomes of care.

TOOLS FOR WOUND STATUS ASSESSMENT

There are few tools available that encompass multiple wound characteristics to evaluate overall wound status and healing. Most of the tools currently available focus on pressure ulcer assessment. The Sessing Scale, the Wound Healing Scale, the Sussman Wound Healing Tool, the Pressure Sore Status Tool, and the Pressure Ulcer Scale for Healing (PUSH) are the available instruments for pressure sore assessment.[34-38] The Pressure Ulcer Scale for Healing and the Pressure Sore Status Tool are discussed here.

The Pressure Ulcer Scale for Healing Tool

Most recently, the National Pressure Ulcer Advisory Panel (NPUAP) reviewed the currently available instruments and concluded there was a need for an instrument that better met criteria for measuring and predicting healing in pressure sores. The outgrowth of a task force with the mandate to develop a tool to measure and predict healing in pressure ulcers is the Pressure Ulcer Scale for Healing (PUSH) tool (see Appendix #37). The PUSH tool incorporates surface area measurements, exudate amount, and surface appearance. These characteristics were chosen based on principal component analysis to define the best model of healing.[38]

The Pressure Ulcer Scale for Healing (PUSH) was developed using principal components analysis to identify key descriptors that are predictive of healing. The authors suggest that content validity, correlational validity, prospective validity, and sensitivity to change can be met by the proposed tool. The model identified the items on the tool, surface area, exudate amount, and surface appearance, and these items performed similarly in a new sample. The first model of principal components explained 55 percent to 60 percent of the variance at weeks 0 through week 8. Reliability and replication in a larger sample are underway.[38] The PUSH tool can offer a quick assessment to predict healing outcomes.

The Pressure Sore Status Tool

The Pressure Sore Status Tool (PSST) (Figure 13-3) developed in 1990 by Bates-Jensen, evaluates 13 wound characteristics with a numerical rating scale and rates them from best to worst possible for the characteristic.[39] The PSST incorporates the necessary indices

Instructions for use

General Guidelines:
Fill out the attached rating sheet to assess a pressure sore's status after reading the definitions and methods of assessment described below. Evaluate once a week and whenever a change occurs in the wound. Rate according to each item by picking the response the best describes the wound and entering that score in the item score column for the appropriate date. When you have rated the pressure sore on all items, determine the total score by adding together the 13-item scores. The HIGHER the total score, the more severe the pressure sore status. Plot total score on the Pressure Sore Status Continuum to determine progress.

Specific Instructions:

1. **Size:** Use ruler to measure the longest and widest aspect of the wound surface in centimeters; multiply length $\times$ width.

2. **Depth:** Pick the depth, thickness, most appropriate to the wound using these additional descriptions:
   1. tissues damaged but no break in skin surface.
   2. superficial, abrasion, blister or shallow crater. Even with, &/or elevated above skin surface (e.g., hyperplasia).
   3. deep crater with or without undermining of adjacent tissue.
   4. visualization of tissue layers not possible due to necrosis.
   5. supporting structures include tendon, joint capsule.

3. **Edges:** Use this guide:
Indistinct, diffuse	= unable to clearly distinguish wound outline.
Attached	= even or flush with wound base, *no* sides or walls present; flat.
Not attached	= sides or walls *are* present; floor or base of wound is deeper than edge.
Rolled under, thickened	= soft to firm and flexible to touch.
Hyperkeratosis	= callous-like tissue formation around wound & at edges.
Fibrotic, scarred	= hard, rigid to touch.

4. **Undermining:** Assess by inserting a cotton tipped applicator under the wound edge; advance it as far as it will go without using undue force; raise the tip of the applicator so it may be seen or felt on the surface of the skin; mark the surface with a pen; measure the distance from the mark on the skin to the edge of the wound. Continue process around the wound. Then use a transparent metric measuring guide with concentric circles divided into 4 (25%) pie-shaped quadrants to help determine percent of wound involved.

5. **Necrotic Tissue Type:** Pick the type of necrotic tissue that is *predominant* in the wound according to color, consistency and adherence using this guide:
☐ White/gray non-viable tissue	= may appear prior to wound opening; skin surface is white or gray.
☐ Non-adherent, yellow slough	= thin, mucinous substance; scattered throughout wound bed; easily separated from wound tissue.
☐ Loosely adherent, yellow slough	= thick, stringy, clumps of debris; attached to wound tissue.
☐ Adherent, soft, black eschar	= soggy tissue; strongly attached to tissue in center or base of wound.
☐ Firmly adherent, hard/black eschar	= firm, crusty tissue; strongly attached to wound base *and* edges (like a hard scab).

FIGURE 13-3 Pressure Sore Status Tool. **A.** Instructions for use. **B.** Pressure Sore Status Tool.

6. **Necrotic Tissue Amount:** Use a transparent metric measuring guide with concentric circles divided into 4 (25%) pie-shaped quadrants to help determine percent of wound involved.

7. **Exudate Type:** Some dressings interact with wound drainage to produce a gel or trap liquid. Before assessing exudate type, gently cleanse wound with normal saline or water. Pick the exudate type that is *predominant* in the wound according to color and consistency, using this guide:

    Bloody = thin, bright red
    Serosanguineous = thin, watery pale red to pink
    Serous = thin, watery, clear
    Purulent = thin or thick, opaque tan to yellow
    Foul purulent = thick, opaque yellow to green with offensive odor

8. **Exudate Amount:** Use a transparent metric measuring guide with concentric circles divided into 4 (25%) pie-shaped quadrants to determine percent of dressing involved with exudate. Use this guide:

    □ None = wound tissues dry.
    □ Scant = wound tissues moist; no measurable exudate.
    □ Small = wound tissues wet; moisture evenly distributed in wound; drainage involves ≤ 25% dressing.
    □ Moderate = wound tissues saturated; drainage may or may not be evenly distributed in wound; drainage involves > 25% to ≤ 75% dressing.
    □ Large = wound tissues bathed in fluid; drainage freely expressed; may or may not be evenly distributed in wound; drainage involves > 75% of dressing.

9. **Skin Color Surrounding Wound:** Assess tissues with 4 cm of wound edge. Dark-skinned persons show the colors "bright red" and "dark red" as a deepening of normal ethnic skin color or a purple hue. As healing occurs in dark-skinned persons, the new skin is pink and may never darken.

10. **Peripheral Tissue Edema:** Assess tissues within 4 cm of wound edge. Non-pitting edema appears as skin that is shiny and taut. Identify pitting edema by firmly pressing a finger down into the tissues and waiting for 5 seconds, on release of pressure, tissues fail to resume previous position and an indentation appears. Crepitus is accumulation of air or gas in tissues. Use a transparent metric measuring guide to determine how far edema extends beyond wound.

11. **Peripheral Tissue Induration:** Assess tissues within 4 cm of wound edge. Induration is abnormal firmness of tissues with margins. Assess by gently pinching the tissues. Induration results in an inability to pinch the tissues. Use a transparent metric measuring guide with concentric circles divided into 4 (25%) pie-shaped quadrants to determine percent of wound and area involved.

12. **Granulation Tissue:** Granulation tissue is the growth of small blood vessels and connective tissue to fill in full thickness wounds. Tissue is healthy when bright, beefy red, shiny and granular with a velvety appearance. Poor vascular supply appears as pale pink or blanched to dull, dusky red color.

13. **Epithelialization:** Epithelialization is the process of epidermal resurfacing and appears as pink or red skin. In partial thickness wounds it can occur throughout the wound bed as well as from the wound edges. In full thickness wounds it occurs from the edges only. Use a transparent metric measuring guide with concentric circles divided into 4 (25%) pie-shaped quadrants to help determine percent of wound involved and to measure the distance the epithelial tissue extends into the wound.

© 1990 Barbara Bates-Jensen

FIGURE 13-3 (*Continued*)

PRESSURE SORE STATUS TOOL

Name_____

Complete the rating sheet to assess pressure sore status. Evaluate each item by picking response that best describes the wound and entering the score in the item score column for the appropriate date.

Location: Anatomic site. Circle, identify right **(R)** or left **(L)** and use "**X**" to mark site on body diagrams:

_____ Sacrum & coccyx   _____ Lateral ankle
_____ Trochanter   _____ Medial ankle
_____ Ischial tuberosity   _____ Heel   Other Site

Shape: Overall wound pattern; assess by observing perimeter and depth.
Circle and *date* appropriate description:

_____ Irregular   _____ Linear or elongated
_____ Round/oval   _____ Bowl/boat
_____ Square/rectangle   _____ Butterfly   _____ Other Shape

Item	Assessment	Date	Date	Date
		Score	Score	Score
1. Size	1 = Length × width < 4 sq cm 2 = Length × width 4–16 sq cm 3 = Length × width 16.1–36 sq cm 4 = Length × width 36.1–80 sq cm 5 = Length × width > 80 sq cm			
2. Depth	1 = Non-blanchable erythema on intact skin 2 = Partial thickness skin loss involving epidermis &/or dermis 3 = Full thickness skin loss with damage/necrosis of subcutaneous tissue; may extend to, not through underlying fascia; &/or mixed partial & full thickness &/or tissue obscured by granulation tissue 4 = Obscured by necrosis 5 = Full thickness skin loss with extensive destruction, tissue necrosis or damage to muscle, bone or supporting structures			
3. Edges	1 = Indistinct, diffuse, none clearly visible 2 = Distinct, outline clearly visible, attached, even with wound base 3 = Well-defined, not attached to wound base 4 = Well-defined, not attached to base, rolled under, thickened 5 = Well-defined, fibrotic, scarred or hyperkeratotic			
4. Under-mining	1 = Undermining < 2 cm in any area 2 = Undermining 2–4 cm involving < 50% wound margins 3 = Undermining 2–4 cm involving > 50% wound margins 4 = Undermining > 4 cm in any area 5 = Tunneling &/or sinus tract formation			
5. Necrotic Tissue Type	1 = None visible 2 = White/grey non-viable tissue &/or non-adherent yellow slough 3 = Loosely adherent yellow slough 4 = Adherent, soft, black eschar 5 = Firmly adherent, hard, black eschar			
6. Necrotic Tissue Amount	1 = None visible 2 = < 25% of wound bed covered 3 = 25% to 50% of wound covered 4 = > 50% and < 75% of wound covered 5 = 75% to 100% of wound covered			

FIGURE 13-3   (*Continued*)

Item	Assessment	Date	Date	Date
		Score	Score	Score
7. Exudate Type	1 = None or bloody 2 = Serosanguineous: thin, watery, pale red/pink 3 = Serous: thin, watery, clear 4 = Purulent: thin or thick, opaque, tan/yellow 5 = Foul purulent: thick, opaque, yellow/green with odor			
8. Exudate Amount	1 = None 2 = Scant 3 = Small 4 = Moderate 5 = Large			
9. Skin Color Surrounding Wound	1 = Pink or normal for ethnic group 2 = Bright red &/or blanches to touch 3 = White or grey pallor or hypopigmented 4 = Dark red or purple &/or non-blanchable 5 = Black or hyperpigmented			
10. Peripheral Tissue Edema	1 = Minimal swelling around wound 2 = Non-pitting edema extends < 4 cm around wound 3 = Non-pitting edema extends ≥ 4 cm around wound 4 = Pitting edema extends < 4 cm around wound 5 = Crepitus &/or pitting edema extends ≥ 4 cm			
11. Peripheral Tissue Induration	1 = Minimal firmness around wound 2 = Induration < 2 cm around wound 3 = Induration 2–4 cm extending < 50% around wound 4 = Induration 2–4 cm extending ≥ 50% around wound 5 = Induration > 4 cm in any area			
12. Granulation Tissue	1 = Skin intact or partial thickness wound 2 = Bright, beefy red; 75% to 100% of wound filled &/or tissue overgrowth 3 = Bright, beefy red; < 75% & > 25% of wound filled 4 = Pink, &/or dull, dusky red &/or fills ≤ 25% of wound 5 = No granulation tissue present			
13. Epithelialization	1 = 100% wound covered, surface intact 2 = 75% to < 100% wound covered &/or epithelial tissue extends > 0.5cm into wound bed 3 = 50% to < 75% wound covered &/or epithelial tissue extends to < 0.5cm into wound bed 4 = 25% to < 50% wound covered 5 = < 25% wound covered			
TOTAL SCORE				
SIGNATURE				

PRESSURE SORE STATUS CONTINUUM

1   *13*   23   33   43   53   *65*

◄───►

Tissue Wound   **Wound**
Health Regeneration   **Degeneration**

Plot the total score on the Pressure Score Status Continuum by putting an "**X**" on the line and the date beneath the line.
Plot multiple scores with their dates to see-at-a-glance regeneration or degeneration of the wound.
© 1990 Barbara Bates-Jensen

FIGURE 13-3 (*Continued*)

for pressure ulcer assessment, provides for quantification of observations, and allows for tracking the condition of the ulcer over time. The PSST is recommended for use as a method of assessment and monitoring of pressure ulcers. The PSST is a pencil and paper instrument comprised of 15 items: location, shape, size, depth, edges, undermining, necrotic tissue type, necrotic tissue amount, exudate type, exudate amount, surrounding skin color, peripheral tissue edema, peripheral tissue induration, granulation tissue, and epithelialization. Two items are nonscored items, location and shape. The remaining 13 are scored items and each appears with characteristic descriptors rated on a Likert scale (1 = best for that characteristic and 5 = worst attribute of the characteristic). The PSST is meant to be used once a pressure ulcer has developed, it is not a risk assessment tool. It is recommended that the pressure ulcer be scored initially for a baseline assessment and at regular intervals to evaluate therapy. Once a lesion has been assessed for each item on the PSST, the 13 item scores can be added to obtain a total score for the wound. The total score can then be monitored to see-at-a-glance regeneration or degeneration of the wound. Total scores range from 13 (skin intact but always at risk) to 65 (profound tissue degeneration). Each of the items on the tool is discussed later.

A modified Delphi technique using a multidisciplinary 20-member panel was used to develop the characteristics and each item on the tool.[40] The PSST was further evaluated for content validity using a 9-member judge panel of experts in the wound healing and pressure ulcer field.[37] Content validity was established for each individual item on the tool and for the total tool with the judge panel.[40] Concurrent validity was evaluated in a long term care setting and involved comparing medical record documentation of pressure ulcer stage with the PSST depth item for a Pearson product moment correlation coefficient of $r = 91$ ($p = .001$).[41] In a later study, the total PSST score was compared to recorded stage of the wound and findings revealed a relatively strong positive relationship between the two scores (Pearson product moment correlation $r = .55$, $p = .001$).[42] The study demonstrated little difference between the mean PSST scores of stage I versus stage II ulcers and for stage III versus stage IV ulcers but significant difference between stage I and II versus stage III and IV ulcers (stage I and II mean PSST score 23.35 versus stage III and IV mean PSST score 31.83; $p < .001$).

Reliability of the PSST has been evaluated in an acute care setting with ET (enterostomal therapy) nurses (nurses with additional training in wound care) and in long-term care using a variety of health care professionals and one ET nurse expert in wound assessment.[37, 41] Interrater reliability ranged from $r = .915$ ($p =$

.0001) for the ET nurses to 0.78 percent agreement for various health care providers. The PSST is the most widely used of the instruments available and forms the framework for the discussion on wound characteristic assessment.

WOUND CHARACTERISTICS ASSESSMENT

Pressure ulcer assessment must encompass a composite of wound characteristics. A single characteristic cannot provide the data necessary to determine the adequacy of the treatment plan or allow for monitoring progress or degeneration of the wound. The indices for pressure ulcer assessment include all of the following: location, size of the ulcer, stage or depth of tissue involvement, condition of the wound edges and presence of undermining or tunneling, necrotic tissue characteristics, exudate characteristics, surrounding tissue conditions, and wound healing characteristics of granulation tissue and epithelialization.

Location

Assess the location of the pressure ulcer by identifying where the lesion occurs on the patient's anatomy. Use of a body diagram may be helpful. The sacral and coccyxgeal area is the most common area for pressure sores, and more severe pressure ulcers often occur over the greater trochanter. There are very few pressure sores on the hips—usually someone has mislabeled the lesion—it most often is the greater trochanter that caused the pressure ulcer.

Shape

As wounds heal, they often begin to assume a more regular, circular or oval shape. The shape also helps to determine the overall size of the wound. If the wound is a crater or hole, remember the shape should then be a three-dimensional shape, like bowl or boat shaped. Butterfly-shaped wounds occur in the sacral and coccyxgeal area and are wounds with mirror images on each side of the gluteal fold. To determine the shape of the pressure ulcer, evaluate the perimeter of the wound. Is the wound circular or oval? As previously stated, as wounds heal, they begin to achieve a circular or oval shape.

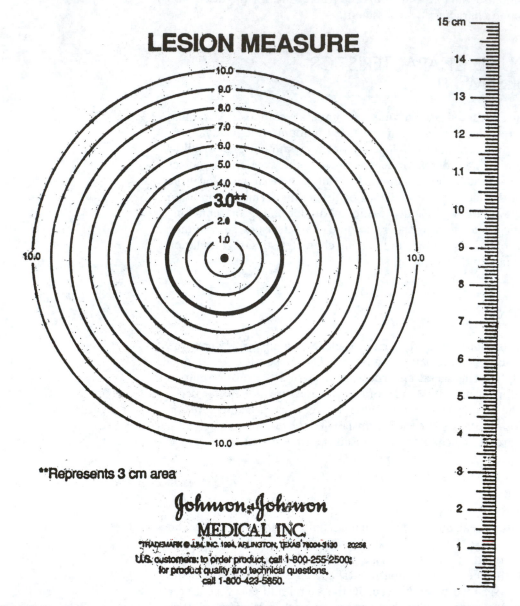

FIGURE 13-4   Example of measuring guide with concentric circles and centimer ruler for wound measurements.

Size

A transparent measuring guide should be used to measure the longest aspect and perpendicular widest aspect of the wound surface *that is visible,* in centimeters, multiply the length by the width to determine the surface area of the wound. Figure 13-4 shows a typical transparent measuring guide and the wound stick. These devices can be useful in obtaining accurate and meaningful measurements. It can be difficult to determine where to measure size on some wounds because the edge of the wound can be hard to visualize. This is a skill that simply takes some practice. The measurements will be more reliable if one looks for the longest portion and the perpendicular widest portion of the wound. In butterfly-shaped wounds measure the longest and widest portion of each wing of the butterfly.

Depth

Pick the depth of tissue layers involved with the wound or the thickness of the wound most appropriate using the 4-stage system presented earlier and the additional guidelines on the PSST.

Measure the depth of the wound using a cotton-tipped applicator. Insert the applicator in the deepest portion of the wound, mark the applicator with a pen and measure the distance from tip to the mark using a metric measuring guide.

Edges

The edges of the wound are one of the most important characteristics of the wound. The wound edges can be a window to the history and health of the wound. When assessing edges, look for how clear and distinct the wound outline appears. If the edges are indistinct and diffuse, there are areas where the normal tissues blend into the wound bed and the edges are not clearly visible. Edges that are even with the skin surface and the wound base are edges that are attached to the base of the wound. This means the wound is flat, with no appreciable depth. Well-defined edges are clear, distinct and can be outlined on a transparent piece of plastic easily. Edges that are not attached to the base of the wound, imply a wound with some depth of tissue involvement. The wound that is a crater or bowl/boat shape is a wound with edges that are not attached to the wound base. The wound has walls or sides. There is depth to the wound. As the wound ages, the edges become rolled under and thickened to palpation. The edge achieves a unique coloring due to hemosiderin staining (see Figure 13-5, color plate 2). The pigment turns a grey or brown color in both dark- and light-skinned persons. Wounds of long duration may continue to thicken, with scar tissue and fibrosis developing in the wound edge causing the edge to feel hard, rigid, and indurated. Hyperkerotosis is the callous-like tissue that can form around the wound edges on neuropathic lesions. Evaluate the wound edges by visual inspection and palpation.

Undermining

Undermining and tunneling are the loss of tissue underneath an intact skin surface. Undermining usually involves a greater percentage of the wound margins with more shallow length than tunneling. Undermining usually involves subcutaneous tissues and follows the fascial planes next to the wound. An undermined area can be likened to a cave, whereas a tunnel is more like a subway. Tunneling usually involves a small percentage of the wound margins, is narrow and quite long, and seems to have a destination.

Assessment for undermining should be done by inserting a cotton-tipped applicator under the wound edge; advancing it as far as it will go without using undue force; raising the tip of the applicator so it can be seen or felt on the surface of the skin; marking the surface with a pen; measuring the distance from the mark on the skin to the edge of the wound (see Figure 13-5, color plates 3 and 4). This process should be continued all around the wound. A transparent metric measuring guide with concentric circles divided into quadrants helps to determine percent of wound involved.

Necrotic Tissue Characteristics

Necrotic tissue should be assessed for the color, consistency, and adherence to the wound bed. The predominant characteristic present in the wound should be chosen. Necrotic tissue type changes as it ages in the wound, as debridement occurs, and as further tissue trauma causes increased cellular death. There are two main types of necrotic tissue: slough and eschar. Slough generally indicates less severity than eschar. Slough usually appears as a yellow to tan, mucinous or stringy material that is nonadherent or loosely adherent to the healthy tissues of the wound bed. Nonadherent is defined as appearing scattered throughout the wound. It looks as if the tissue could be easily removed with gauze. Loosely adherent refers to tissue that is attached to the wound bed. It is thick and stringy and can appear as clumps of debris attached to wound tissue.

Eschar signifies deeper tissue damage. Eschar can be black, grey, or brown in color. Eschar is usually adherent or firmly adherent to the wound tissues and can be soggy and soft or hard and leathery in texture. A soft, soggy eschar is usually strongly attached to the base of the wound but may be lifting from and loose from the edges of the wound. Hard, crusty eschars are strongly attached to the base and the edges of the wound. Hard eschars are often mistaken for scabs. Sometimes, nonviable tissue appears prior to a wound appearing. This can be seen on the skin as a white or grey area on the surface of the skin. The area usually demarcates within a couple of days and the wound appears and interrupts the skin surface.

Evaluating the amount of necrotic tissue present in the wound is one of the easier characteristics to assess. Use a transparent measuring guide with concentric circles divided into quadrants and lay this over the wound. Look at each quadrant and judge how much necrosis is present. Add up the total percentage from the judgments of each quadrant and this determines the percent of the wound involved. The length and width of the necrosis (to determine surface area) can also be measured.

Exudate Characteristics

Evaluating exudate type can be tricky because of the moist wound healing dressings used on most wounds. Some dressings interact with wound drainage to produce a gel or fluid and others trap liquid and drainage at the wound site. Before assessing exudate type, the wound needs to be gently cleansed with normal saline or water and evaluate fresh exudate. The predominant exudate type is selected according to color and consistency. A wound with necrotic tissue present will almost always have an odor.

Exudate amount can be difficult to accurately assess for the same reasons it is difficult to determine the type of exudate in the wound. Moist wound healing dressings interact with wound drainage to trap drainage at the wound site. Others absorb varying amounts of exudate. The amount of exudate in the wound can be judged by observing two areas: the wound itself and the dressing used on the wound. The wound should be observed for moisture, dessication, exudate and whether the drainage has spread throughout the wound. Clinical judgment determines the moisture present in the wound environment. The dressing should be evaluated for how much it interacts with or is "used up" by exudate.

Surrounding Tissue Characteristics

The tissues surrounding the wound are often the first indication of impending further tissue damage. Color of the surrounding skin can indicate further injury from pressure, friction, or shearing. Assess the tissues within 4 cm of wound edge. Dark-skinned persons show the colors "bright red" and "dark red" as a deepening of normal ethnic skin color or a purple or blacker hue. As healing occurs in dark-skinned persons, the new skin is pink and may never darken. In both light- and dark-skinned patients, new epithelium must be differentiated from tissues that are erythemic. To assess for blanchablity, press firmly on the skin with a finger, lift the finger, and look for "blanching," or sudden whitening of the tissues followed by prompt return of color to the area. Nonblanchable erythema signals more severe tissue damage.

Edema in the surrounding tissues will delay wound healing in the pressure ulcer. It is difficult for neoangiogenesis, or the growth of new blood vessels into the wound, to occur in edematous tissues. Tissues within 4 cm of the wound edge should be assessed. Nonpitting edema appears as skin that is shiny and taut, almost glistening. Pitting edema can be identified by firmly pressing a finger down into the tissues and waiting for 5 seconds. On release of pressure, tissues fail to resume previous position and an indentation appears. Crepitus is accumulation of air or gas in tissues. Measure how far edema extends beyond the wound edges.

Induration is a sign of impending damage to the tissues. Along with skin color changes, induration is an omen of further pressure induced tissue trauma. Induration is an abnormal firmness of tissues with margins. Palpation and gently pinching the tissues can determine where the induration starts and where it ends. Induration results in an inability to pinch the tissues. It is usual to feel slight firmness at the wound edge itself. Normal tissues feel soft and spongy, induration feels hard and firm to the touch.

Healing Characteristics

Granulation tissue is a marker of wound health. It signals the proliferative phase of wound healing and usually heralds the eventual closure of the wound. Granulation tissue is the growth of small blood vessels and connective tissue into the wound cavity. It is more observable in full thickness wounds because of the tissue defect that occurs with full thickness wounds. In partial thickness wounds, granulation tissue can occur so quickly and in concert with epithelialization so as to make it unobservable in most cases. The granulation tissue is healthy when bright, beefy red, shiny and granular with a velvety appearance. The tissue looks "bumpy" and may bleed easily. Unhealthy granulation tissue due to poor vascular supply appears as pale pink or blanched to dull, dusky red color. Usually, the first layer of granulation tissue to be laid down in the wound is pale pink and as the granulation tissue deepens and thickens, the color becomes the bright, beefy red color (see Figure 13-5, color plate 5).

It is much easier to judge what percent of the wound has been filled with granulation tissue if there is a history with the wound. If the wound is followed by the same person over multiple observations, it is simple to judge the amount of granulation tissue present in the wound. If the initial observation of the wound was done by a different observer or if the data are not available, best judgment to determine the amount of tissue present should be used.

Epithelialization is the process of epidermal resurfacing and appears as pink or red skin. Visualizing the new epithelium takes practice. In partial thickness wounds, it can occur throughout the wound bed as well as from the wound edges. In full thickness wounds, epidermal resurfacing occurs from the edges only, usually after the wound has almost completely filled with granulation tissue. A transparent measuring guide helps determine percent of wound involved and to measure the distance the epithelial tissue extends into the wound. Clinical judgment forms the foundation for determining treatments and for evaluating effectiveness of therapy.

ASSESSMENT OF TREATMENT RESPONSE

The PSST tool allows for temporal tracking of individual characteristics as well as the total score. Each characteristic is assessed as previously described and given a value from the Likert scale, thus the scores can be monitored for improvement or deterioration in each characteristic. Additionally, the 13-item scores can be summed and the total tracked over time to determine the wound status. This quantification of observations not only allows for monitoring individual items and total score but also groups of characteristics. The characteristics of necrotic tissue type and amount and exudate type and amount can be tracked to evaluate debridement or infection management.

Another benefit associated with the assignment of numerical values to items on the tool is the ability to set realistic goals. Clinical experience shows that not all pressure ulcers heal and certainly not always in the same setting. The PSST allows for more realistic goal setting as appropriate to the health care setting and the individ-

A general rule for evaluating treatment response is that if there is no change in the wound status in 2 weeks, the treatment should be changed, the total patient reevaluated in light of underlying risk factors, or the wound reassessed for a more appropriate treatment.

ual patient and pressure ulcer. For example, the patient with a large necrotic full-thickness ulcer in acute care will probably not be in the facility long enough for the wound to actually heal, however, the tool would enable health care providers to set smaller goals, such as, the wound will decrease in type and amount of necrotic tissue. In some instances, a pressure ulcer may never heal because of host factors or other circumstances, so the goal might be to maintain the total wound score between 20 and 22.

Use of the PSST or a similar instrument should enhance communication between health care providers involved in pressure ulcer care. By providing a framework for assessment and documentation with an attempt at quantification, the communication process becomes more meaningful. An objective method of assessing pressure ulcers and monitoring changes over time allows for evaluation of the therapeutic plan of care, and can be used to guide and direct therapy. This is particularly true with the movement into a managed care environment. For example, if a specific treatment modality is in use and the patient's wound status as determined with the PSST has not changed in 2 weeks, reevaluation of the plan of care is warranted. Use of the PSST may uncover other outcome criteria that will help identify critical attributes during the course of healing. Finally, in a manner similar to the one suggested for risk assessment scores, aggressiveness of treatment intervention could be stratified based on severity of wound status or PSST score.

The PSST has been fully automated with the Braden Scale for Risk Assessment as the Wound and Skin Intelligence System (WSIS). The WSIS incorporates graphic capabilities and tracking ability for all 13 pressure ulcer assessment items for monitoring progress or deterioration of the pressure ulcers. The WSIS captures related risk factor data and evaluates the overall wound status in relationship to risk factor data as well as the assessment data discussed. The system uses relational databases and provides ongoing monitoring capabilities for determining changes in pressure ulcer status over time, produces essential documentation, and automatically reminds users when additional assessments should be completed.

The Wound and Skin Intelligence System

Documentation of pressure sore status and healing is notoriously poor.[43] Documentation is required for reimbursement of specific therapies in use to support the healing of the wound. Using any of the pencil and paper instruments as a form for assessment of pressure sore wound healing has the advantage of providing a means for documentation that is simple and time effective. Paper assessment forms can be entered into the patient's medical record. Paper forms, such as skin care flow sheets in long-term care facilities, provide other examples of documentation formats. Long narrative notes are rarely kept together in an organized manner for easy retrieval of ulcer information. Monitoring data using narrative notes or skin care flow sheets is problematic. It is often difficult and time consuming to analyze the information and determine quickly whether or not the interventions in use are effective. The PSST has the advantage of including a scale at the bottom of the paper form for entering the total wound score to see at a glance the health or degeneration of the wound. The PUSH tool has an area to graph results to see progress at a glance. All paper forms, however, have disadvantages.

Manual tools can provide significant information regarding pressure sore wound healing as well as a method of documenting findings. Yet, as data accumulate over time, any pencil and paper tool is susceptible to the same problems that afflict most documentation systems; the available information soon overcomes the health care providers's ability to interpret and use the findings. Automation of tools should be the next logical step. The Wound and Skin Intelligence System (WSIS) is an automated version of the PSST tool and as such, increases the health care provider's ability to synthesize and act on large volumes of wound assessment data. The purpose of the WSIS is for clinical assessment, management, and documentation, and provision of feedback based on aggregate data within the system and monitoring progress.[41] Data are collected routinely (usually weekly) using the pencil and paper version of the PSST and then transferred to the computerized file by the nurse or designated clerk. Patient files consist of demographic and clinical data, treatment information, and agency and facility and staff data.[41] Relational databases archive facility, patient, treatment, background, and assessment data. Methods to insure validity of data include use of a fixed format screen and prevention of data entry that is illogical. Fixed format screens "walk" the user through data entry with specific sequences required in specific order of entry. Out-of-range values and certain illogical entries are not permitted, for instance a wound could not be entered as covered with necrotic tissue and then have no necrotic tissue type entered.

The system allows for easy data input and a variety of graphic and reporting capabilities. Users enter the relevant characteristics of the patient including demographic data, risk factor and nutritional data, medical and nursing diagnoses, and support surface and topical treatment data. Prevention and treatment care plans are provided to the user based on data entered for the individual patient and wound and using the Agency for Health Care Policy and Research (AHCPR) guidelines for pressure ulcer treatment and prevention as a base.

Initial and follow-up wound assessment data are entered, and from these data, the computer automatically tracks and graphically displays changes in the PSST total and individual scores over time. The system also tracks and monitors the pattern in the scores for the 13 items on the assessment tool. The ability to visually determine general and specific changes in wound status over time and relate these changes to interventions has been greatly aided by the database system.[41] Methods of recording assessment data should allow for tracking of each assessment item and promote quantification of observations for easy examination of changes in the ulcer status. Reports using the total PSST score can also be used to produce outcome data.

The programming within the WSIS allows for benchmarking with other geographical regions, other facilities of the same size and type, and even other countries. Cost benefit analysis and reports of prevalence and incidence and trends are also available.

Like most computer systems, the WSIS does not save time for health care providers in data entry; the real time savings comes from the availability of generating reports using the data entered into the system. Indeed, the changes in pressure ulcer treatment for the future may be based on access to databases with ability to follow general guidelines and not necessarily access to high technology or advanced wound treatments.

SUMMARY

Although the focus of this chapter is on assessment of the pressure ulcer wound, it is important to remember that the wound does not occur in isolation but is an extension of the individual. Thus, pressure ulcer assessment involves a comprehensive assessment approach including a focused history and physical examination, specific attention to laboratory and diagnostic data, a pain assessment, and the wound assessment for the purposes of providing baseline data for future comparison and for determining wound severity. Assessment requires thoughtful attention to the patient's history and physical examination. The history and physical examination should provide a foundation for examination of the wound itself by providing data on potential comorbidities that can influence the healing process. Disease states or conditions that affect tissue perfusion and oxygenation are prime factors for impairments in wound healing. Immunocompromised patients, diabetic patients, and those with frank infection are also in need of special attention in order for healing to be optimal. Pain assessment is important for determining adequate pain relief interventions and for evaluating pain response throughout treatment.

A thorough history, physical examination, and pain assessment provide the context for the wound assessment. Wound assessment can be performed for different reasons. The initial assessment determines the severity and etiology of the tissue insult and is often used as the baseline for comparison of later wound assessment data. The initial assessment determines the severity of the tissue insult and often prescribes treatment interventions. Subsequent assessments are used to predict and monitor healing or deterioration of the wound. Finally, assessment data is often used to monitor response to treatment interventions.

Multiple wound characteristics are assessed as the best method of meeting all the goals of assessment. Assessment of wound characteristics includes examination of wound size, stage or classification of the wound, wound depth, would edges and undermining, surrounding tissue characteristics, necrotic tissue characteristics, exudate characteristics, and presence of healing characteristics of granulation tissue and epithelialization. Prediction of healing is another facet of wound assessment and perhaps the future for wound assessment. Although still in the early stages of investigation, several markers for predicting healing have been identified by researchers. Most notably, the rate of surface area decrease is predictive of time to complete healing. Markers of a 39 percent reduction in surface area at 2 weeks and an overall decrease in size plus a decrease in net PSST score identified wounds that proceeded to complete healing and 50 percent healed significantly faster than other wounds.

Accurate and meaningful documentation of assessment data is critical to valid interpretation of progress. Use of a tool to organize assessment and document findings is beneficial in clinical practice. Several tools for wound assessment are presented, with the PSST the most widely used of the instruments. Although the tools have been developed for use with pressure ulcers, use with other chronic wounds may also be beneficial. Assessment data allows clear communication about the wound among health care providers, provides for continuity in the plan of care, and allows evaluation of treatment modalities in a timely fashion.

An automated system, such as the WSIS, will have significant regulatory implications. Third party payers and managed care groups are looking for the most cost-effective methods of treating chronic wounds. Use of a quantifiable, evidence-based tool can assist the health care provider in proving the effectiveness of a chosen therapy plan, explain the course of the wound more clearly to payers, and provide rationale for therapy decisions, thus expediting reimbursement in particular cases.

Use of this tool, or a similar evidence-based tool, can improve health care provider communication, the generalizability of research studies, allow discrimination in studies, dealing with treatment modalities, and can help to improve understanding of wound healing in pressure ulcers. It can provide increased sensitivity, allowing greater precision and clarity in studies related to the treatment and development of pressure ulcers. An instrument that is sensitive to change in wound status will be helpful in the development of critical pathways for pressure ulcers and is useful as an outcome measure. The ability of computer programs, such as the WSIS, to assist with large volumes of data hold potential promise for future developments that will give health care providers tools for better decision making.

REFERENCES

1. Clarke M, Kadhom HM. The nursing prevention of pressure sores in hospital and community patients. *J Adv Nurs.* 1988;13(3):365–373.
2. Barczak CA, Barnett RI, Childs EJ, Bosley LM. Fourth national pressure ulcer prevalence survey. *Adv Wound Care.* 1997;10(4):18–26.
3. Oot-Girimini BA, Bidwell FC, Heller NB, Parks ML, Wicks P, Williams PM. Evolution of skin care: pressure ulcer prevalence rates pre/post intervention. *Decubitus.* 1989;2(2):54–55.
4. Langemo DK, Olson F, Hunter S, Burd C, Hansen D, Cathcart-Silberberg T. Incidence of pressure sores in acute care, rehabilitation, extended care, home health, and hospice in one locale. *Decubitus.* 1989;2(2):42–47.
5. Young L. Pressure ulcer prevalence and associated patient characteristics in one long term care facility. *Decubitus.* 1989;2(2):52.
6. Brandeis GH, Morris JN, Nash DJ, Lipsitz LA. A longitudinal study of risk factors associated with formation of pressure ulcers in nursing homes. *J Am Geriatr Soc.* 1994;42(4):388–393.
7. Oot-Girimini BA. Pressure ulcer prevalence, incidence and associated risk factors in the community. *Decubitus.* 1993;6(5):24–32.
8. Powell JW. Increasing acuity of nursing home patients and the prevalence of pressure ulcers: a ten year comparison. *Decubitus.* 1989;2(2):56–58.
9. Miller H, Delozier J. *Cost Implications of the Pressure Ulcer Treatment Guideline.* Columbia, MD: Center for Health Policy Studies. Contract No. 28-91-0070. Sponsored by the Agency for Health Care Policy and Research; 1994:17.
10. Meehan M. Multisite pressure ulcer prevalence survey. *Decubitus.* 1990;3(4):14–17.
11. Maklebust J, Sieggreen M. *Pressure Ulcers: Guidelines for Prevention and Nursing Management, 2nd ed.,* Springhouse, PA: Springhouse Corporation; 1996.

12. Allman RM, Laprade CA, Noel LB, et al. Pressure sores among hospitalized patients. *Ann Inter Med.* 1986;105(3):337–342.

13. Maklebust J, Magnan, MA. Risk factors associated with having a pressure ulcer: a secondary analysis. *Adv Wound Care.* 1994;7(6): 25–42.

14. Bergstrom N, Braden B. (1992). A prospective study of pressure sore risk among institutionalized elderly. *J Am Geriatri Soc.* 1992;40(8): 747–758.

15. Pinchcofsky-Devin GD, Kaminski MV. Correlation of pressure sores and nutritional status. *J Am Geriatr Soc.* 1986;34(6):435–440.

16. Berlowitz DR, Wilking SV. Risk factors for pressure sores: a comparison of cross-sectional and cohort-derived data. *J Am Geriatr Soc.* 1989;37(11):1043–1050.

17. Gosnell DJ. Pressure sore risk assessment: a critique Part I of the Gosnell scale. *Decubitus.* 1989;2(3):32–38.

18. Guralnik JM, Harris TB, White LR, Coroni-Huntley JC. Occurrence and predictors of pressure sores in the National Health and Nutrition Examination survey follow-up. *J Am Geriatr Soc.* 1988;36(9):807–812.

19. Maklebust J, Bruckhorst L, Crachiolo-Caraway A et al. Pressure ulcer incidence in high risk patients managed on a special three-layered air cushion. *Decubitus.* 1988;1(4):30–40.

20. Norton D, McLaren R, Exton-Smith NA. *An Investigation of Geriatric Nursing Problems in Hospitals.* London: National Corporation for the Care of Old People; 1962.

21. Panel for the Prediction and Prevention of Pressure Ulcers in Adults. *Pressure Ulcers in Adults: Prediction and Prevention. Clinical Practice Guideline,* No. 3. Rockville, MD.: Agency for Health Care Policy and Research; U.S. Dept. of Health and Human Services publication AHCPR 92-0047; 1992.

22. Spector WD. Correlates of pressure sores in nursing homes: evidence from the national medical expenditure survey. *J Invest Dermatol.* 1994;102(6):42S–45S.

23. Anderson TP, Andberg, MM. Psychosocial factors associated with pressure sores. *Arch Phy Med Rehabil.* 1979;60(8):341–346.

24. Braden BJ, Bergstrom N. A conceptual schema for the study of etiology of pressure sores. *Rehabil Nurs.* 1987;12(1):8–12.

25. Bergstrom N, Demuth PJ, Braden, BJ. A clinical trial of the Braden Scale for Predicting Pressure Sore Risk. *Nurs Clini North Am.* 1987;22(2):417–428.

26. Braden BJ, Bergstrom N. Clinical utility of the Braden Scale for predicting pressure sore risk. *Decubitus.* 1989;2(3):44–51.

27. Bergstrom N, Braden B, Kemp M, Champagne M, Ruby E. Multisite study of incidence of pressure ulcers and the relationship between risk level, demographic characteristics, diagnoses, and prescription of preventive interventions. *J Am Geriatr Soc.* 1996;44(1):22–30.

28. Norton D. Calculating the risk: reflections on the Norton scale. *Decubitus.* 1989;2(3):24–31.

29. Wound and Skin Intelligence System, ConvacTec, Princeton, NJ, 1998.

30. Bergstrom N, Braden BJ, Boynton P, Bruch S. (1995). Using a re-search-based assessment scale in clinical practice. *Nurs Clin North Am.* 1995;30(3):539–551.

31. Xakellis GC, Frantz RA, Arteaga M, Nguyen M, Lewis A. A comparison of patient risk for pressure ulcer development with nursing use of preventive interventions. *J Am Geriatr Soc.* 1992;40(12);1250–1254.

32. Van Rijswijk L. Full-thickness pressure ulcers: patient and wound healing charcteristics. *Decubitus.* 1993;6(1):16–30.

33. Van Rijswijk L, Polansky M. Predictors of time to healing deep pressure ulcers. *Ostomy/Wound Management.* 1994;40(8):40–50.

34. Ferrell BA, Artinian BM, Sessing D. The Sessing Scale for assessment of pressure ulcer healing. *J Am Geriatr Soc.* 1995;43:37–40.

35. Krasner D. Wound Healing Scale, version 1.0: a proposal. *Adv Wound Care.* 1997;10(5):82–85.

36. Sussman C, Swanson G. Utility of the Sussman Wound Healing Tool in predicting wound healing outcomes in physical therapy. *Adv Wound Care.* 1997;10(5):74–77.

37. Bates-Jenesn BM, Vredevoe DL, Brecht ML. Validity and reliability of the Pressure Sore Status Tool. *Decubitus.* 1992;5(6):20–28.

38. Thomas DR, Rodeheaver GT, Bartolucci AA. et al. Pressure Ulcer Scale for Healing: derivation and validation of the PUSH tool. *Adv Wound Care.* 1997;10(5):96–101.

39. Bates-Jensen B. New pressure ulcer status tool. *Decubitus.* 1990; 3(3):14–15.

40. Bates-Jensen B. The Pressure Sore Status Tool: an outcome measure for pressure sores. *Top Geriatr Rehabil.* 1994;9(4):17–34.

41. Bates-Jensen BM, McNees P. Toward an intelligent wound assessment system. *Ostomy/Wound Management.* 1995;(41)7A:80–87.

42. Bates-Jensen BM, McNees P. The Wound Intelligence System: early issues and findings from multi-site tests. *Ostomy/Wound Management.* 1996;(42)7A:1–7.

43. Pieper B, Mikols C, Mance C, Adams W. Nurses' documentation about pressure ulcers. *Decubitus.* 1990;3(1):32–34.

PREOPERATIVE ASSESSMENT

CAROL M. ASHTON

GENERAL CONSIDERATIONS

Changes in demographics, expectations that high levels of physical function can be enjoyed well into the ninth decade, and improvements in surgical and anesthetic practice have led to large increases in the frequency of surgery in elders. Table 14-1 shows the most commonly performed inpatient operations in elders. These are the operations that health care providers performing preoperative assessments should know the most about. Increasingly, minor procedures such as surgical treatment of cataract, carpal tunnel release, and repair of groin hernias are performed in ambulatory settings, a particularly beneficial arrangement for elders as it allows them to avoid the considerable psychological and physiologic stresses of hospitalization.

Decisions about surgery involve a decision-making *team* and a decision-making *process*. Because of his or her role in providing information about the risks and benefits of the courses of action open to a particular patient, the health care provider is a critical member of the decision-making team. The consultant's role begins with an assessment of the patient and requires a literature-based knowledge of the risks and benefits associated with the planned procedure and its alternatives. He or she must also know which risks

The Agency for Health Care Policy and Research (AHCPR) was renamed in December 1999.
This agency is now known as the Agency for Healthcare Research and Quality (AHRQ).

TABLE 14-1. TOP 25 OPERATIONS PERFORMED ON AN INPATIENT BASIS ON PEOPLE OVER AGE 65 YEARS IN THE UNITED STATES, 1991

OPERATION (ICD-9 CODE)	NUMBER OF PROCEDURES PERFORMED
Transurethral prostatectomy (60.2)	258,000
Bypass anastomosis for heart revascularization (36.1)	206,000
Cholecystectomy (51.2)	185,000
Hip Replacement (81.51, 81.52, 81.53)	174,000
Partial excision of large intestine (45.7)	139,000
Operations on lens (13)	135,000
Knee replacement (81.54, 81.55)	132,000
Percutaneous transluminal coronary angioplasty (36.01, 36.02, 36.05)	130,000
Hernia repair (53)	127,000
Lysis of peritoneal adhesions (54.5)	92,000
Mastectomy (85.4)	58,000
Endarterectomy of extracranial vessels of head and neck (38.12)	51,000
Hysterectomy (68.4, 68.5)	50,000
Operations on retina, choroid, vitreous, and posterior chamber of eye (14)	49,000
Colostomy (46.1)	39,000
Exploration and decompression of spinal canal structures (03.0)	37,000
Control of hemorrhage and suture of ulcer of stomach or duodenum (44.4)	33,000
Resection of abdominal aorta with replacement (38.44)	30,000
Operations on appendix (47)	30,000
Heart valve replacement (35.2)	28,000
Above-knee amputation (84.17)	26,000
Open reduction and internal fixation of fracture of femur (79.35)	20,000
Excision of lung and bronchus (32)	21,000
Below-knee amputation (84.15)	16,000
Complete nephrectomy (55.5)	15,000

Source: Graves, EJ. Detailed diagnoses and procedures, National Hospital Discharge Survey, 1991. National Center for Health Statistics. *Vital Health Stat.* 1994;13(115).

can be reduced and how to reduce them. This chapter addresses preoperative assessment and risk reduction in noncardiac surgery. Perioperative care and the approach to acute problems developing during the operative stay will not be covered. The reader should refer to standard cardiology texts for specialized information about assessing an elder for cardiac surgery.

Decisions and Decision Makers

The patient is the one who is "on the wrong end of the diagnosis," and only the patient can fully appreciate how the problem is affecting his or her lifestyle. The decision about whether or not to proceed with surgery should rest with the individual facing the procedure and his or her surgeon. The primary health care provider serves in a consultative capacity to both, and to the anesthesiologist as well. All parties need to understand two things: first, the courses of action that are open to the patient, and second, the risks and benefits associated with each course. In many cases, the surgeon and the health care provider cannot lay out all the possible courses of action without talking to each other: a written referral or consultation note, no matter how complete, may not suffice.

Surprisingly, misperceptions about surgical risk are common among surgeons, anesthesiologists, and medical consultants alike. A 1985 survey of family or general physicians and general surgeons who were members of the Washington State Medical Association showed that only 27 percent of respondents accurately estimated the risk of death or a major complication for ten common procedures.[1] Twenty-six percent underestimated the risk, 27 percent overestimated it, and 21 percent said they had no knowledge. In helping a patient to decide which course of action has the greatest possibility of benefit and the least possibility of harm, information and recommendations should be based on evidence from the literature and not just personal clinical experience.

Special effort is required to respect an elder's autonomy in decisions about surgery. Many elders have sensory or cognitive deficits that interfere with their ability to receive and process information. Also, many trust that "doctor knows best," and will follow recommendations without an understanding of risks, benefits, and alternatives. They will follow recommendations for *inaction* as well as action. At times, elders are needlessly denied surgical relief of their problems simply on the basis of age. Ageism is the explanation in some cases. More often, surgical treatment is advised against because it is perceived as too risky. In truth, many gaps exist in the literature, and the risks and benefits of many surgical procedures in elders are simply not yet known.

Anesthesia and Surgery in the 21st Century

In current practice, preoperative assessment consists of estimating the risk of certain *postoperative* complications rather than the risk of *intraoperative* catastrophes. Improvements in surgical and anesthetic techniques have almost eliminated the latter. A study of 163,240 anesthetic administrations at a Virginia university hospital between 1969 and 1983 showed that 449 intraoperative cardiac arrests occurred, a rate of 3 per 1000.[2] A substantial proportion of these occurred in patients who were brought to the operating room in a moribund state, emergency surgery being the only hope for their life-threatening condition.

Advances in medical science have expanded treatment options for problems prevalent among elders. Safe and effective nonsurgical or minimally invasive treatments are available for an increasing number of problems. For example, until recently, open or transurethral prostatectomy was the only treatment option available for a man with prostatism. The operative mortality with transurethral prostatectomy is low (1 percent or less), but 5 percent to 10 percent of men will experience an early or late postoperative complication, such as urinary tract infection or urethral stricture, and 75 percent will have retrograde ejaculation.[3] The range of effective alternatives now includes watchful waiting (symptoms of prostatism improve in four out of ten men even without therapy), medical therapy with androgen-deprivation agents or alpha-adrenergic antagonists, or minimally invasive procedures such as transurethral incision of the prostate. The medical consultant conducting a preoperative assessment should make sure that he or she understands and has enumerated all courses of action available for the patient at hand. Only then does the calculation of risks and benefits begin.

Calculating Risk: Benefit Ratios

A helpful way to frame the consideration of risks and benefits associated with a given surgical course of action is to ask the question, is this quality-of-life surgery or quantity-of-life surgery? This over-simplifies the situation, but it clarifies the overall goal of the operation and helps the patient and consultant to determine the level of the risk of death or serious morbidity that they are willing to accept to achieve it. Most people are willing to accept higher levels of risk if the planned operation has a reasonable chance of lengthening life. With quality-of-life surgery, patients vary widely and unpredictably in the amount of operative risk they will accept, probably because only the patient can know how much their dysfunction or problem is adversely affecting the quality of their life. For example, one in ten patients has a serious but nonfatal complication after elective closure of an end-colostomy.[4] If one had an end colostomy, would he or she choose to undergo a colostomy closure?

The consultant physician must understand the expected benefits of the planned procedure. If the surgery is for an oncologic problem, is it being undertaken for cure, staging, or control of local disease? If for cure, how many patients surviving the procedure live at least 5 years? For example, lobectomy for lung cancer is associated with an operative mortality rate of at least 6 percent (mortality is substantially higher for pneumonectomy; Table 14-2). One of four patients undergoing lung resection for cancer lives at least 5 years after the operation. If the surgery is to restore function rather than to lengthen life, for example, knee replacement, what proportion of patients actually have improved function postoperatively, what is the magnitude of the improvement, and how long does it last?[5] For any given patient, the appeal and justification for a surgical procedure is based upon the gap between the probability of significant benefit and the improbability of significant harm.

When the planned operation is life-saving, that is, no nonsurgical alternatives exist and the patient will die without the operation, the *level* of operative risk is irrelevant. The role of the medical consultant in such cases is to determine *how operative risk can be reduced.* Consider, for example, a 70-year-old otherwise healthy woman who is diagnosed with a potentially resectable esophageal carcinoma. Before she was diagnosed, she lost 35 pounds; she lost an additional 15 during her preoperative radiotherapy. A course of perioperative total parenteral nutrition will reduce her risk of operative mortality immeasurably more than a cardiac workup.[6]

Most cases are not so clear cut, and the decision to pursue a surgical intervention will rest, to some extent, on the level of operative risk. The risk of death or a nonfatal complication relates not only to the patient's characteristics but also to the proficiency of the surgical team, nursing staff, and other providers in the hospital. Table 14-2 shows the operative mortality rates observed in U.S. Medicare beneficiaries undergoing selected operations. These rates, derived from large population-based (rather than hospital-based) series, represent a statistical average. The risk of any particular patient may be higher or lower. Valid population-based postoperative morbidity rates are harder to obtain. Data derived from Medicare statistical files will be underestimates; complications are significantly under-reported in claims data. Published complication rates are usually derived from primary data collection studies involving one or a few hospitals or one or a few surgeons. Published figures are probably lower than what would be observed in most hospitals in the U.S., because hospitals with low rates are more likely to report their data. A useful rule is that for every fatal complication, three to six nonfatal complications occur. Consultants performing preoperative assessments will find complications data from their own hospital most applicable; such data are increasingly available.

			TABLE 14-2. THIRTY-DAY MORTALITY RATES FOR SELECTED OPERATIONS		
OPERATION	DATA SOURCE	OBSERVATION YEARS	30-DAY MORTALITY (PERCENT)		
Transurethral prostatectomy			(Numerators and denominators not given, but BPH cohort N = 218,127 and cancer cohort N = 34,319)		
				BPH	Cancer
	Medicare files (20% sample)	1984–1990	Age 65–69	0.4	1.0
			Age 70–74	0.7	1.0
			Age 75–79	1.1	1.7
			Age 80–84	1.9	2.3
			Age 85+	3.5	3.6
Heart revascularization	Medicare files	1987–1990	Age 65–74	13,024/263,403	(5.0)
			Age 75–79	5,244/70,861	(7.4)
			Age 80+	2,504/23,620	(10.6)
			Men 65+	12,229/239,783	(5.1)
			Women 65+	8,622/118,102	(7.3)
Coronary angioplasty	Medicare files	1987–1990	Age 64–74	4,097/164,466	(2.5)
			Age 75–79	1,943/42,246	(4.6)
			Age 80+	1,498/19,203	(7.8)
			Men 65+	3,890/129,675	(3.0)
			Women 65+	3,657/96,240	(3.8)
Elective total hip replacement	Medicare files (5% sample)	1983–1985	Age 65–74	13/2,462	(0.5)
			Age 75–84	19/1,946	(1.0)
			Age 85+	9/240	(3.8)
			Men 65+	17/1,637	(1.0)
			Women 65+	24/3,011	(0.8)
Repair of hip fracture	Medicare files (5% sample)	1986–1989	(Total number of patients with fracture: 26,443; all but 2064 had operative repair. Age-specific counts and rates not given.)		
			Men 65+	11	
			Women 65+	6	
Colectomy for colon cancer	Medicare files (5% sample)	1983–1985	Age 65–74	58/2,216	(2.6)
			Age 75–84	131/2,490	(5.3)
			Age 85+	74/795	(9.3)
			Men 65+	139/2,406	(5.8)
			Women 65+	136/3,095	(4.4)
Carotid endarterectomy	Medicare files	1985–1989	Age 65–74	3,610/156,636	(2.3)
			Age 75–85	3,387/86,993	(3.9)
			Age 85+	416/8,057	(5.2)
			Men 65+	4,458/150,422	(3.0)
			Women 65+	3,041/116,374	(2.6)

continued

TABLE 14-2. THIRTY-DAY MORTALITY RATES FOR SELECTED OPERATIONS

OPERATION	DATA SOURCE	OBSERVATION YEARS	30-DAY MORTALITY (PERCENT)		
Elective abdominal aortic aneurysm repair	Medicare files (5% sample)	1983	(In-hospital mortality)		
			Age 65–74	2/51	(3.9)
			Age 75–84	2/31	(6.5)
Lumbar spine surgery	Medicare files	1986	(In-hospital mortality)		
			Men 65+	766/14,726	(0.52)
			Women 65+	729/19,692	(0.37)
Radical prostatectomy for prostate cancer	Medicare files (20% sample)	1984–1990	Age 65–69	59/5,331	(1.1)
			Age 70–74	32/3,982	(0.8)
			Age 75–79	16/1,131	(1.4)
			Age 80+	7/154	(4.6)
Lung resection for lung cancer	Medicare files (5% sample)	1983–1985	(Pneumonectomy)		
			Age 65–74	10/121	(8.3)
			Age 75+	9/34	(26.5)
			Men age 65+	17/114	(14.9)
			Women age 65+	2/41	(4.9)
			(Lobectomy or less)		
			Age 65–74	48/776	(6.2)
			Age 75+	27/342	(7.9)
			Men age 65+	57/703	(8.1)
			Women age 65+	18/415	(4.3)

Sources:
Lu-Yao GL, Barry MJ, Chang CH, Wasson JH, Wennberg JE. Transurethral resection of the prostate among Medicare beneficiaries in the United States: time trends and outcomes. *Urology.* 1994;44:692–698.

Peterson ED, Jollis JG, Bebchuk JD, DeLong ER, Muhlbaier LH, Mark DB, Pryor DB. Changes in mortality after myocardial revascularization in the elderly. The national Medicare experience. *Ann Intern Med.* 1994;121:919–927.

Whittle J, Steinberg EP, Anderson GF, Herbert R, Hockberg MC. Mortality after elective total hip arthroplasty in elderly Americans. Age, gender, and indication for surgery predict survival. *Clin Orthoped Rel Res.* 1993;295:119–126.

Lu-Yao GL, Baron JA, Barrett JA, Fisher ES. Treatment and survival among elderly Americans with hip fractures: a population-based study. *Am J Public Health.* 1994;84:1287–1291.

Whittle J, Steinberg EP, Anderson GF, Herbert R. Results of colectomy in elderly patients with colon cancer, based on Medicare claims data. *Am J Surg.* 1992;163:572–575.

Hsia DC, Krushat WM, Moscoe LM. Epidemiology of carotid endarterectomies among Medicare beneficiaries. *J Vasc Surg.* 1992;16:201–208.

Richardson JD, Main KA. Repair of abdominal aortic aneurysms. A state wide experience. *Arch Surg.* 1991;126:614–616.

Oldridge NB, Yuan Z, Stoll JE, Rimm AR. Lumbar spine surgery and mortality among Medicare beneficiaries, 1986. *Am J Public Health.* 1994;84:1292–1298.

Lu-Yao GL, McLerran D, Wasson J, Wennberg JE. An assessment of radical prostatectomy. Time trends, geographic variation, and outcomes. *JAMA.* 1993;269:2633–2636.

Whittle J, Steinberg EP, Anderson GF, Herbert R. Use of Medicare claims data to evaluate outcomes in elderly patients undergoing lung resection for lung cancer. *Chest.* 1991;100:595–596.

A surgical intervention has other undesirable features in addition to the risk of dying and the risk of a nonfatal complication. One of these is the length of time convalescence will take. Patients often ask, "How long will I be in the operating room?" and "How long will I be in the hospital?," but do not ask "How long will it take until I am back to my usual level of energy and activity?." Little is known about postoperative convalescence in elders. Clinical experience is that it may take 3 months or more for the patient to return to his or her baseline vigor and activity level after a major operation. This may be an important consideration for the elder who is deciding about quality-of-life surgery and who has a coexisting condition likely to limit longevity to a few years.

Deferral of surgery also has risks and benefits. What needs to be factored into the watchful waiting equation is the likelihood that the patient's problem will at some point develop into a situation requiring emergency surgery. Emergency operations are much riskier than elective ones. For example, emergency intra-abdominal or abdominal wall surgery in the elderly is associated with mortality rates of 20 percent to 30 percent.[7] Unfortunately, knowledge of the natural history of common conditions such as hernias and asymptomatic cholelithiasis is incomplete, and the patients who will develop urgent problems cannot be distinguished from those who will coexist peacefully with their conditions.

Anesthesia in Elders

Because of age-related changes in volume of distribution, metabolism, and elimination of drugs, doses of anesthetics, analgesics, and sedatives must be reduced in elders. Even with reduced drug doses, postanesthesia awakening is often delayed. The choice of anesthesia type may be curtailed in elders. For example, in up to 10 percent of elders, attempts to perform a subarachnoid block fail and general anesthesia must be used instead.

Does anesthetic technique matter? Only randomized controlled trials give valid data on this question, and such studies are uncommon. Available data suggest that patients undergoing procedures with local anesthesia or peripheral nerve blocks have fewer problems with nausea, drowsiness, and unstable gait in the immediate postoperative period than patients having spinal or general anesthesia, and they appear to have fewer cardiorespiratory complications as well. Judicious use of sedating agents in the operating room can relieve the patient's anxiety, provide some analgesia, and produce amnesia for the administration of the block itself as well as the performance of the operation. Monitoring is enhanced as the anesthesiologist has the opportunity to interact with a sedated but responsive patient. Nevertheless, these techniques have their own disadvantages and will not be appropriate for every patient.

If local anesthesia or a peripheral nerve block is not feasible, is spinal or epidural anesthesia safer than general anesthesia? Some physiologic data suggest that spinal anesthesia *would* be safer. For example, spinal (or other regional) anesthesia avoids the brief, but at times extreme, hemodynamic response to laryngoscopy during intubation of the trachea. It also reduces the endocrine–metabolic–catabolic response to surgical stress, which is mediated by the hypothalamic–pituitary–adrenal axis, the renin–angiotensin axis, and the sympathetic nervous system; may have beneficial effects on immune function; and may improve blood flow in the vessels of the lower extremities. Many studies have tried to determine whether these physiologic differences translate into better outcomes for patients given a spinal anesthetic, but in most, the selection bias resulting from nonrandom assignment of patients undermines the validity of the findings. At this time, available data do not permit a firm conclusion that spinal anesthesia is associated with better outcomes than general anesthesia.

The ultimate decision about anesthetic technique should be left up to the anesthesiologist. The medical consultant should notify the anesthesiologist and surgeon directly if the patient's status is so impaired that an elective procedure should be foregone entirely if local anesthesia or a peripheral nerve block cannot be used.

FIRST-LINE RISK ASSESSMENT TOOLS

The preoperative assessment has two purposes. The first is to determine what conditions the patient has that will place him or her at an increased risk of perioperative complications. The second is to develop strategies that minimize the risk of complications and maximize the chances for a good outcome. At the conclusion of the assessment, the health care provider must synthesize the information and answer five questions: (1) What is the patient's overall physical status and level of physical functioning? (2) What is the level of cognitive function? (3) Which organ systems are normal, normal but with diminished reserve due to aging, or abnormal because of disease? (4) How severely dysfunctional is the diseased organ system(s), and is it possible, feasible, and necessary to correct the dysfunction preoperatively? (5) What perioperative therapeutic maneuvers will reduce the risk of a postoperative complication? A consultation explicitly addressing these five points is much more helpful to the surgical team than one with terms like "high risk" or "low risk." Since "high" and "low" mean different things to different people, these terms impede rather than enhance communication. Moreover, the consultation provides a blueprint for action should postoperative problems arise.

History and Physical Examination

The foundation of the preoperative assessment is a comprehensive history and physical examination, supplemented by some special physical examination maneuvers and selected diagnostic tests. Table 14-3 shows areas of special emphasis.

Areas of concentration during the interview include habitual use of cigarettes, alcohol, and drugs; daily exercise routines; functional status; and social support systems. Levels of alcohol consumption should be noted, as alcohol withdrawal can be a cause of postoperative delirium. Polypharmacy is prevalent in elders and a careful drug ingestion history is critical, for prescribed as well as over-the-counter medications. If the patient is taking oral anticoagulants, the indication for the therapy must be ascertained, because that will influence decisions about the use of intravenous heparin in the immediate perioperative period.[8] Drug allergies and past anesthesia problems should be noted. The patient should be questioned about his or her daily exercise program and activity level. The diagnosis of rheumatoid arthritis should be noted. The prevalence of cervical instability is very high in patients with rheumatoid arthritis, and the anesthesiologist will need to avoid hyperextension

---

TABLE 14-3. AREAS OF SPECIAL EMPHASIS DURING PREOPERATIVE EVALUATION

History
  Current medications, including over-the-counter preparations
  Drug allergies
  Activity level and daily exercise program
  Functional status, including performance of instrumental and personal
    activities of daily living
  Past anesthetic problems and operative complications
  Coexisting illnesses, including rheumatoid arthritis
  Tobacco use
  Illicit drug use
  Social support systems and plans for postoperative convalescence
Physical examination
  Supine and standing blood pressure measurements
  Body weight
  Cough test
  Walk test (selected patients) with pre- and post-measurement of heart
    rates
  Mental status examination
  Screening test for depression (selected patients)

of the neck during tracheal intubation so that compression of the upper spine does not occur. Needs and plans for social support during postoperative convalescence should be discussed. Formal assessment of instrumental activities of daily living (IADLs); (home management activities such as shopping and doing housework) and, with more impaired patients, activities of daily living (ADLs); (personal care activities such as bathing and dressing) will provide information especially useful in planning for the postoperative convalescence.

The physical examination should include measurement of supine and standing blood pressure. Postural hypotension is extremely common in elders. Up to 25 percent of elders have a fall exceeding 20 mm Hg in their systolic blood pressure when they change from the supine to the standing position. Postural hypotension in elders is attributable to drugs, age-related deterioration in cardiovascular reflexes, and diseases such as diabetes. Though its association with postoperative complications has not been evaluated, in some patients, postural hypotension is a marker for impaired cardiovascular reserve. Nursing staff must exercise special vigilance in the postoperative period when they assist the elder to ambulate, as postural hypotension can lead to falls.

Body weight should be measured. In patients with heart failure, a notation should be made of the patient's "dry" weight, so it can serve as a target weight in the postoperative period. Some of the hormonal responses to surgery and anesthesia cause the kidneys to retain salt and water. Fluid retention in conjunction with generous intravenous fluid administration in the perioperative period can lead to pulmonary edema in patients with heart failure. Body weight is a more accurate estimate of fluid overload than intake and output disparities.

Exercise capacity should be estimated. An inverse relationship exists between exercise capacity and the risk for a poor outcome with surgery. With patients whose physical abilities are uncertain, a 6-minute walking test can provide an objective estimate of physical status and exercise capacity.[9] The test is conducted in a level corridor of known length. The patient is instructed to cover as much ground as possible in the time allotted. At the end of the test, the distance walked is tallied. Normal participants can walk about 750 yards in 6 minutes. Timed walking tests have been used to assess exercise capacity in patients with chronic obstructive lung disease, heart failure, and arthritis. The distance walked in 6 minutes correlates with exercise capacity as determined by oxygen consumption during maximal treadmill exercise. Patient reports of functional status, flows and volumes on pulmonary function tests, and echocardiographic or radionuclide estimates of left ventricular ejection fraction correlate very poorly with objectively measured exercise capacity. For example, fewer than half the patients known to have a left ventricular ejection fraction under 30 percent report dyspnea on exertion. A timed walking test will give a more precise estimate of exercise capacity than these, and can be administered by nursing personnel in the hall outside the examining room. Its value is enhanced by pre- and post-test measurements of heart rate, particularly in patients with bradycardia whose heart rate response to exercise is unknown.

Another useful addition is the cough test.[10] It was common wisdom as early as 1950 and is still true today that a patient with a preoperative bronchitis is likely to develop atelectasis or pneumonia postoperatively, and that pulmonary complications are unlikely in the patient without bronchorrhea, even if lung disease is present. The cough test provides information that cannot be obtained from the history, the lung examination, or spirometry. Most patients underestimate the amount of sputum they produce, and most patients with bronchitis do not have abnormal adventitious sounds on lung auscultation. Flows and volumes may be normal or abnormal in the patient with chronic bronchitis. To perform the cough test, the examiner stands at a normal conversational distance and instructs the patient to cough vigorously. The normal cough is a single blast and is not self-propagating. The abnormal cough can be wet or dry and mildly, moderately, or severely abnormal. A dry cough is a voluntary cough that results in a paroxysm of dry or hoarse coughing without a deliberate effort behind each blast. A wet cough is mildly abnormal if rhonchi (heard without a stethoscope) disappear immediately without obvious expectoration or swallowing; moderately abnormal if the adventitious sounds disappear only after repeated coughs and obvious expectoration or swallowing; and severely abnormal if the adventitious sounds persist after prolonged, vigorous coughing. The cough test should be used to identify patients who will benefit from a program of perioperative pulmonary toilet. A survey of the literature suggests that the cough test may be a better predictor of postoperative pulmonary complications after abdominal surgery than preoperative spirometry.[11]

In patients who seem to have cognitive impairment, a formal mental status examination, perhaps using a test like the Folstein Mini-Mental State Examination, is helpful. Results can serve as a baseline should postoperative delirium develop. A screening test for depression can also be useful, because depression can retard postoperative recovery.

FIRST-LINE DIAGNOSTIC TESTS: BLOOD AND URINE TESTS, CHEST RADIOGRAPHY, AND THE ELECTROCARDIOGRAM

There is much more opinion and tradition than evidence about which screening tests are needed preoperatively, for elders as well as younger patients. Consequently, instead of individualizing the preoperative testing regimen, the same set of tests is ordered for all patients, and much unnecessary testing is done. Although it is difficult for any one member of the team to go against established practice, team members can come to consensus and develop logical, evidence-based algorithms for preoperative screening that maximize usefulness and minimize costs. These algorithms are most successful when they are developed on the local level by teams consisting of surgeons, anesthesiologists, and primary health care providers.

Screening—testing asymptomatic people for clinically significant silent disease—is not the main consideration here. Most patients referred for a preoperative assessment have medical problems and will have already been seen by the surgeon if not the anesthesiologist. Most will arrive with some test results in hand. A preoperative test ordered by the consultant is justified if it (1) assesses the status of an established or suspected condition, the status of which cannot be reliably known from the interview and the examination; (2) assesses the biochemical derangements that can result from drugs the patient is taking; (3) measures a blood or serum level of a drug that can cause perioperative complications, for example, digoxin, theophylline, or lithium; (4) has at least a modest likelihood of uncovering a clinically silent and correctable condition, which in the short term substantially increases the likelihood of a perioperative complication or in the long term, will threaten function or longevity; or (5) establishes a useful baseline in the patient in whom perioperative problems are anticipated. The consultant can minimize costs by individualizing preoperative testing strategies. A test that does not satisfy one of the five criteria is an unnecessary one. The recency of tests is another consideration. Some data suggest that there is no added value in repeating tests if values obtained in the prior 4 months were normal.[12]

Are Risk Indexes Useful?

Several preoperative risk classification schemes have been developed, for example the time-honored American Society of Anesthesiologists' Physical Status classification,[13] the Cardiac Risk Index developed by Goldman and associates,[14] one for patients facing peripheral vascular surgery by Eagle and colleagues,[15] and one predicting perioperative myocardial infarction by Ashton and colleagues.[16] These are given in Tables 14-4 through 14-7. Worsening scores generally correspond to an increased likelihood of complications on average, but no index is able to make precise predictions for an individual.

Various uses for these indices have been proposed. Surgeons and anesthesiologists might use them to distinguish patients who

TABLE 14-4. FORTY-EIGHT-HOUR OPERATIVE MORTALITY RATES ACCORDING TO THE PHYSICAL STATUS CLASSIFICATION SYSTEM[a]

PHYSICAL STATUS CLASS[b]	NUMBER OF ANESTHETIC PROCEDURES	DEATHS [NUMBER (PERCENT)]
I. Normal healthy patients	50,703	43 (0.1)
II. Patients with mild to moderate systemic disease	12,601	34 (0.3)
III. Patients with severe systemic disease that limits activity but is not incapacitating	3,626	66 (1.8)
IV. Patients with an incapacitating systemic disease that is a constant threat to life	850	66 (7.8)
V. Moribund patients not expected to survive 24 hours with or without operation	608	57 (9.4)

[a]Classification system used by the American Society of Anesthesiologists; data from 11 U.S. Naval Hospitals in mid 1960s.

[b]Emergency and elective cases are grouped together.

TABLE 14-5. THE CARDIAC RISK INDEX[a]

COMPONENTS OF THE INDEX	POINTS
Age >70 years	5
Myocardial infarction in past 6 months	10
S_3 gallop or jugular venous distension	11
Important valvular aortic stenosis	3
Cardiac rhythm other than sinus or atrial premature contractions on last ECG	7
>5 Ventricular premature contractions per minute anytime before operation	7
Poor general status ($Po_2 < 60$ or $Pco_2 > 50$ mm Hg, $K^+ < 3.0$ or $HCO_3^- < 20$ mEq/L, BUN > 50 or creatinine > 3.0 mg/d, abnormal SGOT, signs of chronic liver disease, or bedridden from noncardiac causes)	3
Intraperitoneal, intrathoracic, or aortic operation	3
Emergency operation	4
Total Possible	53

POSTOPERATIVE OUTCOMES ACCORDING TO POINT SCORE

CLASS (NUMBER OF PATIENTS)	POINT TOTAL	NUMBER (PERCENT) OF PATIENTS WITH CARDIAC DEATH OR NONFATAL CARDIAC COMPLICATIONS
I (537)	0–5	5/537 (0.9)
II (316)	6–12	21/316 (6.7)
III (130)	13–25	18/130 (13.9)
IV (18)	≥26	14/18 (77.8)

[a]Developed by Goldman and associates in the mid 1970s.

Abbreviations: K^+, potassium; HCO_3, bicarbonate; SGOT, serum glutamic oxaloacetic transaminase; and BUN, blood urea nitrogen.

TABLE 14-6. INCIDENCE OF CARDIAC COMPLICATIONS AFTER PERIPHERAL VASCULAR SURGERY ACCORDING TO A RISK STRATIFICATION SCHEME	
RISK STRATUM (NUMBER)	NUMBER (PERCENT) WITH POSTOP CARDIAC COMPLICATIONS[a]
No clinical predictors present (64)	2 (3.1)
1 or 2 clinical predictors but no thallium redistribution on dipyridamole/ thallium test (62)	2 (3.2)
1 or 2 clinical predictors plus thallium redistribution (54)	16 (29.6)
3 or more clinical predictors (20)	10 (50.0)

[a]Unstable angina, pulmonary edema, myocardial infarction, or cardiac death.

Clinical predictor variables: Q wave on ECG, age > 70, angina history, history of ventricular ectopy requiring treatment, and diabetes requiring treatment.

[15]Developed by Eagle and Associates (late 1980s).

would benefit from a preoperative medical evaluation from those who would not. Consultants might use them to guide decisions about selecting patients for advanced preoperative cardiac testing. To the consultant, however, their greatest usefulness—and they are extremely useful in this regard—is to serve as checklists of factors which, if corrected, can lower perioperative risk. They should not be used as a basis on which to deny surgery. Point scores cannot be used as decisional fulcrums by responsible surgeons and anesthesiologists. It is difficult to see how writing a point score on a consultation enhances the value of a preoperative medical assessment.

TWO COMMON PROBLEMS IN ELDERS: HYPERTENSION AND DIABETES

The medical consultant is sure to encounter hypertension and diabetes in elders facing surgery because of the high prevalence of these conditions. Data from the 1990 U.S. National Health Interview Survey showed that hypertension affects 354 per 1000 people aged 65 to 74 years and 392 per 1000 of those over age 75 years. Diabetes affects 102 per 1000 in the 65 to 74 age group, and 80 per 1000 of those over 75. Although it is unclear whether either of these conditions *per se* increases the risk of preoperative complications, they cause or predispose to other conditions that do. For example, both hypertension and diabetes are risk factors for atherosclerosis, and coronary atherosclerosis is a risk factor for ischemic postoperative complications such as myocardial infarction.

TABLE 14-7. INCIDENCE OF PERIOPERATIVE INFARCTION, CARDIAC MORTALITY, AND ALL-CAUSE MORTALITY ACCORDING TO A PREOPERATIVE RISK STRATIFICATION SCHEME

DESCRIPTION OF STRATA	ESTIMATED PREVALENCE OF CORONARY ARTERY DISEASE (percent)	OBSERVED MYOCARDIAL INFARCTION RATE [n of n (percent)]	CARDIAC DEATH RATE [n of n (percent)]	OVERALL DEATH RATE [n of n (percent)]
High risk for myocardial infarction: patients with coronary artery disease: history of MI or ECG evidence of MI, typical angina pectoris, angiographically documented significant coronary artery disease, or history of coronary bypass surgery	Nearly 100	13 of 319 (4.1)	7 of 319 (2.3)	13 of 319 (4.1)
Intermediate risk: patients without evident coronary artery disease but with atherosclerotic disease elsewhere: history of stroke, previous or planned vascular surgery, carotid bruit, transient ischemic attack, claudication, or atypical chest pain	30 to 70	2 of 260 (0.8)	1 of 260 (0.4)	9 of 260 (3.5)
Low risk: patients without evident atherosclerotic disease but who are either older than 75 years or who have a high atherogenic risk factor profile; based on age, gender, smoking, blood pressure, glucose tolerance, and cholesterol; patients who have a ≥15% likelihood of a cardiac event within 6 years	5 to 30	0 of 256 (0)	1 of 256 (0.4)	8 of 256 (3.1)
Negligible risk: patients without evident atherosclerosis and with low atherogenic risk factor profiles	Almost 0	Not known[a]	0 of 652 (0)	8 of 652 (1.2)

[a]Electrocardiograms, creatine kinase MB values, and daily postoperative surveillance for infarction were not done in this group. Only the occurrence of and cause of death were tabulated.

Abbreviations: ECG, electrocardiogram; MI, myocardial infarction.

[16]Developed by Ashton and Associates (late 1980s)

Hypertension

People with isolated, reasonably well-controlled high blood pressure do not seem to be at increased risk for perioperative complications. Hypertensive patients who do not have clinically apparent heart disease (by history, physical examination, or electrocardiogram) have a negligible risk of perioperative cardiac complications, even with major surgery, and sophisticated preoperative cardiac testing is not warranted.[16] The hypertensive patient with cardiac disease, renal insufficiency, and a severely limited activity level does have an increased risk of postoperative mortality.[17] The drugs used to treat hypertension can cause intravascular volume deficits and electrolyte abnormalities, and these should be diagnosed and treated before surgery. Stroke with nonneurologic, noncardiac surgery is extremely rare, even in hypertensive elderly patients with overt cerebrovascular disease,[18] and no special preoperative evaluation of the cerebral circulation is indicated. Hypertensive patients, even those who are well controlled, are prone to intraoperative blood pressure lability.

Uncontrolled hypertension, sometimes severe, is a common discovery during a preoperative examination of an elderly patient. If the surgery is elective, it is preferable to defer the procedure for several weeks until the blood pressure is acceptable and the antihypertensive regimen is stable. The choice of antihypertensive regimen should be based on the presence or absence of end-organ damage and the urgency of surgery. Hypertensive emergencies (new or progressive end-organ damage in conjunction with marked elevation of blood pressure) should be treated with parenteral agents; this of course requires hospitalization. Hypertensive urgencies (marked blood pressure elevation without end-organ damage) can be treated with regimens that lower blood pressure over several hours, for example, oral clonidine loading. More important than rapid control is long-term control of the blood pressure. Poorly controlled hypertensive patients can have a higher incidence of postoperative complications. Elevated blood pressure increases myocardial oxygen demand and could increase the risk of perioperative myocardial ischemia.

Antihypertensive medications should generally be continued throughout the perioperative period, unless the patient has a complication that threatens intravascular volume or the integrity of the cardiovascular system. During the preoperative assessment, patients receiving diuretics as antihypertensive agents should have their supine and standing blood pressure measured as a check of volume status. Also, serum potassium should be checked preoperatively. Thiazide and loop diuretics can cause hypokalemia, whereas angiotensin-converting-enzyme inhibitors and potassium-sparing diuretics can cause hyperkalemia.

Diabetes

Studies have shown that complications, especially wound infections, are more common in diabetic patients than in nondiabetic patients. Diabetics with hyperglycemia have impaired collagen synthesis and leukocyte function, both of which predispose to surgical wound problems. The vascular, neurologic, and renal sequelae of diabetes predispose to postoperative cardiac complications and deterioration in renal function. If the first-line preoperative assessment tools do not detect any evidence of atherosclerosis or renal disease, no further preoperative testing is warranted.

Oral hypoglycemic agents can be a source of perioperative complications. Until recently, only sulfonylureas were used as oral hypoglycemics in the United States. They can cause hypoglycemia in the patient who is fasting or who has a poor postoperative food intake. Of all the sulfonylureas, chlorpropamide has the longest half-life (>30 hours) and the longest duration of action (60 to 72 hours). The second generation sulfonylureas, glipizide and glyburide, have a duration of action of up to 24 hours.[19] Consequently, sulfonylureas should be omitted for 24 hours or longer before surgery. Recently, metformin, a biguanide, was approved for use in the United States as an oral hypoglycemic. Metformin should be discontinued 48 hours before surgery. Lactic acidosis is a very rare complication of metformin use; it is associated with a 50 percent mortality rate.[20] If perioperative hyperglycemia develops while oral hypoglycemics are being held, patients can be treated with sliding-scale insulin. Numerous protocols for partial-dose insulin or continuous insulin infusion have been proposed for intra- and perioperative care of the insulin-requiring diabetic patient.[21] None of these regimens appears to be superior in terms of patients' outcomes, however.

Poorly controlled diabetes predisposes to prerenal azotemia in the postoperative period because glucosuria induces osmotic diuresis, urinary losses of sodium and water, and volume depletion. The elderly diabetic patient undergoing surgery thus faces a triple threat to renal function: prerenal azotemia occurring against a background of diabetic nephropathy and age-related diminution in glomerular filtration rate.

RISK OF CARDIAC COMPLICATIONS

Perioperative cardiac complications consist of myocardial infarction, unstable angina, pulmonary edema, dysrhythmias, and infective endocarditis. The latter is a rare complication that can be prevented with prophylactic antibiotics. The regimens recommended by the American Heart Association[22] vary according to the type of cardiac abnormality and the nature of the procedure.

Average rates of perioperative myocardial infarction with noncardiac procedures are given in Table 14-8. With current anesthetic

TABLE 14-8. INCIDENCE RATES OF PERIOPERATIVE MYOCARDIAL INFARCTION (MI) WITH NONCARDIAC SURGERY

OPERATION	AVERAGE MYOCARDIAL INFARCTION RATE (percent)
Transurethral resection of prostate	<1
Cataract extraction	<1
Intrathoracic and upper abdominal procedures	6
Elective major orthopedic procedures	2
Carotic endarterectomy	4
Repair of nonruptured infrarenal aortic aneurysm	7
Vascular surgery of lower extremity	4
Amputation of lower extremity	8

As reported in recent literature.

practices, pre-existing coronary artery disease seems to be a *sine qua non* for the development of a perioperative infarction.[23] Even so, perioperative infarction is a rare event with minor procedures such as cataract extraction and transurethral surgery, despite the high prevalence of coronary artery disease in those surgical populations. Vascular surgery carries the highest risk for perioperative infarction, up to 15 percent in some series. General and orthopedic surgery have intermediate rates. About 30 percent of perioperative infarcts are fatal.

The risk of cardiac complications is a function of the nature of the patient's pre-existing heart disease, the severity of the resultant dysfunction, and the type of the operation. Heart disease can be broadly classified as involving the coronary circulation (coronary atherosclerosis), the valves, the cardiac muscle, or the conduction system. Of course, two or more can coexist in a given patient, and one dysfunction can be secondary to another (e.g., a dilated cardiomyopathy resulting from ischemia). The health care provider will almost always be able to characterize the nature of the patient's heart disease using the first-line assessment tools. In many cases, those first-line tools will also be able determine the severity of the resultant dysfunction. Some patients will need to undergo specialized testing.

Two professional groups have published narrative and algorithmic guidelines for perioperative cardiovascular evaluation for noncardiac surgery.[24, 25] These are extremely helpful; however, they cannot substitute for a thoughtful diagnostic and treatment plan developed by a thorough medical consultant (see Figures 14-1 and 14-2).

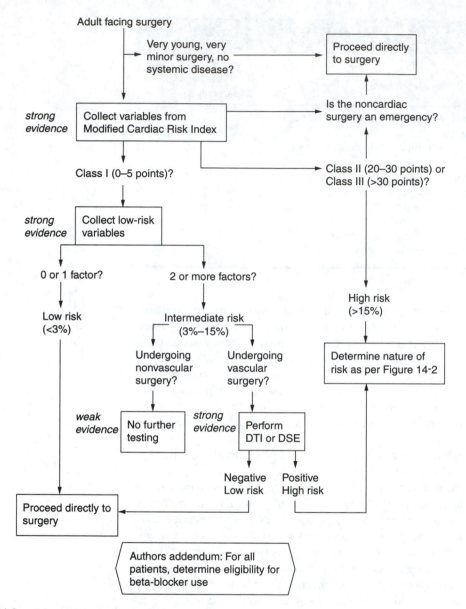

FIGURE 14-1 Algorithm for risk assessment and management of patients at low or intermediate risk for perioperative cardiac events. (Reproduced, with permission, from American College of Physicians. Guidelines for assessing and managing the perioperative risk from coronary artery disease associated with major noncardiac surgery. *Ann Intern Med.* 1997;127(4):311.)

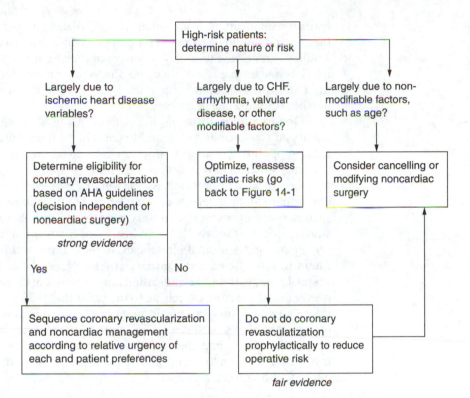

FIGURE 14-2   Algorithm for risk assessment and management of patients at high risk for perioperative cardiac events. (Reproduced, with permission, from American College of Physicians. Guidelines for assessing and managing the perioperative risk from coronary artery disease associated with major noncardiac surgery. *Ann Intern Med.* 1997;127(4):311.)

Preoperative Cardiac Testing

The topic of cardiac testing before noncardiac surgery is one for which numerous and often conflicting opinions abound but little evidence exists from well-designed, empiric studies.[26] The problem exists because physicians do not know how to act on the results of the tests when they receive them. No randomized trials have been performed to evaluate the efficacy and safety of the interventions purported to reduce the risk of perioperative cardiac complications with noncardiac surgery. Proposed interventions include the use of certain drugs intraoperatively, preoperative angioplasty, preoperative coronary artery bypass, the use of intraoperative left ventricular assist devices, or even, postoperative monitoring in the intensive care unit. The morbidity and mortality risks of some of these interventions exceed, on average, the risk of a perioperative cardiac complication. Consequently, specialized preoperative cardiac testing should be reserved for patients whose clinical condition would warrant such testing *if they were not facing surgery.* Specialized cardiac testing is not indicated unless the current condition of the patient is such that cardiac tests would be warranted even if he/she were not facing surgery.

One exception to this is the patient facing abdominal aortic aneurysm repair or aortofemoral bypass. In such patients, specialized preoperative testing is informative because the prevalence of coronary atherosclerosis is very high and the first-line assessment tools do not yield an accurate assessment of the presence or absence of coronary atherosclerosis or its severity. Many patients requiring such surgery have overt coronary atherosclerosis. Among those who do not, that is, who have no history of myocardial infarction, no angina, and a normal electrocardiogram, about a third will be found to have significant coronary atherosclerosis of at least one vessel. Lower extremity claudication limits activity in these patients, preventing them from exercising to the point that they would experience angina. Moreover, aortic aneurysm repair and aortofemoral bypass procedures require cross-clamping of the aorta during surgery. This sudden impedance to left ventricular outflow increases myocardial oxygen demand and can be tolerated poorly in the patient with coronary stenosis.

Coronary Artery Disease

In the patient with coronary artery disease, further preoperative testing is not generally necessary if the patient (1) has a remote history of myocardial infarction (at least 3 months) but is now asymptomatic; or (2) has chronic, stable exertional angina. Patients with newly discovered angina or an anginal pattern that is worsening or poorly controlled, should be treated with the appropriate medications and evaluated using a noninvasive estimate of coronary flow reserve such as stress thallium scintigraphy or stress echocardiography. (Coronary flow reserve is the difference between the coronary flow at rest and during maximal coronary vasodilatation.) Patients who are unable to exercise can undergo testing with a pharmacologic agent such as dipyridamole or adenosine, or in the case of echocardiography, dobutamine. Some may then be referred on for coronary angiography. Angiography may reveal that the patient fits into a category of patients in whom longevity will be improved by angioplasty or coronary artery bypass surgery. In such patients, the surgical problem takes a back seat until the cardiac problem is treated.

Aortic Stenosis

Aortic stenosis is an established risk factor for cardiac complications with operative procedures. Longstanding obstruction to left ventricular outflow and its attendant compensatory mechanisms limit the patient's ability to tolerate the tachyarrhythmias and blood pressure changes that can occur perioperatively. The early compensatory mechanism is the development of left ventricular hypertrophy. Myocardial oxygen demand is increased by the hypertrophied muscle mass, the increase in left ventricular systolic pressure needed to overcome the outflow obstruction, and the prolongation of left ventricular ejection time. Myocardial oxygen supply is compromised because an increase in left ventricular diastolic pressure can decrease the perfusion pressure across the coronary bed, which can result in subendocardial ischemia. Moreover, atherosclerosis of the epicardial coronaries often coexists with aortic stenosis.

Careful anesthetic management can reduce the risk of perioperative complications in the patient with aortic stenosis. It is, therefore, important for the surgical team to know whether or not aortic stenosis is present before the patient reaches the operating room. If the first-line assessment tools lead the medical consultant to suspect aortic stenosis, Doppler echocardiography can estimate its severity by examining the valve area and the transvalvular aortic gradient.

In the patient with aortic stenosis, operative risk with noncardiac surgery is a function of the degree of symptomatology of the valve disease, the degree of left ventricular systolic and diastolic impairment, the severity of the outflow obstruction, the nature of the operation, and the anesthetic technique. The literature indicates that in certain patients, especially those with preserved left ventricular systolic function, careful perioperative care can keep the incidence of cardiac complications low, even if the aortic stenosis is severe.[27] In patients whose longevity would clearly be improved by valve replacement, the noncardiac procedure should be deferred. In still others, balloon valvuloplasty may be an option. Though generally only a temporizing measure because its favorable effects on hemodynamics are short-lived, and restenosis occurs rapidly, it may reduce the risk of perioperative cardiac complications in patients who are not candidates for valve replacement.

Heart Failure

Heart failure is one of the strongest risk factors for perioperative cardiac complications with noncardiac surgery. It is quite prevalent among American elders, and its prevalence has increased as the death rate from acute myocardial infarction has decreased. In 1995, heart failure accounted for 6.5 percent of all hospital stays provided to the nation's 29 million fee-for-service Medicare beneficiaries. It is not uncommon that the initial diagnosis of heart failure is made at the time of a preoperative assessment.

Heart failure is a clinical syndrome that occurs when the cardiac output is insufficient to meet the body's needs. Its symptoms include dyspnea on exertion, decreased exercise tolerance, fatigue, orthopnea, paroxysmal nocturnal dyspnea, lower extremity edema, abdominal complaints, and in elders, mental status changes. Dyspnea on exertion, usually the earliest symptom of heart failure, is a symptom that is found frequently during preoperative assessments. Yet it is nonspecific, and can result from several noncardiac causes as well. The first-line assessment tools will usually be able to determine the likely explanation for dyspnea on exertion. If the cardiovascular examination reveals elevated jugular venous pulses, an S_3 gallop, and a laterally displaced apical impulse, the most likely diagnosis is heart failure. A national expert panel has recommended that such patients undergo echocardiography or radionuclide ventriculography to assess left ventricular ejection fraction, as the history and physical cannot reliably distinguish heart failure resulting from systolic dysfunction from that resulting from diastolic dysfunction, valvular heart disease, or other causes.[28] This is particularly true in elders. These distinctions are important because treatment differs. For example, several of the pharmacologic agents useful in systolic dysfunction (i.e., digoxin, nitrates, and angiotensin converting enzyme inhibitors) can actually worsen heart failure due to diastolic dysfunction. Elective surgery should be deferred for patients with newly diagnosed heart failure until the etiology and contributing factors (e.g., thyroid disease, anemia) are understood and the patient is well compensated on a stable medication regimen.

Patients who come to preoperative assessment with a known diagnosis of heart failure should be well compensated and at their dry weight at the time they are sent to surgery. At their "dry weight," a heart failure patient has normal jugular venous pressures, no S_3, no pedal edema, and an exercise capacity as good as can be achieved. Repeating echocardiographic or radionuclide ventriculography preoperatively in patients who have undergone past testing has little value. The left ventricular ejection fraction tells nothing about the degree of compensation. This must be determined by history and physical examination (the only alternative is to insert a pulmonary artery catheter and plot left ventricular function curves). Simply having the left ventricular ejection fraction in the chart when the patient is sent for surgery does not reduce the risk of perioperative cardiac complications. If test results will not or cannot influence therapy or decision making, then testing is a waste of resources.

Conduction Disorders

Atrial fibrillation is the most common chronic disorder of the cardiac rhythm and is observed in about 5 percent of elders. Most elders with atrial fibrillation have organic heart disease. If atrial fibrillation is detected for the first time at the preoperative assessment, elective surgery should be deferred until the etiology of the arrhythmia has been established (e.g., hyperthyroidism), decisions about cardioversion and antiembolic therapy have been made, and the ventricular rate controlled. A rapid ventricular rate can lead to heart failure, ischemia, and hypotension perioperatively. Atrial fibrillation with a slow ventricular rate not attributable to drugs is considered to be indicative of sick sinus syndrome; further evaluation is mandatory, as this disorder commonly requires permanent pacemaker insertion. Atrial flutter is much less common than atrial fibrillation. Seldom chronic, it is usually paroxysmal.

Of the atrioventricular blocks, 3rd-degree AV block, though rare, has serious implications both in the short term for elective surgery and over the long term. It can be an incidental finding on the preoperative electrocardiogram, but more commonly is symptomatic, with about half the patients reporting syncope or near syncope. Pacemaker insertion is usually required. Second-degree AV block is rare and usually asymptomatic. Pacemaker insertion is usually not required. First-degree AV block is observed in up to 10 percent of elderly patients. It is of no clinical consequence.

Sick sinus syndrome (or sinus node dysfunction) is an uncommon condition. It is usually symptomatic, and usually requires permanent pacemaker insertion. Sick sinus syndrome is actually a collection of arrhythmias, including sinus pauses, sinoatrial exit block, chronic or paroxysmal atrial fibrillation, paroxysmal atrial flutter, and some types of supraventricular tachyarrhythmias. The so-called brady-tachy syndrome is considered to be a variant. If discovered at the time of a preoperative assessment, surgery should be deferred until it is certain that the cardiac rhythm is hemodynamically stable.

Bundle branch blocks are another relatively common conduction disorder in elders. Organic cardiac disease is much more likely to be present when left bundle branch block is observed than with right bundle branch. Even when bifascicular block is present (the most common combination is right bundle branch block with left anterior fascicular block), progression to more advanced block is rare. Temporary pacemaker insertion for prophylaxis during noncardiac surgery is no longer thought to be necessary.

Atrial premature contractions are commonly observed on 12-lead electrocardiograms in elders. They merit no attention if no organic cardiac disease is present. Similarly, ventricular premature contractions are present in up the three quarters of elders. These are usually isolated and asymptomatic. Those causing syncope and near syncope require full evaluation before elective surgery is undertaken. Some patients may require suppressive therapy; this is an area of controversy.

If a permanent pacemaker is present, its function should be evaluated in the weeks prior to noncardiac surgery. The operating room team should be notified so that a magnet is available to change the pacemaker from a demand to a fixed rate mode if need be, and so that precautions can be taken with regard to placement and operation of the electrocautery unit.

RISK OF PULMONARY COMPLICATIONS

The overall frequency of postoperative pulmonary complications is thought to rival, if not exceed, that of cardiac complications, but precise estimates are difficult to obtain because of definitional and ascertainment differences among studies. Pulmonary complications are most common after thoracic and intra-abdominal operations. The most common pulmonary complications are atelectasis and pneumonia. One recent, well-designed study documented a 15 percent incidence of these after abdominal surgery involving visceral manipulation (i.e., not abdominal wall or groin hernia repair).[29] Atelectasis occurs because of under-ventilation and/or the pooling of secretions in dependent regions of the lung (rarely, due to malpositioning of the endotracheal tube intraoperatively). Infection can occur if the atelectatic areas are not reexpanded promptly. Atelectasis or pneumonia can lead to respiratory failure (an arterial PO_2 <60) and ventilator dependence. Pleural effusions are common after intra-abdominal procedures; they are not considered complications. Postoperative adult respiratory distress syndrome, which is due to a noncardiogenic pulmonary edema, is a very rare postoperative complication; its incidence appears to be decreasing even further. The fat embolism syndrome is an uncommon complication of fracture of long bones. It is a rare occurrence after total hip arthroplasty. Fat deposition in the lungs can cause a full-blown adult respiratory distress syndrome, and most of the fatalities from fat embolism occur from respiratory failure. Clinically significant pneumonitis due to aspiration of gastric contents is quite uncommon; it is seen most often in patients who need emergency surgery and come to the operating room with a full stomach. In patients undergoing general, orthopedic, or urologic surgery who are not treated with prophylactic subcutaneous heparin perioperatively, the frequency of fatal pulmonary embolism secondary to deep venous thrombosis is 0.5 percent to 1 percent, and of nonfatal pulmonary embolism, about 2 percent; prophylactic heparin can prevent half of these.[30]

The risk for pulmonary complications is a function of the nature of the patient's pre-existing lung disease, the amount of secretions produced by the tracheobronchial tree, the severity of chronic gas exchange derangements, the location of the incision and its proximity to the diaphragm, the breaching of the lung's mechanical barriers to infection by tracheal intubation and mechanical ventilation, and respiratory depression secondary to anesthesia and analgesic agents. All chronic lung diseases increase the risk for postoperative pulmonary complications. The conditions most often encountered include chronic obstructive lung disease (chronic bronchitis and emphysema), reactive airways disease, the restrictive diseases, and obstructive sleep apnea. Upper abdominal surgery carries the highest risk for complications (after, of course, lung resective surgery.) Vital capacity is reduced after surgery on the upper abdomen, due to pain as well as a pain-independent suppression of diaphragmatic function. Shallow respirations and infrequent sighing predispose to atelectasis. Laparascopic cholecystectomy may not be a good alternative to the open procedure in patients with chronic lung disease. The procedure requires insufflation of a large amount of CO_2 into the peritoneal cavity, which compromises diaphragmatic excursion. Moreover, because CO_2 is so soluble in blood and so rapidly diffused across the peritoneum, the arterial P_{CO_2} can rise, causing hypercarbia and acidosis.

The first-line assessment tools, including the cough test and the 6-minute walking test, will reliably indicate whether significant chronic lung disease is present and will provide a good estimate of mechanical ventilatory capacity. The function of the lung is gas exchange, however, and blood gas derangements cannot be reliably detected by history and physical examination. Patients with moderate to severe chronic lung disease should have their arterial blood gases measured as part of the preoperative assessment. Noninvasive measurement of O_2 saturation is not sufficient, because arterial P_{CO_2} levels must be known. Chronic CO_2 retention is a marker for increased all-cause mortality postoperatively; some pulmonologists believe that only life-saving surgery should be performed in patients with chronic CO_2 retention.

Preoperative Spirometry

Spirometry, which measures air flows and volumes, is greatly over-utilized in the preoperative setting. Occasionally, the first line-assessment tools will fail to reveal the cause of dyspnea on exertion. The consultant may find spirometry diagnostically helpful in such patients. The only patients in whom preoperative spirometry is unequivocally useful *in a predictive sense* are those facing lung resection. The decision to proceed with resection is based, in part, on estimates of what ventilatory capacity will be after lung resection. Those estimates are based on preoperative spirometry and other tests of ventilation and perfusion.

Otherwise, preoperative spirometry is of uncertain value. Does spirometry provide relevant diagnostic information over and above that obtained by the first-line assessment tools? Usually not. Will the decision to operate or not to operate be based on the test results? Not if the surgery is life-saving. If the operation is to restore function, perhaps it should not be done if the patients' chronic lung disease is what most limits exercise capacity. Will test results influence anesthesia technique? Since there is no reliable evidence that anesthetic technique influences the risk of postoperative pulmonary complications, why not just proceed based on the assumption that lung disease is present? Can the test predict more accurately than the health care provider which patients are most likely to have postoperative pulmonary complications? No; the actual values for flows and volumes do not discriminate levels of risk well. Can the test save money or enhance safety by identifying patients who will benefit from prophylaxis against pulmonary complications? No; the only prophylaxis shown to be effective is a program of perioperative incentive spirometry and pulmonary toilet,[29] a program so cheap and harmless that it can performed on all patients.

Risk Reduction

Smokers who abstain for 8 weeks or more reduce their chances of a postoperative pulmonary complication to levels near those of nonsmokers. Patients who have been taking long-term oral corticosteroids will need intravenous steroids in the immediate perioperative period. Atelectasis is avoided or reversed by a program of deep breathing and sputum mobilization consisting of early ambulation, coughing and deep breathing, incentive spirometry, and in some patients, inhaled bronchodilator. Elders will benefit from learning this program a week or two before admission for surgery. Prophylaxis against thromboembolic disease using heparin, warfarin, or mechanical means is part of the standard of care for all lower extremity joint replacement operations and most other major operations.

RISK OF POSTOPERATIVE DELIRIUM

Postoperative delirium is an acute, temporary deterioration in cognitive status characterized by fluctuating levels of consciousness and inattention occurring shortly after an operation. Patients who develop postoperative delirium have a longer hospital stay and a greater risk of other sorts of postoperative complications. It is a common occurrence in elders but its precise incidence is uncertain.[31] Based on patients' self-report, the incidence is surprisingly high. Six of ten patients relate that they experienced cognitive difficulties during their early postoperative course.

Risk factors include advanced age, preoperative cognitive impairment (dementia or depression), use of anticholinergic drugs, and alcohol abuse. Anesthetic technique does not seem to be a strong factor. A clinical prediction rule for postoperative delirium was developed in a recent study.[32] Seven factors were found to be independently associated with postoperative delirium: age over 70 years; alcohol abuse; poor cognitive status; poor functional status; abnormal preoperative serum sodium, potassium, or glucose; noncardiac thoracic surgery; and aortic aneurysm surgery. These factors should be evaluated during the preoperative assessment. Reversible problems, such as electrolyte abnormalities, should be corrected preoperatively. Patients and families should be cautioned that a brief cognitive decline may occur in the early postoperative period (see Chapter 20).

Factors Independently Associated with Postoperative Delirium

- Age over 70 years
- Alcohol abuse
- Poor cognitive status
- Poor functional status
- Abnormal preoperative serum sodium, potassium, or glucose
- Noncardiac thoracic surgery
- Aortic aneurysm surgery

RISK OF URINARY TRACT COMPLICATIONS

The most common postoperative complications involving the urinary tract include acute renal failure, urinary retention, and urinary tract infection. The actual incidence of these complications in elders has not been tabulated, but clinical observation indicates they occur quite frequently. Frequency varies by type of operation. Acute oliguric or nonoliguric renal failure is seen most commonly with cardiac and vascular operations. Mild or moderate deterioration in renal function, usually transitory, is often seen postoperatively in elderly patients regardless of the type of operation.

Many endogenous and exogenous threats to renal function are present in the elderly patient facing surgery. Factors threatening

Threats to Intravascular
Volume

- Change in body composition with loss of muscle mass and adipose tissue gain
- Decline in glomerular filtration rate
- Decline in kidney's ability to conserve water
- Decline in kidney's ability to conserve salt
- Decreased fluid intake due to decline in thirst perception

intravascular volume and predisposing to prerenal azotemia include the fasting state, the purges and bowel preparations required before some operations, and the fluid losses associated with the surgical problem, which may include vomiting, nasogastric suction, third-space sequestration, or hemorrhage. These are superimposed upon five age-related changes that impair the ability of elders to respond to a threat to intravascular volume: (1) a change in body composition with loss of muscle mass and gain of adipose tissue, which leads to a decrease in total body water; (2) a decline in glomerular filtration rate; (3) a decline in the kidney's ability to conserve water; (4) a decline in the kidney's ability to conserve salt; and (5) decreased fluid intake because of a decline in thirst perception. Moreover, many elders use diuretics and drugs with adverse effects on the kidney such as nonsteroidal anti-inflammatory agents. Background diabetic or hypertensive nephropathy can complicate matters further. Fractures, orthopedic procedures, and the restraints required in some patients with postoperative delirium "trap" the patient in bed and limit voluntary ingestion of fluids.

In assessing the elderly patient for surgery, renal function should be evaluated by a check of blood urea nitrogen and serum creatinine. A urinalysis and examination of urinary sediment should be performed. If renal insufficiency is newly diagnosed, elective surgery should be deferred until its severity and etiology can be determined by means of the standard evaluation of renal function and structure. When renal insufficiency is severe, the assistance of a nephrologist may be necessary in the perioperative period. Urinary tract infections should be treated before surgery, particularly when the operation involves placement of a prosthetic material. Men should be questioned about lower tract obstructive symptoms; benign prostatic hyperplasia places them at risk for acute urinary retention postoperatively.

REFERENCES

1. Kronlund SF, Phillips WR. Physician knowledge of risks of surgical and invasive diagnostic procedures. *West J Med.* 1985;142(4):565–569.
2. Keenan RL, Boyan P. Cardiac arrest due to anesthesia. A study of incidence and causes. *JAMA.* 1985;253(16):2373–2377.
3. Oesterling JE. Benign prostatic hyperplasia. Medical and minimally invasive treatment options. *N Engl J Med.* 1995;332(2):99–109.
4. Wong RW, Rappaport WD, Witzke RB, Putnam CW, Hunter GC. Factors influencing the safety of colostomy closure in the elderly. *J Surg Res.* 1994;57(2):289–291.
5. Callahan CM, Drake BG, Heck DA, Dittus RS. Patient outcomes following tricompartmental total knee replacement. *JAMA.* 1994;271(17):1349–1357.

6. Detsky AS, Baker JP, O'Rourke K, Goel V. Perioperative parenteral nutrition: a meta-analysis. *Ann Intern Med.* 1987;107(2):195–203.

7. Greenburg AG, Saik RP, Coyle JJ, Peskin GW. Mortality and gastro-intestinal surgery in the aged: elective vs. emergency procedures. *Arch Surg.* 1981;116(5):788–791.

8. Kearon C, Hirsch J. Management of anticoagulation before and after elective surgery. *N Engl J Med.* 1997;336(21):1506–1511.

9. Lipkin D, Scriven A, Crake T, Poole-Wilson PA. Six-minute walking test for assessing exercise capacity in chronic heart failure. *BMJ.* 1986;292(8 Mar):653–655.

10. Greene BA, Berkowitz S. The preanesthetic induced cough as a method of diagnosis of preoperative bronchitis. *Ann Intern Med.* 1952;37(11):723–732.

11. Lawrence VA, Page CP, Harris GD. Preoperative spirometry before abdominal operations. A critical appraisal of its predictive value. *Arch Intern Med.* 1989;149(2):280–285.

12. MacPherson DS, Snow R, Lofgren RP. Preoperative screening: value of previous tests. *Ann Intern Med.* 1990;113(12):969–973.

13. Vacanti CJ, VanHouten RJ, Hill RC. A statistical analysis of the relationship of physical status to postoperative mortality in 68,388 cases. *Anesth Analg.* 1970;49(4):564–566.

14. Goldman L, Caldera DL, Nussbaum SR, et al. Multifactorial index of cardiac risk in noncardiac surgical procedures. *N Engl J Med.* 1977;297(16):845–850.

15. Eagle KA, Cooley CM, Newell JB, et al. Combining clinical and thallium data optimizes preoperative assessment of cardiac risk before major vascular surgery. *Ann Intern Med.* 1989;110(11):859–866.

16. Ashton CM, Petersen NJ, Kiefe CI, Wray NP, Dunn JK, Wu L. The incidence of perioperative myocardial infarction with noncardiac surgery. *Ann Intern Med.* 1993;118(7):504–510.

17. Browner WS, Li J, Mangano DT, for the Study of Perioperative Ischemia Research Group. In-hospital and long-term mortality in male veterans following noncardiac surgery. *JAMA.* 1992;268(1):228–232.

18. Ropper AH, Wechsler LR, Wilson LS. Carotid bruit and the risk of stroke in elective surgery. *N Engl J Med.* 1982;307(22):1388–1390.

19. Halter JB, Morrow LA. Use of sulfonylurea drugs in elderly patients. *Diabetes Care.* 1990;13(suppl. 2):86–92.

20. Bailey CJ, Turner RC. Metformin. *N Engl J Med.* 1996;334(9):574–579.

21. Schiff RL, Emanuele MA. The surgical patient with diabetes mellitus: guidelines for management. *J Gen Intern Med.* 1995;10(3):154–161.

22. Dajani AS, Bisno AL, Chung KJ, et al. Prevention of bacterial endocarditis. Recommendations by the American Heart Association. *JAMA.* 1990;264(22):2919–2922.

23. Ashton CM. Perioperative myocardial infarction with noncardiac surgery. *Am J Med Sci.* 1994;308(1):41–48.

24. American College of Physicians. Guidelines for assessing and managing the perioperative risk from coronary artery disease associated with major noncardiac surgery. *Ann Intern Med.* 1997;127(4):309–312.

25. American College of Cardiology/American Heart Association Task Force. Guidelines for perioperative cardiovascular evaluation for noncardiac surgery. *J Am Coll Card.* 1996;27(4):910–948.

26. Mangano DT, Goldman L. Preoperative assessment of patients with known or suspected coronary disease. *N Engl J Med.* 1995;333(26): 1750–1756.

27. O'Keefe JH, Shub C, Rettke SR. Risk of noncardiac surgical procedures in patients with aortic stenosis. *Mayo Clin Proc.* 1989; 64(4):400–405.

28. Konstam M, Dracup K, Baker D, and the members of the Heart Failure Guideline Panel. Heart failure: evaluation and care of patients with left-ventricular systolic dysfunction. *Clinical Practice Guideline,* no. 11. AHCPR Pub. No. 94-0612. Rockville, MD: Agency for Health Care Policy and Research, PHS, USDHHS, June; 1994.

29. Hall JC, Tarala R, Harris J, Tapper J, Christiansen K. Incentive spirometry versus routine chest physiotherapy for prevention of pulmonary complications after abdominal surgery. *Lancet.* 1991;337(Apr 2):953–956.

30. Collins R, Scrimgeour A, Yusuf S, Peto R. Reduction in fatal pulmonary embolism and venous thrombosis by perioperative administration of subcutaneous heparin. Overview of results of randomized trials in general, orthopedic, and urologic surgery. *N Engl J Med.* 1988;318(18):1162–1173.

31. Dyer CB, Ashton CM, Teasdale TA. Postoperative delirium. A review of 80 primary data collection studies. *Arch Intern Med.* 1995;155(Mar 13):461–465.

32. Marcantonio ER, Goldman L, Mangione CM, et al. A clinical prediction rule for delirium after elective noncardiac surgery. *JAMA.* 1994;271(2):134–139.

PAIN

BRUCE A. FERRELL

Pain is a common problem in elders. Population-based studies have estimated that the prevalence of pain complaints may be as high as 25 percent to 50 percent of community-dwelling elders.[1-2] Among nursing home residents, the prevalence is even higher and has been reported to be as high as 45 percent to 80 percent.[3-4] Studies have also suggested that pain is often under recognized and under treated.[4-6] The consequences of pain are also common. Depression, decreased socialization, sleep disturbance, impaired ambulation, slow rehabilitation, and adverse effects from multiple drug prescriptions have all been associated with pain in elders.[1]

Pain is an unpleasant sensory and emotional experience.[7] It is a universal human discomfort derived from sensory stimuli and modified by individual memory, expectations, and emotions. Unfortunately, there are no reliable biologic markers of pain. Thus, the most accurate evidence for the existence of pain is the patient's description, interpretation, and self-report.[8]

Pain assessment is the most important part of pain management. Accurate pain assessment is important to identify the underlying cause, choose the most effective management strategy, evaluate the effectiveness of treatment, and maximize outcomes. Compared to younger populations, older people can present unique challenges to pain assessment. For example, elders often exhibit

The Agency for Health Care Policy and Research (AHCPR) was renamed in December 1999.
This agency is now known as the Agency for Healthcare Research and Quality (AHRQ).

altered presentations of common illness, multiple potential sources for pain, as well as sensory and cognitive impairment, making accurate pain assessment more difficult. Recent publication and acceptance of clinical practice guidelines for pain assessment and management have made pain assessment and essential part of all health care.[9-12] This chapter discusses salient principles of pain assessment and measurement, with special emphasis on important issues that apply especially to elders.

CLASSIFICATION OF PAIN

Individual pain experiences are quite variable in description, as are underlying diseases, and responses to treatment. For understanding and treating pain, several classification schemes have been proposed. The distinction between acute and chronic pain can help set the tone for diagnostic evaluation as well as urgency for treatment of remedial or life-threatening conditions. For chronic pain, understanding and identifying pathophysiologic mechanisms that produce pain can be essential in the approach to long-term treatment.

Acute Versus Chronic Pain

For diagnostic purposes, it can be helpful to categorize pain as acute or chronic. Acute pain is usually defined by its distinct onset, obvious source, and relatively short duration. It is often self-limited with rapid diagnosis and effective remedy of the underlying cause. Acute pain can be associated with autonomic nervous system signs such as tachycardia, diaphoresis, mild hypertension, or temperature elevation. Acute pain often implies the existence of acute injury such as trauma, ischemia, or inflammation. More importantly, acute pain can indicate the existence of remedial disease, which if not diagnosed accurately and treated appropriately, might result in loss of life or serious disability. For this reason, acute pain should often trigger an emergent search for diagnosis and definitive treatment of the underlying cause.

Chronic pain is often categorized by its long duration and association with chronic conditions. Examples include pain associated with osteoarthritis, back disease, diabetic neuralgia, and postherpetic neuralgia. There are usually no physiologic signs of pain, other than longstanding functional and psychological responses to chronic disease. The identification of chronic pain usually requires a broad approach to assessment and treatment that does not usually require emergency diagnosis and treatment.

In reality, chronic pain is not always easy to describe and has led to considerable difficulty in classification and treatment. A universally acceptable definition for chronic pain remains problematic. For some conditions, chronic pain is defined arbitrarily as pain that lasts longer than 3 or 6 months, or beyond an expected time frame for healing. An example might be a traumatic neuropathy that persists beyond the expected time frame for healing other tissues. For some conditions, it is recognized from the onset that healing may never occur. In these cases, definition of chronic pain has become synonymous with the underlying disease. Examples might include cancer pain or diabetic neuropathy, considered chronic pain syndromes by definition regardless of the onset or duration. In many cases, chronic pain is understood as persistent pain that is not amenable to routine pain control methods. Such conditions are considered chronic pain only after several attempts at treatment have failed. Finally, chronic pain can also be defined by recurrent attacks of acute pain associated with conditions such as osteoarthritis, headaches, or vascular insufficiency. Because there are many differences in what may be regarded as chronic pain, care must be taken to carefully diagnose underlying diseases and understand the natural history of pain associated with these chronic disease states. For a more detailed description, the reader is encouraged to study the classification of chronic pain by the International Association for the Study of Pain.[7, 8]

Finally, a variety of successful new approaches to pain management have made the distinction between acute and chronic pain less important for pain treatment decisions. Strategies such as fast-acting oral medications, infusion technology, and sustained-release drugs have found widespread use in chronic as well as acute pain situations. Thus, the distinction between acute and chronic pain has become less important for treatment purposes.

Pathophysiology of Pain

For making decisions regarding pain relief strategies, classifying chronic pain in terms of pathophysiology can be helpful.[9] Treatment strategies targeted specifically to underlying pain mechanisms are more likely to be effective. For example, nociceptive pain typically responds well to most analgesic medications. In contrast, effective strategies for neuropathic pain can include nontraditional analgesic medications such as antidepressants, anticonvulsants, or local anesthetics. Indeed, pathophysiologic pain mechanisms of pain generation have been identified for many chronic pain syndromes. Although it is beyond the scope of this chapter to describe the pathophysiology of every pain syndrome, most can be classified

TABLE 15-1. PATHOPHYSIOLOGIC CLASSIFICATION OF CHRONIC PAIN

I. Nociceptive Pain
  Trauma (fractures, strain, tears)
  Burns
  Mechanical stretch and tissue deformity (tumor bulk)
  Arthropathies (rheumatoid arthritis, osteoarthritis, gout, post-
    traumatic arthropathies, mechanical neck and back syndromes)
  Myalgia (myofascial pain syndromes, muscle spasm)
  Skin and mucosal ulcerations
  Nonarticular inflammatory disorders (polymyalgia rheumatica)
  Ischemic disorders
  Visceral pain (pain of internal organs and viscera, cancer)
II. Neuropathic Pain
  Peripheral nervous system
   Post-herpetic neuralgia
   Trigeminal neuralgia
   Painful diabetic neuropathy
   Postamputation pain (phantom limb)
   Nerve infiltration by cancer (bracheoplexis or femeroplexis syn-
     dromes)
  Central nervous system
   Post-stroke pain ("central pain")
   Myelopathic/radiculopathic pain (e.g., spinal stenosis, arach-
     noiditis, root sleeve fibrosis)
  Sympathetic nervous system
   Reflex sympathetic dystrophy
   Causalgia-like syndromes (complex regional pain syndromes)
III. Mixed or Undetermined Pathophysiology
  Chronic recurrent headaches (tension headaches, migraine head-
    aches, mixed headaches)
  Vasculopathic pain syndromes (painful vasculitis)
IV. Psychologically Mediated Pain Syndromes
  Somatization disorders
   Hysterical reactions

into four broad categories. An outline of this classification system with examples are shown in Table 15-1. Nociceptive pain can be visceral (related to internal organs and viscera) or somatic (related to body walls and the musculoskeletal system) and is most often derived from stimulation of pain receptors.[13] Nociceptive pain can arise from tissue inflammation, mechanical deformation, ongoing injury or destruction. Examples include inflammatory or traumatic arthritis, myofascial pain syndromes, and ischemic disorders. Neuropathic pain results from a pathophysiologic process that involves the peripheral or central nervous system.[14] Examples include trigeminal neuralgia, post-herpetic neuralgia, post-stroke "central" or "thalamic pain," and post-amputation "phantom limb" pain.[15] Mixed or unspecified pain is often regarded as having mixed or unknown mechanisms. Examples include recurrent headaches and some vasculitic pain syndromes. Treatment of these syndromes is more unpredictable, and may require various trials of different or combined approaches. Finally, when psychological factors are judged to play a major role in the onset, severity, exacerbation, or maintenance of pain, this is described as psychologically mediated pain.[16] Examples include somatoform disorders such as conversion hysterical syndromes.[17] These patients can benefit from specific psychiatric treatments, but traditional medical interventions for analgesia are not indicated.

PAIN HISTORY AND PHYSICAL EXAMINATION

History

Assessment of pain should begin with a thorough history to help establish the medical diagnosis and form a baseline description of pain experiences. Pain treatment is most successful when the underlying cause of pain is identified and treated definitively. Past medical and surgical history is important in order to focus on coexisting disease and medication use. A review of systems should include emphasis on the musculoskeletal and nervous system because of the frequency with which problems often arise in these systems. Any history of trauma should be thoroughly investigated because even minor trauma can result in occult fractures and other injuries in frail elders. In this setting, care must be taken to avoid attributing acute pain to preexisting conditions. Making this problem worse is the fact that chronic pain can fluctuate with time. Injuries due to trauma as well as acute inflammatory arthritis such as gout or calcium pyrophosphate crystal disease, can be easily overlooked in this setting. Only astute questioning and comprehensive evaluation can help avoid these pitfalls.[18]

Elders often use a variety of words to describe pain. Many do not use the word "pain" but they refer to the problem as "hurting," "aching," "burning," or other descriptive terms. Health care providers should probe for and use these descriptive terms in the initial assessment and during subsequent follow-up evaluations.

To elicit a specific description of pain, the history should include the questions: what, when, where, and how.

The mnemonic, "OLD CART," can be useful in taking the pain history.
Onset
Location
Duration
Characteristics
Aggravating factors
Relieving factors
Treatments

Physical Examination

A thorough physical examination should be performed and findings should confirm any suspicions suggested by the history. Because of the frequency with which problems are often identified, the physical examination should probably concentrate on the musculoskeletal and nervous systems. Palpation should be performed for tender points of inflammation, muscle spasm, and trigger points. Inspection and observation for deformities such as scoliosis, kyphosis, abnormal posture, joint alignments, and gait disturbances should be conducted. Joint range of motion and reproduction of aggravating movements are helpful in identifying disabilities often associated with pain and the need for rehabilitation.[19] A systematic neurologic examination is also important. A search for sensory deficits, weakness, and muscle atrophy can confirm suspicions of neuropathic mechanisms of pain. Signs of autonomic neuropathies should also be elicited, such as mottled skin in a denervated extremity, the presence of a Charcot joint, orthostatic hypotension accompanied by a failed heart rate response, and disorders of gastric emptying or incontinence. These signs can imply the existence of reflex sympathetic dystrophy or sympathetically maintained pain syndromes.[14–15]

Functional Status

It is important to assess the patient's functional status to identify self-care deficits and formulate treatment interventions that maximize independence and enhance quality of life. Functional status can also represent an important outcome for assessment of overall pain management. Assessment of functional status includes information obtained in the history and physical examination as well as information that can be obtained by use of one or several functional status scales validated in elders. Activities of Daily Living (see Appendix #24),[20, 21] the Functional Independence Measure (FIM) (see Appendix #15),[22] the Arthritis Impact Scale (AIMS),[23] or the Sickness Impact Profile[24] are examples of functional status scales that can be helpful. Similarly, it can be helpful to include performance-based measures of functional status such as the Tinetti Gait Evaluation (POMA) (see Appendix #36),[25] the timed Get Up and Go Test,[26] or the Six-Minute Walk test.[27] These observed performance measures can provide more accurate information than self-reported questionnaires.

Psychological and Social Assessment

A brief psychological and social evaluation is important for comprehensive assessment of elders with pain. Depression, anxiety, social isolation, and disengagement are common in this population.[28] Parmelee and associates, clearly show a statistically significant correlation between pain and depression in elders, even when controlling for self-reported health and functional status.[29] Therefore, assessment should at least include a screen for depression and social networks. Depression can be screened for using a variety of instruments or questionnaires that have been validated in elders. These might include the Geriatric Depression Scale (GDS) (see Appendix #16)[30] or the Center for Epidemiologic Studies Depression Scale (CES-D) (see Appendix #7).[31] Social networks should be explored for availability and involvement of family and other caregivers. Ferrell and colleagues have shown that family and informal caregivers are often involved and can have substantial impact on overall pain management.[32-33] Evaluation of caregivers is particularly necessary when high-tech pain management strategies are contemplated, such as continuous analgesic infusions. Some pain management strategies can place substantial demands on caregivers resulting in the need for frequent transportation and work absence, not to mention technical training and abilities.

Psychological evaluation should also include consideration of anxiety and coping skills. Anxiety is common among patients in pain. This often requires additional time and frequent reassurance from health care providers. Indeed, chronic pain often requires effective coping skills for anxiety and other emotional feelings.[34] For those with significant psychiatric problems, referral for formal psychiatric evaluation and management may be necessary. In these patients, specific counseling, supportive group therapy, biofeedback, or some psychoactive medications may be necessary for developing and maintaining coping strategies, as well as management of major psychiatric complications.

Pain Assessment Scales

A variety of qualitative and quantitative scales are available to help assess and measure pain. Figure 15-1 provides a form that can be adapted to record qualitative and quantitative information from the pain history and physical examination, as well as assessments of mood, functional status, and overall pain.[9, 11] Such charts help organize necessary information for medical–legal reasons as well as communication with consultants and other health care team members. Indeed, the form can be used to summarize initial pain evaluation on admission to health care facilities as well as to summarize pain consultation at any time during the course of the illness.

Formal pain scales have been devised to help categorize and quantify pain problems. These instruments can be grouped into multidimensional and unidimensional pain scales. Since there are no objective biologic markers for pain, validity of pain scales is largely based on face value, concurrence with other known scales,

Date: _____   Medical Record Number _____

Patient's Name _____

Medications:

Problem List:
_____   _____
_____   _____
_____   _____
_____   _____

Pain Description

Pattern: Constant   Intermittant

Duration: _____   Location: _____
_____

Pain Intensity:
0 1 2 3 4 5 6 7 8 9 10
None   Moderate   Severe

Character:
Lancinating   Burning   Stinging
Shooting   Tingling   Radiating

Worst Pain in Last 24 hours:
0 1 2 3 4 5 6 7 8 9 10
None   Moderate   Severe

Other Descriptors:
_____
_____
_____
_____

Mood: _____

Depression Screening Score: _____

Gait and Balance

Score: _____
Exacerbating Factors:
_____
_____

Impaired Activities:
_____
_____
_____

Relieving Factors:
Quality: _____
_____
_____

Sleep

Bowel Habits: _____
_____

Other Assessments or
Comments: _____
_____
_____

Most Likely Cause of
Pain: _____

Plans: _____
_____
_____
_____

FIGURE 15-1   Geriatric pain assessment.

and experience in many populations over several years. In general, multidimensional scales with multiple items often result in more stable measurement and evaluation of pain in several domains. For example, the McGill Pain Questionnaire has been shown to capture pain in terms of intensity, affect, sensation, location, and several other domains that are not possible to evaluate with a single question. At the same time, multidimensional scales are often long, time consuming, and can be difficult to score at the bedside, making them difficult to use in a clinical setting. Table 15-2 describes some available multi-item pain scales along with advantages and disadvantages offered by the scales. Unfortunately, little has been published on the psychometric properties of these tools evaluated specifically in elders.

TABLE 15-2. SUMMARY OF MULTIDIMENSIONAL PAIN SCALES

INSTRUMENT	DESCRIPTION	TARGET	VALIDITY	RELIABILITY	ADVANTAGES	DISADVANTAGES	REFERENCES
McGill Pain Questionnaire	Subjects asked to identify words descriptive of individual pain from 78 words grouped in 20 categories; plus 4 other items (including a 5-point word descriptive scale of pain intensity at the moment [PPI] scored separately	All pain	Good	Good	Multidimensional, extensively studied over a long time; may discriminate between types of pain	Long, difficult to score	Melzack, 1975[35]
Short-Form McGill Pain Questionnaire	Fifteen words scored on Likert scale; plus a visual analog and PPI scales.	All pain	Good	Good	Shorter than original McGill; not studied as deeply as original	May not discriminate between pain types	Melzack, 1987[36]
Wisconsin Brief Pain Inventory	Sixteen-item scale; items scored separately	Cancer pain	Good	Good	Multidimensional	Studied largely in cancer pain	AHCPR Cancer Pain Guidelines[11]
Memorial Sloan Kettering Pain Scale	Four-word descriptor scales	Cancer pain	Good	Good	Multidimensional	Studied largely in cancer pain	Fishman, et al, 1987[37]
Roland and Morris Disability Questionnaire	Twenty four items scored yes or no	Back pain	Good	Good	Specific for back pain	May not be generalizable to other pain syndromes	Waddell, et al[38]
Hurley Discomfort Scale	Designed to score discomfort behaviors in patients with severe Alzheimer's disease	Acute pain	Probably fair	Reasonable	Does not rely on self-report	Relys on behavioral observation	Hurley, et al[39]
Osteoarthritis Pain Behavior Observation System	Designed to score position, movement, and behavior among adults	Osteoarthritis of knee	Compared to 0–10 scale $r = .45$	Test–retest over 10 weeks $r = .53$	Does not rely on verbal ability	Limited to osteoarthritis of knee	Keefe, et al[40]

Of recent interest in the management of elders, Hurley and colleagues have developed a discomfort scale for patients with dementia of the Alzheimer's type (DS-DAT).[39] This scale consists of 9 items scored by a trained examiner after observation of a noncommunicative patient. Behavioral observations include breathing, vocalization, facial expression, body language, and restlessness scored on Likert scales. In preliminary testing[39] and at least one clinical trial,[41] the scale demonstrated reasonable reliability and stability over time. Unfortunately, the scale requires substantial skill and training to administer and probably remains a research tool at this time.

Unidimensional scales have found widespread use for clinical evaluation of pain intensity in many settings. Although limited largely to the evaluation of pain intensity alone, unidimensional scales are easy to administer and require little time, training, or experience to get reasonably valid and reliable results.[42] Table 15-3 describes some of the available unidimensional instruments with advantages and disadvantages for use in elders. It is important to remember that each of these are usually obtained when referenced in the "here and now." The interviewer may frame the question or instrument as: "How much pain are you having right now?" Alternatively, the interviewer can frame the question as: "How much pain have you had over the last week?" or "On average, how much pain have you had over the last month?" The latter questions require more integration of memory over time and can be more difficult for patients. Recent studies of elders, especially

TABLE 15-3. SUMMARY OF UNIDIMENSIONAL PAIN SCALES

SCALE	DESCRIPTION	VALIDITY	RELIABILITY	ADVANTAGES	DISADVANTAGES	REFERENCES
Visual Analog	100-mm Line; vertical or horizontal	Good	Fair	Continuous scale	Requires pencil and paper	Clinical Practice Guidelines[9-11]
Present Pain Intensity	Six-point 0–5 scale with word descriptors (subscale of McGill Pain Questionnaire)	Good	Fair	Easy to understand; word anchors decrease clustering toward middle of scale	Usually requires visual cue	Melzack, 1975[35]
Graphic Pictures	Happy faces; others	Fair	Fair	Amusing	Requires vision and attention	Herr, et al[43]
Sloan Kettering Pain Card	Seven words randomly distributed on a card	Good	Fair	Ease of administration	Requires visual cue	Ferrell, et al[3]
Verbal 0–10 Scale	On a scale of zero to ten, if 0 means no pain and 10 means the worst pain you can imagine, how much is your pain now?	Good	Fair	Probably easiest to use	Requires hearing	Ferrell, et al[3]

those with cognitive impairment, have shown that pain reports are influenced by pain at the moment and cognitive impairment.[44]

Finally, in a clinical setting, it may be useful to evaluate "pain at the moment" with the frequent use of a unidimensional scale. Figure 15-2 provides an example of a medical chart form that can

Date: _____   Medical Record Number _____

Patient's Name _____

Pain Medications and Directions:

_____

_____

_____

Pain Scale Used* _____

Date	Time	Pain Intensity*	Activity	Action	Results

*Choose an appropriate scale, indicate which scale is being used, and use the same scale for each assessment.

FIGURE 15-2   Chronic pain record.

be used to record frequent assessment of pain intensity similar to the frequent measurement of vital signs. Even though pain experiences often wax and wane over several minutes or hours, frequent assessment can be more valid and reliable than memory of events over time. This is especially true for those with mild to moderate cognitive impairment.[3]

PAIN ASSESSMENT IN THE COGNITIVELY IMPAIRED

Cognitive impairment is a common problem among elders that can present substantial challenges to pain assessment. It has been estimated that as many as 50 percent of elders in long-term care institutions may have significant cognitive impairment as a result of stroke, Alzheimer's disease, and other dementing illnesses.[3] Parmelee and colleagues, in a study of 750 residents of a long-term care facility, reported that pain reports from persons with mild to moderate cognitive impairment were no less valid that those from patients with normal cognitive function.[45] More recently, Weiner and associates supported these observations and provided data to suggest that pain reports from these patients with mild to moderate cognitive impairment are indeed, reliable (or stable over time) as well.[44] Studies have shown that using commonly available tools such as those described in Table 15-3 are feasible for use in most patients with cognitive impairment.[3] Thus most elderly patients with mild to moderate cognitive impairment appear to have the capacity to report pain accurately and reliably using commonly available instruments.

For clinical purposes, it is important to remember that these persons also have a variety of other disabilities in addition to cognitive impairment. Low vision, hearing deficits, motor weakness due to stroke, arthritis, and slow mentation all make administration of pain scales more difficult. Therefore, choosing an appropriate pain scale requires choosing scales tailored for a patient's individual disabilities. If the patient is hard of hearing, a verbal scale may not be very appropriate. If the patient is blind, a scale that requires visual cues is inappropriate. In this case, it is important to always use the same scale for each individual during subsequent evaluations.

Patients with severe cognitive impairment may present substantial challenges, for which no generalizable methods for pain assessment have been identified. Although it has often been assumed that those in deep coma do not experience pain, it is not clear that such brain damage necessarily results in complete anesthesia. Patients with "locked in syndrome" (having intact perception and cognitive function but no purposeful motor function and no means of communication) may suffer severely. Unfortunately, no reliable methods exist to assess pain in these individuals. Health care providers must be aware of these situations and provide analgesia empirically, at least during procedures or for conditions known to be uncomfortable or painful. More often, the majority of those with severe cognitive impairment can and do make their needs known through simple yes and no answers communicated in various ways. Indeed, those with profound aphasia can often provide accurate and reliable answers to yes and no questions when confronted by a sensitive and skilled interviewer. For these patients, it is important for health care providers to be creative in establishing communication methods for the purposes of pain assessment.

Using Proxies in Pain Assessment

Although pain is an individual experience, the use of family and caregivers in the assessment of pain can sometimes be helpful.[46] Among patients with cognitive impairment, the history is often entirely obtained from family or close caregivers. Family and caregivers are an excellent source of qualitative information about general behavior, medication usage, actions that seem to reduce pain, and actions that seem to aggravate pain. It is important to remember, however, that family and caregivers are limited in their interpretation of events and behaviors. In fact, data have suggested that when it comes to estimating pain intensity, proxies are not always very accurate or reliable. Our studies in elderly cancer patients suggest that caregivers often overestimate pain intensity and pain distress.[32] It is often very distressing to family and other caregivers who feel helpless in managing severe pain. Both physicians and nurses have been found to underestimate pain as well as provide inadequate pain medication.[5, 45] In the final analysis, family and caregivers can be an important source of qualitative information, but they probably should not be relied on entirely for quantitative assessment of pain intensity or distress, especially among those patients able to communicate their pain experiences.

SUMMARY

Pain assessment has reached a high level of sophistication as described in a variety of clinical practice guidelines recently published. Pain in elders can present unique challenges to assessment, including a high prevalence of multiple sources of pain and frequent disabilities such as hearing impairment, blindness, and cognitive impairment, which can make pain assessment more difficult. Accurate pain assessment relies on an accurate medical history and physical examination as well as other diagnostic acumen leading to a definitive diagnosis of medical problems underlying the pain complaint. Evaluation of physical function, psychosocial function, and the character of the pain are helpful to identify complications of pain, need for rehabilitation, and to establish outcome goals of overall pain management. Fortunately, a variety of pain scales are valid and reliable for assessment and measurement of pain in elders, including those with mild to moderate cognitive impairment.

Additional research is still needed. An objective biologic marker for pain has yet to be identified and remains a "holy grail" in pain research. A definition of significant pain remains problematic despite the universality of pain and the means to quantify it. Therefore, we are lacking a valid definition of significant pain.

Nonetheless, assessment of pain remains the most important determinant of successful pain management. Pain assessment should be a routine part of comprehensive geriatric assessment. If comfort and control of pain are a central goal in geriatric medicine, accurate and reliable pain assessment must become standard practice in all geriatric settings.

REFERENCES

1. Ferrell BA. Pain management in elderly people. *J Am Geriatr Soc.* 1991;39:64–73.
2. Helm RD, Gibson SJ. Pain in the elderly. In: Jensen JS, Turner JA, Wiesenfeld-Hallin Z, ed. *Proceedings of the 8th World Congress on Pain, Progress in Pain Research and Management,* vol. 8. Seattle: IASP Press; 1997:
3. Ferrell BA. Pain in cognitively impaired nursing home residents. *J Pain Symptom Manage.* 1995;10(8):591–598.
4. Fox PL, Raina P, Jadad A. Prevalence and treatment of pain in older adults in nursing homes and other long-term care institutions: A systematic review. *Canadian Medical Assoc Journal (CMAJ)* 1999; 160(3):329–33.
5. Ferrell BA, Ferrell BR, Osterweil D. Pain in the nursing home. *J Am Geriatr Soc.* 1990;38:409–414.
6. Bernabei R, Gambassi G, Lapane K, et al. Management of pain in elderly patients with cancer. SAGE Study Group. Systematic Assessment of Geriatric Durg Use Via Epidemiology. *JAMA.* 1998; 279(23):1877–1882.
7. Merskey H, Bogduk N, eds. *Classification of Chronic Pain,* 2nd ed. Seattle: IASP Press; 1994.
8. Turk DC, Melzack R. The measurement of pain and the assessment of people experiencing pain. In: Truk DC, Melzack R, eds, *Handbook of Pain Assessment.* New York: Guilford Press; 1992:3–12.
9. American Geriatric Society Panel on Chronic Pain in Older Persons. The management of chronic pain in older persons. *J Am Geriatr Soc.* 1998;46:635–651.

10. Car DB, Jacox AK, Chapman CR, et al. *Acute Pain Management: Operative or Medical Procedures and Trauma.* Clinical Practice Guideline No. 1. AHCPR Pub. No 92-0032. Rockville, MD: Agency for Health Care Policy and Research, Public Health Service, U.S. Department of Health and Human Services, Feb 1992.

11. Jocox A, Car DB, Payne R, et al. *Management of Cancer Pain.* Clinical Practice Guideline No. 9. AHCPR Publication No. 94-0592. Rockville, MD: Agency for Health Care Policy and Research, U.S. Department of Health and Human Services, Public Health Service, March 1994.

12. Bigos S, Bower O, Braen G, et al. *Acute Low Back Problems in Adults.* Clinical Practice Guideline, No. 14, AHCPR Publication No. 94-0642. Rockville, MD: Agency for Health Care Policy and Research, U.S. Department of Health and Human Services, Public Health Service, December 1994.

13. Myer RA, Campbell JN, Rija SN. Peripheral and neural mechanisms of nociception. In: Wall PD, Melzack R, eds, *Textbook of Pain,* 3rd ed. New York: Churchill Livingstone; 1994:13–44.

14. Bennett GF. Neuropathic pain. In: Wall PD, Melzack R, eds, *Textbook of Pain,* 3rd ed. New York: Churchill Livingstone; 1994:201–224.

15. Lipman AG. Analgesic drugs for neuropathic and sympathetically maintained pain. *Clin Geriatr Med.* 1996;12(3):501–515.

16. Craig KD. Emotional aspects of pain. In: Wall PD, Melzack R, eds, *Textbook of Pain,* 3rd Ed. New York: Churchill Livingstone; 1994:261–274.

17. American Psychiatric Association. *Diagnostic and Statistical Manual of Mental Disorders,* 4th ed. (DSM-IV). Washington, DC: American Psychiatric Association; 1994.

18. Ferrell BA. Pain management. In: Hazzard WR, Blass JP, Ettinger WH, Halter JB, Ouslander JG, eds, *Principles of Geriatric Medicine and Gerontology,* 4th ed. New York: McGraw-Hill; 1999;413–433.

19. Nishikawa ST, Ferrell BA. Pain assessment in the elderly. Clin Geriatr Issue Long Term Care. 1993;1(4):15–28.

20. Katz S, Ford AB, Moskowitz RW, et al. Studies of illness in the aged. The index of ADL: a standardized measure of biological and psychosocial function. *JAMA.* 1963;185:914–919.

21. Lawton MP, Brody EM. Assessment of older people: self-maintaining and instrumental activities of daily living. *Gerontologist.* 1969; 9:179–186.

22. Kieth RA, Granger CV, Hamilton BB, Sherwin FS. The functional independence measure: a new tool for rehabilitation. *Adv Clin Rehabil.* 1987;1:6–18.

23. Meenan RF, Mason JH, Anderson JJ. AIMS2. The content and properties of a questionnaire. *Arthritis Rheum.* 1992;35(1):1–10.

24. Bergner M, Bobbitt, RA, Carter WB, Gibson BS. The sickness impact profile: development and final revision of a health status measure. *Med Care.* 1981;19:787–805.

25. Tinetti M. Performance oriented assessment of mobility problems in elderly patients. *J Am Geriatr Soc.* 1986;14:61–65.

26. Podiasdlo D, Richardson S. The timed "Up & Go": a test of basic functional mobility for frail elderly persons. *J Am Geriatr Soc.* 1991;39:142–148.

27. Ferrell BA, Josephson KR, Pollan AM, et al. A randomized trial of walking versus physical methods for chronic pain management. *Aging.* (Milano) 1997;9:99–105.

28. Kerns RD, Jacob MC. Assessment of the psychosocial context of the experience of pain. In: Turk DC, Melzack R, eds, *Handbook of Pain Assessment.* New York: Guilford Press, 1992.

29. Parmelee PA, Katz IR, Lawton MP. The relation of pain to depression among institutionalized aged. *J Gerontol.* 1991;46:15–21.

30. Yessavage JA, Brink T, Rose TL, et al. Development and validation of a geriatric depression screening scale: a preliminary report. *J Psychiatry Res.* 1983;17:37–49.

31. Fadloff LS. The CES-D Scale. A self report depression scale for research in the general population. *Appl Psychol Meas.* 1977;1: 385–401.

32. Ferrell BR, Ferrell BA, Rhiner M, Grant M. Family factors influencing cancer pain. *Postgrad Med J.* 1991;67 (suppl 2):S64–S69.

33. Ferrell BR, Ferrell BA, Ahn C, Tran K. Pain management for elderly patients with cancer at home. *Cancer.* 1994;74(suppl 7): 2139–2146.

34. Keefe FJ, Beaupre PM, Weiner DK, Seigler IC. Pain in older adults: a cognitive-behavioral perspective. In: Ferrell BR, Ferrell BA, eds, *Pain in the Elderly.* Seattle: IASP Press; 1996;11–19.

35. Melzack R. The McGill Pain Questionnaire: major properties and scoring methods. *Pain.* 1975;1:277–299.

36. Melzack R. The short-form McGill Pain Questionnaire. *Pain.* 1987;30:191–197.

37. Fishman B, Pasternak S, Wallenstein SL, Houde RW, Holland JC, Foley KA. The Memorial Pain Assessment Card: A valid instrument for the evaluation of cancer pain. *Cancer.* 1987;60(5):1151–1158.

38. Waddell G, Turk DC. Clinical assessment of low back pain. In: Turk DC, Melzack R, eds, *Handbook of Pain Assessment.* New York: Guilford Press; 1992;15–36.

39. Hurley AC, Volicer BJ, Hanrahan PA, Houde S, Volicer V. Assessment of discomfort in advanced Alzheimer patients. *Res Nurs Health.* 1992;15:369–377.

40. Keefe FJ, Williams DA. Assessment of pain behaviors. In: Turk DC, Melzack R, eds, *Handbook of Pain Assessment.* New York: Guilford Press; 1992.

41. Fabiszewski KL, Volicer B, Volicer L. Effect of antibiotic treatment of outcomes of fevers in the institutionalized Alzheimer patients. *JAMA.* 1990;263:3168–3172.

42. Downie WW, Leathan PA, Rhind VM, Writht V, Banco JA, Anderson JA. *Ann of Rheum Dis.* 1978;37:378–381.

43. Herr KA, Mobily PR, Kohour FJ, Sagenaar D. Evaluation of the Faces Pain Scale for use with the elderly. *Clin J Pain.* 1998;14:1–10.

44. Weiner DK, Peterson BL, Logue P, Keefe FJ. Predictors of self-report in nursing home residents. *Aging Clin Exper Res.* 1998;10:411–420.

45. Parmelee AP, Smith BD, Katz IR. Pain complaints and cognitive status among elderly institutional residents. *J Am Geriatr Soc.* 1993;41:517–522.

46. O'Brien J, Francis A. The use of next-of-kin to estimate pain in cancer patients. *Pain.* 1988;35:171–178.

47. Camp DL. A comparison of nurses' recorded assessments of pain as described by cancer patients. *Cancer Nurs.* 1988;11(4):237–243.

SLEEP

CATHY A. ALESSI

Sleep problems are very common in elders. Over half of all elders complain about their sleep, and one third report having chronic problems with sleep.[1] In addition, one half of community-dwelling elders use either over-the-counter or prescription sleeping medications.[2,3] Two thirds of residents in long-term care facilities have problems with sleep and many of them are prescribed sleeping medications.[4,5] Many factors may contribute to sleeping problems in elders, such as age-related changes in sleep, changes in lifestyle, bereavement, medications, and coexisting illnesses. In addition, most primary sleep disorders increase in prevalence with age.[6,7]

The health care provider must be knowledgeable in the assessment of sleep because problems with sleep can adversely affect quality of life in elders and can be associated with increased morbidity and mortality. This chapter discusses important issues in the recognition and evaluation of sleep problems in elders, including the basic aspects of normal sleep, the changes in sleep that are common in elders, the differential diagnosis of sleep problems, and the indications for referral to a sleep laboratory.

NORMAL SLEEP

Sleep can be described in several ways, including sleep pattern, sleep structure, and subjective report of the sleeper. Sleep pattern and sleep structure are usually determined with monitoring in a sleep laboratory with concurrent measurement by electroencephalography (EEG), electromyography (EMG), and electrooculography (EOG), in addition to other measures. Subjective reporting of sleep is usually assessed with questionnaires.

Sleep pattern is defined as the amount and timing of sleep an individual experiences. On average, adults under the age of 60 years sleep about 7 hours during a period of 7.5 hours spent in bed, although this varies considerably. They may have a couple awakenings during the night, of which they may or may not be aware. Time to fall asleep (sleep latency) varies, but is usually less than 15 to 20 minutes in "normal" sleepers.

Sleep structure is a description of the stages of sleep. The two general stages of sleep are rapid-eye-movement (REM) sleep and nonrapid-eye-movement (NREM) sleep. REM sleep is characterized by EEG activation, low or absent muscle tone on EMG, and bursts of rapid eye movement on EOG. During REM sleep, there are increased oxygen requirements, increased autonomic activity, and dreaming. Four stages of NREM are described. Stage 1 is the transitional period between wakefulness and sleep. Stage 2 is a deeper stage of sleep, with characteristic sleep spindles and K complexes on the EEG. Stages 3 and 4 are the deepest stages of sleep and are categorized by high-amplitude delta-wave (slow-wave) EEG activity. During a night of sleep, a person passes through cycles of various stages of NREM and REM sleep.

Subjective report of sleep in normal sleepers can include occasional difficulty falling asleep or staying asleep. These are universal and normal experiences, particularly during periods of stress. It is when these symptoms become persistent and/or intrude into daytime functioning that a sleep problem is suspected. In addition, some people appear to sleep less than average with no problems with daytime sleepiness or functioning; they have been termed natural "short sleepers."

> Subjective report of sleep in normal sleepers can include occasional difficulty falling asleep or staying asleep. When these symptoms become persistent and/or intrude into daytime functioning, a sleep problem should be suspected.

CHANGES IN SLEEP WITH AGE

> Age-related changes in sleep pattern include decreased sleep efficiency, similar or decreased total sleep time, increased sleep latency, earlier bedtime and earlier morning awakening, more arousals during the night, and more daytime napping.

Age-related changes have been demonstrated in sleep pattern, structure, and subjective report; although studies have had conflicting results. Commonly described changes in sleep pattern with age include decreased sleep efficiency (time asleep divided by time in bed), similar or decreased total sleep time, increased sleep latency (time to fall asleep), earlier bedtime and earlier morning awakening, more arousals during the night, and more daytime napping.[6,8] Despite these findings, healthy elders do not have more daytime sleepiness and have as regular a daily lifestyle as younger adults.[9]

Reported age-related changes in sleep structure vary, but common findings include decreased REM latency (i.e., earlier onset of REM) and decreased total REM sleep but no change or a decrease in percentage of REM sleep.[10,11] Elders have more equal distribution of REM sleep throughout the night, whereas younger people have longer periods of REM sleep as the night progresses. They also have a decrease in spindles and K complexes on EEG during sleep.[12] There is a decrease in stage 3 and stage 4 sleep with age, with stages 1 and 2 increasing or remaining the same (Figure 16-1). The decline in deep sleep seems to begin in early adulthood and progresses throughout life. In very old people (over age 90), stages 3 and 4 may disappear completely.[13]

Subjective report of sleep by elders reflects these age-related changes in sleep pattern and structure. Older people typically describe increased difficulty in falling asleep, more awakenings during the night, and early morning awakening.[14,15] Difficulty maintaining sleep is one of the most commonly reported sleep complaints

> With increasing age, there are some changes in REM sleep and a decrease in stage 3 and 4 sleep (deep sleep).

> Elders typically report earlier sleep time, increased difficulty in falling asleep, more awakenings during the night with difficulty maintaining sleep, early morning awakening, and more daytime naps.

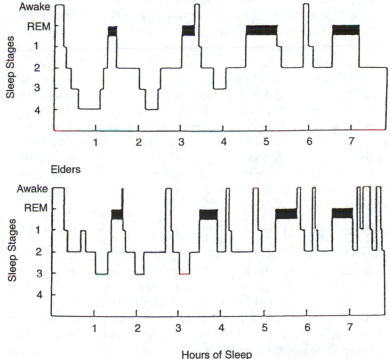
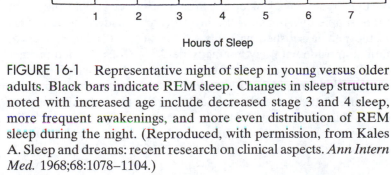

FIGURE 16-1 Representative night of sleep in young versus older adults. Black bars indicate REM sleep. Changes in sleep structure noted with increased age include decreased stage 3 and 4 sleep, more frequent awakenings, and more even distribution of REM sleep during the night. (Reproduced, with permission, from Kales A. Sleep and dreams: recent research on clinical aspects. *Ann Intern Med.* 1968;68:1078–1104.)

among elders. In addition, they often report more daytime naps, shorter nighttime sleep with more wakefulness, and earlier sleep hours. In healthy older normal sleepers, daytime napping is not associated with difficulty in nighttime sleep.[16, 17] Conversely, elders with difficulty sleeping at night who take naps during the day may benefit from a decrease in their daytime napping.

The significance of these reported changes in sleep with age is unclear. There is some evidence that elders need less sleep, although establishing need for sleep is difficult.[18] After a period of sleep deprivation, they do show less daytime sleepiness, less evidence of decline in performance measures, and recover their normal sleep structure more quickly than younger people.[19] Elders, however, do have more sleep disturbance with jet lag and shift work, but this may reflect physiologic changes in circadian rhythm with age. In addition, it is not clear to what extent changes in sleep are due to changes of normal aging or to pathologic changes from other processes. In studies comparing good sleepers to poor sleepers, poor sleepers take more medications, make more physician visits, and have poorer self-ratings of health. In addition, chronologic age *per se* does not seem to correlate with higher prevalence of poor sleep. Poor sleep is associated with physical illness, inactivity and bedrest, medication use, alcohol use, and conditions such as chronic pain, nighttime urination, headache, gastrointestinal illness, bronchitis and asthma, diabetes, cardiac disease, and menopausal symptoms. In addition, psychologic factors may play a role, such as depression, change in lifestyle, and anxiety, in addition to lack of social support. Bereavement can also play a role in sleep disturbance. In addition, some previously reported changes in sleep with age may be secondary to unrecognized primary sleep disorders.

ASSESSMENT OF SLEEP IN ELDERS

Recommended Screening Questions

1. Satisfaction with sleep
2. Daytime fatigue and sleepiness
3. Complaints by a bed partner

People may not report sleep complaints unless specifically queried by their health care provider. To aid in screening elders for sleep problems, the National Institutes of Health Consensus Statement on the Treatment of Sleep Disorders of Older People suggested three simple questions for the health care provider, including: (1) Is the person satisfied with his or her sleep? (2) Does sleep or fatigue intrude with daytime activities? (3) Does the bed partner or do others complain of unusual behavior during sleep, such as snoring, interrupted breathing, or leg movements?[20] A positive response to these questions should trigger a more detailed history of the sleep complaint. Transient sleep problems (e.g., less than 2 to 3 weeks) are usually situational; persistent sleep problems are often more serious and require more detailed evaluation.

History, Physical Examination, and Simple Laboratory Testing

The initial and subsequent office evaluations of a patient with sleep complaints can be rather lengthy. To obtain a careful description of the sleep complaint, it can be helpful to have the patient keep a sleep log in which, each morning, he or she records time in bed, estimated amount of sleep, number of awakenings, time of morning awakening, and any symptoms that occurred during the night. An example of a sleep log is in Appendix #42. This should be supplemented by information from the spouse, bed partner, or others who may have observed unusual symptoms during the night. Sleep questionnaires are available to help obtain additional information to guide further testing and treatment.[21]

The spouse, bed partner, or others can be important sources of information for unusual symptoms during the night.

The history should also screen for treatable medical conditions that can contribute to sleep difficulty. These include pain from arthritis and other conditions, paresthesias, cough, dyspnea from cardiac or pulmonary illness, gastroesophageal reflux, and nighttime urination.[10, 11] In elders, nighttime urination can be associated with increased sleep disorders, poorer quality of sleep, increased thirst (particularly at night), and increased fatigue in the daytime. Certain medications and other agents taken near bedtime can exacerbate symptoms, such as diuretics or stimulating agents (e.g., caffeine, sympathomimetics, and bronchodilators). Alcohol can also be problematic. Elders with poor sleep should be instructed to avoid nighttime alcohol, because although alcohol causes an initial drowsiness, it can impair sleep later in the night. Certain medications can induce nightmares and impair sleep, such as some antidepressants, antiparkinson agents, and antihypertensives (e.g., propranolol). Sedating medications (e.g., antihistamines, anticholinergics, and sedating antidepressants) should be given at bedtime rather than during the day, if possible. Depression is a common cause of sleep disorder and should be considered. Other psychosocial problems to consider include stress, anxiety, bereavement, loss of social supports, and lifestyle changes such as retirement. Finally, a disruptive nighttime environment may contribute to poor sleep. This can be particularly true in the acute hospital and the nursing home, where medical illness and psychosocial factors are often also contributory.

The focused physical examination will depend on evidence from the history. For example, reports of painful joints should be followed by a careful examination of the affected areas. Reports of nocturia disrupting sleep should be followed by evaluation for cardiac, renal, or prostatic disease, or other conditions such as diabetes. Careful mental status testing is also indicated in most cases. Simple laboratory testing should be guided by findings from

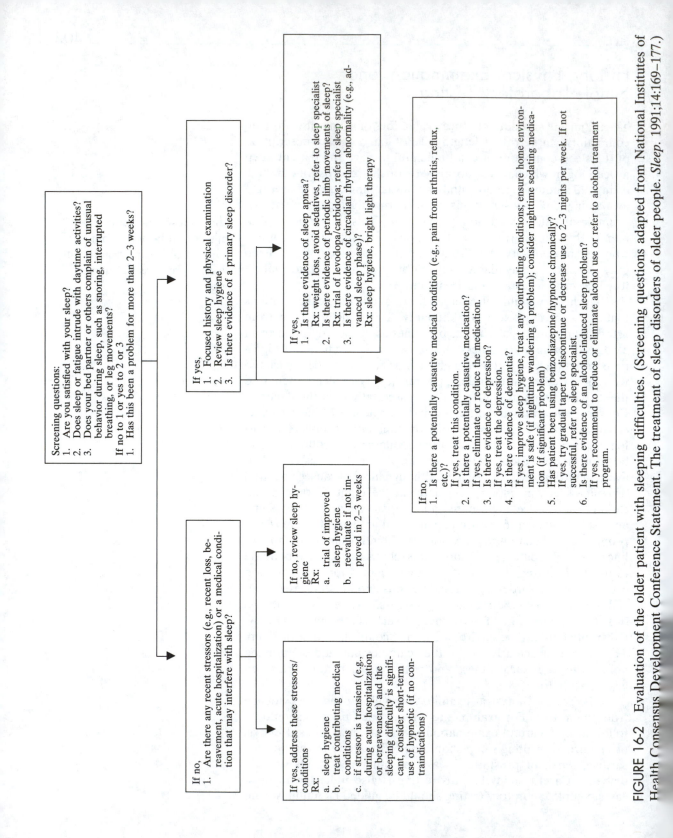

FIGURE 16-2 Evaluation of the older patient with sleeping difficulties. (Screening questions adapted from National Institutes of Health Consensus Development Conference Statement. The treatment of sleep disorders of older people. *Sleep.* 1991;14:169–177.)

TABLE 16-1. COMMONLY RECOMMENDED MEASURES TO IMPROVE SLEEP HYGIENE

Maintain a regular rising time
Maintain a regular sleeping time, but do not go to bed unless sleepy
Decrease or eliminate naps, unless necessary part of sleeping schedule
Exercise daily, but not immediately prior to bedtime
Use bed for sleeping only (i.e., do not read or watch television in bed)
Relax mentally prior to sleep, do not use bedtime as worry time
If hungry, have a light snack before bed (unless there are symptoms of gastroesophageal reflux or medically contraindicated) but avoid heavy meals at bedtime
Limit or eliminate alcohol, caffeine, and nicotine, especially prior to bedtime
Wind down prior to bedtime, and maintain a routine period of preparation for bed (e.g., washing up, going to the bathroom, etc.)
Control the nighttime environment with comfortable temperature, quiet, and dark
Trial of a familiar background noise (e.g., fan or other appliance or a "white noise" machine)
Wear comfortable bed clothing
If unable to fall asleep within 30 minutes, get out of bed and perform soothing activity such as soft music or light reading (but avoid exposure to bright light during these times)
Get adequate exposure to bright light during the day

the history and physical examination. Figure 16-2 outlines a suggested approach to the evaluation of sleeping difficulties in elders.

If the initial history and physical examination do not suggest a serious underlying cause for the sleep problem, a trial of improved sleep hygiene is the best first approach. Commonly recommended measures are listed in Table 16-1. Behavioral techniques, such as relaxation therapy can be effective and help avoid hypnotic medications. If the patient takes daytime naps, it is important to clarify if these are needed rest periods for the individual, or are due to inactivity, boredom, or daytime sedating medications. It is important to explain to the person that daytime naps will decrease nighttime sleep.

SPECIFIC SLEEP DISORDERS

Classification of Sleep Disorders

Sleep problems can be classified in various ways. The *1990 International Classification of Sleep Disorders (ICSD) Diagnostic and Coding Manual* listed 84 sleep disorders with detailed descriptions and

The two main symptoms of sleeping problems to distinguish are insomnia (difficulty in initiating and maintaining sleep, DIMS) and hypersomnolence (disorders of excessive daytime sleepiness, DOES).

diagnostic criteria.[22] A summary of these categories is shown in Table 16-2. The ICSD also includes a differential diagnosis listing of sleep disorders that cause the two main sleep symptoms, insomnia and excessive sleepiness, and those that produce other symptoms. Many sleep disorders, however, can produce either insomnia or excessive sleepiness, so there is considerable overlap of conditions listed under these two main symptoms. In 1994, *The Diagnostic and Statistical Manual of Mental Disorders,* 4th ed (DSM-IV) was released, which included another system of classifying sleep disorders (Table 16-3).[23] It is helpful to be aware of these classifications in order to follow the growing literature on sleep disorders. A third classification of sleep disorders, which has been widely used in the past, is the *Diagnostic Classification of the Sleep and Arousal Disorders* (DCSAD), published by the Association of Sleep Disorders Centers in 1979. Four main categories of sleep problems were listed in the DCSAD, including (1) disorders of initiating and maintaining sleep (DIMS, or insomnia); (2) disorders of excessive somnolence (DOES, or hypersomnolence); (3) disorders of the sleep–wake schedule; and (4) dysfunctions associated with sleep, sleep stages, or partial arousals (parasomnias).

Classically, it is taught that insomnia is due to psychiatric, medical, or neurologic illness and hypersomnolence is associated with primary sleep disorders such as sleep-related respiratory disorders (sleep apnea). All three classification systems mentioned previously, however, (ICSD, DSM-IV, and DCSAD) reveal significant overlap of conditions that can cause insomnia or hypersomnolence. In a large study of patients of all ages referred to sleep disorder centers, DIMS was most commonly due to psychiatric illness, psychophysiologic problems, drug and alcohol dependence, and restless legs syndrome; and DOES was most commonly due to sleep apnea, periodic leg movements, or narcolepsy. Patients referred to sleep centers are a select population, however, and the most common causes of excessive sleepiness in the community are probably chronic insufficient sleep (either voluntarily or due to work schedules), or medical, toxic, and environmental conditions. Therefore, although determining whether the patient's primary sleep complaint is insomnia or hypersomnolence is important in initially determining the most likely etiologies, there is considerable overlap between conditions that cause these symptoms. The health care provider should not rule out a primary sleep disorder in the patient presenting with insomnia, and similarly should probably not refer every patient with daytime sleepiness to a sleep laboratory. See Appendix #14 for an example of a questionnaire to screen for daytime sleepiness.

TABLE 16-2. SUMMARY OF THE 1990 INTERNATIONAL CLASSIFICATION
OF SLEEP DISORDERS (ICSD)

1. Dyssomnias = disorders that produce either difficulty initiating or maintaining sleep or excessive sleepiness
   A. *Intrinsic sleep disorders* = disorders that originate within the body (e.g., psychophysiological insomnia, obstructive and central sleep apnea syndrome, periodic limb movement disorder, restless legs syndrome, etc.)
   B. *Extrinsic sleep disorders* = disorders that originate or develop from causes outside the body (e.g., inadequate sleep hygiene, environmental sleep disorder, hypnotic- or stimulant-dependent sleep disorder, etc.)
   C. *Circadian rhythm sleep disorders* = disorders related to the timing of sleep within the 24-hour day (e.g., time zone change/jet lag, shift work, irregular sleep–wake pattern, etc.)
2. Parasomnias = disorders of arousal, partial arousal, and sleep stage transition, that intrude into the sleep process and are not primarily disorders of sleep and wake states, per se
   A. *Arousal disorders* = manifestations of partial arousal that occur during sleep (e.g., confusional arousals, sleepwalking, sleep terrors)
   B. *Sleep–wake transition disorders* = disorders that occur mainly during the transition from wakefulness to sleep or from one sleep stage to another (e.g., rhythmic movement disorder, sleep starts, sleep talking, nocturnal leg cramps)
   C. *Parasomnias usually associated with REM sleep* = have their onset during REM sleep (e.g., nightmares, sleep paralysis, sleep-related painful erections, etc.)
   D. *Other parasomnias* = do not fall into one of the above categories (e.g., sleep bruxism, sleep enuresis, primary snoring, etc.)
3. Medical/psychiatric sleep disorders = medical or psychiatric disorders that have either sleep disturbance or excessive sleepiness as a major feature
   A. *Associated with mental disorders* (e.g., psychosis, mood disorder, anxiety disorder, panic disorder, alcoholism)
   B. *Associated with neurologic disorders* (e.g., cerebral degenerative disorder, dementia, parkinsonism, etc.)
   C. *Associated with other medical disorders* (sleeping sickness, nocturnal cardiac ischemia, chronic obstructive pulmonary disease, sleep-related asthma, sleep-related gastroesophageal reflux, peptic ulcer disease, fibrositis)
4. Proposed sleep disorders = disorders for which there is insufficient information available to confirm unequivocal existence of the disorder (e.g., short sleeper, long sleeper, etc.)

> **TABLE 16-3.** CLASSIFICATION OF SLEEP DISORDERS BY THE DIAGNOSTIC AND STATISTICAL MANUAL OF MENTAL DISORDERS, 4TH EDITION (DSM-IV)
>
> 1. Primary sleep disorders = disorders which arise from endogenous abnormalities in sleep–wake generating or timing mechanisms, often complicated by conditioning factors
>   A. *Dyssomnias* = abnormalities in the amount, quality or timing of sleep (e.g., primary insomnia, primary hypersomnia, narcolepsy, breathing-related sleep disorder, circadian rhythm sleep disorder)
>   B. *Parasomnias* = abnormal behavioral or physiologic events occurring in association with sleep, specific sleep stages, or sleep–wake transitions (e.g., nightmare disorder, sleep terror disorder, sleepwalking disorder)
> 2. Sleep disorder related to another mental disorder = a prominent complaint of sleep disturbance that results from a diagnosable mental disorder but that is sufficiently severe to warrant independent clinical attention (may be insomnia or hypersomnia)
> 3. Sleep disorder due to a general medical condition = a prominent complaint of sleep disturbance that results from the direct physiologic effects of a general medical condition on the sleep–wake system (may be insomnia, hypersomnia or parasomnia)
> 4. Substance-induced sleep disorder = prominent complaints of sleep disturbance that result from the concurrent use, or recent discontinuation of use, of a substance including medications (may be insomnia, hypersomnia, or parasomnia)

Sleep Disorders in Older People

The most common sleep problems in elders are limited in number, and the health care provider who is knowledgeable about these conditions can identify, diagnose, manage, and, if appropriate, refer the patient to a sleep specialist.

PSYCHIATRIC DISORDERS

Psychiatric disorders (particularly depression) are the most common etiology of sleep problems in community-dwelling elders presenting with insomnia.

Most studies report that psychiatric disorders are the etiology of sleep problems in over half of patients presenting with DIMS. This is particularly true for depression, where early morning awakening is the most characteristic pattern, although other changes in sleep can be seen, such as increased sleep latency and more nighttime wakefulness.[24] These changes may not be present or can be less marked in depressed individuals not seeking medical care. Conversely, sleep disturbance in elders who are not currently depressed can be an important predictor of future depression. In depressed older patients with sleep disturbance, treatment of depression can also improve the sleep abnormalities. Several studies have found changes in sleep EEG towards a more normal sleep structure with antidepressant medications, which some authors suggest indicates that antidepressant drug efficacy may depend to some extent on regulation of sleep and changes in REM-sleep regulation.

Bereavement can also effect sleep. Bereavement without major depression is not associated with significant changes in sleep measures, but people with bereavement and depression have identical sleep patterns to those found in major depression.[25] These sleep abnormalities improve with treatment of depression.

Anxiety and stress can also be associated with sleeping difficulty, usually difficulty with initiating sleep or perhaps, early awakening. Patients may have difficulty falling asleep because of excessive worrying at bedtime.

DRUG AND ALCOHOL DEPENDENCY

Drug and alcohol use are thought to account for 10 percent to 15 percent of cases of DIMS. Chronic use of sedatives can lead to light, fragmented sleep. Most sleeping medications, when used chronically, lead to tolerance and the potential for increasing doses. When individuals who chronically use sleeping medications suddenly stop the drug, they may have an associated rebound insomnia that leads to restarting the medication.

Alcohol abuse is often associated with lighter and shorter duration of sleep. In addition, some persons attempt to self-treat their sleeping difficulties with alcohol. As mentioned previously, however, although alcohol causes an initial drowsiness, it can impair sleep later in the night. Finally, it is important to remember that sedatives and alcohol can worsen sleep apnea, and these respiratory depressants should be avoided in elders with documented or suspected sleep apnea.

> Although alcohol (e.g., a nightcap) causes an initial drowsiness, it can impair sleep later in the night and actually interfere with sleep.

MEDICAL PROBLEMS

Medical problems can be the cause or an aggravating factor in sleep difficulties. Chronic pain at night is a very common medical cause, particularly in older patients with arthritis. Assessment and management of the painful condition is the appropriate approach in these individuals. Other common medical etiologies of poor sleep in elders are paresthesias, cough, dyspnea from cardiac or pulmonary illness, gastroesophageal reflux, and nocturia. Additional medical problems to consider are described in the discussion of the history and physical examination.

SLEEP DISORDERED BREATHING (SLEEP APNEA)

Excessive daytime sleepiness (DOES) is a common complaint in the patient with sleep apnea (periodic reductions in ventilation during sleep). Various terms have been used for this syndrome (e.g., sleep-related breathing disorder, sleep-disordered breathing), but sleep apnea remains the term used by most health care providers. Sleep apnea can be characterized as central (simultaneous cessation of breathing effort and nasal and oral airflow), obstructive (thoracic respirations persist without normal airflow), or mixed. In sleep laboratories, evidence of obstructive sleep apnea is more commonly seen than central. Patients with obstructive sleep apnea usually present with hypersomnolence and are typically unaware of the frequent arousals associated with reductions in ventilation. Patients are often obese and may have morning headache and personality changes. Other frequently reported changes in cognition and thinking include poor memory, confusion, and irritability. Other symptoms of sleep apnea that can be helpful in recognizing this syndrome, and may be noted by a bed partner, include loud snoring, cessation of breathing, and choking sounds during sleep.

The reported prevalence of sleep apnea among older persons varies from 20 percent to 70 percent, depending on the population studied.[26] The lower prevalence rates are probably more valid estimates for the general aged population. The prevalence of sleep apnea increases with age. Sleep apnea is very common among patients referred to sleep centers for evaluation of daytime sleepiness, reportedly occurring in 70 percent of such patients at one center. The most important predictor of sleep apnea is large body mass. Other reported predictors identified in community-dwelling elders include falling asleep at inappropriate times, male gender, and napping. The use of alcohol within 2 hours of bedtime has also been identified as a predictor.[10, 11, 27] Alcoholism is an important risk factor for sleep apnea, and sleep-disordered breathing is a significant contributor to sleep disturbance in male alcoholics over age 40 years. Finally, there appears to be an association between sleep apnea and dementia. One nursing home study found that sleep apnea was associated with dementia, and the sleep disorder was positively correlated with the severity of dementia.[28] Another study, however, concluded that sleep-disordered breathing in Alzheimer's patients is mild and not associated with mental status or behavioral changes.[29]

The importance of mild degrees of sleep-disordered breathing in elders is unclear. One study found no association between mild or moderate sleep-disordered breathing and subjective sleep–wake disturbance.[30] The long-term consequences of asymptomatic sleep-disordered breathing are also unclear.[31, 32, 33]

Patients suspected of having sleep apnea should be referred to a sleep laboratory for evaluation, and if the diagnosis is documented, a trial of treatment. An example of a questionnaire to

Sleep apnea usually presents as daytime sleepiness in an obese male with loud snoring, cessation of breathing, and choking sounds during sleep; perhaps with morning headache and personality changes.

Respiratory depressants, such as sedatives and alcohol, can worsen sleep apnea, and should be avoided in elders with documented or suspected sleep apnea.

screen for sleep apnea is included in Appendix #39. There is some evidence that older patients can tolerate the main treatment of obstructive sleep apnea, nasal continuous positive airway pressure (CPAP), as well as middle-aged patients. Unfortunately, there may be prejudice among health care providers against the use of nasal CPAP in older patients, perhaps due to assumptions that the treatment will not be tolerated or successful in this population.

PERIODIC LEG MOVEMENTS IN SLEEP

Periodic leg movements in sleep (PLMS, or nocturnal myoclonus) is a condition of debilitating, repetitive, stereotypic leg movements occurring in NREM sleep. The leg movements occur every 20 to 40 seconds and can last hours or even much of the night, and each movement can be associated with an arousal. The occurrence of PLMS seems to increase with age.[34] One study found evidence of PLMS in over one third of community-dwelling elders.[7] Correlates of PLMS included dissatisfaction with sleep, sleeping alone, and reported kicking at night. Some authors have suggested that the high prevalence of PLMS with age is associated with delayed motor and sensory latencies noted on nerve conduction testing. PLMS may present as difficulty maintaining sleep or excessive daytime sleepiness. A bed partner may be aware of the leg movements, or these movements may remain occult until identified in a sleep laboratory. This condition is often best documented in a sleep laboratory.

RESTLESS LEGS SYNDROME

The restless legs syndrome (RLS) is a condition of an uncontrollable urge to move the legs at night. The symptoms can also involve the arms. The patient usually reports this symptom, and the diagnosis is made based on the patient's description of symptoms. The sleep complaint is usually difficulty in initiating sleep, and these individuals may not be able to get to sleep until very late in the evening or early morning. There may be a family history of the condition and, in some cases, an underlying medical disorder seems associated (e.g., renal, neurologic, or cardiovascular disease). The prevalence of RLS also increases with age.[6, 27] Many patients with RLS will also have periodic limb movements of sleep. The symptoms of RLS can be very distressing to the patient, but can respond to simple therapy, particularly antiParkinson's medications (e.g., a nighttime dose of carbidopa/levodopa). Unfortunately, some patients describe a shift of their symptoms to daytime hours with successful treatment of their symptoms at night.

Most sleep disorders, such as sleep apnea, periodic leg movements in sleep, and restless legs syndrome, increase in prevalence with increasing age.

DISTURBANCES IN THE SLEEP–WAKE CYCLE

Disturbances in the sleep–wake cycle can be transient, as in jet lag, or associated with an obvious cause (e.g., shift work). Some patients have persistent disturbance with either a delayed sleep-phase (fall asleep late and awaken late) or an advanced sleep-phase (fall asleep early and awaken early). Some patients have persistent sleep-phase disturbance, where circadian rhythms and sleeping period have become completely desynchronized (e.g., persons who are always asleep during the day and awake at night), or have irregular sleep–wake cycles and very disjointed sleep habits. It is unclear to what degree, if any, that changes in sleep pattern in elders (such as increased daytime napping and disrupted nighttime sleep) are due to alterations in the circadian rhythm.[35,36] Results have been mixed, but several studies have shown age-related decreases in hormonal levels and evidence of earlier circadian rises in certain hormones, suggesting age-related alteration in circadian rhythm.

People with a significant sleep-phase cycle disturbance should be referred to a sleep laboratory for evaluation. Two conditions in elders where sleep–wake disturbance are common include dementia and delirium. Additional sleep complaints in both conditions can include increased nighttime awakenings, nighttime wandering, and nighttime agitation.

SPECIAL ISSUES RELATED TO SLEEP IN ELDERS

Changes in Sleep With Dementia

Described changes in sleep with dementia include more sleep disruption and nighttime arousals, further decreases in stage 3 and 4 sleep, perhaps a decrease in REM sleep, disturbances of the sleep–wake cycle, and the phenomenon of "sundowning."

Most studies of sleep in dementia have focused on Alzheimer's disease (AD). Unfortunately, the baseline slowing of EEG activity often seen with dementia can cloud the distinction between sleep versus wakefulness and various stages of NREM sleep. Changes in sleep with dementia have been described. Demented patients have more sleep disruption and arousals, lower sleep efficiency, higher percentage of stage 1 sleep, and decreases in stage 3 and 4 sleep compared to nondemented older people (see Chapter 21). Some authors have noted a decreased percentage of sleep spent in REM, but this has not been reported in all studies. Of interest, recent studies suggest that older demented individuals actually have less sleep disturbance than older depressed persons. In fact, some suggest that sleep disturbance may be an indicator of depression as the diagnosis in persons with cognitive impairment, and sleep EEG can be a diagnostic tool in distinguishing major depression from dementia.[37] Disturbances of the sleep–wake cycle are common with dementia, resulting in daytime sleep and nighttime wakefulness. "Sundowning," the term commonly used to describe a worsening of confusion in the evening or night in persons with dementia, is likely to have a neurologic basis.[38]

Snoring

Although not considered a sleep disorder, chronic snoring has received increased attention in the literature. Over 60 percent of men over 60 years of age snore. Habitual loud snoring has been associated with increased risk of heart disease and hypertension, anxiety, dreaming, and stroke.[39, 40] In the older patient who snores, it is important to consider the diagnosis of sleep apnea; report of daytime sleepiness and the presence of other risk factors should increase suspicion for sleep apnea. Measures that can help habitual loud snorers include weight loss if overweight, abstinence from alcohol or other sedatives (e.g., benzodiazepines and antihistamines) prior to sleep, and measures to avoid supine sleeping (e.g., taping a tennis ball to the back of their sleeping attire). In the absence of sleep apnea, contributing conditions to consider include allergies, nasal pathology, or nasopharyngeal enlargement. Several intranasal sprays are available if allergic rhinitis is contributing to snoring (e.g., intranasal steroid or cromolyn sprays). Patients with suspected structural problems may need referral to an ear, nose, and throat specialist.

There is recent evidence that in some people, snoring in the absence of apnea can lead to disruption of sleep. The condition of increased ventilatory effort during sleep resulting in repetitive arousals from sleep (in the absence of apnea or hypopnea) has been termed the upper airway resistance syndrome (UARS).[41] This nonapneic snoring can be eliminated with nasal CPAP, but this remains a primarily investigational treatment for this condition and there are no clear guidelines for use of nasal CPAP in this population.

Sleep in Nursing Home Residents

Studies of sleep in nursing home residents have demonstrated marked disruption in sleep with frequent arousals during the night.[42, 43] In addition, sleep-related problems are a common reason for institutionalization. Up to 70 percent of caregivers report that nighttime difficulties played a significant role in their decision to institutionalize, often because the sleep of the caregiver was being

Potential causes of impaired sleep in nursing home residents include multiple illnesses, psychoactive medications, debility and inactivity, increased prevalence of sleep disorders, and environmental factors.

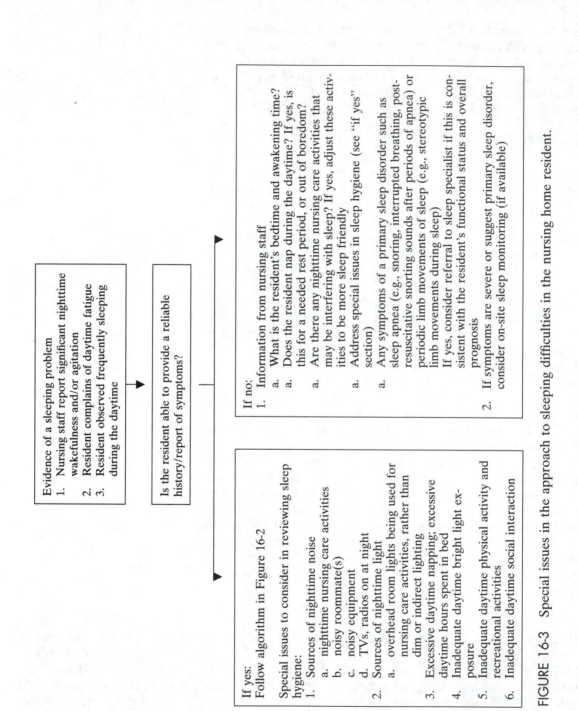

Evidence of a sleeping problem
1. Nursing staff report significant nighttime wakefulness and/or agitation
2. Resident complains of daytime fatigue
3. Resident observed frequently sleeping during the daytime

Is the resident able to provide a reliable history/report of symptoms?

If yes:
Follow algorithm in Figure 16-2

Special issues to consider in reviewing sleep hygiene:
1. Sources of nighttime noise
   a. nighttime nursing care activities
   b. noisy roommate(s)
   c. noisy equipment
   d. TVs, radios on at night
2. Sources of nighttime light
   a. overhead room lights being used for nursing care activities, rather than dim or indirect lighting
3. Excessive daytime napping; excessive daytime hours spent in bed
4. Inadequate daytime bright light exposure
5. Inadequate daytime physical activity and recreational activities
6. Inadequate daytime social interaction

If no:
1. Information from nursing staff
   a. What is the resident's bedtime and awakening time?
   a. Does the resident nap during the daytime? If yes, is this for a needed rest period, or out of boredom?
   a. Are there any nighttime nursing care activities that may be interfering with sleep? If yes, adjust these activities to be more sleep friendly
   a. Address special issues in sleep hygiene (see "if yes" section)
   a. Any symptoms of a primary sleep disorder such as sleep apnea (e.g., snoring, interrupted breathing, post-resuscitative snorting sounds after periods of apnea) or periodic limb movements of sleep (e.g., stereotypic limb movements during sleep)
   If yes, consider referral to sleep specialist if this is consistent with the resident's functional status and overall prognosis
2. If symptoms are severe or suggest primary sleep disorder, consider on-site sleep monitoring (if available)

FIGURE 16-3 Special issues in the approach to sleeping difficulties in the nursing home resident.

disrupted.[44] Once in the nursing home, many residents sleep much during the day and have frequent awakenings during the night. One study of nursing home residents found that the average duration of sleep episodes during the night was only 20 minutes.[45] Common conditions in nursing home residents that may contribute to these sleep difficulties included multiple physical illnesses, psychoactive medications, debility and inactivity, increased prevalence of sleep disorders, and environmental factors such as nighttime noise, light, and disruptive nursing care activities.[46] The lack of bright light exposure during the day may also be a factor. A study of nondemented community-dwelling elders with sleep maintenance insomnia found that timed exposure to bright light in the evening was associated with improvement in several sleep parameters.[47] Another study in institutionalized demented residents with sleep and behavior problems found that morning bright light exposure was associated with better nighttime sleep and less daytime agitation.[48] Social interaction can be another factor affecting sleep in the nursing home. One study of residents with dementia and behavioral problems found that a program of social interaction with nurses was effective in reducing behavioral problems and sleep–wake rhythm disorders in 30 percent of the participants. Figure 16-3 illustrates a suggested approach to the evaluation of sleeping difficulties in the nursing home resident.

INITIAL MANAGEMENT AND INDICATIONS FOR REFERRAL

The appropriate treatment of sleep problems must be guided by knowledge of likely etiology(ies) and potential contributing factors. It is not appropriate to start an elder with sleep complaints on a sedative hypnotic agent without a careful clinical assessment to identify the cause. Sedative hypnotics have a documented association with falls, hip fracture, and daytime carryover symptoms in elders.[27] Transient, situational insomnia can respond to improvement in sleep hygiene (Table 16-1). One recent randomized, controlled trial on the treatment of late-life insomnia demonstrated that both behavioral treatment (i.e., cognitive-behavior therapy) and drug therapy were effective, but long-term results were better with behavioral therapy.[49] Short-term use of hypnotic medications may be appropriate in some cases of transient, situational insomnia, particularly during bereavement, acute hospitalization, and other periods of temporary acute stress. The health care provider should not withold treatment in these situations if it is clearly indicated. In the patient with chronic insomnia, it is imperative the health care provider rule out primary sleep disorders and review medica-

It is not appropriate to start an older patient on a sedative-hypnotic agent without some assessment of the sleep complaint.

tions and other medical conditions that may be contributory. A circadian rhythm abnormality should also be considered, particularly the advanced sleep-phase syndrome, where the person goes to bed early in the evening and awakens early in the morning. This syndrome is extremely common in elders, and evidence suggests that bright light exposure in the evening can help alleviate this syndrome.[50] Even short durations of bright light (e.g., in the morning) have been shown to improve sleep complaints in healthy elders.[51]

Indications for referral for polysomnography include suspicion for a primary sleep disorder such as sleep apnea or periodic leg movements, or for chronic insomnia where etiology is unclear.

Polysomnography is indicated when the health care provider is suspicious of primary sleep disorders such as sleep apnea or PLMS. Even if symptoms of these conditions are not evident, some authors recommend polysomnography prior to embarking on chronic treatment of insomnia with sleeping medications in elders in whom primary sleep disorders are so common. Such testing is sometimes cost-prohibitive and not always readily available.

Methods to measure sleep other than traditional polysomnography in a sleep laboratory have been developed and are being used more extensively in studies of sleep in elders. For example, the wrist actigraph is a device that estimates sleep versus wakefulness based on wrist activity.[52] One study demonstrated that the wrist actigraph is sensitive enough to assess the efficacy of treatment interventions in elders with insomnia. Another nonintrusive measure of sleep that has been developed for home sleep monitoring is a pressure-sensitive pad that reports signals from respiration and movement. Observational sleep assessment methods have been developed; in particular, an observational tool for detecting sleep problems and sleep-related breathing disorders has been used successfully in nursing home residents in the research setting.[53] Finally, ambulatory monitoring devices are available (e.g., which measure pulse oximetry, heart rate, respirations, and nasal airflow to screen for evidence of sleep apnea) and are being used more extensively in both the clinical and research settings.

PROGNOSIS OF SLEEP PROBLEMS IN ELDERS

Some studies attempted to address the prognosis of sleep problems in older people. One longitudinal study found that insomnia was a strong predictor of death and nursing home placement in older men, but in women, insomnia was only a borderline predictor of mortality and not associated with nursing home placement.[54] Other studies suggested an association between use of medication for sleep and excess mortality in elders, but self-medication to promote sleep may be an epidemiologic marker for elders with high morbidity and mortality.[55] The association between sleeping difficulties and development of cognitive dysfunction is unclear.

Sleep-disordered breathing has significant long-term complications, and a high level of respiratory disturbance with sleep apnea is a strong predictor of mortality in elders. The natural history of mild sleep disordered breathing in elders is unknown. There is some evidence, however, that mild sleep disordered breathing in community-dwelling elders is not associated with progression of symptoms over time and is not associated with cognitive dysfunction or impaired daytime functioning.

Despite the growing literature on the frequency and nature of sleep problems in elders, current practice lags behind treatment recommendations. Surveys show that generalists often obtain inadequate history in patients with insomnia and often resort to use of psychoactive medications, even when nonpharmacologic therapies might be more effective. A study of experienced geriatricians also found deficiencies in the care of patients with sleep disorders.[56] Half of the study sample did not perform a comprehensive sleep history in the patients. In patients with sleep complaints, these geriatricians usually attributed the problem to secondary conditions, rarely diagnosed primary sleep disorders, and seldom obtained polysomnography. This study, and others, suggest that there is a great need for improved education in the diagnosis and management of sleep problems in elders.

REFERENCES

1. Hohagen F, Kappler C, Schramm E, et al. *Acta Psychiatr Scand.* 1994;90:102–108.
2. Pressman MR, Fry JM. What is normal sleep in the elderly? *Clin Geriatr Med.* 1988;4:71–81.
3. Moran MG, Thompson TL, Nies AS. Sleep disorders in the elderly. *Am J Psychiatry.* 1988;145:1369–1378.
4. James DS. Survey of hypnotic drug use in nursing homes. *J Am Geriatr Soc.* 1985;33:436–439.
5. Alessi CA, Schnelle JF, Traub S, Ouslander JG. Psychotropic medications in incontinent nursing home residents: association with sleep and bed mobility. *J Am Geriatr Soc.* 1995;43:788–792.
6. Prinz PN, Vitiello MV, Raskind MA, Thorpy MJ. Geriatrics: sleep disorders and aging. *N Engl J Med.* 1990;323:520–526.
7. Ancoli-Israel S, Kripke DF, Mason W, et al. Sleep apnea and periodic leg movements in an aging sample. *J Gerontol.* 1985;40:419–425.
8. Ancoli-Israel S. Epidemiology of sleep disorders. *Clin Geriatr Med.* 1989;5:347–362.
9. Reynolds CF, Jennings JR, Hoch CC, et al. Daytime sleepiness in healthy "old old": a comparison with young adults. *J Am Geriatr Soc.* 1991;39:957–962.

10. Bliwise DL. Sleep in normal aging and dementia. *Sleep.* 1993; 16:40–81.

11. Dement W, Richardson G, Prinz P, Carskadon M, Kripke D, Czeisler C. Changes of sleep and wakefulness with age. In: Finch DE, Schneider EL, eds., *Handbook of the Biology of Aging,* 2nd ed. New York: Von Norstrand Reinhold Co; 1985:692–717.

12. Hirshkowitz M, Moore CA, Hamilton CR, Rando KC, Karacan I. Polysomnography of adults and elderly: sleep architecture, respiration and leg movements. *J Clin Neurophysiol.* 1992;9:56–62.

13. Wauquier A, van Sweden B, Lagaay AM, Kemp B, Kamphuisen HAC. Ambulatory monitoring of sleep-wakefulness patterns in healthy elderly males and females (> 88 years): the "Senieur" protocol. *J Am Geriatr Soc.* 1992;40:109–114.

14. Habte-Gabr E, Wallace RB, Colsher PL, et al. Sleep patterns in rural elders: demographic, health and psychobehavioral correlates. *J Clin Epidemiol.* 1991;44:5–13.

15. Gislason T, Reynisdottir H, Kristbjarmarson H, Benediktsdottir B. Sleep habits and sleep disturbances among the elderly—an epidemiological survey. *J Int Med.* 1993;234:31–39.

16. Bliwise NG. Factors related to sleep quality in healthy elderly women. *Psychol Aging.* 1992;7:83–88.

17. Metz ME, Bunnell DE. Napping and sleep disturbances in the elderly. *Fam Pract Res J.* 1990;10:47–56.

18. Bonnett MH. Recovery of performance during sleep following sleep deprivation in older normal and insomniac adult males. *Perceptual Motor Skills.* 1985;60:323–334.

19. Bonnett MH. The effect of sleep fragmentation on sleep and performance in younger and older subjects. *Neurobiol Aging.* 1989;10: 21–25.

20. National Institutes of Health Consensus Development Conference Statement: the treatment of sleep disorders of older people. *Sleep.* 1991;14:169–177.

21. Buysse DJ, Reynolds CF, Monk TH, Hoch CC, Yeager AL, Kupfer DJ. Quantification of subjective sleep quality in healthy elderly men and women using the Pittsburgh Sleep Quality Index (PSQI). *Sleep.* 1991;14:331–338.

22. Diagnostic Classification Steering Committee, Thorpy MJ, Chairman. *ICSD—International Classification of Sleep Disorders: Diagnostic and Coding Manual.* Rochester, MN: American Sleep Disorders Association; 1990.

23. American Psychiatric Association. Sleep disorders. *Diagnostic and Statistical Manual of Mental Disorders,* 4th ed. Washington, DC: American Psychiatric Association; 1994:551–607.

24. Rodin J, McAvay G, Timko C. Depressed mood and sleep disturbances in the elderly: a longitudinal study. *J Gerontol.* 1988;43:45–52.

25. Reynolds CF, Hoch CC, Buysse DJ, et al. Electroencephalographic sleep in spousal bereavement and dereavement-related depression of late life. *Biol Psychiatry.* 1992;31:69–82.

26. Ancoli-Israel S, Kripke DF, Klauber MR, Mason WJ, Fell R, Kaplan O. Sleep-disordered breathing in community-dwelling elderly. *Sleep.* 1991;14:486–495.

27. Gottlieb GL. Sleep disorders and their management: special considerations in the elderly. *Am J Med.* 1990;88:29S–33S.

28. Ancoli-Israel S, Klauber MR, Butters N, Parker L, Kripke DF. Dementia in institutionalized elderly: relation to sleep apnea. *J Am Geriatr Soc.* 1991;39:258–263.

29. Hoch CC, Reynolds CF, Nebes RD, et al. Clinical significance of sleep-disordered breathing in Alzheimer's disease: preliminary data. *J Am Geriatr Soc.* 1989;37:138–144.

30. Knight H, Millman RP, Gur RC, et al. Clinical significance of sleep apnea in the elderly. *Am Rev Respir Dis.* 1987;136:845–850.

31. Phillips BA, Berry DT, Schmitt FA, Magan LK, Gerhardwtein DC, Cook YR. Sleep-disordered breathing in the healthy elderly. Clinically significant? *Chest.* 1992;101:345–349.

32. Ancoli-Israel S, Kripke DF, Klauber MR, et al. Morbidity, mortality and sleep-disordered breathing in community dwelling elderly. *Sleep.* 1996;19:277–282.

33. Hayward L, Mant A, Hewitt H, et al. Sleep disordered breathing and cognitive function in a retirement village population. *Age Ageing.* 1992;21:121–128.

34. Buysse DJ, Reynolds CF, Kupfer DJ, et al. Clinical diagnoses in 216 insomnia patients using the International Classification of Sleep Disorders (ICSD), DSM-IV and ICD-10 categories: a report from the APA/NIMH DSM-IV Field Trial. *Sleep.* 1994;17:630–637.

35. Pollak CP, Perlick D, Linsner JP. Daily sleep reports and circadian rest-activity cycles of elderly community residents with insomnia. *Biol Psychiatry.* 1992;32:1019–1027.

36. Buysse DJ, Monk TH, Reynolds CJ, Mesiano D, Houck PR, Kupfer DJ. Patterns of sleep episodes in young and elderly adults during a 36-hour constant routine. *Sleep.* 1993;16:632–637.

37. Bahro M, Riemann D, Stadtmuller G, Berger M, Gattaz WJ. REM sleep parameters in the discrimination of probable Alzheimer's disease from old-age depression. *Biol Psychiatry.* 1993;34:482–486.

38. Vitiello MV, Bliwise DL, Prinz PN. Sleep in Alzheimer's disease and the sundown syndrome. *Neurology.* 1992;42(suppl. 6):83–93.

39. Zaninelli A, Fariello R, Boni E, Corda L, Alicandri C, Grassi V. Snoring and risk of cardiovascular disease. *Int J Cardiol.* 1991; 32:347–352.

40. Palomaki H, Partinen M, Erkinjuntti T, Kaste M. Snoring, sleep apnea syndrome and stroke. *Neurology.* 1992;42(suppl):75–81.

41. Strollo PJ, Sanders MH. Significance and treatment of nonapneic snoring. *Sleep.* 1993;16:403–408.

42. Ancoli-Israel S, Parker L, Sinaee R, Fell RL, Kripke DF. Sleep framentation in patients from a nursing home. *J Gerontol.* 1989; 44:M18–M21.

43. Bliwise DL, Bevier WC, Bliwise NG, Edgar DM, Dement WC. Systematic 24-hour behavioral observations of sleep and wakefulness in a skilled-care nursing facility. *Psychol Aging.* 1990;5:16–24.

44. Pollak CP, Perlick D, Linsner JP, et al. Sleep problems in the community elderly as predictors of death and nursing home placement. *J Comm Health.* 1990;15:123–135.

45. Schnelle JF, Ouslander JG, Simmons SF, Alessi CA, Gravel MD. Nighttime sleep and bed mobility among incontinent nursing home residents. *J Am Geriatr Soc.* 1993;41:903–909.

46. Schnelle JF, Ouslander JG, Simmons SF, et al. The nighttime environment, incontinence care, and sleep disruption in nursing homes. *J Am Geriatr Soc.* 1993;41:910–914.

47. Campbell SS, Dawson D, Anderson MW. Alleviation of sleep maintenance insomnia with timed exposure to bright light. *J Am Geriatr Soc.* 1993;41:829–836.

48. Mishima K, Okawa M, Hishikawa Y, Hozumi S, Hori H, Takahashi K. Morning bright light therapy for sleep and behavior disorders in elderly patients with dementia. *Acta Psychiatr Scand.* 1994;89:1–17.

49. Morin, CM, Colecch C, Stone J, Sood R, Brink D. Behavioral and pharmacological therapies for late-life insomnia. *JAMA.* 1999; 281:991–999.

50. Cooke KM, Kreydatus MA, Atherton A, et al. The effects of evening light exposure on the sleep of healthy elderly women expressing sleep complaints. *J Behav Med.* 1998;21:103–114.

51. Kohsaka M, Fukuda N, Kobayashi R, et al. Effects of short duration morning bright light in healthy elderly. II: sleep and motor activity. *Psychiatry Clin Neurosci.* 1998;52:252–253.

52. Hauri PJ, Wisbey J. Wrist actigraphy in insomnia. *Sleep.* 1992; 15:293–301.

53. Cohen-Mansfield J, Waldhorn R, Werner P, Billig N. Validation of sleep observations in a nursing home. *Sleep.* 1990;13:512–525.

54. Pollak CP, Perlick D. Sleep problems and institutionalization of the elderly. *J Geriatr Psychiatry Neurol.* 1991;4:204–210.

55. Rumble R, Morgan K. Hypnotics, sleep, and mortality in elderly people. *J Am Geriatr Soc.* 1992;40:787–791.

56. Haponik EF. Sleep disturbances of older persons: physician's attitudes. *Sleep.* 1992;15:168–172.

CONSTIPATION, DIARRHEA, AND FECAL INCONTINENCE

C. BREE JOHNSTON / MARY KANE GOLDSTEIN / GEORGE TRIADAFILOPOULOS

Bowel disorders are common in elders. In this chapter, we discuss the clinical manifestations and assessment of constipation, diarrhea, and fecal incontinence in elders. As in all areas of geriatric medicine, the patient's goals and values must be taken into account before any evaluation of a clinical complaint is undertaken. For example, in some patients, a limited assessment or an empiric treatment regimen will be more appropriate to the patient's goals and value system. These comments on treatment are not meant to be comprehensive; rather, they highlight a few areas that are pertinent to assessment issues or that the authors feel are of critical importance.

CONSTIPATION

Constipation is one of the most common complaints that a health care provider will encounter among elders and requires a systematic approach.

Definition

The definition of constipation is not standard. Normal stool frequency varies according to diet, activity, and other factors. In Western countries, it appears that approximately 95 percent to 99 percent of people have between three bowel movements per day and three per week.[1,2] Generally, if a patient reports rare defecation (less than three times per week), hard stool consistency, sense of incomplete evacuation, or straining upon defecation more than 25 percent of the time, the diagnosis of constipation would be made with confidence.[2]

Prevalence

The prevalence of constipation is difficult to estimate because of lack of a consistent definition. A number of epidemiologic studies have found that self-report of constipation increases with age; however, many elders who self-report constipation have normal bowel habits as defined by objective criteria.[3] In both nursing home and community-dwelling elders, laxative use is common, even among people who are not constipated. Among nursing home residents in one study, 50 percent used laxatives, 47 percent self-reported constipation, but only 62 percent of that group met study criteria for symptomatic constipation.[4]

Risk Factors

Many of the risk factors for constipation are prevalent in the older population. The National Health and Nutrition Evaluation Survey and Epidemiologic Follow Up Survey indicates that risk factors for constipation include advanced age, female gender, black race, decreased activity, low income, low education level, and depression.[3] Other studies also correlated psychological distress with increased complaints of constipation; whether increased complaints correspond to increased rates of constipation remains to be determined. The use of multiple medications, low caloric intake, and the presence of multiple chronic illnesses have also been identified as risk factors.[1,4] The role of fiber in constipation is complex; although a low fiber diet is commonly identified as a risk factor for constipation and epidemiologic data support this view, some studies have failed to bear this out.

Neurologic disorders, including Parkinson's disease and diabetic neuropathy, can lead to constipation by altering bowel motility and causing decreased mobility. Acute hospitalization commonly results in constipation due to a variety of factors, including bedrest.

Clinical Manifestations

A patient's complaint can consist of a reduction in stool frequency, straining in defecation, or a sensation of incomplete evacuation. Specific symptoms can give a clue to the underlying cause. In general, any change in bowel habits can be a sign of colon cancer, and should be taken seriously. A constricting tumor can cause a decrease in the caliber of the stool; a rectal tumor or fissure can be associated with straining or tenesmus. A decrease in stool frequency or bulk can be due to decreased oral intake secondary to systemic illness rather than primary bowel pathology, and can coexist with weight loss, anorexia, and other symptoms that point to an underlying cause. Medications, bedrest, neuromuscular disorders, or any factors that decrease bowel motility will increase the stool's exposure time to the resorptive surface of the colon and can result in smaller harder stools.

Pain, straining, or discomfort on defecation can suggest dyschezia (disordered defecation) as the primary cause of constipation. Such patients have a neuromuscular cause, such as pelvic floor dyssynergia (inappropriate contraction of the puborectalis or external anal sphincter during defecation) or an anorectal disorder, such as fissure, tumor, hemorrhoid, or prolapse. Dyschezia may or may not be associated with infrequent defecation.

Diverticular disease is clinically silent in 80 percent to 85 percent of cases, but can be associated with both constipation and pain. Metabolic disorders, such as hypothyroidism and hypercalcemia, can cause constipation and can be associated with other clinical manifestations.

Complications

Constipation can result in a variety of untoward consequences. Fecal impaction can result from prolonged stasis of stool in the colon and rectum. The elder with fecal impaction can present with pain, cramping, fever, urinary or fecal incontinence, diarrhea, or delirium. Severely impaired or bedbound patients with neuromuscular disorders and chronic constipation are at risk for volvulus, most commonly of the sigmoid colon. This complication should be suspected when a patient develops sudden abdominal distention, cramping, vomiting, and obstipation.

Other complications associated with constipation include urinary incontinence, chronic abdominal pain, hemorrhoids, and syncope or other cardiovascular complications precipitated by straining.

Who to Assess

Any patient who presents with constipation deserves some degree of clinical assessment, if only to confirm or exclude the diagnosis. For those patients in whom the diagnosis is confirmed, further assessment should be performed if consistent with the overall goals of care.

How to Assess

A thorough history detailing change in bowel habits, stool frequency, consistency, and straining should always be the first step in confirming or excluding the diagnosis of constipation. Constipation is a subjective complaint, and the patient's perceptions of what is normal or pathologic can differ significantly from the health care provider's. These perceptions should be explored openly. If the patient and health care provider are not in agreement about the goals of evaluation and therapy, both parties are likely to become frustrated, and time and health care resources may be wasted. It is important for the health care provider to address the patient's concerns, even when the bowel frequency is technically within the normal range. When the history is not clear, the patient or caregiver should be asked to keep a record. This is particularly important when the patient has dementia.

The history should focus on factors that might contribute to constipation (Table 17-1), particularly medications (Table 17-2), lack of fiber in the diet, previous or recent abdominal surgery, inactivity, and diseases that might cause delayed bowel transit time (e.g., Parkinson's disease or autonomic neuropathy). The time of onset of constipation is important. Long-standing constipation is usually functional in origin. In contrast, recent onset of painful constipation implies the presence of organic pathology, such as rectal carcinoma.

TABLE 17-1. COMMON CAUSES OF CONSTIPATION
Metabolic: hypothyroidism, hypokalemia, hypercalcemia
Retentive: anal fissure, proctitis
Pharmacologic: See Table 17-2
Neuromuscular: spinal cord injury, scleroderma, Parkinson's disease
Psychogenic: depression, preoccupation with bowels
Obstructive: colon cancer, stricture
Dietary: low fiber, low caloric intake, or low fluid intake
Functional: immobility, poor toileting facilities

TABLE 17-2. COMMON DRUGS CAUSING CONSTIPATION

Opiates
Phenothiazines
Tranquilizers
Tricyclic antidepressants
Calcium channel blockers
Beta-blockers
Anticholinergics
Bismuth, iron, calcium, aluminum

A general physical and rectal examination are always warranted. The health care provider should focus the general examination on the patient's general appearance, looking specifically for signs of wasting and the patient's degree of self-care. Signs of hypothyroidism or malnutrition should be sought. The head and neck examination should particularly focus on dentition, as inadequate dentition or poor fitting dentures can correlate with poor caloric intake leading in turn, to constipation. The cardiac and lung examinations are important in excluding other significant disease, which may lead to immobility.

The abdominal examination should focus on the presence of surgical scars and hernias, areas of tenderness, bowel sounds, and palpation for excessive amounts of stool in the colon or other masses. Rectal examination is critical. Visual inspection may reveal prolapse, hemorrhoids, or fissures. Digital examination should assess anal sphincter tone, anorectal tenderness, masses, the presence and degree of impaction, and the contractility of the anal sphincters and puborectalis muscle. By placing the patient in the lateral decubitus position and asking the patient to strain or bear down, the health care provider may be able to bring out subtle prolapse, internal hemorrhoids, or lack of descent or ballooning of the perineum, which is indicative of pelvic floor dysfunction. The examiner can detect puborectalis muscle dysfunction by asking the patient to expel the index finger during digital rectal exam. Lack of motion is abnormal. Occult blood can be checked, although trauma from the examination and lack of dietary preparation can increase the rate of false positive results. Anoscopy is easily performed in the clinic, and can help further identify hemorrhoids, fissures, or other anorectal pathology.

The neurologic examination should first identify the presence or absence of systemic neurologic disease (e.g., Parkinson's, autonomic neuropathy) that might be etiologically related to the cause of constipation. The anal wink and bulbocavernosus reflexes help determine sacral neurologic function. Finally, the mental status examination will determine the reliability of the historian and the possible presence of dementia.

A complete blood count, glucose, electrolytes, calcium, and thyroid-stimulating hormone tests will identify those persons with anemia or the rare person with an endocrine or metabolic disorder, and should be considered a standard part of the workup.

Further assessment depends on the features of the case, but at a minimum, flexible sigmoidoscopy should be considered. The procedure requires no sedation, minimal bowel preparation with a laxative and an enema before the procedure, and can be performed in the office setting with the patient in the left lateral decubitus position. Sigmoidoscopy is generally safe and well tolerated in elders and allows the distinction between organic and functional causes of constipation. It can reveal melanosis coli—a dark pigmentation of the bowel wall that indicates chronic laxative abuse—or other pathology such as colorectal cancer, diverticular or ischemic stricture, or extrinsic compression by a pelvic tumor.

For constipation of less than 2 years' duration, unexplained change of bowel habits, anemia, bleeding, or any clinical suspicion of a more proximal organic stenosis (cancer or stricture), colonoscopy is generally indicated. Compared to barium enema plus sigmoidoscopy, colonoscopy carries the advantage of allowing polypectomy, biopsy, and direct visualization of the entire length of large bowel. Colonoscopy requires sedation, however, and has a higher complication rate than sigmoidoscopy alone. For some patients, such as a patient in whom sedation is undesirable, the combination of sigmoidoscopy and barium enema will be more appropriate. Clinical judgment and patient preference should guide the decision of which diagnostic approach to employ.

In most cases, instituting a bowel program and monitoring its effects is the next step, as described in Table 17-3. True treatment failure will be observed in only 1 percent of patients; only 10 percent of patients in one highly selected referral population were refractory to treatment.[2] If the bowel program fails to correct constipation, further testing is warranted.

The next step in most cases is performing a radiopaque marker transit test. In this test, a gelatin capsule containing a number of radiopaque markers is ingested on day 1 and the patient is placed on a fiber enriched diet and no laxatives. On the fifth day, a plain abdominal radiograph is performed and should show passage of 80 percent of the markers if colonic transit time is normal. In this case, the patient may have irritable bowel syndrome, a psychological disorder with fixation about bowel evacuation, or infrequent evacuation without pathology. If more than 20 percent of markers are scattered throughout the colon the diagnosis of "slow transit constipation" can be made. In contrast, the diagnosis of anorectal

TABLE 17-3. LONG-TERM BOWEL PROGRAM
Stop laxatives
Stop offending medications, when possible
Encourage regular time for defecation after a meal
Allow adequate time for defecation
Exercise daily
Add fiber to diet (bran or psyllium)
Take adequate liquids, particularly when taking fiber
Use a stool by toilet/commode to achieve squatting position
Involve both the caregiver and the patient in the plan
If above measures fail, consider:
Increasing fiber to 20–30 grams daily (with fluids)
Using a glycerin suppository after a meal
Adding an osmotic laxative, such as lactulose or sorbitol

dysfunction or dyschezia may be suggested if multiple markers are visualized in the rectosigmoid area.

A history of treatment failure in the setting of excessive straining, finger disimpaction, anorectal pain, incontinence, or failure to respond to enemas suggests a disturbance in anorectal function. A number of physical assessment methods of anorectal function can then be employed. Balloon expulsion, which can be performed by a specialist or motivated primary care practitioner, has been advocated as a good screening test for anorectal dysfunction. The history of abnormal defecation combined with an abnormal balloon expulsion test are reported to be more than 90 percent predictive of an abnormal defecatory process.[2] To perform balloon expulsion, a urinary catheter is placed in the rectum with the balloon inflated to 50 to 60 mL. The patient can be seated on the toilet and asked to expel the balloon. Inability to expel the balloon is indicative of dysfunction.

The approach to further testing is problematic, and depends, in part, on available resources and the cost of testing. Defecation proctography, a radiologic procedure that measures perineal descent and the anorectal angle during rest, squeezing, and straining, is recommended by many experts in the field, although it is unclear how sensitive and specific this test is. Ultrasonography can detect anatomic sphincter defects. No clear "gold standard" examination exists in this area, so the approach is often empiric.

The colonic transit study is simple, safe, repeatable, and low cost. A normal study excludes significant constipation; an abnormal study distinguishes slow transit constipation from dyschezia.

Management Considerations

These comments are not comprehensive; areas that are relevant to assessment or that the authors feel are clinically important are highlighted.

If the patient's history and physical examination indicate the cause of constipation (e.g., hypothyroidism), intervention is straightforward. Every effort should be made to adjust or eliminate medications that may be contributing to the problem. Anticholinergics, narcotics, psychotropics, and calcium channel blockers are common causes of constipation, and should be reduced or eliminated when possible. When no reversible cause of the patient's constipation is found on the initial evaluation, empiric treatment should begin. The first step is to clear an impaction, if present. An irritant laxative such as bisacodyl, water or commercial enema, or oral polyethylene glycol may all be used. It can be necessary to give daily enemas over the course of a week to clear the stasis. During this time, frequent leakage of semiliquid stool and new or worsening fecal incontinence may develop. Both the individual and caregiver should be warned about these effects in advance and should be reassured that these changes are temporary while fecal stasis is being cleared. It is usually possible to manage this procedure and its effects at home, perhaps with the assistance of a visiting nurse, but occasionally, a patient will require admission to a geriatric unit or skilled nursing facility.

Individuals placed on a long-term bowel program should be given the instructions that are listed in Table 17-3. The health care provider should review each step with patients and their families, explaining the instructions and allowing the patient an opportunity to solve problems at each step and find socially and culturally appropriate ways to achieve adherence. If patients are from a particular ethnic group, it is efficient to obtain consultation with a nutritionist and other health care workers who are familiar with the customs of the group.

In the person who has a neuromuscular cause of constipation or megacolon, fiber supplementation is of no value. The most successful approach in these people will be a combination of osmotic agents such as lactulose or sorbitol, suppositories, and enemas once to twice weekly, as well as avoidance of anticholinergic and other constipating medications.

Common Problems in Assessment

Frequently, the health care provider may have difficulty in determining the severity of constipation, and some patients and caregivers have difficulty completing diaries. Perhaps the most common problem in assessment is determining which patients have truly intractable constipation versus inadequate treatment. The radiopaque marker transit study is very useful in assessing the effectiveness of therapy. For the patients with pelvic floor and anorectal dysfunction, assessment instruments and treatment modalities are still controversial and not universally available.

DIARRHEA

Whereas diarrheal illness is recognized as a serious problem in children, it can also be catastrophic in elders. Although the majority of diarrheal deaths occur among those who are older than 75 years, those between 55 and 74 are also at increased risk.[5] Nursing home residents are at particularly high risk of death from diarrheal illness.

Physiologic changes that are common with aging, including a decrease in the thirst mechanism, cardiovascular disease, and decreased concentrating ability of the kidney, make elders particularly vulnerable to the fluid losses that result from diarrhea. The increasing incidence of *Clostridium difficile* colitis is becoming another challenging cause of diarrhea in institutional settings.

Definition

Diarrhea is defined objectively by daily stool weights of more than 300 grams, and is accompanied clinically by an increase in stool water. Clinically, diarrhea can be defined as frequent consecutive liquid stools. Acute diarrhea is defined as diarrhea lasting less than 3 weeks, whereas chronic diarrhea is diarrhea lasting greater than 3 weeks. Dysentery implies the occurrence of frequent expulsion of liquid bloody mucus material with almost no feces, associated with tenesmus, and results from acute distal colitis.

Prevalence

The prevalence of diarrhea among community-dwelling elders is difficult to determine with accuracy. For the nursing home residents, acute diarrheal illnesses appear to have a 24-hour prevalence of less than 2 percent but chronic and epidemic diarrhea may be much more common.

Risk Factors

Diabetic patients, particularly those with neuropathy, are susceptible to diarrhea; the prevalence of diarrhea has been reported in between 8 percent and 22 percent of chronic diabetics.[6] Patients on tube feedings commonly experience diarrhea. Nursing home residents are vulnerable to epidemic outbreaks of infectious diarrhea. Pelvic irradiation can lead to chronic diarrhea.

Clinical Manifestations

Patients present with an increase in stool volume and bulk, usually with an increase in stool frequency and water content. Dehydration and cardiovascular collapse can result from acute or chronic diarrhea, with secondary complications of hypernatremia, hyponatremia, hypokalemia, renal failure, or syncope.

Specific clinical manifestations can indicate the etiology. Bloody diarrhea should suggest mucosal invasion with pathogens such as *Escherichia coli* 0157:H7, *Shigella, Campylobacter, Salmonella,* or inflammation due to ischemia or inflammatory bowel disease. An acute infectious cause of diarrhea is often obvious from its acute onset in association with other symptoms, including nausea and vomiting (with staphylococcal toxin or *Bacillus cereus* infection), malaise, or fever. Infectious diarrhea often occurs in the setting of contact with other ill persons, recent travel, or ingestion of suspect food. *Salmonella* outbreaks are not uncommon in nursing homes and result from ingestion of contaminated poorly cooked foods of animal origin.

In a patient in whom antibiotics were recently used, particulary in an institutional setting, *Clostridium difficile* colitis should be considered first. Clinical features that are strongly associated with *C. difficile* infection include cephalosporin use, prolonged hospital stay (> 15 days), onset of symptoms 6 or more days after the administration of antibiotics, and semiformed stool.[6] Antibiotics can also cause diarrhea by other mechanisms, including stimulating gut motility (e.g., erythromycin).

Fecal impaction is a common cause of acute diarrhea ("pseudodiarrhea" or "overflow diarrhea") in elders and should be suspected in the setting of loose stools preceded by constipation. Fecal incontinence commonly coexists in this setting. Relapsing infections, particularly parasitic, can cause chronic diarrheal syndromes. *Clostridium difficile* colitis can be relapsing as well. Diarrhea is common in diabetic patients, and the history can give a clue to the cause. Such patients, or others with autonomic neuropathy, can develop a copious diarrhea that is often worse at night or with recumbency. Other manifestations of autonomic neuropathy are usually present. Other mechanisms of diarrhea in the diabetic patient that have been found include pancreatic exocrine insufficiency, celiac sprue, intestinal bacterial overgrowth, and colonic dysmotility in association with impaction and overflow diarrhea.[7]

Food additives, caffeine, and alcohol can lead to diarrhea. Osmotically active agents such as sorbitol, a commonly used sweetener for diet foods, can lead to an osmotic diarrhea, and can be one cause of diarrhea in diabetic patients. Carbohydrate malabsorption in elders is often subtle, presenting with cramping, bloating, or flatus, with or without diarrhea. Generalized malabsorption can present with weight loss, diarrhea, steatorrhea, or micronutrient (folate, B_{12}, or vitamin D) deficiency. Causes of malabsorption in elders include bacterial overgrowth due to altered bowel motility, hypochlorhydria, pancreatic disease, or mesenteric ischemia.[8]

Inflammatory bowel disease (IBD) is bimodal in age distribution, with the first peak occurring in the third decade and the second peak occurring between ages 50 and 80 years, most often near the age of 70. Although bleeding is common in IBD, diarrhea may be the sole manifestation in elders. Fever, weight loss, elevated sedimentation rate, and anemia can also be seen.[9]

Bowel ischemia is one of the most serious causes of diarrhea in elders. The diagnosis should be considered in any patient with underlying vascular disease. Colonic ischemia often presents with mild abdominal pain, rectal bleeding, or bloody diarrhea. Patients often have tenderness and guarding on examination. Almost a quarter of patients will have an associated predisposing lesion, such as colon carcinoma, stricture, or fecal impaction. In contrast to colonic ischemia, mesenteric ischemia usually initially presents with abdominal pain and bloating; diarrhea and bleeding are uncommon until late in the course when the patient is generally critically ill.[10]

Who to Assess

Every patient with the complaint of diarrhea needs assessment to determine illness severity and the risk for dehydration. For those who are acutely ill or who develop chronic diarrhea, further assessment is in order.

How to Assess

ACUTE DIARRHEA

The causes of acute diarrhea in elders are listed in Table 17-4 and should be kept in mind during the assessment. Many cases of acute diarrhea are self-limited, and can be managed supportively for 2 to 3 days without instituting a work-up if the patient is not seriously ill.

TABLE 17-4. CAUSES OF ACUTE DIARRHEA IN ELDERS

Fecal impaction

Intestinal infection (*Clostridium difficile, Shigella, Salmonella, Campylobacter, Escherichia coli,* and viral)

Drug-induced (colchicine, misoprostol, magnesium containing antacids, antibiotics, L-dopa, quinidine, theophylline, nonsteroidals, lactulose, and donepezil and other cholinergic agents)

Laxative abuse

Inflammatory bowel disease

Radiation colitis

Intestinal ischemia

In nursing home-dwelling elders, the leading cause of acute diarrhea is *C. difficile* infection.

The first step in the evaluation of the patient with acute diarrhea is always the aggressive assessment of the patient's hydration status and risk for dehydration or electrolyte imbalance based on the volume of diarrheal fluid losses. Also, frank blood in the stools or maroon, black, or occult blood positive stools should be detected as early as possible to develop a treatment plan and arrange for hospitalization when necessary.

The physical examination should focus on the general appearance and presence or absence of fever, pallor, or tachycardia. The orthostatic blood pressure measurement may be the most reliable indicator of significant volume loss, but may not become abnormal until up to 10 percent of circulating blood volume is lost. It can be difficult to interpret because of medication use, prolonged recumbency, or autonomic insufficiency. Other signs, such as poor skin turgor, sunken eyes, or dry mucous membranes, can also be unreliable indicators of hydration status in elders.

The abdominal examination should focus on presence or absence of tenderness, distension, and presence of bowel sounds. Rectal examination can detect fecal impaction, although the absence of stool in the rectal vault does not rule out its occurrence more proximally. A palpable rectal mass in a patient with diarrhea suggests villous adenoma; gross or occult blood and tenderness on rectal exam imply acute or chronic colitis.

Further testing should include a plain abdominal radiograph if fecal impaction is considered likely in the differential diagnosis and to exclude megacolon. If the history and physical examination suggest an inflammatory condition, stool should be obtained for leukocytes and occult blood evaluation. If positive, a stool culture should be obtained. Other screening tests for inflammatory diarrhea have been reported and may be available in some settings.[11] In the setting of recent antibiotic use, institutionalization, or a clinical cluster of cases, a stool sample should be sent for *C. difficile* examination.[6] Generally, tissue culture assay is the most sensitive test available. A number of immunoassays are available, but vary in sensitivity and specificity. Repeat testing within 7 days of a negative test is rarely helpful unless the original test was not a tissue culture assay. If obtaining a stool sample is difficult, rectal swabbing is a relatively easy alternative. A sigmoidoscopy and biopsy will be necessary in the setting of acute diarrhea if the patient is acutely ill and a diagnosis cannot be made by less invasive testing.

CHRONIC DIARRHEA

Chronic diarrhea is defined as diarrhea lasting longer than 3 weeks. As in acute diarrhea, patients with chronic diarrhea can become dehydrated, and assessing volume losses and nutritional status should be done early so that the patient can be maximally supported while the work-up is in progress. Secondary lactase deficiency is common after an episode of acute diarrhea and can prolong the diarrheal syndrome; a period free of dairy products should be instituted early in the evaluation to rule out this common problem. Medications should be thoroughly evaluated, as many drugs can cause diarrhea. Any new or suspect drugs should be eliminated if possible. Occult laxative use should always be considered. Small bowel bacterial overgrowth should be suspected in patients over age 75 years with chronic diarrhea, anorexia, or nausea, but is unusual in younger age groups.[12]

The initial physical examination should focus on signs of systemic illness, malnutrition, dehydration, or anemia. In the diabetic patient, signs of autonomic insufficiency should be sought. As in acute diarrhea, abdominal and rectal examinations are mandatory. Stool should be sent for occult blood, leukocytes, ova and parasites, and *Clostridium difficile* toxin. Stool pH can be tested; a stool pH of less than 5.3 indicates carbohydrate intolerance.[13] In most cases, blood tests should include a CBC with differential, albumin, BUN, creatinine, electrolytes, and thyroid function tests, and in suspected inflammatory bowel disease, a sedimentation rate may be helpful. In cases in which malabsorption is suspected, testing for micronutrient deficiency (e.g., B_{12}) is reasonable.

A number of examinations are useful when occult laxative abuse is suspected. A stool alkalinization assay can be used to detect phenolphthalein, as contained in many nonprescription laxatives (e.g., Correctol, Ex-lax). Urine studies utilizing thin layer chromatography can be used to test for bisacodyl, phenolphthalein, or anthraquinones.

Further evaluation should be guided by the particular clinical features of the case. Visualization is the next step if colonic pathology is suggested by bloody diarrhea or other symptoms, such as tenesmus, abdominal tenderness, and small volume liquid stools.

Small volume diarrhea with tenesmus implies colonic origin; large volume diarrhea with weight loss suggests a small bowel etiology.

Colonoscopy is probably the procedure of choice, as it allows for direct colonic visualization and the ability to obtain biopsy specimens for tissue diagnosis. Sigmoidoscopy can be used initially if the patient is too ill for colonoscopy or to look for melanosis coli. A small bowel series or barium enema can be useful if visualization of the ileocecal valve or proximal colon is desirable.

If steatorrhea is suspected, a plain film to rule out pancreatic calcifications is easy to perform. A 72-hour fecal fat collection is the gold standard for evaluation of steatorrhea, but can be difficult to complete in the elderly. If such a collection seems unrealistic, a qualitative assay for fecal fat with Sudan stain can be used, but loses sensitivity when fecal fat is less than 10 grams in a 24-hour period.[8, 13] A 5-gram D-xylose test with measurement of a one-hour blood xylose level has been validated as test of nutrient malabsorption in elders, and may be more useful than the standard D-xylose urine test. The hydrogen breath test is simple and low cost for diagnosing small bowel bacterial overgrowth syndrome, but its sensitivity can be variable in elders and it is not universally available. In cases of malabsorption in which small bowel pathology (e.g. bacterial overgrowth, lymphoma, Whipple's disease, or giardiasis) is suspected, upper endoscopy with duodenal biopsy may be necessary if other less invasive tests are normal. Upper gastrointestinal series with small bowel follow through or enteroclysis are also helpful in defining mucosal abnormalities, but do not rule out pathology when normal.[8, 13] In the setting of copious watery diarrhea, hypokalemia, and negative laxative screen, further specialized tests can be performed to rule out endocrine secreting tumors.[13]

Common Problems in Assessment

Patients with diarrhea are often quite ill, and completing a workup can be a challenge when frailty and dehydration are present. Therefore, inpatient management and intravenous fluids can be necessary. The assessment of malabsorption can be particularly challenging in elders, as the symptoms and signs can be vague and some diagnostic tests can be difficult to obtain, comply with, or interpret (e.g., 72-hour fecal fat). Given the challenges of evaluating chronic diarrhea, particularly in frail, homebound or nursing home-dwelling elders, instituting empiric therapy without a clear diagnosis is often the most realistic clinical course.

Treatment Considerations

In cases of acute diarrhea, treatment should focus on early and aggressive patient resuscitation with fluids and blood as needed.

Care must be taken to rehydrate with liquids containing the correct electrolyte balance, using a number of homemade or commercially available preparations.

In most cases of diarrhea that are not self-limited, treatment is directed at the underlying etiology. In cases in which no clear etiology is found, however, or in cases in which diabetic diarrhea is present, treatment is geared to maximizing function and minimizing symptoms. Loperamide (nonprescription) and diphenoxylate hydrochloride with atropine (prescription) are useful in suppressing diarrhea resulting from most etiologies. Anticholinergic side effects can be problematic in some patients. For diabetic patients in whom bacterial overgrowth is suspected, a 2-week course of broad-spectrum antibiotics (ciprofloxacin, metronidazole) can be beneficial.

FECAL INCONTINENCE

Few interventions will have a larger impact on a patient and caregiver than the successful evaluation and treatment of fecal incontinence. Often in such patients, even minor therapeutic interventions will yield a major imporovement in quality of life.

Definition

Fecal incontinence is the involuntary leakage of stool. It should not be confused with diarrhea as it can occur in subjects with otherwise normal habits or even in patients with constipation and fecal impaction

Prevalence

The prevalence of fecal incontinence in community-dwelling elders in not well delineated, but may be close to 5 percent. One study of a nursing home population found a prevalence rate of 46 percent. Risk factors include diarrhea, dementia, restricted mobility, and male gender.[14] Heightened caregiver burden, social isolation, and increased rate of institutionalization are some of the potentially devastating consequences of fecal incontinence.

Clinical Manifestations

Normal continence requires the ability to sense rectal filling, the ability of the rectum and colon to store feces, and the ability of the sphincters to prevent unwanted defecation. Manifestations of

TABLE 17-5. CAUSES OF FECAL INCONTINENCE

Fecal impaction
Loss of normal continence mechanism
  Local neuronal damage
  Impaired neurologic control of spinal reflex arc and central inhibition
  Trauma
Problems that overwhelm a normal continence mechanism
  Diarrhea
  Poor access to toileting facilities
  Immobility
Psychological problems
  Severe depression
  Dementia

Adapted, with permission, from Goldstein et al. Fecal incontinence in an elderly man: Stanford University Geriatrics Case Conference. *J Am Geriatr Soc.* 1989; 37:991–1002.

fecal incontinence vary according to the etiology, which are listed Table 17-5. Fecal impaction is a common cause of acute fecal incontinence, and should be suspected in an acutely ill or hospitalized elder. Chronic fecal impaction can lead to chronic fecal soiling. The leaked feces can be hard, soft, or liquid, and reported to the health care provider as diarrhea. The rectum can be filled with small, hard, or soft feces, around which liquid or soft stool may pass. With chronic constipation, the rectum becomes distended, the sphincters lose their normal tone, and the anus can become patulous. Under these conditions, leakage can occur even when neuromuscular mechanisms are intact. Clinically, the patient can present with frequent leakage of stool or with the complaint of diarrhea. Neuronal damage at a low level of the spinal cord can cause an autonomous colon that empties incontinently without warning. A lesion above the sacral segments can produce a "reflex colon," which disrupts the sacral center from the cerebral cortex. Through this mechanism, defecation is involuntary, but fairly effective and complete. Finally, central nervous system disorders can lead to an uninhibited colon, in which defecation occurs by reflex mechanisms, usually after gastrocolic stimulation, (e.g. after breakfast or a cup of coffee).

Local trauma, as it occurs with obstetrical or anorectal surgery, can lead to nerve or muscular damage of the pelvic floor or levator ani muscles. In these disorders, the sphincter tone and normal anorectal angle may be lost. Demented patients can become incontinent due to loss of voluntary control, failure to respond to normal cues, immobility, or difficulty in communicating their needs to caregivers. Depression is usually profound before it will interfere with a patient's desire to maintain continence. Finally, overwhelming diarrhea or acute loss of mobility can lead to fecal incontinence in people with normal neuromuscular continence mechanisms.

Who to Assess

Many patients will not volunteer that they have fecal incontinence. Therefore, the first step in assessment is to ask the patient or caregiver about the existence and magnitude of the problem. Every patient who presents with fecal soiling or lack of bowel control deserves an assessment. In the setting of an acute, self limited illness, the assessment can be abbreviated, focusing on fecal impaction, immobility, or delirium.

How to Assess

The first step in the assessment of fecal incontinence is a complete history, particularly about the onset, frequency, and duration of symptoms. Acute reversible causes, such as fecal impaction, acute diarrheal disorders, or delirium should be readily apparent. The history should also assess if fecal incontinence is spontaneous or induced by increased intra-abdominal pressure, such as coughing or sneezing, and the amount and quality of fecal soiling. The pattern of bowel evacuation prior to the onset of incontinence can provide clues to long-standing laxative abuse or other bowel pathology. Other important associated symptoms to be elicited include pain, cramping, bleeding, tenesumus, and urinary incontinence. The past surgical and obstetrical history can give clues to prior nerve damage, which can sometimes contribute to fecal incontinence years later.

The impact on the patient and caregiver are important to elicit in the history. Often, a new complaint of fecal incontinence drives a caregiver "over the edge" to begin placement proceedings; for the formerly active person, incontinence can lead to decreased activity, social isolation, and depression.

The physical examination focus is similar to that for the patient with constipation (see preceding section). The digital rectal examination can provide information about rectal tone, although this is not predictive of continence. Patients with poor sphincter tone can remain continent, while those with normal tone can become incontinent if the rectal distention is significant enough or other risk factors are present. Other components of the rectal examination, such as rectal sensation and the quality of the anal wink and bulbocavernosus reflexes are particularly important in assessing neurologic function. Impaction does not have to imply hard stool; "soft impaction" can result in the same clinical sequelae.

		Date	Date	Date	Date	Date	Date	Date
Diet								
	Fluids							
	Fiber							
Stool								
Soilage (Y or N)								
Amount								
	Small (S)							
	Large (L)							
Consistency								
	Solid (S)							
	Liquid (L)							
Time								
	Bowel Medications							
	Enema (E)							
	Suppository (S)							
	Oral Medication							
Activity								
	Upright Posture							
	Recumbancy							
	Other							
Urinary Incontinence								

FIGURE 17-1 Incontinence record.

10. Reinus JF, Brandt LJ, Boley SJ. Ischemic diseases of the bowel. *Gastroenterol Clin North Am.* 1990;19:319–343.

11. Miller JR, Barrett LJ, Kotloff K, Guerrant RL. A rapid test for infectious and inflammatory enteritis. *Arch Intern Med.* 1994; 154:2660–2664.

12. Riordan SM, McIver CJ, Wakefield D, Bolin TD, Duncombe VM, Thomas MC. Small intestinal bacterial overgrowth in the symptomatic elderly. *Am J Gastroenterol.* 1997;92:47–51.

13. Donowitz M, Kokke FT, Saidi R. Evaluation of patients with chronic diarrhea. *N Engl J Med.* 1995;332:725–729.

14. Johanson JF, Irizarry F, Doughty A. Risk factors for fecal incontience in a nursing home population. *J Clin Gastroenterol.* 1997;26:156–160.

15. Madoff RD, Williams JG, Caushaj PF. Fecal incontinence. *N Engl J Med.* 1992;326:1002–1007.

OLDER DRIVER ASSESSMENT

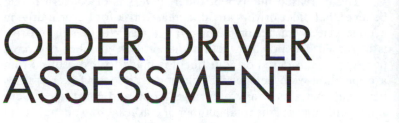

RICHARD MAROTTOLI

Older drivers have been the focus of increased attention for several reasons: the demographic shift toward more older individuals; the perception that older drivers are at greater risk for safety problems such as moving violations or crashes; and the reality that older individuals are more likely than younger individuals to be injured or killed if a crash does occur. A number of questions remain: Is there an older driver "problem"? What resources are available to the health care provider for detection or referral? What can be done with the information once it is obtained? This chapter addresses these issues.

BACKGROUND

As noted, the number of older individuals and the number of older drivers are expected to increase dramatically in the next 25 years. In 1990, individuals age 65 years and older constituted approximately 13 percent of both the United States population and the number of licensed drivers (33 million and 22 million, respectively).[1] It is estimated that by 2020, 17 percent of the population will be age 65 years and older resulting in approximately 50 million persons and 33 million licensed drivers.[1,2] Older drivers will likely constitute an even greater proportion, however, because current figures include many women who never drove, which will not be the case in 2020.[1-3] For instance, in a representative cohort of older individuals in New Haven, Connecticut in 1989, 43 percent of cohort members had never driven and 88 percent of those were women.[3]

The increased number of older drivers is of concern if one believes that older drivers are at increased risk for adverse driving events such as crashes or moving violations. Whether or not risk is increased depends on whether the absolute number of events per year is considered or adjustment is made for exposure. From a population-wide perspective, older drivers have fewer crashes per year than almost any other age group and constitute a very small percentage of the total number of crashes. From an individual perspective, however, when adjusting for the fewer number of miles that elders drive on average in a given year, crash rates per mile driven increase to approach or surpass the otherwise highest risk age group, drivers younger than 25 years old.[4] Compared to younger individuals, crashes sustained by older drivers are more likely to occur at intersections and to involve right of way or traffic sign violations.[4]

In addition to the increasing number of older drivers and the potential increase in adverse events that may result, concern is raised because older drivers are more likely than younger individuals to be injured, hospitalized, and killed as a result of a crash. Barancik and colleagues found that individuals age 75 years and older had almost twice the hospitalization and mortality rates following crashes of any other age group.[5] Thus, motor vehicle trauma represents a potentially preventable cause of morbidity and mortality among elders, as well as the other drivers, passengers, and pedestrians who may be involved.

> Crash rates, per mile driven, increase to approach or surpass the otherwise highest risk age group—drivers younger than 25 years old.

Potential safety concerns must be balanced against an elder's mobility needs, however, and the important role that driving plays in meeting those needs in our society. Although many elders drive less often or fewer miles than they did previously, the vast majority still rely on the automobile as their primary form of transportation.[3,6,7] If limitation or cessation of driving is the recommendation following evaluation, mobility may be further compromised. Thus, it is important to consider mobility needs in the assessment process, and help to plan for the most appropriate transportation methods to meet those needs safely based on an individual's capabilities and circumstances.

ROLE OF THE HEALTH CARE PROVIDER

Why should health care providers get involved in this issue in the first place? This section focuses on two aspects of this question: (1) concern for personal and public safety and the prevention of injury; and (2) the ability to identify factors that place certain older drivers at potential risk for driving problems (other aspects of interest, such as minimization of risk of injury once a crash occurs and the evacuation and treatment of individuals after a crash, are not considered here).

Physician Surveys

Two recent surveys addressed the role of physicians in older driver issues and identified features of current practices and areas that require attention. In a study by Drickamer and Marottoli, 59 percent of 3450 general practitioners, internists, ophthalmologists, neurologists, and neurosurgeons in Connecticut responded to a mailed questionnaire.[8] Of the more than 2000 responding physicians, 77 percent had discussed driving issues with their patients and 14 percent had reported patients to the Department of Motor Vehicles (DMV) in the previous year. Neurologists were more likely to have reported patients to the DMV. This is as expected because reporting individuals with recurrent attacks of epilepsy or loss of consciousness had been mandatory in Connecticut until recently when the statute was changed to state that physicians "may" report an individual with chronic health problems that "will significantly affect the person's ability to safely operate a motor vehicle." Eighty-nine percent of responding physicians felt it was their responsibility to counsel patients about driving and 59 percent felt it was their responsibility to report unsafe drivers to the DMV. Only 9 percent had referred patients to a driver retraining program in the previous year. Regarding the issue of reporting, two different themes emerged from respondents: (1) driving safety is a public health issue and health care providers should report someone they felt to be a danger to themselves or to others; and (2) the determination of driver safety is the responsibility of the state, not health care providers.

These findings are similar to those obtained in a national survey by Miller and Morley of the 5009 physician members of the American Geriatrics Society.[9] Of the 2404 (48 percent) respondents, 89 percent viewed driving as a privilege rather than a right. Eighty-seven percent felt physicians had a responsibility to medically assess their patients' capacity to drive, although only 29 percent were aware of American Medical Association guidelines concerning medical conditions affecting drivers. Twenty-one percent kept a record of patients' driving status, 37 percent had referred one or more patients to their state licensing agency in the previous year, and 12 percent had referred patients to a refresher course.

Both studies demonstrate that the issue of counseling older drivers is raised in the practices of many physicians. The studies suggest that health care providers would benefit from more clear guidelines on what their role should be, however, particularly in terms of which individuals to evaluate, how to evaluate them, and what to do with that information (counseling, retraining, and reporting).

Identification of Risk Factors

The previously discussed studies also help to define the role of the health care provider in this process (for the purposes of this discussion, the term, health care provider, refers to physicians, physician assistants, and nurse practitioners who provide medical care to elders). In relation to driving, the strength of health care providers is their ability to identify (and potentially treat) medical conditions and impairments that can affect driving ability. Other professionals, such as therapists with specialized training in driving assessment or DMV evaluators, are better able to assess the actual effects these conditions or impairments have on driving ability. Thus, one approach to the evaluation process would be to have a two-way referral pattern, with health care providers identifying risk factors among patients that place them at potential risk for driving problems. These patients would then be referred to a therapist who assesses the impact of these risk factors on driving performance and suggests possible corrective measures or adaptive strategies. Some driving assessment programs provide a full range of services including physical examination and the assessment of impairments, determining the impact of these on driving performance, and suggestions of interventions or adaptions to correct or compensate. If interventions fail or are not possible, patients could be counseled to limit or stop driving, or a referral could be made to the DMV for a licensing decision, depending on the reporting requirements of the state or province. On the other hand, elders identified by the DMV as being at risk because of their driving record or licensing test performance can be referred to health care providers to determine if there is a medical reason that is responsible. Indeed, in many areas, approaches like this exist with interaction between health care providers, therapists, and licensing agencies, although often on an informal basis.

Licensing and Reporting

Licensing is a government function. State or provincial motor vehicle departments determine and enforce the criteria for issuing, maintaining, and, ultimately, revoking a license. These criteria vary

TABLE 18-1. STATES, PROVINCES, AND TERRITORIES WITH MANDATORY PHYSICIAN REPORTING	
STATES	PROVINCES AND TERRITORIES
California	British Columbia
Delaware	Manitoba
Nevada	New Brunswick
New Jersey	Newfoundland
Oregon	Northwest Territories
Pennsylvania	Ontario
	Prince Edward Island
	Yukon Territory

Source: Petrucelli E, Malinowski M. Update of medical review practices and procedures in U.S. and Canadian commercial driver licensing programs. *Federal Highway Administration Report.* Washington, DC Publication DTFHG195PO1200. 1997.

across states and provinces, complicating the issue for health care providers who move from one state or province to another. The responsibilities of the health care provider may not be widely publicized and the legal ramifications of reporting or not reporting may not be clear. The relative merits and pitfalls of mandatory versus voluntary reporting are beyond the scope of this chapter. At the very least, health care providers should contact their state's or province's DMV and become familiar with their requirements and recommendations. Table 18-1 provides a summary of the states and provinces with mandatory reporting based on a survey conducted by Petrucelli and Malinowski in 1997.[10]

Incentives and Disincentives

So why should health care providers get involved? Because they are concerned about the health and safety of their patients. If risk factors for driving problems can be identified, it is conceivable that some of these could be correctable or adaptations available, allowing the elder to continue driving as usual. Alternatively, the factors may affect driving performance only under certain conditions, so that restrictions may still allow for a graduated license that permits driving under certain circumstances. If, however, no corrections or adaptations are possible and a person is deemed too unsafe to continue driving, the health care provider is in an ideal position to help counsel patients because of the nature of their relationship and the weight their advice often carries. Health care providers can work with the elder and family or friends to define mobility needs and to identify alternative transportation sources so that activity level and some degree of independence can be maintained.

There are also reasons for not addressing the issue or severely limiting the scope of this interaction. The discussion and evaluation process can place a strain on the health care provider–patient relationship, particularly if reporting to the DMV is involved. Additionally, as noted, it is not always clear which elders to evaluate, how to evaluate them, where to refer them for further assessment, and what to do with the information obtained in this evaluation. The process can be time consuming and confusing. The remainder of this chapter provides a framework for addressing these issues, although there are no definite answers at present and the approach must be tailored to the individual situation.

ASSESSMENT STRATEGIES

This section is divided into three parts. The first describes elements of the history that can be used to determine if there is potential cause for concern. The second describes some of the functional abilities most relevant to driving, how to assess them, and a description of evidence supporting their relationship to driving outcomes. It also provides a brief overview of some of the medical factors that can contribute to risk and where to find more detailed information on these. The third part provides an overview of approaches to the assessment process ranging from measures that can be used in an office setting to those that require specialized equipment or training to administer, some of which are established and others under investigation.

Transportation History

It is important to include questions on transportation and driving in the history to identify potential areas of difficulty.

It is important to include questions on transportation and driving in the history to identify potential areas of difficulty, as well as factors motivating continued driving or use (or lack of use) of alternative sources of transportation. Does the elder drive, how often, under what circumstances, and for what purposes? If not, how does he or she get where he or she needs to go? If he or she drives, has he or she gotten lost, received any moving violations, or had crashes or near misses? If so, what were the circumstances? Is he or she, or family and caregivers, concerned about driving safety and why? In a recent review, Reuben described a sample questionnaire that can be used to obtain this information in an interview or as a self-administered questionnaire (see Appendix #34).[11]

Risk Factor Assessment

FUNCTIONAL ABILITIES

Basically, the act of driving requires the driver to obtain information on the environment, process that information, and act upon it. Obviously, this is a simplified view of a very complex process that will depend on the driver and environment, as well as on how well the systems that obtain, process, and act on information work independently and with each other. For the purposes of this discussion, we focus on: the sensory information obtained; the central processing of, and decision-making based on, this information (cognition); and the peripheral execution of the resulting decision (motor).

Sensory

VISION

MEASURES

There are at least three elements of vision important to the driving task that can be assessed in an office setting: acuity, fields, and contrast sensitivity. Distance acuity can be measured simply using a standard wall chart that has letters of equal contrast that get progressively smaller as one moves down the chart and that is read at a specified distance. Acuity requirements vary by state, but a corrected acuity of 20/40 or better is the most common requirement.[12] Horizontal visual fields can be measured qualitatively in an office by confrontation. While sitting across from the patient, have him or her cover the right eye. Move a pencil or finger from behind his or her left ear slowly across a plane level with the left eye, from the temporal side toward the nasal side until the patient identifies the object; then start on the nasal side and come across the horizontal plane toward the temporal side until the object is identified. Repeat for the other eye. For a more quantitative and thorough assessment, automated perimetry may be required. State requirements for binocular visual fields range from 100 ° to 140 °.[12] Contrast sensitivity assesses the limits at which an individual can detect a difference in contrast between an object and the background. One simple method for assessing this involves reading letters off a chart, such as a Pelli-Robson chart (while available for office use, such charts are expensive).[13] Unlike acuity testing, in this case, the letters stay the same size, but get progressively lighter as one moves down the chart, with contrast sensitivity being the lightest letters a participant can distinguish from the background.

EVIDENCE

Shinar and Schieber describe a consistent, but small association between acuity and crash history in a number of studies.[14] With respect to fields, Johnson and Keltner, in a study of 10,000 individuals applying for relicensure in California, found that elders were more likely to have peripheral field loss, and individuals with peripheral field loss were often unaware of these deficits and were more likely to have a history of crashes or moving violations.[15] Decina and Staplin reviewed 12,400 Pennsylvania drivers at the time of license renewal, comparing their performance on vision tests (binocular static acuity, horizontal visual fields, and contrast sensitivity) with crash history over a 3.67 year period.[16] Failure on any of the three tests combined (static acuity worse than 20/40, horizontal fields less than 140°, and below normal contrast sensitivity) was predictive of crash history for individuals age 66 years and older, whereas the individual tests were not predictive.

HEARING
MEASURES

Screening for hearing deficits can be accomplished with the whisper test, which involves whispering several numbers while standing to the side of the patient and having them repeat the numbers.[17] Alternatively, a hand-held audiometric device that reproduces tones at a range of frequencies can be employed. If a more detailed evaluation is required or if a hearing aid is being considered, referral for formal audiometric testing should be made.

EVIDENCE

Although it is theoretically likely that maximizing both visual and auditory sensory input would be helpful to interpret and act on environmental stimuli, the extent to which hearing deficits may affect the driving safety of elders is not clearly established at present (see Chapter 10).

Cognition

MEASURES

In terms of cognitive functioning, driving is a complex task requiring the individual to efficiently and meaningfully sort and process incoming sensory information, make rapid choices among response alternatives, and react with a coordinated set of motor responses. Global measures of cognitive function have the advantage of being quick and easy to administer. The better ones also sample several domains of cognitive ability. The downside of their brevity and ease of use is that they tend to be somewhat crude measures of cognitive function. Among the most widely used is the Mini-Mental State Examination (MMSE), which takes approximately 5 to 10 minutes to administer and includes items that sample orientation, short term memory, attention/calculation, language, and visual-spatial function (see Appendix #29).[18]

To better understand the nature and extent of cognitive impairment, more detailed testing of specific domains or subcomponents of cognition is necessary. Domains such as attention and visual–spatial function can be particularly relevant to driving. The tests utilized to measure these and other domains or subcomponents, however, may be less accessible to health care providers than global measures and may require training to administer or to score them. In addition, domains often have more than one element. For instance, attention can involve selective attention (the ability to focus on one among several stimuli), divided attention (attending to more than one simultaneously presented stimuli), or attention switching (alternately attending to different stimuli). One simple measure of attention that can be utilized in an office is the digit span, which involves having the subject repeat a series of digits either in the same order (forward) or reversed (normative values are available).[19] Visual–spatial functions also involve a variety of different elements, including the ability to detect and monitor the entire visual field (visual attention), the ability to understand the relationship between different shapes in space, and the ability to create or reproduce figures and designs (construction). Constructional ability may be the easiest of these to assess in the office, asking a patient to copy a design (such as the intersecting pentagons of the MMSE) or to draw a clock.

EVIDENCE

As described by Odenheimer, the MMSE has been associated with driving status and road test performance, but not with crash history.[20] Odenheimer and colleagues found significant correlations between a road test they developed and MMSE scores.[21] Similarly, Fitten and colleagues also found a correlation between the driving test they developed and MMSE scores.[22] Hunt and colleagues, comparing small samples of healthy elderly subjects to those with very mild and mild Alzheimer's disease, found a significant association between another brief global measure, the Short Blessed Test, and an open-road test.[23] Each of these studies also found associations among several individual measures of memory, attention, and visual–spatial function and their respective road tests.

Marottoli and colleagues found one component of the MMSE, design copying, to be one of three factors significantly associated with crashes and moving violations among older drivers in a cohort drawn from the general population.[24] A somewhat longer and more detailed global measure than the MMSE, the Mattis Organic Mental State Screening Examination (MOMSSE),[25] was found by Owsley and colleagues to be one of the two factors most closely associated with crash history in a sample of 53 volunteers from an optometry clinic.[26] The factor most closely associated in that study was a measure of visual attention, the useful field of view.

Motor

MEASURES

Strength and range of motion of the extremities can be assessed by manual muscle testing. Trunk mobility can be assessed qualitatively by having patients turn to look behind them without moving their feet (the examiner should position himself or herself on the side to catch them if they should lose their balance). Neck mobility can be assessed by having the patient try to touch either shoulder with their chin. An examination of peripheral sensation, particularly pin prick and position sense, can be helpful.

EVIDENCE

There is little evidence on the specific role of motor factors and driving history. Little information is also available on the amount of strength and range of motion necessary to operate a vehicle. The United States Public Health Service guidelines suggest a minimum of grade 4/5 strength (complete antigravity and partial resistance) in the right leg and both arms to operate a private vehicle.[27] McPherson and colleagues in a two-phase study, found that range of motion was related to driving performance and that it was possible to increase trunk range of motion and shoulder flexibility through exercise training in a small sample of volunteer older drivers.[28] The improvement in range of motion, however, did not affect performance on a driving test.

Medical Conditions, Medications, and Alcohol Use

A number of medical conditions prevalent among elders can potentially affect driving ability depending on their severity and the ability to control them with treatment or to compensate for the deficits they produce. Among the more common of these are dementia (of all types), stroke, progressive neurologic disorders (such as Parkinson's disease), seizure disorders, syncope, angina, myocardial infarction, arrhythmias, diabetes, sleep disorders, chronic obstructive pulmonary disease, and visual disorders (such as cataracts, glaucoma, macular degeneration, and diabetic retinopathy). In theory, any condition that can chronically or transiently affect visual, cognitive, or motor ability, or their interaction, can potentially affect driving ability. In addition, medications (particularly central-acting ones) and alcohol or illicit substances can adversely affect an individual's ability to drive. Guidelines are available from both the American and Canadian Medical Associations regarding the threshold at which these and other conditions can potentially affect driving and should be referred to if there are questions about individual conditions.[29, 30] State medical advisory boards are also available for consultation. Elders should be warned about potential medication side effects and efforts made to adjust dosing schedules to minimize the effect on driving performance.

Assessment Approaches

This section provides an overview of several measures that either test the functional abilities described previously or their impact on driving performance. Some of these are established elements of the driving evaluation process. Others are newer methods that hold promise, but need to be tested on larger, more representative samples of elders. Their respective roles in the evaluation process need to be determined. These are included to help in understanding what might happen after a referral for driving performance evaluation, as well as newer tests that may eventually help to decide who needs such an evaluation.

IN-OFFICE SCREENING MEASURES

At present, there are no validated measures available to help identify a group at high risk for driving problems that needs to be evaluated further. Two recently described approaches, however, may potentially prove helpful if validated.

Traffic Sign Naming

- **Authors:** Carr, LaBarge, Dunnigan, and Storandt[31]
- **Purpose:** To determine if a simple test of traffic sign naming could distinguish drivers with dementia from healthy elderly control participants

- **Participants:** 66 persons without a diagnosis of dementia and 42 with mild or moderate dementia on the basis of clinical evaluation and cognitive testing, recruited from the Washington University Alzheimer's Disease Research Center Patient Registry.
- **Strengths:** Simple measure; face-validity for relevance to driving task.
- **Weaknesses:** No data presented on relationship to driving performance or crash risk.
- **Scale:** 10 road signs selected from a larger battery of 39 signs based on the ability to discriminate nondemented from mildly to moderately demented persons.
- **Who administers:** Psychometrician.
- **How administered:** 10 second presentation of sign; 2 points for correct naming, 1 point for partially correct, 0 points for incorrect response.
- **Sensitivity, specificity, and positive predictive value (PPV):** Using a cutoff of 9 or less out of 20 correct, sensitivity for identifying subjects with dementia was 74 percent, specificity was 97 percent, and PPV was 94 percent (calculated). In separate studies, both Odenheimer and Hunt have found an association between other measures of traffic sign recognition and driving performance in small samples of subjects.[21, 23]
- **Comments:** Potentially an easy to use measure that merits further testing to determine its ability to identify dementia or to identify crash risk or poor driving performance in a general population.

Clinical Predictors of Crashes, Moving Violations, and Being Stopped by Police

- **Authors:** Marottoli, Cooney, Wagner, Doucette, and Tinetti.[24]
- **Purpose:** Identify factors from examination or history that prospectively predict occurrence of crashes, moving violations, and being stopped by police in 1 year.
- **Participants:** All active drivers ($N = 283$) in a representative cohort of individuals age 72 years and older in New Haven, CT.
- **Strengths:** Simple measures; prospective assessment; general population.
- **Weaknesses:** Modest sample size; limited range of cognitive and visual tests; self-report of adverse driving events; no information on nature of crashes.
- **Scales:** Multivariable analysis identified 3 independent predictors of events: ability to copy a pentagon from MMSE

(correct/incorrect), number of blocks walked in average day (0 versus 1 +), number of foot abnormalities (toenail irregularities, callouses, bunions, toe deformities, scored as present/absent for range of 0–8 both feet combined; 0–2 versus 3 +).

- **Who administers:** Nonmedical personnel can be trained.
- **How administered:** Questions asked, participant examined.
- **Specificity, sensitivity, and PPV:** Not reported; model prediction based on number of risk factors present (if 0 present, 6 percent had events; if 1 factor present, 12 percent had events; if 2 factors present, 26 percent had events; and if all 3 present, 47 percent had events).
- **Comments:** Preliminary study; needs replication in different population, expanded range of measures.

REFERRAL EVALUATION

For some individuals, the decision about whether to recommend continued driving or limitations or cessation will be clear based on the history and examinations as described. For other individuals, the impact of their conditions or functional impairments on driving safety will be less clear, and a more detailed assessment of these abilities or their impact on performance may be warranted.

Measures Requiring Special Equipment: Visual Attention as a Predictor of Crashes

- **Authors:** Ball, Owsley, Sloane, Roenker, and Bruni.[32]
- **Purpose:** To identify visual factors associated with crashes among older drivers.
- **Participants:** Sample of drivers ($N = 294$) drawn from all drivers age 55 years and older in Jefferson County, Alabama; stratified sample to achieve equal numbers in 21 cells according to state-recorded 5-year crash history (0, 1–3, 4 + crashes) and age (55–59, 60–64, 65–69, 70–74, 75–79, 80–84, and 85 + years).
- **Strengths:** Thorough evaluation of visual function.
- **Weaknesses:** Selected sample weighted toward individuals with multiple crashes.
- **Scales:** Primary measure was the Useful Field Of View (UFOV), a measure of visual attention.
- **Who administers:** Not described.
- **How administered:** Utilized UFOV Visual Attention Analyzer, Model 2000; 3 subtests. (1) speed of visual processing: identify target of varying duration in central box; (2) ability to divide attention: identify central target and simultaneously presented peripheral target; (3) selective attention:

central and peripheral target identification, but peripheral target embedded in distracting stimuli.

- **Sensitivity, specificity, and PPV:** A UFOV reduction of more than 40 percent identified individuals with a history of one or more crashes with a sensitivity of 89 percent, specificity of 81 percent, and a PPV of 85 percent (latter calculated from data presented). In a recent publication utilizing the same sample, individuals with a 40 percent or more reduction in UFOV had a relative risk of 2.2 for involvement in a crash in 3 years of prospective follow-up.[33]

Measures Requiring Special Equipment: Driving Advisement System

- **Authors:** Gianutsos, Campbell, Beattie, and Mandriota.[34]
- **Purpose:** To develop a computerized measure that evaluates the cognitive abilities necessary for driving and that could be used to assess and counsel brain-injured drivers.
- **Strengths:** Conceptually simple approach; includes pretest self-appraisal of driving ability.
- **Weaknesses:** Little published data on performance in general older population.
- **Scale:** Driver Advisement System.
- **Who administers:** Trained examiner.
- **How administered:** Participants sit in front of a computer screen attached to a steering wheel and accelerator and brake pedals. Tracking assessed by ability to keep "vehicle" in center of moving schematic roadway on screen (assess speed through course, number of scrapes with side walls, number of times off course entirely); measures of simple, choice, complex reaction time.
- **Sensitivity, specificity, and PPV:** No data presented in the article. A study by Rebok and colleagues found that 10 subjects with Alzheimer's disease exhibited slower reaction times and more pedal selection errors, but little difference in tracking ability or self-ratings of ability, compared to 12 healthy elderly control participants.[35]

SIMULATORS

Simulators typically have the participant seated at a control module that resembles the driver's seat in an automobile. The participant has a steering wheel and accelerator and brake pedals and looks at either a picture screen or video terminal. There are two basic types: interactive and noninteractive. With interactive simulators, the scene changes with driver input to more closely approximate actual driving than noninteractive simulators, where the scene presented does not change with driver input. Traditionally, however, interactive simulators tend to have less realistic scenes depicted (more like a video game than a film), which detracts from their approximation of actual driving. As technology improves, interactive video displays should become more realistic.

Simulators are used to approximate the actual driving experience. The advantage they have over road tests is safety because they do not involve driving an actual vehicle. A variety of parameters can be assessed with a simulator, including reaction times and response to road hazards. Thus, simulators serve as a good initial assessment of performance and as an indicator of whether or not an individual should be tested on the road. Their role in the assessment process may expand as technology improves and more evidence becomes available regarding their applicability.[36]

ROAD TESTS

Road tests provide the most accurate assessment of driving performance because they involve driving an actual vehicle. The major potential problem is safety because, if they are conducted on open roadways, interaction with other vehicles and pedestrians will occur. Consequently, a spectrum of road tests is possible, ranging from closed-course routes (typically a parking lot or closed road where no interaction with traffic is possible) to open road evaluations on actual streets. Closed-course routes assess the ability to maneuver a vehicle isolated from traffic, but yield much less information about how a driver interacts with other vehicles and pedestrians. Open road tests offer information on vehicle maneuvering and traffic interaction, but at the potential expense of safety. One compromise is what can be called a semiopen road test that assesses performance over a road course on a university or hospital campus that offers some, but very limited, interaction with other vehicles and pedestrians. Questions can be raised about how well even open road tests assess driving performance, because one cannot always recreate all the hazards and situations that will arise during normal driving that could potentially tax a driver's ability to safely operate the vehicle. Open road tests, however, are the current gold standard of driving performance evaluation and often, the final arbiter of licensing decisions.

Driving Skills and Age (Miller Road Test)

- **Authors:** Carr, Jackson, Madden, and Cohen.[37]
- **Purpose:** To determine the effect of age on driving performance utilizing a standardized road test.
- **Participants:** Healthy elderly (65+ years), teen-age (18–19 years), and young adult (25–35 years) volunteers.

- **Strengths:** Comparison of healthy elders to young individuals; standardized road test.
- **Weaknesses:** Semiopen course on university campus, not open roads; selected sample; limited to healthy individuals; small sample size.
- **Scale:** Miller Road Test, a standardized test developed by a division of the North Carolina DMV.
- **Who administers:** Driving instructor who underwent a special certification course.
- **How administered:** Five-mile course through a university campus, scored as total score and total number of driving errors (took 30 minutes to complete).
- **Sensitivity, specificity, and PPV:** There was no significant difference in total scores among the three groups, but the elderly drivers had significantly fewer errors than did the two younger groups.

Semiopen Road Test: Dementia

- **Authors:** Fitten, Perryman, Wilkinson, Little, Burns, Pachana, Mervis, Malmgren, Siembieda, and Ganzell.[22]
- **Purpose:** To compare driving performance of individuals with and without a diagnosis of dementia.
- **Participants:** Subjects recruited from a variety of sources: Alzheimer's disease (MMSE $\geq$ 19, N = 13), vascular dementia (MMSE $\geq$ 19, N = 12), diabetes (MMSE $\geq$ 24, N = 15), healthy comparison groups (MMSE $\geq$ 28; 60 + years, N = 24; 20–35 years, N = 16).
- **Strengths:** Multiple comparison groups.
- **Weaknesses:** Small sample size in individual groups; selected sample.
- **Scale:** Sepulveda Road Test.
- **Who administers:** Instructor.
- **How administered:** A 2.7-mile course on the grounds of Sepulveda VA Medical Center, divided into six stages that differed in complexity; scoring criteria created by panel: 0–41 points (higher score better), scored by instructor according to set criteria.
- **Sensitivity, specificity, and PPV:** Total driving scores were significantly lower for both dementia groups than for the three control groups, which did not differ from each other.

Open Road Test

- **Authors:** Odenheimer, Beaudet, Jette, Albert, Grande, and Minaker.[21]

- **Purpose:** To develop a systematic road test that measures the driving skills of elders.
- **Participants:** Convenience sample of 30 licensed drivers over age 60 years chosen to reflect a range of cognitive abilities.
- **Strengths:** Carefully designed open road test.
- **Weaknesses:** Small sample size; nonprobability sample.
- **Scale:** Open road test along a set route of streets near the West Roxbury VA Medical Center.
- **Who administers:** Driving instructor and research rater.
- **How administered:** Ten-mile route through streets near West Roxbury VA including both closed course and in-traffic components (approximately 45 minutes to complete); administered in midafternoon on weekdays. Driving instructor provided global rating of performance; 2 research raters scored 7 closed course and 68 traffic tasks, each task graded as pass/fail; course designed to specifically assess these tasks; graded according to set criteria.
- **Sensitivity, specificity, and PPV:** Instructor's global score was significantly correlated with the independently rated closed-course and in-traffic scores. Road test score was also significantly correlated with performance on a number of cognitive measures including the MMSE, traffic sign recognition, visual and verbal memory, Trail Making Test Part A, and complex reaction time.

SUGGESTED APPROACH

The following is a suggested outline of one way to approach the issue with older drivers. The ability to utilize such an outline will depend on the availability of referral programs in a given area and the ability and willingness to pay for such evaluations either by the individual or third-party payers. A flow chart based on this approach is depicted in Figure 18-1.

1. Raise the issue
   a. Ask if individuals drive, how often, where, and if they have available alternative sources of transportation.
   b. Ask if they are having any problems such as getting lost, moving violations, near misses, and crashes.
   c. Potentially check with family and caregivers about concerns, especially for cognitively impaired individuals who may not be aware of their limitations.
2. Identification of risk factors
   a. Review medical conditions regarding severity, level of control or adaptation; consult available guidelines, if needed.

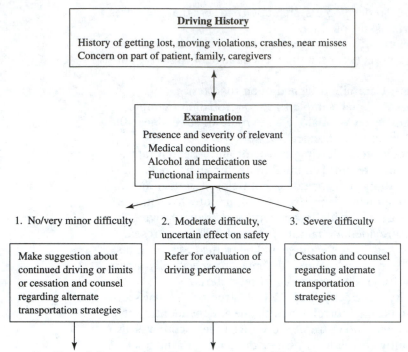

FIGURE 18-1 Flow chart for assessing driver safety.

    b. Assess basic functional abilities that can be addressed in the office or clinic; treat or refer for treatment if possible.

    c. Review medications and alcohol/drug use—adjust medications, dosing schedules, and counsel regarding substance use as appropriate.

    d. Review findings with the individual. For minimally or severely affected elder, the health care provider may be able to stop here. For more questionable cases, refer for further evaluation.

3. Referral for performance evaluation

    a. Find a local program with experience evaluating that particular type of patient.

    b. Obtain results of performance evaluation and recommendations regarding continued driving, treatment options, and adaptive equipment.

4. Discuss options

    a. Review findings and options with the elder and family and caregivers; weigh risks and benefits of intervention options. Document the discussion.

    b. Inform about local alternative transportation options (hospital social work departments, area agencies on aging, chambers of commerce (resources such as an infoline may have such information) if patients need to limit or stop driving.

5. Reporting
   a. Be aware of state or province reporting requirements.
   b. If not mandatory, reporting can be used either as an initial approach or as a back-up option if the elder does not follow your advice and the family is not able or willing to intervene.

Role of the Health Care Team

Depending on the composition of the health care team and individual expertise and interests, it can be helpful and more efficient to divide the responsibilities for different aspects of the assessment process. Health care providers can be responsible for detecting the presence and severity of medical conditions, alcohol and medication use, and functional impairments that affect driving ability. They can also refer patients to various subspecialists for a more detailed evaluation of a given area as needed. Occupational and physical therapists can assess the extent of functional impairments and the availability of adaptive or corrective interventions. Therapists with specialized training in driver assessment can determine the impact of medical conditions and functional impairments on driving performance and make additional recommendations about interventions. Social workers or care managers can assist in obtaining the driving history, assess the concerns of family or caregivers, determine the availability of alternative sources of transportation, and assist in counseling the patient and family about adapting to driving limitations or cessation. The goal is to provide a supportive and therapeutic environment and utilize the particular resources of a health care team to optimize the mobility, independence, autonomy, and safety of elders.

SUMMARY

This chapter provides an understanding of the factors affecting driving ability and examples of the types of measures that can be employed to assess both functional abilities and the effects of those abilities on driving safety. Although not all of these techniques are available or appropriate for in-office evaluation, they illustrate the types of approaches that can be taken. Driving is an important issue to elders and their families because of its association with independence and mobility. Although health care providers may be reluctant to get involved in this issue, they are often in the best position to assess the relationship between medical conditions and functional abilities and if treatments are available. They are also in a position to make referrals to individuals who are able to assess the impact of these conditions or impairments on actual driving performance. Finally, they may be in a position to help elders and their families adjust to the changes that occur if they are forced to limit or stop driving.

REFERENCES

1. Retchin SM, Anapolle J. An overview of the older driver. *Clin Geriatr Med.* 1993;9:279–296.
2. Waller PF. The older driver. *Human Factors.* 1991;33:499–505.
3. Marottoli RA, Ostfeld AM, Merrill SS, et al. Driving cessation and changes in mileage driven among elderly individuals. *J Gerontol B Psychol Sci Soc Sci.* 1993;48:S255–260.
4. Cerrelli E. Older drivers: the age factor in traffic safety. *National Highway Traffic Safety Administration Technical Report.* DOT HS 807 402;1989.
5. Barancik JI, Chatterjee BF, Greene-Cradden YC, et al. Motor vehicle trauma in northeastern ohio. I:Incidence and outcome by age, sex, and road use category. *Am J Epidemiol.* 1986;123:846–861.
6. Jette AM, Branch LG. A ten-year follow-up of driving patterns among the community-dwelling elderly. *Human Factors.* 1992;34: 25–31.
7. Rosenbloom S. Transportation needs of the elderly population. *Clin Geriatr Med.* 1993;9:297–310.
8. Drickamer MA, Marottoli RA. Physician responsibility in driver assessment. *Am J Med Sci.* 1993;306:277–281.
9. Miller DJ, Morley JE. Attitudes of physicians toward elderly drivers and driving policy. *J Am Geriatr Soc.* 1993;40:722–724.
10. Petrucelli E, Malinowski M. Update of medical review practices and procedures in U.S. and Canadian commercial driver licensing programs. *Federal Highway Administration Report.* Washington, DC DTFH6195P01200, 1997.
11. Reuben DB. Assessment of older drivers. *Clin Geriatric Med.* 1993;9:449–459.
12. Keltner JL. Johnson CA. Visual function, driving safety, and the elderly. *Ophthalmology.* 1987;94:1180–1188.
13. Pelli DG, Robson JG, Wilkins AJ. Designing a new letter chart for measuring contrast sensitivity. *Clin Vis Sci.* 1988;2:187–199.
14. Shinar D, Schieber F. Visual requirements for safety and mobility of older drivers. *Human Factors.* 1991;33:507–519.
15. Johnson CA, Keltner JL. Incidence of visual field loss in 20,000 eyes and its relationship to driving performance. *Arch Ophthalmol.* 1983;101:371–375.
16. Decina LE, Staplin L. Retrospective evaluation of alternative vision screening criteria for older and younger drivers. *Acc Anal Prev.* 1993;25:267–275.

17. MacPhee GJ, Crowther JA, McAlpine CH. A simple screening test for hearing impairment in elderly patients. *Age Ageing.* 1988;17: 347–351.

18. Folstein MF, Folstein SE, McHugh PR. Mini-Mental State: a practical method for grading the cognitive state of patients for the clinician. *J Psychiatr Res.* 1975;12:189–198.

19. Wechsler D. *Wechsler Adult Intelligence Scale—Revised Manual.* New York: Psychological Corporation; 1981.

20. Odenheimer GL. Dementia and the older driver. *Clin Geriatr Med.* 1993;9:349–364.

21. Odenheimer GL, Beaudet M, Jette AM, Albert MS, Grande L, Minaker KL. Performance-based driving evaluation of the elderly driver: safety, reliability, and validity. *J Gerontol A Biol Sci Med Sci.* 1994;49:M153–159.

22. Fitten LJ, Perryman KM, Wilkinson CJ, et al. Alzheimer and vascular dementias and driving. *JAMA* 1995;273:1360–1365.

23. Hunt L, Morris JC, Edwards D, Wilson BS. Driving performance in persons with mild senile dementia of the Alzheimer's type. *J Am Geriatr Soc.* 1993;41:747–753.

24. Marottoli RA, Cooney LM, Wagner DR, Doucette J, Tinetti ME. Predictors of automobile crashes and moving violations among elderly drivers. *Ann Intern Med.* 1994;121:842–846.

25. Mattis S. Mental status examination for organic mental syndrome in the elderly patient. In: Bella L, Karasu TB, eds, *Geriatric Psychiatry.* New York: Oxford University Press, 1976;77–121.

26. Owsley C, Ball K, Sloane ME, Roenker DL, Bruni JR. Visual/cognitive correlates of vehicle accidents in older drivers. *Psychol Aging.* 1991;6:403–415.

27. Stock MS, Light WO, Douglass JM, Burg FD. Licensing the driver with musculoskeletal difficulty. *J Bone Joint Surg.* 1970;52A:343–346.

28. McPherson K, Ostrau A, Shaffron P. *Physical Fitness and the Aging Driver* (phase 2). Washington, DC: AAA Foundation for Traffic Safety; 1989.

29. Doege TC, Engelberg AL, eds. *Medical Conditions Affecting Drivers.* Chicago: American Medical Association; 1986.

30. Canadian Medical Association. *Physicians' Guide to Driver Examinations,* 5th ed. Ottowa, Ontario: CMA; 1991.

31. Carr DB, LaBarge E, Dunnigan K, Storandt M. Differentiating drivers with dementia of the Alzheimer type from healthy older persons with a traffic sign naming test. *J Gerontol A Biol Sci Med Sci.* 1998;53A:M135–139.

32. Ball K, Owsley C, Sloane ME, Roenker DL, Bruni JR. Visual attention problems as a predictor of vehicle crashes in older drivers. *Invest Ophthalmol Vis Sci.* 1993;34:3110–3123.

33. Owsley C, Ball K, McGwin G, et al. Visual processing impairment and risk of motor vehicle crash among older adults. *JAMA.* 1998;279:1083–1088.

34. Gianutosos R, Campbell A, Beattie A, Mandriota F. The driving advisement system: a computer-augmented quasi-simulation of the cognitive prerequisites for resumption of driving after brain injury. *Assist Technol.* 1992;4:70–86.

35. Rebok GW, Keyl PM, Bylsma FW, Blaustein MJ, Tune L. The effects of Alzheimer disease on driving-related abilities. *Alzheimer Dis and Assoc Dis.* 1994;8:228–240.
36. Cox DJ, Taylor P, Kovatchev B. Driving simulation performance predicts future accidents among older drivers. *J Am Geriatric Soc.* 1999;47:381–382.
37. Carr D, Jackson TW, Madden DJ, Cohen HJ. The effect of age on driving skills. *J Am Geriatr Soc.* 1992;40:567–573.

CHAPTER 19

DEPRESSION

IRA M. LESSER / CAROL BANYAS

The assessment of depression in a patient is an essential, though often overlooked, component of a comprehensive evaluation. In an elder, this assessment can be more complicated than that which occurs in a younger person because of the many physical, social, psychological, and spiritual changes associated with aging. Depression in elders can present as a primary problem, can be caused by medical illness, or can be a reaction to medical problems. In any case, if depression is left untreated, it can result in severe consequences, such as increased morbidity from the medical illness, decreased quality of life, and suicide. The following vignettes illustrate the complexities of recognizing depression in elders.

The actual assessment of depression in clear-cut cases is not necessarily difficult or time consuming; however, typically, there are medical comorbidities and social factors that make this task more complex. "Masked depressions," where the most prominent symptoms are somatic and the affective aspect of depression less apparent, and diagnosing depression amidst true medical illness, present significant diagnostic challenges to the health care provider. This chapter focuses on depressive illness in elders, covering the diagnostic criteria; prevalence; risk factors; clinical presentations; differential diagnosis with disorders of cognition, as well as other psychiatric and medical disorders; and techniques of assessing depression and suicidality.

Vignette: I have lived a full life. I was a good husband for 57 years, I worked hard all my life, I watched my children and my grandchildren and my great grandchildren grow up and do well. I am proud of how I lived my life. Most of my friends have died. I can barely walk because of the pain in my knees and my dizziness. What do I have to live for? I am not afraid of dying.

—97-year-old man living in a retirement hotel

Vignette: What I have begun to discover is that, mysteriously and in ways that are totally remote from normal experience, the gray drizzle of horror induced by depression takes on the quality of physical pain. But it is not an immediately identifiable pain like that of a broken limb. It may be more accurate to say that despair owing to some evil trick played on the sick brain by the inhabiting psyche, comes to resemble the diabolical discomfort of being imprisoned in a fiercely overheated room.[1]

These vignettes raise questions such as those listed in Table 19-1.

The evaluation of depression in elders needs to be a high priority. Unrecognized depression is costly on several fronts: it decreases the quality of life for the elder and for his or her family; it increases medical morbidity and perhaps, mortality; it leads to excessive use of medical services; and it is associated with suicide. There are, however, impediments to the successful assessment of depression.[2,3,4] Potential problems with the assessment process can be divided into those associated with the patient, the health care provider, and the system. Of course, these all interact with each other in a dynamic way.

The elderly patient may not be comfortable discussing his or her feelings or acknowledging the depression. This can be particularly true when the elder is of a different ethnic group than the health care provider. Alternatively, the elder may focus exclusively

Unrecognized depression:
Decreases quality of life
Increases medical morbidity
Leads to excessive use of medical services
Is associated with suicide

TABLE 19-1. QUESTIONS TO ASK WHEN ASSESSING DEPRESSION

Understandable sadness and age appropriate concerns?
Depressive symptoms or full-blown syndrome?
Physical disorder?
Mental disorder?
Will it resolve on its own?
Will this person make a suicide attempt?
Should it be treated, and if so, how?

upon somatic complaints, making recognition of depression difficult. Accurately recognizing depression in the patient who has multiple medical problems, is receiving multiple medications, and/or has cognitive impairment presents a challenge. The elder in a long-term care facility, who likely is ill and cognitively impaired, is particularly difficult to evaluate. We provide guidelines to help in these situations, but nevertheless, recognition can be difficult.

The health care provider must deal with his or her own attitudes toward elders and understand his or her own view of what constitutes normal aging. Depression is not a normal part of aging and should not be thought of as such. Ageist attitudes on the part of health care providers often impede the recognition of depression. Such statements as, "I would be depressed if I had these problems" or, "What more do you expect in this situation" reflect inappropriate attributions to the elder. Therapeutic nihilism should not be part of the geriatric evaluation process. Although the dictum "Do no harm" should always be kept in mind, this should not prevent health care providers from treating depression, even in old and frail patients.

The health care system, with its fragmentation, economic and time constraints, and reimbursement strategies, mitigates against a comprehensive psychological and psychosocial evaluation of an elder. Extra efforts to develop multidisciplinary geriatric assessment teams are one way to counteract this system bias. Also, as training in geriatrics and geriatric psychiatry becomes more popular, and more research funds are available for studies in geriatrics, the situation will likely improve.

DESCRIPTION OF THE PROBLEM

Definitions

The assessment of mood in the elderly patient needs to address the questions raised in the previous discussion. Initially, one must determine whether the behavioral and psychological symptoms or complaints are part of normal experience, or are they indicative of a mood disorder. Sadness is a normal *affect,* often seen in response to psychosocial events and should not be pathologized. Elders, in particular, are subject to a wide array of stressors, including serious losses (e.g., loss of health, function, status, friends, mates, etc.). The appropriate response to these losses may be a disturbance in mood with tearfulness, withdrawal, loss of interest in activities, sleep disturbance, and so forth. Usually, sadness in response to an event is time-limited and does not greatly interfere with functioning.

The diagnostic criteria for mood disorders in elders do not differ from those that are used for younger depressed patients. The symptom picture can differ, however, with elders complaining more of somatic symptoms, and often demonstrating more apathy and amotivational states than younger depressed patients. The *Diagnostic and Statistical Manual of Mental Disorders,* 4th ed.[5] provides operational criteria for diagnosing psychiatric disorders. For a diagnosis of a *major depressive episode (MDE)*, one needs to have five (or more) of the symptoms listed in Table 19-2.

These symptoms must be present most of the time, nearly every day for a minimum period of 2 weeks. The symptoms must represent a change from a previous level of functioning and cause significant distress or impairment in function. The presence of a specific precipitant is important to note, but its presence or absence is not considered when making the diagnosis of MDE. If the depressive syndrome occurs within 2 months of the death of a close person, however, it is more appropriately considered as bereavement.

Less severe states of depression, where the person may not have sufficient symptoms or be depressed for sufficient time to meet criteria for MDE, are actually much more prevalent than MDE in elders. These are subsyndromal states, or minor depression. A DSM-IV proposed set of diagnostic criteria for minor depression include two or more (but less than five) of the symptoms listed for major depression, being present for at least 2 weeks, and causing some impairment. In lieu of using the term minor depression (which has not been officially recognized), the most appropriate diagnostic category for these symptoms are Depression, Not Otherwise Specified (NOS). Recent studies suggest that minor depression may be prodromal for major depression, further implying that they are not benign states.[6, 7]

TABLE 19-2.   SYMPTOMS FOR A DIAGNOSIS OF A MAJOR DEPRESSIVE EPISODE

1. A feeling of sadness, being "down" or "blue"
2. A loss of interest in all or almost all usual activities
3. Appetite change, with weight gain or loss
4. Sleep disturbance, with insomnia or hypersomnia
5. Evidence for physical agitation or retardation
6. Fatigue or loss of energy
7. Feelings of worthlessness, self-reproach, inappropriate or excessive guilt
8. Difficulty with concentration, thinking, or making decisions
9. Preoccupation with death or suicidal thoughts

Five or more of the symptoms must be present, with at least one being item 1 or 2.

When milder depressions become chronic, with symptoms present most of the time for over 2 years, and the depressed mood is accompanied by two or more of the following: poor appetite or overeating, sleep disturbance, low energy or fatigue, low self-esteem, poor concentration or trouble making decisions, and a feeling of hopelessness, a diagnosis of *dysthymic disorder* can be made. Often, episodes of MDE are superimposed upon a dysthymic disorder, a condition referred to as double depression.

Frequently, people's reaction to a stressful event can lead to symptoms of depression that are not severe enough or do not last long enough to meet criteria for MDE. An *adjustment disorder with depressed mood* is a short-term maladaptive reaction to an identified psychosocial stressor where the presenting symptoms are those of a mild depression. For example, the predominant manifestations may be depressed mood, tearfulness, and hopelessness, but they are not present most of the time, most of the day. Adjustment disorders are expected to remit if the stress can be alleviated or the person can adjust to the stress. On the other hand, stressors can be ongoing (e.g., taking care of an ill spouse), and the symptoms can persist. If the number of symptoms exceeds the threshold for MDE and they last more than 2 weeks, a diagnosis of MDE is made regardless of the presence of the identifiable stressor.

After establishing the presence of a depression, it is important to ascertain if there are psychotic symptoms. Questions relating to delusional thoughts, particularly somatic delusions and auditory hallucinations must be asked. These questions often need to be asked of collaterals (e.g., family, friends, nursing home staff, etc.) because the elder may hide the delusions due to embarrassment or be guarded and suspicious about sharing them. This is a very important part of the diagnostic evaluation because the presence of a psychotic component to the depression will lead to a different treatment strategy.

Although it is relatively rare to have an onset of mania late in life, questions about current or past manic symptoms are important, because the diagnosis of bipolar disorder will alter the treatment. DSM-IV defines a manic episode as a distinct period of abnormally and persistent elevated, expansive or irritable mood, with at least three (or four if the mood is irritable) of the following: (1) inflated self-esteem or grandiosity; (2) decreased need for sleep; (3) more talkative or pressured speech; (4) flight of ideas or the feeling that one's thoughts are racing; (5) distractibility; (6) increase in goal-directed behavior; and (7) excessive involvement in activities that have a high potential of leading to negative consequences. If these criteria are met, last for 1 week or more (or any duration if the patient is hospitalized), and cause impairment in occupational or social pursuits, a manic episode can be diagnosed. If there is only one manic episode or if there have been depressive episodes prior to the current manic episode, the diagnosis will be *bipolar disorder*.

Although not a part of official DSM-IV nomenclature, the concept of primary or secondary mood disorders can be a useful one. Primary refers to the mood disorder occurring first temporally and secondary refers to the mood disorder occurring after either a medical illness or another psychiatric disorder. Particularly in elders, mood disorders can be a result of medical illness. The term *mood disorder due to a general medical condition* is used to indicate that the depression, for example, is due to hypothyroidism. For this diagnosis to be made, there must be corroborative evidence from history and physical and/or laboratory examinations that the mood disturbance is the direct physiologic consequence of the medical condition. Finally, and again frequently seen in elders, are cases where depression can be a result of taking physician- or self-prescribed medications or of drug–drug interactions. A *substance-induced mood disorder* can be the appropriate diagnosis in this instance.

Prevalence

The prevalence of depressive symptoms (minor depression or depression, NOS) is much higher than that of the full depressive syndrome. Estimates of the prevalence of significant dysphoric feelings in elders residing in the community are as high as 15 percent, with an even greater prevalence in medically ill populations.[6] In a large community-based epidemiologic study (Epidemiologic Catchment Area Study),[8] however, the 1-year prevalence rate of MDE was approximately 1.4 percent and the lifetime prevalence was 2 percent. To health care providers working with elders, these numbers seem to be low. Some methodologic issues related to how these data were collected can help to address this discrepancy.[6] Older individuals tend to under-report psychiatric symptoms and this introduces a bias in case identification. Elders may focus more upon their somatic symptoms, even when these symptoms are part of the depression and were not present before the depression. This suggests the possibility of a "cohort effect" whereby older people, as a group, may report symptoms differently than do younger generations. This possibility needs to be kept in mind when evaluating an elder. The comorbidity with cognitive disorders (discussed more fully as follows) can also make it more difficult to identify depression in elders. On the other side of the argument, the prevalence may indeed be lower in elders because of a postulated cohort effect, whereby recent generations are more vulnerable to depression than previous generations. Although the data are somewhat scanty, and methodologic problems abound, it appears that elders from minority groups demonstrate a slightly lower prevalence of MDE than do Caucasians.

Risk Factors

The major risk factors for developing depression in older age groups can be viewed from a number of perspectives. As discussed in this chapter, a very important and well-established risk factor for depression in elders is comorbid medical illness. Women and the oldest old (older than 85 years) probably are at higher risk. Elders who are single have a substantially higher risk of depression compared to those with a partner. Social isolation either by virtue of living alone or the result of severe sensory deficits increases the vulnerability to depression. Another risk factor is the older adult who functions as a caregiver (i.e., providing care for an impaired adult such as a spouse with dementia). It has been reported that more than 50 percent of principal caregivers for patients with Alzheimer's Disease become clinically depressed.[9] Related to this, but much broader, is the well-known relationship of a wide variety of recent (and even remote) adverse life events being related to the onset of depression.

There also have been attempts to identify risk factors leading to depression for older adults who have been admitted to long-term care facilities.[10] A multivariate model was able to correctly classify those who developed depression with 90 percent accuracy. The items considered in the model were: coping with admission to the facility, life satisfaction at admission, affective symptoms, health status, friends in the facility, and change in affective symptoms after admission to the facility.

Bereavement is a risk factor for depression, and attempts have been made to identify those factors related to bereavement that are most associated with depression. Understandably, most widows and widowers experience intermittent depressive symptoms as part of their grief process. In the DSM-IV, a diagnosis of MDE is not made if the symptoms are present up to 2 months after the death of a loved one; in this instance, a diagnosis of bereavement can be made. It has been shown, however, that as many as 14 percent of bereaved individuals meet criteria for MDE 2 years after they lost their spouse.[11] Like depression in general, persistent depression after bereavement is more likely if the patient has a past and/or a family history of depression, significant alcohol consumption, and comorbid medical illnesses.

There has been little study of personality factors or personality disorders that are risk factors for depression in elders. It has been suggested that older patients with recurrent depressions have more life-long personality difficulties than patients with late-onset depression. This also holds true for those whose depression is comorbid with an anxiety disorder.[12,13] One difficulty in assessing personality disorders in depressed patients is to disentangle "state" versus "trait" phenomena. More work needs to be done before one can say which personality traits or disorders are true risk factors for the development of depression.

On the positive side, social support seems to be a protective factor, decreasing the risk of depression. This includes the number and structure of the social network available, the actual support (financial, practical items), and the perception of this support. Participation in religious activities also may exert a protective effect (see Chapters 4 and 26).

One also needs to consider that depression, itself, is a risk factor for physical illness and poor outcome. A number of studies have shown that depressive symptoms in elders leads to decreased quality of life, increased utilization of medical resources, increased morbidity and even mortality.[14] This underscores the need for improved recognition and treatment.

WHO AND HOW TO ASSESS

Assessment of Mood

Screening questions related to mood; interest in activities including, hobbies, work, and sexual activity; appetite; sleeping patterns; cognition; and thoughts about death should be part of every comprehensive evaluation of an elder who is seeking care. If suspicions are raised by this screen, a more detailed evaluation is required.

The clinical interview is fundamental to establishing the diagnosis of depression in elders. Unfortunately, in a busy office practice, health care providers often fail to ask the necessary questions, and consequently, the diagnosis is missed. If possible, both the elder and the family members should be included in the interview process. This not only helps in eliciting historical information, but aids in education about depression and adherence to a specific treatment plan. Sensitive interviewing techniques are important to help identify depression in elders. Elders might avoid using words like "depression" and instead, will talk about their physical condition. The interviewer should try to focus on behavioral aspects such as what activities can be accomplished, what enjoyment is found in life, and outlook on life and the future. Examples of

TABLE 19-3. QUESTIONS THAT CAN BE ASKED TO ELICIT DEPRESSIVE SYMPTOMS	
Dysphoria	Have you been feeling sad, blue, down in the dumps?
Anhedonia	What do you do to enjoy yourself?
	Has your interest in usual activities changed any?
	Do you enjoy being with your children and grandchildren?
Agitation/Retardation	Are your physical movements slowed down or sped up?
Concentration	Can you follow what you are reading watching on TV?
Self-esteem	Have you been down on yourself lately?
	Do you feel bad about things you have done or have not done?
Suicidal ideation	How does the future look to you?
	Do you sometimes feel like life is not worth living?
	Do you ever wish you were dead?
	Do you ever have thoughts about hurting or killing yourself?

questions that may be asked to elicit these symptoms are seen in Table 19-3.

Although we believe that direct clinical assessment is the most important and accurate method of identifying depression, there are several screening instruments that can aid the health care provider in identifying those elders who may be at risk for depression and for whom a more detailed interview is clearly warranted. Two self-rating scales, the Beck Depression Inventory (BDI)[15] and the Geriatric Depression Scale (GDS)[16] (see Appendix #s 5 and 16) have been well validated in elderly populations, are easily administered, and could serve as screening instruments. Both pose disadvantages for frail elderly patients with cognitive impairment, however, so that their use in institutionalized elders is limited. Another widely used instrument, the Hamilton Depression Scale[17] is less of a diagnostic instrument, but measures the severity of depression. It is completed by health care providers and could serve as a measure of response to treatment.

Recently introduced aids to assessment include screening questionnaires. These are designed for use in primary care settings and alert the health care provider to follow up more thoroughly on specific areas of concern. These can be administered either in paper-and-pencil format or in computer form. Examples of these include the PRIME-MD (Primary Care Evaluation of Mental Disorders[18]) and the SDDS-PC (Symptom Driven Diagnostic System—Primary Care).[19] Both of these instruments screen for common mental disorders, including depression, anxiety disorders, and substance abuse, which often occur in patients seeing primary care providers. Answers to the screening questions are available so that definitive questions leading to a variety of diagnoses can be pursued. Experts have found the CES-D to be a useful tool to screen groups for the presence of depression (see Appendix #7).[20, 21]

Assessment of Cognition

The screening and assessment of cognition is another important component of the evaluation. A number of screening tools for cognitive impairment have been developed, and perhaps the most commonly used is the Mini-Mental State Examination (MMSE) (see Appendix #29).[22] The MMSE assesses orientation, attention, calculation, immediate and short-term recall, language, and the ability to follow simple commands. A maximum score is 30 points; scores below 24 are suggestive of cognitive deficits (although such factors as age, ethnicity, language, and attention need to be taken into consideration). The depressed elder in an outpatient setting who does not have significant independent brain pathology usually does not score in the dementia range. Because there often is considerable medical comorbidity, however, nondemented, depressed elders may score below 24, although rarely in the single digit or low teens. These lower scores are almost certainly reflective of a dementia. Scores in the moderately impaired range can be indicative of either cognitive impairment associated with depression, an independent cognitive disorder, or a combination of both. Intellectual functions such as memory do decline with normal aging, so care must be taken to distinguish age-related memory impairment from loss due to a disease process such as dementia. Other screening instruments for cognitive impairment are discussed more fully elsewhere in this book. More thorough neuropsychological test batteries can be necessary to establish the severity of the impairment and whether it is more reflective of a dementia or of the milder memory impairment seen in patients with depression.

Assessment of Functional Capacity

An important component of a comprehensive assessment is the functional status screening. Functional assessment means what a person can or cannot do. The most common scales to measure function are the activities of daily living (ADLs) (see Appendix

#24)[23] and the instrumental activities of daily living (IADLs) (see Appendix #25).[24] The ADLs assess the basic activities (bathing, dressing, transferring, continence, and feeding). The IADLs augment this basic information with more complex tasks important for independent living in the community such as the ability to use the telephone, shop, prepare food, and so forth. These evaluations are necessary to complete in order to assess how much independence can be tolerated or what additional plans need to be made to optimize community living.

Assessment of Comorbid Medical Conditions

If through screening there is a suspicion of depression or a diagnosis of depression is made, further evaluation regarding etiology must be conducted. A review of prescribed and over-the-counter medications is crucial. Because elders are likely to have concomitant medical illnesses for which they are taking medications, they are vulnerable to the development of depressive symptoms as side effects of medications. In fact, this is a major cause of depression in elders. Nutritional assessment, food preferences, ethnic foods, and eating habits also should be assessed in relation to body weight. Social isolation and the need for support systems should be evaluated, and physical limitations assessed so that physical or occupational therapies can be considered.

From what has been discussed previously, it should be apparent that, in addition to a complete history, a physical and neurologic examination (with attention to sensory deficits), including cognitive screening, is required on all patients. Diagnostic procedures to be considered should include an electrocardiogram, complete blood count, urinalysis, T_3, T_4, TSH, B_{12} and folate levels, glucose, electrolytes, BUN, creatinine, liver function tests, and syphilis serology. Somewhat more controversial is whether neuroimaging, particularly CT or MRI scanning, should be done routinely. Clearly, intracranial pathology (e.g., tumors, cysts, subdural hematomas, etc.) can present with behavioral symptoms that include depression. Cerebral atrophy and ventricular dilatation may be present, but these are rather nonspecific findings. The cost–benefit analysis of doing anatomic imaging in this population has not been determined. Consideration might be given to an imaging study in new onset cases of depression, when the behavior changes are rapid and/or accompanied by bizarre or psychotic symptoms, or when the depression is refractory to treatment. Functional imaging such as SPECT or PET are not recommended as routine evaluations, although there is active research being conducted to see if blood

An important risk factor for depression in elders is comorbid medical illness.

flow studies can help in distinguishing patterns of cerebral hypoperfusion indicative of differing types of dementia and late-life depression.[25, 26]

DIFFERENTIAL DIAGNOSIS

The differential diagnosis within the class of mood disorders follows
the previous discussion regarding the nature and severity of the
symptoms, their time course or chronicity, the presence or absence
of manic episodes or psychosis, and the presence of medical illness
or medications as causative factors.

Cognitive impairment and depressed mood are two symptoms
in elders that often co-occur and present one of the challenges in
differential diagnosis. Primary depression in elders can be accompanied by cognitive deficits, and the term "depressive pseudodementia" has often been applied in this situation. There has been discomfort with this term, however, as the dementia is real, and can persist
even if the depression is successfully treated. In fact, studies indicate
that even when the cognitive deficits that accompany the depression
improve as the depression is successfully treated, those patients
who had cognitive impairment are at a significantly higher risk for
the development of a progressive dementia several years later.[27]
Recent data from our research group and others has indicated that,
at least in a mild to moderately depressed group of elders who
are in good physical health, the cognitive deficits accompanying
primary MDE are relatively mild, and the more severe deficits are
seen in those patients who have accompanying structural brain
disease (e.g., white matter hyperintensities seen on MRI).[28, 29] Studies of this nature have led to the concept of vascular depression,
whereby cerebrovascular disease is presumed to be a etiologic
factor in some cases of depression presenting later in life.[30] Current
work is trying to establish the validity of this concept, its cognitive
correlates, and its relationship to treatment outcome.

On the other hand, primary degenerative dementias often
present with depression early in the course, especially as the individual becomes increasingly aware of his or her cognitive deficits.
In various studies, up to 40 percent of patients with Alzheimer's
disease (AD) have an accompanying depression, and at least an
equal or higher percent is found in those patients with a frontotemporal dementia (FTD). The depression in Alzheimer's disease is
reported to be fluctuating over time and not of the same melan-
cholic character as that often seen in major depression without
cognitive impairment.[31] Also, data suggest that depression may be
a risk factor for the development of dementia and depression in

patients with dementia confers an additional burden of disability to patients.[32, 33]

Recent interest in the behavioral aspects of damage to frontal and temporal lobes of the brain has led to more awareness that FTD may be associated with many behaviors similar to those seen in depression. Conversely, cerebral blood flow (CBF) studies suggest that older patients with MDE have lowered CBF in these same anatomic areas.[25] Damage to these areas of the brain, whether anatomic or functional, may lead to affective symptoms. In the case of FTD, there can be altered personality traits such as loss of social skills, poor judgment, behavioral disinhibition leading to antisocial behaviors, strange and remote affect, and development of eccentric ideas. These can precede the cognitive deficits by several years. The older depressed patient usually shows less dramatic changes in prior personality function than those seen in patients with FTD. In AD, the memory, language, and visuospatial skill impairments are usually seen first. Major personality changes, as seen in FTD, are more rare in AD, although withdrawal, apathy, and depression may present early in the course of the disorder (see Chapter 21).

Potential factors that lead the examiner to consider depression rather than dementia as the major diagnosis include: a recurrence of a previous depression, feelings of worthlessness and guilt, suicidal thoughts, and a family history of depression. On the other hand, severe memory impairment, language disturbances, confusional episodes, outbursts related to frustration over not being able to accomplish a desired goal, and progressive impairment all are more associated with degenerative dementias.

A detailed discussion of other dementia syndromes, such as dementia with Lewy bodies and subcortical dementias (e.g., Huntington's, Parkinson's, progressive supranuclear palsy, AIDS) is beyond the scope of this chapter. Each of these, by virtue of the anatomic areas they affect, can be accompanied by mood syndromes. Evaluation should be guided by the primary physical findings.

The differentiation of depression from dementias becomes more difficult when one considers the oldest old, particularly those residing in long-term care facilities. In fact, the results of studies using psychometric and neuroimaging evaluations were unable to differentiate patients who had previously been diagnosed with a primary depression or a primary dementia.

If psychotic symptoms are identified, they can be a component of dementia, a mood disorder, or can be indicative of another psychiatric disorder in elders. *Schizophrenic disorders* (either early or late-onset) present with predominant psychotic symptoms, more of a formal thought disorder (derailment of speech, misuse of words), disorganized behavior, and often more bizarre delusions (delusions of thoughts being planted into one's head or of thoughts being taken out of one's mind). Confusion with depression can occur with what are called the negative symptoms of schizophrenia (avolition, amotivation, anergia, affective flattening) and with catatonic behavior, which may be confused with severe psychomotor retardation. In schizophrenia, there is usually a lengthy downward course without return to previous function, whereas in depression, an episodic course is more commonly seen. When schizophrenic disorder presents in late life, there may not be as pronounced a thought disorder as seen in younger schizophrenic patients. The prominence of the mood symptoms and the time course should help to distinguish these disorders. *Delusional disorders* also can present in elders. Here, the delusions are prominent, hallucinations and formal thought disorder are usually absent, and mood symptoms are not prominent.

In primary mood disorders, there often is an admixture of depression and anxiety symptoms. Distinguishing this from a primary anxiety disorder can be difficult. In general, the rates of anxiety disorders in elders, particularly late-onset anxiety disorders (with the exception of phobic disorders), are relatively low. Some studies estimate that at least one-quarter of elderly depressed patients have an accompanying anxiety disorder. The most frequent comorbid disorders are *phobias* and *generalized anxiety disorder* (GAD). GAD is a chronic condition where excessive worry about multiple spheres is accompanied by physical symptoms such as restlessness, fatigue, muscle tension, poor sleep, irritability, and trouble concentrating. Obviously, there is overlap with depressive symptomatology. *Panic disorder* is seen more rarely in the elderly than in younger patients and is less likely to be comorbid with depression in this group. Because elders are vulnerable to suffering severe traumas (being victimized, robbed, etc.), they may be at risk for *post-traumatic stress disorder*. Careful questioning about the precipitants preceding the change in behavior can help to elicit the traumatic experience and clarify the diagnosis. Nightmares and flashbacks about the event are usually present, as is hyperarousal and withdrawal from situations which remind the individual of the trauma. These symptoms are not typically part of a depressive illness. Investigations of frail elders residing in long-term care facilities have found extremely high (80 percent) rates of comorbidity between anxiety and depressive symptoms, making the differential diagnosis in this situation very difficult or impossible.

An area that often is overlooked in relation to the elderly is *alcohol and substance abuse*. It is estimated that up to 10 percent of elderly men (and probably a higher prevalence in medically hospitalized men) and almost 2 percent of women meet criteria for alcohol dependence. Mood disturbances, cognitive problems, falls, and erratic behavior can all be indications of alcohol abuse. Careful questioning of the patient and collaterals, along with active medical evaluation, must be carried out to diagnose this problem. Alcohol use also is a risk factor for suicide attempts. Substance abuse, at least with illegal substances, is considerably lower in elders than in younger patients. Iatrogenic substance dependence and dependence on over-the-counter preparations, however, are significant problems in elders. Benzodiazepines and drugs with anticholinergic properties are especially troublesome and can lead to states that can be confused with depression. Careful medication histories and having the patient bring all their medications (prescribed and home remedies) to the evaluation often is necessary. Another potentially important issue, and one which is probably seen more in minority elderly, is the use of herbal remedies. Many of these herbs have central nervous system (CNS) activity, and either by themselves or by interaction with prescribed medications, can lead to depression, psychosis, and confusional states.

The onset of preoccupation with health in elders is typically more related to realistic medical concerns or to depression than to one of the somatoform disorders (e.g., *hypochondriasis,* which more often is a long-standing pattern). Hypochondriasis is defined as a disorder where the key symptoms are a preoccupation with the idea that one has a serious disease based upon a misperception of bodily symptoms, and preoccupation with this idea despite evidence to the contrary. The belief is not held with delusional intensity, that is, the elder can entertain the notion that his or her belief may not be valid, yet is held for at least 6 months. Depression often occurs in the context of hypochondriasis, as well as in *pain disorder,* another of the somatoform disorders. The main differential point is the pervasiveness of the mood symptoms (depression, loss of interest, decreased self-worth); neurovegetative symptoms are seen in MDE but are not a major component of the somatoform disorders. On the other hand, when the differential is difficult, it may be best to proceed as if the patient had a depression because its treatment is more effective than that for somatoform disorders, and the somatic symptoms may be alleviated as the depression improves. This can be best understood as a masked depression, whereby the somatic symptoms (often without true physiologic pathology) are the most prominent complaint; again, this presentation may be more likely to occur in elders.

The distinction between depression and *bereavement* is discussed elsewhere in this chapter. Although many of the elements are similar, depression is more often associated with feelings of low self-worth, guilt, and nihilism. It is very difficult to put a time limit on when bereavement should end, particularly elders who may have been married for decades and then lost their sole companion. Nevertheless, if the symptoms are severe, debilitating, and last for months after the death, serious consideration should be given to a depressive illness.

Additional Comorbid Medical Illnesses

Multiple medical illnesses can present with symptoms of depression (Table 19-4). Some of these (e.g., hypothyroidism) can produce symptoms of depression directly, whereas for other disorders (e.g., myocardial infarction), the depression can result from the psychological impact of the illness. Perhaps most commonly, health care providers see elders who have existing chronic medical illness and some behavioral element that could be a component of the medical illness or a symptom of depression. Complicating the problem is the bidirectional nature of this interaction: depression can be a result of medical problems or can worsen the symptoms and course of medical illness.[34, 35] Because of this interplay, recognizing depression amid medical illness can be quite problematic. Several paradigms have been suggested as a means of dealing with symptoms that could be reflective of depression: (1) count the symptom as

TABLE 19-4. MEDICAL ILLNESSES ASSOCIATED WITH DEPRESSION

Cardiovascular disorders	Neoplastic disorders
Congestive heart failure	Carcinoma of the pancreas
Myocardial infarction	CNS neoplasms
Hypertension	Remote effect of other neoplasms
Endocrine disorders	Neurologic disorders
Hypothyroidism	Cerebral infarction
Hyperthyroidism	Parkinson's disease
Hyperparathyroidism	Huntington's disease
Hypercortisolism	Dementia
Addison's disease	Amyotrophic lateral sclerosis
Diabetes mellitus	Multiple sclerosis
Infectious disorders	Other disorders
Influenza	Pain
Hepatitis	Anemia
Epstein-Barr virus	Rheumatoid arthritis
Pneumonia	
Metabolic disorders	
Electrolyte imbalance	
Dehydration	
Renal disease	
Dialysis	

part of depression only if it is judged to be part of the mood disorder (etiological approach); (2) count all symptoms regardless of presumed etiology (inclusive approach); (3) use a list that eliminates potentially confounding neurovegetative and somatic items (exclusive approach); and (4) construct a symptom list that replaces the neurovegetative and somatic items with additional affective or cognitive items (substitutive approach).[33] Although there has not been adequate study of these different approaches in a research context, it would appear that in clinical practice using the broadest approach (the inclusive approach) would miss the fewest cases of true depression.

When the symptoms of depression begin abruptly, an acute medical illness or medication side effect should be suspected. For example, an elder who over the course of several days is noted to be withdrawn, apathetic, eating poorly, and perhaps confused, needs to be evaluated for dehydration and/or electrolyte disturbance. On the other hand, symptoms of depression that are more chronic and accompany a known medical illness may be seen more as a reaction to the disability, pain, and psychological losses related to the primary illness.

In addition, there are certain specific medical conditions, many of them disorders of the CNS, where there is a very high prevalence of depression. Estimates are that up to 50 percent of patients who suffer a stroke develop symptoms of depression, either acutely or within 1 year of the stroke. This post-stroke depression syndrome has been reported most commonly when the infarction was in the frontal pole (perhaps more often the left frontal area). Investigators have indicated that the depression is independent of the degree of disability, and clinical trials of antidepressants have proved promising.[36] Other CNS illnesses with a high prevalence of depression (up to 50 percent) are Parkinson's and Huntington's disease.

Although no etiologic link has been established, it has been shown that depressed patients with cardiac disease have higher mortality rates than those without cardiac illnesses. There is a particularly high prevalence of depression post-myocardial infarction. A variety of endocrinopathies have been associated with depression, highlighting the interplay that hormonal dysregulation has with mood and behavior.

The other illness listed in Table 19-4 usually have additional physical signs and symptoms to alert the clinician to where the primary pathology lies. As a general rule, however, the first onset of depression in someone over 60 years old should arouse suspicions that there may be an accompanying medical illness.

In addition to the association of medical illness and depression, there are multiple medications that can cause or worsen depressive symptoms. The major classes of medications responsible for this are: antihypertensives (methyldopa, reserpine, beta-blockers, and clonidine), CNS active agents (alcohol, benzodiazepines, barbiturates, L-dopa, amphetamines, and cocaine withdrawal), steroids, analgesics (narcotic and nonsteroidal antiinflammatory), antineoplastic agents, and antiulcer medications (cimetidine, ranitidine). Other classes of medications also can cause depression as can the interaction of different medications.

Suicide

A tragic outcome for elders is suicide. Unfortunately, this happens more frequently than might be predicted. The suicide rate for elders is about 50 percent higher than the rate for the nation as a whole. In 1988, the national rate for suicide was 12.4 per 100,000 population, whereas for those above age 65 years, it was 21.0 per 100,000, and for those in the 80 to 84 year range, it was 26.5 per 100,000.[37, 38, 39] For men, suicides continue to rise each decade until at least the ninth decade, whereas for women suicide increases until about the seventh decade and then declines somewhat. Caucasian men are most at risk, and reports indicate that more than three quarters of these men had visited a primary care physician within a month of their suicide.[38]

The suicide rate for elders is about 50 percent higher than the rate for the nation as a whole.

Despite increasing interest in suicide in elders, it remains difficult to identify a specific pattern associated with either making a suicide attempt or completing suicide. Many of the factors related to suicide in elders are similar to those for younger people, although the age-specific response to these factors can differ. Depression specifically, as well as other psychiatric disorders, are clearly risk factors for making a suicide attempt. This underscores the great importance of determining the level of depression in elders. Some psychosocial factors associated with suicide in elders include: social isolation, bereavement, lack of financial resources (especially recent financial setbacks), recent retirement, and strain in relations with relatives. Those who have had a chronic and unremitting depression and those who have made suicide attempts in the past are at greater risk. Comorbid medical illness and reduced cognitive function are risk factors, as is comorbid alcohol and substance abuse. In contrast to younger people who commit suicide, elders who kill themselves have a lower rate of previously attempted suicide, demonstrate more mood disorder, and tend to use more lethal means than younger people.

Every elder who is evaluated for behavioral disturbance should be asked questions related to suicide. This is imperative for those elders in whom depressive illness is suspected. These questions can be asked in the context of taking the history and should be asked in a straightforward manner. The myth that mentioning suicide may give the patient an idea to hurt themselves has no basis. The questions need to be direct. For example, "Have you been feeling so down that you are thinking about not wanting to go on living, hurting, or killing yourself?" "What kind of thoughts about hurting or killing yourself have you had?" "How would you do it?" It is necessary to establish what kind of a plan the patient has and whether the means to accomplish it are available (e.g., is there a gun in the house, do they have stockpiles of medications). Eliciting information from collateral sources can be of tremendous benefit, particularly if the patient is reluctant to discuss the plans. If the health care provider asks these questions, there must be a plan to act on the answers. Removal of the immediate means to hurt oneself, increased supervision, and inpatient hospitalization are among the choices.

There are cases where the wish to die is very strong, but the means of harming oneself are less overt. Examples include not taking necessary medication, starving oneself, and engaging in risk-taking behavior. These behaviors need to be evaluated, and if they represent a change for the patient and accompany other symptoms of depression, they should be considered as covert suicidal behavior, and aggressive plans to protect the individual must be taken.

Assessment in Long-Term Care Facilities

The prevalence of depression in nursing homes has been estimated as being as high as 25 percent with an annual incidence of about 14 percent.[40] There are multiple unique problems in the screening, recognition, and treatment of depression in long-term care settings.[41, 42, 43] Although it may appear to be reasonable to attribute depression in long-term care patients to a self-limited adjustment disorder, there is evidence that symptoms are more likely to be persistent. How well the elder can adapt and the elder's ability to appraise his or her environment are important to evaluate. If the demands of the environment are too great or if the demands are too few, the elder's condition may decline.

Assessment of depression for nursing home patients can be difficult and often may be missed because it presents in atypical fashion. Initially, depression may be unrecognized because many staff members attribute any changes in affect or mood to a normal consequence of being placed in a long-term facility. The elder who also has cognitive impairment can present a particular challenge, as he or she may not be able to articulate what he or she is feeling and cannot complete the self-rating scales discussed previously.

Also, depression that presents with physical symptoms (e.g., weight loss, sleep disturbance, somatization, and cognitive slowing) may be interpreted as a natural progression of the patient's dementia and again, can go unrecognized and untreated. Severe pain states also complicate the assessment of depressed mood (see Chapter 15).

Depression also can present primarily as social withdrawal and may not be brought to the attention of a physician because staff members may view this behavior as normal or, at the very least, as not bothersome. On the other hand, depression also can present with agitation, yelling, screaming, and other disruptive behaviors. This presentation, quite disturbing to staff members, may be misdiagnosed and improperly treated with neuroleptics and/ or benzodiazepines when, in actuality, the patient may need an antidepressant. A major concern is that as few as 10 percent of nursing home residents who suffer from depression are treated with antidepressants; a larger percentage receive neuroleptics or benzodiazepines, and most receive no treatment at all.[41]

SUMMARY

The assessment of depression in elders needs to be carried out on multiple levels, with consideration to psychological, medical, neurologic, social, spiritual, and cultural spheres. A multidisciplinary approach typically is the most comprehensive way to successfully complete the evaluation. Throughout the evaluation, respect for the dignity of the patient must be maintained. This includes balancing the need for privacy and confidentiality of the information elicited versus sharing crucial information (e.g., suicide plans) with family, and respecting the patient's need to not disclose shameful information. Ideally, an ongoing rapport with the patient and family will facilitate this process.

Although this chapter is not designed to discuss treatment strategies, we want to state strongly that there are very effective treatment modalities for the elder with depression, and serious consequences to leaving these disorders untreated.[44] Treatments include the full range of antidepressants, psychotherapy (both more traditional and brief, focused psychotherapies), group therapy and self-help groups, bereavement groups, day hospitals and socialization centers, inpatient care, and electroconvulsive therapy. The choice of which modalities to choose will depend a great deal on the results of the comprehensive assessment of the patient, his or her family and support system, their functional capacities, and the available resources. Most studies report that treatment results for elders is somewhat similar to those for younger people, and therefore, every effort should be made to treat depression when recognized.

REFERENCES

1. Styron W. *Darkness Visible.* New York: Random House, Inc.; 1990:50.
2. Reynolds CF. Recognition and differentiation of elderly depression in the clinical setting. *Geriatrics.* 1995;50(suppl. 1):S6–S15.
3. Conn DK, Steingart AB. Diagnosis and management of late life depression: a guide for the primary care physician. *Int J Psychiatry Med.* 1997;27:269–281.
4. Lasser R, Dukoff R, Sunderland T. Diagnosis and treatment of geriatric depression. *CNS Drugs.* 1998;9:17–30.
5. American Psychiatric Association. *Diagnostic and Statistical Manual of Mental Disorders,* 4th ed. (DSM-IV). Washington, DC: American Psychiatric Association; 1994.
6. Blazer DG. Is depression more frequent in late life? An honest look at the evidence. *Am J Geriatr Psychiatry.* 1994;2:193–198.
7. Meyers BS. Epidemiology and clinical meaning of "significant" depressive symptoms in later life: the question of subsyndromal depression. *Am J Geriatr Psychiatry.* 1994;2:188–192.
8. Robins LN, Regier DA. *Psychiatric Disorders in America: The Epidemiologic Catchment Area Study.* New York: The Free Press; 1991.
9. Cohen D, Eisdorfer C. Depression in family members caring for a relative with Alzheimer's disease. *J Am Geriatr Soc.* 1988;36:885–889.
10. Foster JR, Cataldo JK. Prediction of first episode of clinical depression in patients newly admitted to a medical long-term care facility: findings from a prospective study. *Int J Geriatr Psychiatry.* 1992;8:297–304.
11. Zisook S, Shuchter S. Major depression associated with widowhood. *Am J Geriatr Psychiatry.* 1993;1:316–326.
12. Abrams RC, Rosendahl E, Card C, Alexopoulos GS. Personality disorder correlates of late and early onset depression. *J Am Geriatr Soc.* 1994;42:727–731.
13. Kunik ME, Mulsant BH, Rifai AH, et al. Personality disorders in elderly inpatients with major depression. *Am J Geriatr Psychiatry.* 1994;1:38–45.
14. Bruce ML, Seeman TE, Merrill SS, Blazer DG. The impact of depressive symptomatology on physical disability: MacArthur studies of successful aging. *Am J Public Health.* 1994;84:1796–1799.
15. Beck AT, Ward C, Mendelson M, Mock J, Erbaugh J. An inventory for measuring depression. *Arch Gen Psychiatry.* 1961;4:561–571.
16. Yesavage J, Brink T, Rose T, et al. Development and validation of a geriatric depression screening scale: a preliminary report. *J Psychiatr Res.* 1983;17:37–49.
17. Hamilton M. Development of a rating scale for primary depressive illness. *Br J Soc Psychol.* 1967;6:278–296.
18. Spitzer RL, Williams JB, Kroenke K, et al. Utility of a new procedure for diagnosing mental disorders in primary care: the PRIME-MD 1000 study. *JAMA.* 1994;272:1749–1756.

19. Broadhead WE, Leon AC, Weissman MM, et al. Development and validation of the SDDS-PC Screen for multiple mental disorders in primary care. *Arch Fam Med.* 1995;4:211–219.

20. Irwin M, Artin KH, Oxman MN. Screening for Depression in the Older Adult: Criterion Validity of the 10-Item Center for Epidemiological Studies Depression Scale (CES-D), *Arch Intern Med.*, 1999;159:1701–1704.

21. American Medical Directors Association. Depression, Clinical Practice Guideline, 1996.

22. Folstein MF, Folstein SE, McHigh PR. Mini-Mental State: a practical method for grading the cognitive state of patients for the clinician. *J Psychiatr Res.* 1975;12:185–198.

23. Katz S, Ford A, Moskowitz RW, Jackson BA, Joffe MW. Studies of illness in the aged. The Index of ADL. *JAMA.* 1963;185:914–919.

24. Lawton MP, Brody E. Assessment of older people: self-maintaining and instrumental activities of daily living. *Gerontologist.* 1969; 9:179–186.

25. Lesser IM, Mena I, Boone KB, Miller BL, Mehringer CM, Wohl M. Reduction in cerebral blood flow in older depressed patients. *Arch Gen Psychiatry.* 1994;51:677–686.

26. Miller BL, Chang L, Oropilla G, Mena I. Alzheimer's disease and frontal lobe dementias. In: Coffey CE, Cummings JL, eds, *Textbook of Geriatric Neuropsychiatry.* Washington DC: American Psychiatric Press, Inc.; 1994:390–404.

27. Alexopoulos GS, Meyers BS, Young RC, Mattis S, Kakuma T. The course of geriatric depression with "reversible dementia": a controlled study. *Am J Psychiatry.* 1993;150:1693–1699.

28. Lesser IM, Boone KB, Mehringer CM, Wohl M, Miller BL, Berman N. Cognition and white matter hyperintensities in older depressed patients. *Am J Psychiatry.* 1996;153:1280–1287.

29. Miller DS, Kumar A, Yousem DM, Gottlieb GL. MRI high-intensity signals in late-life depression and Alzheimer's disease: a comparison of subjects without major vascular risk factors. *Am J Geriatr Psychiatry.* 1994;2:332–337.

30. Alexopoulos GS, Meyers BS, Young RC, Campbell S, Silbersweig D, Charlson M. "Vascular depression" hypothesis. *Arch Gen Psychiatry.* 1997;54:915–922.

31. Devanand DP, Jacobs DM, Tang MX, et al. The course of psychopathologic features in mild to moderate Alzheimer disease. *Arch Gen Psychiatry.* 1997;54:257–263.

32. Devanand DP, Sano M, Tang MX, et al. Depressed mood and the incidence of Alzheimer's disease in the elderly living in the community. *Arch Gen Psychiatry.* 1996;53:175–182.

33. Forsell Y, Winblad B. Major depression in a population of demented and nondemented older people: prevalence and correlates. *J Am Geriatr Soc.* 1998;46:27–30.

34. Katz I. On the inseparability of mental and physical health in aged persons: lessons from depression and medical comorbidity. *Am J Geriatr Psychiatry.* 1996;4:1–16.

35. Lyness JM, Bruce ML, Koening HG, et al. Depression and medical illness in late life: report of a symposium. *J Am Geriatr Soc.* 1996;44:198–203.

36. Robinson RG, Starkstein SE. Current research in affective disorders following stroke. *J Neuropsychiatry Clin Neurosci.* 1990;2:1–14.

37. McIntosh JL. Older adults: The next suicide epidemic? *Suicide Life Threat Behav.* 1992;22:322–332.

38. Schneider LS, Reynolds CF, Lebowitz BD, Friedhoff AJ. *Diagnosis and Treatment of Depression in Late Life: Results of the NIH Consensus Development Conference.* Washington, DC: American Psychiatric Press, Inc.; 1994.

39. Bharucha A, Satlin A. Late-life suicide: a review. *Harvard Rev Psychiatry.* 1997;5:55–65.

40. Katz IR, Parmelee PA. Depression in elderly patients in residential care settings. In: Schneider LS, Reynolds CF, Lebowitz BD, eds. *Diagnosis and Treatment of Depression in Late Life: Results of the NIH Consensus Development Conference.* Washington, DC: American Psychiatric Press, Inc.; 1994:437–461.

41. Samuels SC, Katz I. Depression in the nursing home. *Psychiatric An.* 1995;25:419–424.

42. Masand PS. Depression in long-term care facilities. *Geriatrics* 1995; 50(suppl 1):S16–S24.

43. Rosen J, Mulsant BH, Pollock BG. Depression in the nursing home: risk factors and interventions. *Nursing Home Med.* 1997;5:156–165.

44. Stoudmire A. Recurrence and relapse in geriatric depression: a review of risk factors and prophylactic treatment strategies. *J Neuropsychiatry and Clin Neurosci.* 1997;9:208–221.

DELIRIUM

JOSEPH FRANCIS

Acute illness, drug toxicity, surgery, and other physiologic stressors commonly produce acute confusion in older patients. Delirium is now the preferred term for this complex phenomenon that threatens life and independence and increases the costs of illness for elders. Health care providers must detect delirium rapidly and uncover its causes accurately and efficiently. Because delirium is so pleomorphic and underlying etiologies virtually endless, the quarry can be elusive and the quest frustrating and expensive. This chapter outlines principles that make the task easier.

DESCRIPTION OF THE PROBLEM

Definitions

Throughout the history of medicine, health care providers have observed dramatic cognitive and behavioral changes in the setting of acute illness. Over 30 terms have been used for this phenomenon, which made the topic itself a cause of confusion! Beginning in 1980 with the *Diagnostic and Statistical Manual,* 3rd ed. (DSM-III), the American Psychiatric Association specified criteria for the nosology of delirium. The current version, DSM-IV, outlines four cardinal features of delirium (Table 20-1) which form the current working definition.[1] One advantage of DSM-IV is its emphasis on core features of delirium identified in recent studies of older patients. DSM also avoids ambiguous terms (e.g, clouding of con-

TABLE 20-1. DSM-IV CRITERIA FOR DELIRIUM

Disturbance of consciousness (i.e., reduced clarity of awareness of the environment) with reduced ability to focus, sustain, or shift attention.

Change in cognition (such as memory deficit, disorientation, language disturbance) or the development of a perceptual disturbance that is not better accounted for by a preexisting, established, or evolving dementia.

The disturbance develops over a short period of time (usually hours to days) and tends to fluctuate over the course of the day.

There is evidence from the history, physical examination, or laboratory findings that the disturbance is caused by the direct physiological consequences of a general medical condition, by an intoxicating substance, by medication use, or by more than one etiology.

sciousness) that have not been standardized among health care providers.

Using clear diagnostic criteria is extremely important. Health care providers fail to recognize nearly 70 percent of the cases of delirium, not because they miss confusion, but because they wrongly attribute it to normal aging or to other conditions such as depression or dementia.[2] Many health care providers also expect delirium to present with agitation or psychosis, features which are not part of its definition and which occur infrequently among older patients. Additionally, they fail to assess the patient for attention, cognition, and time course, which are the cardinal features of the disorder.

Prevalence

Studies using DSM criteria show that 10 percent to 15 percent of elders enter the hospital with established delirium and that an additional 5 percent to 30 percent become delirious during their hospital stay.[3] Delirium also complicates approximately 10 percent of general surgery, 30 percent of open-heart surgery, and 50 percent of hip fracture repair.[4] These startling figures identify delirium as one of the most common adverse outcomes of illness in older patients, as well as a leading iatrogenic complication.

Less is known about the prevalence of delirium in outpatient or in long-term care settings. Delirium appears to be less likely where there is less underlying illness or superimposed physiologic stress. For instance, delirium is uncommonly reported after outpatient procedures such as lens replacement performed for cataracts in healthy elders. In nursing homes, delirium often complicates a pre-existing dementia, which makes it harder to recognize. One study estimated that 9 percent of all nursing home residents, and 16 percent of residents on dementia special care units, met criteria for delirium.[5]

Risk Factors

Delirium is more likely to occur in severely ill patients, patients with advanced age, patients receiving psychoactive medication, and those with impaired physical or cognitive function. Recent prospective studies[6] identified and validated factors predicting delirium in clinical settings (Table 20-2). Dementia is one of the strongest and most consistent risk factors for delirium: 25 percent to 50 percent of delirious patients have underlying dementia, and the presence of dementia increases the risk of delirium by two- to three-fold.[3] Patients experiencing delirium often have evidence of other chronic brain diseases such as Parkinson's disease or stroke, which can cause immobility or cognitive impairment and increase the risk for delirium.

Whether comorbid psychiatric illness other than dementia increases the risk for delirium is uncertain. Patients with depression, paranoid personality, psychosis, or adjustment problems have been reported to have increased risk of postoperative delirium, but premorbid psychiatric symptoms could not be ascertained with assurance in these studies. Most recent studies have not found significant correlations between delirium and psychiatric illness other than dementia.

Recognizing risk factors for delirium and addressing them through standardized interventions (e.g., encouragement of oral

Dementia greatly increases delirium risk.

TABLE 20-2.   RISK FACTORS FOR DELIRIUM IDENTIFIED IN RECENT STUDIES

Advanced age
Dementia or prior cognitive impairment
Impaired physical function
Severe illness
Fever or infection
Use of narcotics or sedatives
Fluid and electrolyte abnormality
Fracture
Immobility
Alcoholism
Anticholinergic drugs
Depression
Visual impairment
Hearing impairment

intake of fluids to correct dehydration, provision of visual aids or amplification to those with sensory impairment) has been demonstrated to reduce the incidence and duration of delirium among hospitalized elders.[7]

Clinical Manifestations

DSM-IV criteria form a practical way to understand the manifestations of delirium. Each criterion, along with its associated manifestations, is discussed in depth as follows.

DISTURBANCE OF CONSCIOUSNESS

Delirium results from a diffuse disturbance of brain function, and one of its first manifestations is a change in level of awareness and ability to focus, sustain, or shift attention. This can present as a change in the level of consciousness. Patients with delirium can appear drowsy, lethargic, or even semicomatose. The opposite extreme, hypervigilance, can occur in cases of alcohol or sedative drug withdrawal. If awake and calm, delirious patients appear distractable, or may need to be redirected many times in order to maintain a conversation.

> Health care providers who are unaware of the possibility of delirium may consider the patient a "poor historian" or "uncooperative."

IMPAIRMENT OF COGNITION AND PERCEPTION

Delirious persons have cognitive impairment and perceptual problems that cannot be explained by a prior or progressing dementia. Because the cognitive manifestations can resemble those of dementia, knowledge of the patient's baseline level of functioning is important. Among the possible manifestations of delirium are short-term memory deficits, disorientation, misinterpretations of the surrounding environment, and language problems. Common language difficulties include problems with writing, incoherent or irrelevant speech, and perseverations. Delirious patients may misidentify the health care provider or believe that objects or shadows in the room represent a person. Vague delusions of harm often accompany these misperceptions. Visual and tactile hallucinations, although they are among the most dramatic features of the perceptual disturbance of delirium, are relatively uncommon.

> People who learned English as a second language may revert to the language of their birth when delirious.

ACUTE ONSET AND FLUCTUATING COURSE

Chronology is a key feature that distinguishes delirium from other mental disorders. Delirium is acute (defined in DSM-IV as hours to days) and varies over the course of a day (typically being worse at night). Patients with delirium can be lucid during morning rounds even if combative or confused the night before, so health care providers must rely on more than just a single point assessment if they are not to miss the problem.

Not only can consciousness and cognition fluctuate, but so can emotional state and psychotic features. The fleeting character of the affective and psychotic features helps health care providers to distinguish delirium from primary mood or thought disorders. Psychomotor activity also can show extreme variation, with patients appearing hyperactive one moment, then withdrawn and hypoactive the next. In the face of such variability, it is hard to subclassify delirium based on its appearance.

One aspect of chronology no longer required in the definition of delirium is prompt reversibility. Although the disturbance of consciousness and cognition is potentially correctable when delirium is promptly recognized and its underlying cause effectively treated, a complete return to baseline may take weeks or months, or never occur at all.[8]

> Delirium can be irreversible if not promptly diagnosed and treated.

MEDICAL ETIOLOGY

Patients with delirium are sick. Although delirium has been described as "brain failure," usually its cause lies outside of the central nervous system (CNS). Lists of conditions reported to cause delirium have been published; the more extensive tend to resemble the contents of an entire medical textbook, but the typical precipitants are those common conditions listed in Table 20-3. Often, several illnesses are identified in elders that can potentially precipitate a mental change.[9]

TABLE 20-3. MEDICAL CONDITIONS COMMONLY CAUSING DELIRIUM

Fluid and electrolyte disturbances
  Dehydration
  Hyponatremia or hypernatremia
Infections
  Urinary tract
  Respiratory tract
  Skin and soft-tissue
Drug toxicity
Metabolic disorders
  Hypoglycemia
  Hypercalcemia
  Uremia
  Hepatic insufficiency
Low perfusion states
  Shock
  Heart failure
Withdrawal from alcohol, sedatives

In surgical patients, delirium appears to result not so much from the stress of surgery itself, but rather from complications such as wound infection, hypoxia, drug toxicity, blood loss, undertreated pain, or cardiac decompensation. Inhaled anesthetic agents do not appear to cause delirium any more frequently than epidural or regional anesthesia.[10]

Drug toxicity accounts for a large proportion of cases; the list of potential agents is exhaustive,[11] but those most commonly associated with delirium are listed in Table 20-4.

One challenge with delirium is that patients often do not look "sick." Acute confusion may be the earliest, or only, manifestation of serious illness such as sepsis or myocardial infarction. More typical manifestations of illness, such as fever, chest pain, or dyspnea, may be absent because of impaired immune response or inability to effectively communicate symptoms. There is little correlation between the underlying cause of delirium and its clinical manifestations, although hyperactive delirium is more likely to be seen with febrile conditions and alcohol withdrawal.

> Delirium can be a presenting finding of acute myocardial infarction in some older patients.

Serious underlying illness makes delirium a medical emergency. Short-term mortality is high—approximately 14 percent at 1 month and 22 percent at 6 months following a diagnosis of delirium, an increase of over 2-fold compared with patients without delirium.[12]

Other complications also occur. Patients with delirium typically have prolonged hospitalizations and generate higher costs than comparable patients without delirium. Many patients with

TABLE 20-4. DRUGS COMMONLY ASSOCIATED WITH DELIRIUM
Medications with anticholinergic effects
Tricyclic antidepressants
Antipsychotics
Antihistamines
Antiarrhythmics
Ophthalmic preparations
Antispasmodics
Antiparkinson agents
Over-the-counter sleep and allergy drugs
Other medication classes
Sedative-hypnotics
Anticonvulsants
Steroids
Nonsteroidal antiinflammatory drugs
Salicylates
H_2-receptor blockers
Narcotics
Dopaminergic agents
Cardiac drugs (digoxin, lidocaine)

delirium never are able to return home, but require institutional care after their acute illness. One study showed that delirium placed patients at risk for losing independence as long as 2 years after the event.[13] The reason for this poor long-term prognosis is not clear, but may reflect underlying frailty, early dementia, or persistent cognitive effects of delirium itself.

OTHER MANIFESTATIONS

Although DSM-IV makes no mention of sleep disturbance, a reversed sleep–wake cycle is often found in delirious patients. Nighttime often represents the period of greatest arousal and agitation, with daytime consumed by drowsiness or lethargy that health care providers may mistakenly attribute to simple fatigue. So striking is this sleep disturbance that it was once felt that sleep deprivation itself caused delirium. Recent investigations have shown the contrary is true—insomnia results from, and is often the first manifestation of, delirium due to another medical condition. Many other conditions (acute illness, pain, dementia), however, disturb sleep in elders, so this finding has less diagnostic value than the core features emphasized in DSM-IV.

In addition to insomnia, other prodromal features of delirium can include difficulty concentrating, anxiety, restlessness, irritability, hypersensitivity to lights and sounds, and vivid dreams or nightmares. Patients able to recall this phase of their delirium attest to feeling intense fear and other emotions.

Delirium is common in elders with underlying chronic disease, the group most prone to functional decline during hospitalization. Acute urinary incontinence and loss of the ability to perform basic self-care tasks often complicate delirium. The medical complications of immobility, such as falling, aspiration pneumonia, and skin breakdown, occur more frequently in patients with delirium, often as a result of the use of chemical or physical restraints.

The physical signs of delirium can include autonomic nervous system activation (tachycardia, sweating, flushing, dry mouth, and dilated pupils), but these responses are typically blunted or absent in older patients, even those experiencing alcohol or sedative-drug withdrawal. Nonrhythmic muscle jerking (myoclonus) and flapping motions of an outstretched, dorsiflexed hand (asterixis) are common features of delirium caused by metabolic disturbances.

WHO TO ASSESS

Cost-effective care of elders requires targeting assessment to the high-risk patients and efficient screening.[14] Because 1 in 3 hospitalized elders may develop delirium, brief screening should be mandatory in all such patients. The older and sicker the patient, the closer one should look; risk factors in Table 20-3 can be used to focus these extra efforts. Other target groups for special attention include patients with hip fractures and those known to have dementia or other brain diseases.

It is important to suspect delirium whenever subtle changes in behavior are noticed. Drowsiness, irritability, tangential speech, and mild disorientation must not be "normalized" as part of the patient's age or illness, but should be considered important clues that prompt a more complete assessment. Active listening is particularly important: family and caregivers who complain that the patient "isn't himself" must be taken seriously.

HOW TO ASSESS

Examinations

IDENTIFYING DELIRIUM

The diagnosis of delirium requires careful observation of the patient's present abilities plus some knowledge of the patient's past level of functioning. The best approach to bedside screening has not been determined, but recent studies identifying high rates of delirium shared several features. First among these is use of firm diagnostic criteria. A second feature is a structured evaluation to uncover findings that satisfy these criteria. This generally involved a bedside interview that included a screening instrument for cognitive impairment, such as the Mini-Mental State Exam (MMSE) (see Appendix #29), and brief assessment of attention. A third feature is interviewing family informants, nursing staff, and other involved caregivers to establish baseline functioning and identify fluctuations. Perhaps the most important determinants of success were the high index of suspicion for delirium and input from all available sources of information.[15]

All members of the treatment team should observe the patient for symptoms and signs of delirium so fluctuations won't be missed.

Translating research into practice involves balancing exactness with practicality. Busy health care providers are less concerned about psychometric issues but also cannot afford to miss delirium. Unfortunately, no single screening instrument can take the place of an astute clinical evaluation. Table 20-5 outlines one possible approach which the author has found useful.

UNCOVERING A CAUSE

Once a diagnosis of delirium is established, there must be a search for underlying causes (the plural here is important). Because prompt treatment is needed to reverse the effects of delirium, rapid

TABLE 20-5. IMPROVING RECOGNITION OF DELIRIUM IN OLDER PATIENTS

1. Maintain a high index of suspicion
   Do not treat lethargy or tangential speech as "normal"
   When in doubt, presume delirium
2. Perform cognitive testing (MMSE, digit span) on initial encounter
   and whenever a change is suspected
   Observing performance is more important than calculating "score"
3. Look for clues in conversation
   Distractibility
   Perseveration
   Incoherent responses
4. Interview capable informants (family members and caregivers)
   Be an active listener
   Take subtle changes seriously
5. Use a team approach
   Actively solicit evidence of behavior change
   Review nursing notes for after-hours confusion
   Educate all team members about delirium
6. Focus on key features (CAM algorithm, Appendix #12)
   Does nurse or family member report acute change and fluctuating
     course?
   Did the patient have difficulty focusing attention during the in-
     terview?
   Was the patient's thinking disorganized or incoherent, such as ram-
     bling or irrelevant conversation, unclear or illogical flow of ideas,
     or unpredictable switching from subject to subject?
   Was the patient's level of consciousness abnormal?

diagnosis is preferred, and therapy should not be delayed because of diagnostic uncertainties. A prudent approach is to use a stepwise evaluation (Table 20-6), starting with quick, basic tests meant to uncover the most likely etiologies, reserving more sophisticated or time-consuming testing based on clinical suspicion and the patient's response to initial therapy.[14]

Although most authorities recommend starting with a comprehensive history and physical, this often proves difficult in the confused and uncooperative patient. It is more important to do a focused assessment, the components of which (and potential pitfalls) are summarized in Table 20-7.

A very effective step in evaluating confusion is reviewing the medication list. A trial of eliminating unnecessary medication serves both a diagnostic and therapeutic purpose. When a certain class of drug is essential, substituting an alternative with less delirium-inducing potential is wise. For example, morphine can be substituted for meperidine. Among antibiotics, quinolones can produce more acute confusion than other agents.

TABLE 20-6. STEPWISE EVALUATION OF DELIRIUM

1. Perform a focused history and physical
2. Review all current medications
    Trust no category of drugs
    Eliminate the nonessential, substitute alternatives
3. Order basic laboratory studies
    Complete blood count
    Electrolytes, creatinine, blood urea nitrogen
    Calcium
    Urinalysis
4. Consider further testing based on results of basic evaluation and response to initial therapy
    Chest x-ray; selected cultures
    Drug levels; toxicology screens
    Pulse oximetry or arterial blood gases
    Serum B_{12}, thyroid function tests, liver enzymes
    Electrocardiogram
    Brain imaging
    Lumbar puncture
    EEG

Be wary as well of unseen medications. Over-the-counter drugs, drugs prescribed by other physicians, or drugs belonging to other household members can be a potential cause of delirium. Asking the family to clean out the medicine cabinet and bring the contents for review can prove useful.

The neurologic exam is helpful in identifying those patients with delirium who need immediate neuroimaging. Unfortunately, its value in the assessment of delirium has had little study. Because many items of the classic neurologic exam have shown poor inter-rater reliability (e.g., plantar and deep-tendon reflexes) or are difficult in uncooperative patients (e.g., sensory testing), a standardized neurologic examination for the delirious patient should emphasize level of consciousness and unambiguous cranial nerve and motor deficits. Testing of visual fields should be attempted whenever possible; hemianopsia may be the only clue of a posterior cortical strokes presenting as delirium with no motor findings.[16]

Instruments and Tools

COGNITIVE SCREENING INSTRUMENTS

Structured cognitive tests such as the MMSE can identify cognitive impairment missed by health care providers doing unstructured evaluations, but this data comes from settings where dementia,

Table 20-7. Focused Physical Examination for Delirium	
COMPONENT	COMMENTS AND PITFALLS FOR ELDERS
Temperature	Can be < 101°F in serious infections; an increase in temperature > 2.4°F is a more sensitive indicator
Heart rate	Tachycardia can be absent in older patients with alcohol/sedative drug withdrawal or anticholinergic intoxication
Respiratory rate	Tachypnea can be a sensitive indicator of pneumonia
Visual and auditory acuity	Impairment is common and can contribute to confusion
Visual fields	Homonymous hemianopsia is a subtle sign of posterior cortical stroke presenting with delirium
Nuchal rigidity	Less specific and sensitive for meningitis in elders
Lung auscultation	Basilar crackles can signify atelectasis, not pneumonia; consolidation infrequent in older patients with pneumonia
Abdominal palpation	Peritoneal signs often absent in intra-abdominal sepsis; rule out fecal impaction and urinary retention if mass is felt
Neurologic examination	Many components (Babinski, sensory examination) have poor reliability in uncooperative patients; focus on gait, pupillary responses, eye movements, and muscle strength.
Skin and soft tissues	Turgor is not always reliable measure of hydration; check all pressure-prone areas for breakdown and infection

rather than delirium, is the sought-after condition. The MMSE and similar tests have less value for following patients with delirium. Performance scores cannot distinguish between delirium and dementia, except in those circumstances when baseline testing has been performed. Test–retest reliability is poorer in delirious participants compared with demented persons, the result of inability to follow directions, drowsiness, and the fluctuating nature of delirium. The behavioral problems that accompany delirium often correlate poorly with cognitive testing scores. Finally, a "normal" score may lull health care providers into complacency when other factors would still indicate the ongoing presence of delirium.

Nonetheless, cognitive screening tests are still useful in the assessment of delirium. Delirium is more likely than dementia if the attention wanders or commands have to be repeated multiple

The MMSE provides more than just a score; how the patient does the test is just as important.
The score will not distinguish delirium from dementia
A cut-off point of 24 will miss mild cases of delirium

times. The nature of the errors can also be diagnostic. In demented patients, wrong answers are still related to the correct ones; delirious patients, rather than showing "near misses," often produce an incoherent jumble or totally unrelated responses, perhaps because the question is misperceived; perseverations also are more common. Such global impressions can be quite valuable: in one study, an examiner's rating of "accessibility" during administration of the MMSE had greater sensitivity (90 percent) and specificity (95 percent) for delirium than the MMSE score, and was less subject to influence from age or educational level.[15]

SIMPLE TESTS OF ATTENTION

Several short tests of attention can be useful at the bedside, especially in the serial assessment of patients with delirium.[17] These include the attention component of the MMSE (serial 7s or backwards spelling), sentence writing, trailmaking tests, and digit span. Occasionally, these tests detect impairment that is not evident in casual conversation or even on other cognitive tasks. One of the easiest bedside tests is the digit span, in which one asks the patient to listen carefully to and then repeat a series of numbers presented at a rate of per 1 second, starting with a two-number sequence and increasing to up to 7 digits.

Quick tip: Because a normal digit span is 7, ask patients to repeat a telephone number (but do not pause between the third and fourth digits).

Tests of attention are far from perfect, so must be used along with clinical judgment in order to arrive at a diagnosis of delirium. Some tests, such as Trailmaking Test B, are difficult for acutely ill patients, and visual and musculoskeletal impairments can impair performance and confound their interpretation. Easier tests can be considerably less sensitive to mild or fluctuating impairment. In one study, digit span had a low sensitivity (30 percent) to delirium, although specificity was quite high (90 percent) when a cutpoint of 5 digits was used.[15] Simple tests of attention share the same problem as cognitive screens: a single test will not measure change from baseline or detect fluctuation. Nonetheless, brief tests of attention can be useful for busy health care providers, especially when performed serially.

OBSERVER-BASED DIAGNOSTIC INSTRUMENTS

The literature now contains at least 20 instruments designed to evaluate confusional states, including cognitive screening tests, diagnostic tests that operationalize DSM criteria, and scales that are used to rate the severity of the disturbance. Only three tests have been validated specifically for use in delirium and for their ability to distinguish delirium from dementia.[18–20] These are described in Table 20-8.

All of these observer-based instruments are designed to be completed following a standardized evaluation, including interview

			SEPARATES	
		PERFORMANCE	DEMENTIA	
		COMPARED	FROM	TIME NEEDED
INSTRUMENT	DESCRIPTION	WITH PSYCHIATRIST	DELIRIUM	(MINUTES)
Confusion Assessment Method (CAM)	Diagnostic algorithm applied after interview with Mini-Mental State Examination by trained lay or clinical interviewer; nurse or family also interviewed	Sensitivity 46%–100% Specificity 90%–95%	Yes	10
Delirium Rating Scale	Ten-item scale completed after thorough psychiatric assessment	No overlap in scores between delirium and control patients	Yes	30 or longer
Delirium Symptom Interview	Structured interview assessing cognition and other symptoms	Sensitivity 90% Specificity 80%	Not assessed	15 or longer

TABLE 20-8. OBSERVER-RATED INSTRUMENTS USED TO ASSESS DELIRIUM

of the patient and caregivers. Training is required for all. The need for clinical acumen varies from the highly structured Delirium Symptom Interview (DSI),[19] designed for administration by a lay interviewer, to the unstructured Delirium Rating Scale (DRS),[20] which is meant to be completed after a psychiatrist's detailed assessment. The length of both the DSI and DRS limits their efficiency for repeated screening of at-risk patients; they are most appropriate when evaluating behavioral changes noted by staff members or caregivers.

By far, the most tested and user-friendly instrument for screening for the presence of delirium is the Confusion Assessment Method (CAM).[18] This scale operationalizes core criteria from DSM-III-R and uses a simplified diagnostic algorithm (see Appendix #12) that takes little time to complete. Health care providers can easily be trained to use the CAM, whose flexible structure is adaptable to many settings. The CAM is easily incorporated into the medical record as a "geriatric vital sign"; such a daily reminder can enhance health care provider recognition of confusion. The CAM appears to have better sensitivity and specificity for delirium than cognitive screening instruments, since it was designed to incorporate information from all available sources.

According to the CAM, delirium is present if there is:
Acute onset and fluctuating course PLUS
Inattention PLUS
Either disorganized thinking or altered level of consciousness

Special Procedures and Tests

LABORATORY STUDIES

Laboratory tests for delirium are listed in Table 20-6. Because of their expense or the time needed to obtain results, they should be targeted based on the results of the initial clinical examination. Unless a cause is obvious on this evaluation, a limited number of basic studies are indicated. Drug levels should be ordered where appropriate; however, many agents can cause delirium in older patients even when present in "therapeutic levels."

LUMBAR PUNCTURE

Although elders with bacterial meningitis are more likely than the young to present with delirium rather than the classic triad of fever, headache, and meningismus, this is still an uncommon cause of delirium. Nuchal rigidity, when present, does not increase the likelihood of meningitis. Cervical arthritis, or other neurologic illness, can mimic this finding in up to one third of acutely ill elders without meningitis. In febrile elders with delirium, routine evaluation of the cerebrospinal fluid is usually not necessary if other infectious foci are evident.[21]

NEUROIMAGING

Neuroimaging should be obtained immediately if there is a new focal neurologic finding or recent head trauma, but should be used selectively in other situations. Head CT abnormalities are common in patients with delirium, even when focal signs are absent, but often reflect predisposing rather than acute, treatable lesions.[22] If the initial evaluation discloses an obvious treatable disturbance, and the patient improves with initial treatment, neuroimaging is probably not warranted.

ELECTROENCEPHALOGRAPHY

Electroencephalography (EEG) has a long tradition of use in delirium; slowing of the dominant posterior alpha rhythm and the appearance of abnormal theta-and delta-wave activity have been recognized for decades as reliable indicators of delirium. In cases of alcohol withdrawal, a fast EEG pattern may be seen. Rarely, however, is the EEG needed to make a diagnosis of delirium, for the clinical criteria are quite sensitive themselves. Also, a single EEG in a patient with mild delirium may not show clearly abnormal findings. A very small percentage of delirious patients can have acute, fluctuating confusion due to nonconvulsive status epilepticus. An EEG can be considered in patients with a history of prior seizures or patients showing subtle rhythmic motor disturbances, or automatisms for whom other causes of delirium have been ruled out.

FORESTALLING FUNCTIONAL DECLINE

Elders experiencing delirium are vulnerable for functional decline as a result of aspects of acute hospital care that immobilize patients and discourage independence. These complications may occur regardless of the nature of the underlying illness and despite its successful treatment. Delirium can be the event that ushers in a "cascade" of progressive functional loss. Careful attention to maintaining mobility, skin integrity, continence, adequate bowel evacuation, and self-care skills can forestall some of the functional decline associated with acute illness. The need for comprehensive assessment of the health and physical function of patients with delirium does not end with discharge from the hospital, since functional and cognitive deficits often persist once the acute illness has resolved.

Patients at risk for delirium should be targeted for special interventions, (e.g., geriatric units, team consultations, or restorative nursing protocols) to prevent further cognitive or functional decline.

COMMON PROBLEMS IN ASSESSMENT

The Patient with Dementia

A common challenge for health care providers is assessing the demented patient presenting with altered behavior. Psychotic or depressive features can be seen in 30 percent to 40 percent of patients with Alzheimer's disease. Adjustment reactions to the loss of abilities, sudden environment changes (the so-called catastrophic reaction), and superimposed visual or auditory impairment, can produce such behavioral change. An estimated 10 percent of persons with primary degenerative dementia are believed to have Lewy-body type degeneration, which presents with early psychotic features and an abrupt, often fluctuating course (in contrast to delirium, fluctuations occur over weeks to months) that potentially can be mistaken for delirium. As important as these considerations are, superimposed medical illness or drug toxicity so often causes altered behavior in demented persons, that a wise principle is to first rule out delirium.

Many older patients with dementia show predictable behavioral deterioration in the evening hours (sundowning), particularly in institutional settings. Although sometimes considered synonymous with delirium, sundowning is usually seen among demented patients who are medically stable or who have had a recent environmental change. Little is known about the causes of sundowning, but worsening evening behavior in such instances may reflect impaired sleep regulation (a common complication of dementing illness) or nocturnal factors in the institutional environment (e.g., shift changes, fewer nurses) that reduce the staff members' ability to effectively handle agitation. Again, it is prudent to perform an initial evaluation for delirium for the sundowning patient, particularly if this is an unexplained departure from established behavioral patterns. For further details on sleep evaluation, see Chapter 16.

When in doubt, presume delirium!

Persistent Delirium

Although reversibility was once a key feature in the definition of delirium, recent investigations have highlighted the persistence of delirium, often for many months after its onset. In some cases, it appears that acute illness "unmasked" a dementia that was not recognized by caregivers. For others, precipitants of delirium (thiamine deficiency, hypoxia, hypoglycemia) may have caused irreversible brain damage leading to dementia. Finally, it is not uncommon for hospitalized patients to experience a cascade of iatrogenic complications; these can potentially maintain a state of delirium even when the initial inciting event has been treated. One source of such iatrogenic persistence of delirium can be the use of chemical and physical restraints to manage agitated behaviors while the underlying cause is being treated.

The approach to the patient whose delirium persists after correction of obvious underlying medical disturbances is first to search for co-occurring conditions. These include acute CNS lesions, unrecognized drug toxicity or withdrawal, ongoing or new infections (e.g., recurrent aspiration pneumonia), intermittent hypoxia or hypoperfusion, or metabolic disturbances missed during initial evaluation (e.g., occult hypoglycemia). Second-tier tests are useful but should not be invoked in "shotgun" fashion; diagnostic efforts should still follow clinical suspicion.

Zeal to uncover an etiology must be tempered by knowledge of the patient's underlying functional status and the desire to avoid iatrogenic harm. For some patients who are in the terminal stages of irreversible disease (including end-stage dementia), a palliative approach may be more appropriate than aggressive medical intervention. Even when disease is not terminal, there may be situations where it is most appropriate to manage the persistently delirious patient in a supportive, restorative environment that avoids chemical and physical restraints and allows gradual recovery of cognitive and physical functions.

Preterminal Delirium

There appears to be a close association between delirium and uncontrolled pain. Thirty to eighty percent of cancer patients experience delirium in the week before death; similar rates can occur in other terminal conditions. Even if death is predictable and imminent, it is still important for health care providers to recognize and treat delirium. The experience of delirium can create a nightmarish terror for patients or produce a pattern of crescendo pain. Although a comprehensive search for underlying medical problems may not be appropriate in all such patients, delirium should never be discounted. The appropriate use of analgesics, sedatives, and antipsychotics to manage symptoms of mental distress is appropriate to attain comfort in the final days.

SUMMARY

Delirium is a medical emergency with a high rate of mortality prevalent among elders admitted to the hospital. The diagnosis of delirium should be suspected in all acute confusional states with a fluctuating course. The diagnosis is made clinically. Prevention of delirium is possible, recognizing risk factors and intervening early to treat underlying causes.

REFERENCES

1. American Psychiatric Association. *Diagnostic and Statistical Manual of Mental Disorders,* 4th ed. Washington, DC: American Psychiatric Association; 1994.
2. Farrell KR, Ganzini L. Misdiagnosing delirium as depression in medically ill elderly patients. *Arch Intern Med.* 1995;155:2459–2464.
3. Francis J. Delirium in older patients. *J Am Geriatr Soc.* 1992;40: 829–838.
4. Dyer CB, Ashton CM, Teasdale TA. Postoperative delirium: a review of 80 primary data-collection studies. *Arch Intern Med.* 1995;155: 461–465.
5. Fries BE, Mehr DR, Schneider D, et al. Mental dysfunction and resource use in nursing homes. *Med Care.* 1993;31:898–920.
6. Inouye SK, Viscoli CM, Horwitz RI, et al. A predictive model for delirium in hospitalized elderly medical patients based on admission characteristics. *Ann Intern Med.* 1993;119:474–481.
7. Inouye SK, Bogardus ST, Charpentier PA, et al. A multicomponent intervention to prevent delirium in hospitalized older patients. *N Engl J Med.* 1999;340:669–676.
8. Levkoff SE, Evans DA, Liptzin B, et al. Delirium: the occurrence and persistence of symptoms among elderly hospitalized patients. *Arch Intern Med.* 1992;152:334–340.
9. Francis J, Martin D, Kapoor WN. A prospective study of delirium in hospitalized elderly. *JAMA* 1990;263:1097–1101.
10. Williams-Russo P, Sharrock NE, Mattis S, Szatrowski TP, Charlson ME. Cognitive effects after epidural versus general anesthesia in older adults: a randomized trial. *JAMA* 1995;274:44–50.
11. Francis J. Drug-induced delirium: diagnosis and treatment. CNS Drugs. 1996;5:103–114.
12. Cole MG, Primeau FJ. Prognosis of delirium in elderly hospital patients. *Can Med Assoc J.* 1993;149:41–46.

13. Francis J, Kapoor WN. Prognosis after hospital discharge of older medical patients with delirium. *J Am Geriatr Soc.* 1992;40:601–606.

14. Inouye SK. The dilemma of delirium: clinical and research controversies regarding diagnosis and evaluation of delirium in hospitalized elderly medical patients. *Am J Med.* 1994;97:278–288.

15. Pompei P, Foreman M, Cassel CK, et al. Detecting delirium among hospitalized older patients. *Arch Intern Med.* 1995;155:301–307.

16. Benbadis SR, Sila CA, Cristea RL. Mental status changes and stroke. *J Gen Intern Med.* 1994;9:485–487.

17. Strub RL, Black FW. *The Mental Status Evaluation in Neurology,* 2d ed. Philadelphia: FA Davis Co; 1985.

18. Trzepacz PT, Baker WB, Greenhouse J. A symptom rating scale for delirium. *Psychiatry Res.* 1988;23:89–97.

19. Albert MS, Levkoff SE, Reilly C, et al. The delirium sympton interview: an interview for the detection of delirium symptoms in hospitalized patients. *J Geriatr Psychiatry Neurol.* 1992;5:14–21.

20. Inouye SK, van Dyck CH, Alessi CA, et al. Clarifying confusion: the Confusion Assessment Method, a new method for detection of delirium. *Ann Intern Med.* 1990;113:941–948.

21. Warshaw G, Tanzer F. The effectiveness of lumbar puncture in the evaluation of delirium and fever in the hospitalized elderly. *Arch Fam Med.* 1993;2:293–297.

22. Naughton BJ, Moran M, Ghaly Y, Michalakes C. Computed tomography scanning and delirium in elder patients. *Acad Emerg Med.* 1997;4:1107–1110.

DEMENTIA

JEFFREY KAYE / RICHARD CAMICIOLI

The diagnosis and assessment of dementia requires a unique combination of clinical skills. These skills include a thorough knowledge base of cognitive and behavioral neuroscience as well as the ability to conduct a productive clinical interview with a confused patient and his or her distraught relative. In this chapter, pragmatic approaches to these and other challenges facing the health care provider are given to help frame the context of the assessment of dementia. The starting point for the assessment is a clinical concern of cognitive or functional impairment either initiated by the patient, the family, or the health care provider.[1] How to proceed or even whether to initiate a thorough evaluation depends largely on the health care provider's concept or definition of dementia, and his or her values regarding the merits of making a diagnosis. Although a number of guidelines and consensus statements regarding dementia assessment have appeared,[2,3] many patients with cognitive impairment remain undiagnosed.[4] Although strict definitions of the dementias have clear utility for the well-established case or in the research clinic, they may be less easily applied in many clinical settings, such as the earlier stages of cognitive decline.

The Agency for Health Care Policy and Research (AHCPR) was renamed in December 1999.
This agency is now known as the Agency for Healthcare Research and Quality (AHRQ).
This reader is encouraged to refer to Chapters 3, 19 and 20 in order to fully benefit from this chapter.

DESCRIPTION OF THE PROBLEM

Definitions

Dementia is defined by the presence of acquired impairment in memory and in at least one other cognitive domain in association with functional decline.

Probably the most widely quoted definition of dementia is derived from the *Diagnostic and Statistical Manual of the American Psychiatric Association* (DSM-IIIR and DSM-IV).[5] This definition encompasses the key feature that first must be established for the diagnosis of dementia: multiple spheres of cognitive impairment must be involved (Table 21-1). Virtually all definitions of dementia follow this general rule.[6] The character of the cognitive impairment and the number of cognitive domains affected vary. For the common dementias, notably Alzheimer's disease the loss of memory function, operationally considered the inability to recall new information (short-term memory) and old information (long-term memory) is in evidence. In disorders such as the frontotemporal dementias,[7,8] in which the frontal lobes of the brain are primarily affected, the health care provider will be misled if memory function is expected to distinctly fail or be impaired early on. Because all dementias begin regionally in the brain, all cognitive domains are rarely uniformly affected. Thus, the dementias are initially relatively focal disorders that, with progression, lead to increasingly severe deficits in an initial cognitive or behavioral domain with later extension to involve other areas of the brain and the functions they subserve. Depending on the sensitivity of the detection methods and the number of functions assessed, a diagnosis of dementia may or may not be made. This is why the initial detection of deficits in more than one sphere of cognitive function becomes somewhat arbitrary depending on the number of domains assessed and the degree of difficulty of the cognitive tests. Moreover, because of the potential for focal onset, the insistence on memory impairment as a necessary condition for the diagnosis of dementia can lead to misdiagnosis

---

TABLE 21-1. COGNITIVE DOMAINS AFFECTED IN DEMENTIA

Memory
At least one or more of the following must be present.
 Aphasia: Disturbance in language not related to mechanical aspects of speech.
 Apraxia: Failure to carry out motor tasks, despite intact basic motor and sensory function.
 Agnosia: Failure to recognize or identify objects despite intact basic sensory function.
 Disturbance of executive functioning: Impaired planning, organizing, sequencing, and abstract reasoning.

Adapted from DSM-IV.

when other cognitive areas are first affected. This can occur as an atypical presentation of a common dementia, such as Alzheimer's disease,[9, 10] that usually first affects memory.

Since the most common dementias demonstrate memory impairment early on, this becomes a key focus of any assessment. In addition to the memory loss, there is at least one other ability that demonstrates impaired function. Disturbances of language function, visuospatial perception, learned motor skills (apraxia), abstract reasoning, judgment, and problem solving are most common. Many formal definitions and experienced health care providers also include personality change as a "cognitive" deficit consistent with dementia. Behavioral changes are important to include in the spectrum of symptoms of dementia as these are often present early and noted especially by the family. These symptoms are derived from the history and might not be apparent on formal testing.

There is an important element of timing in defining dementia. The memory and cognitive deficits must be new, that is, an acquired change from a previously established level of cognitive function, to distinguish dementia from mental retardation syndromes. Dementia is a persistent disorder that must be distinguished from acute confusional states such as delirium and seizures, which present with major fluctuations in levels of consciousness, onset over a short period, and often an underlying cause.[11] Dementia with Lewy bodies is characterized by fluctuations in cognitive function in the absence of delirium.[12] The ICD-10 coding of dementia requires the dementia syndrome to be present for at least 6 months to qualify as a persistent disorder,[13] whereas other classification systems do not delineate a specific time limit. Selection of diagnostic criteria will influence the prevalence of dementia in a given population or diagnosis in an individual patient.[14] Selection criteria in clinical trials can affect the generalizability of the results.[15]

There is a common acknowledgment that the cognitive disturbance characteristic of dementia must interfere with social and occupational function, as stipulated in the DSM criteria. When cognitive deficits are of sufficient severity to tax the elder's social support system or individual compensation strategies, the diagnosis of dementia is straightforward. Although functional decline can sometimes precede the development of dementia,[16] it often lags behind objective signs of cognitive impairment. Clearly, some elders will initially work and function adequately despite detectable cognitive deficits. Early on, such individuals will not meet the functional status decline criteria for the diagnosis of dementia if one strictly requires deterioration in the ability to perform activities of daily living (ADLs).

Dementia can be classified into three broad categories: dementias with clinical or laboratory evidence of other medical disease (e.g., hypothyroidism, B_{12} deficiency, or diabetes), dementias with neurologic signs without obvious medical disease (e.g., parkinsonism, cerebral infarctions, and brain tumor), and dementias without distinctive neurologic signs or evidence of neurologic or medical disease (e.g., Alzheimer disease, frontotemporal dementias, and depression). This classification scheme is based more on the common clinical presentations of dementia than on the particular system or region of the brain that is affected. In subsequent sections, more specific definitions of individual dementing disorders within these broad categories will be given in the context of the assessment.

Prevalence and Risk Factors

The diagnostic assessment is best informed by an understanding of the most likely circumstances in which a particular dementia will occur. The likely diagnosis is arrived at based on the age- and gender-specific prevalence (number of people with the disorder in the population being examined) of various dementias in a given clinical setting. The differential diagnosis in a 40-year-old man should evoke a different set of possibilities as opposed to an 80-year-old woman. The prevalence of dementia in various populations is subject to considerable variability. This is due, in part, to variations in the criteria used to establish the diagnosis.[17] Recently, however, there has been some adoption of relatively uniform criteria, which has allowed for the cross-comparison or pooling of data to generate consistent prevalence estimates. Prevalence is influenced by incidence (number of cases occurring in a population per unit time) and by survival after the time of diagnosis, which might also explain some differences between studies. The prevalence of dementia according to DSM-III diagnostic criteria increases exponentially, doubling every 5 years between the ages of 60 and 84 and then leveling off somewhat after 85 years. This translates into a prevalence of approximately 6 percent between the ages of 60 and 84, whereas in those age 85 or older, the prevalence is considerably higher at about 33 percent.[18] Some community surveys applying a screening test for cognitive impairment find that cognitive impairment consistent with dementia may be present in up to 50 percent of those over age 85.[19] Certain settings, such as nursing homes, are likely to have a much higher prevalence of people with dementia than in the general community.

Aside from the major influence that age plays on dementia prevalence, there are other risk factors that also increase the likelihood of developing dementia.[20–22] Risk factors are best identified from incidence studies, which allow for their identification prior to the development of dementia, thereby avoiding biases such as differential survival and forgetfulness at the time of risk assessment. Many of these are associated with the two major causes of dementia in those over age 65: Alzheimer's disease and dementia secondary to cerebrovascular disease. In the latter case, those risks associated with stroke or cerebrovascular disease[23, 24] are generally believed to be associated with vascular dementia, although only age is clearly established. A history of transient ischemic events, stroke, hypertension, cigarette smoking, diabetes, or low education have all been associated with vascular dementia. Unequivocal risk factors for Alzheimer's disease, aside from age itself, are family history of dementia, one of several identified gene mutations, and the apolipoprotein E genotype (Table 21-2). Female gender, low education, and depression are additional risk factors, while estrogen use and nonsteroidal anti-inflammatory agent use appear to be protective factors.[25]

Three known genetic mutations occurring on three separate chromosomes (chromosomes 1, 14, 21) cause Alzheimer's disease.[26] The mutation on chromosome 21 is in the gene coding for the amyloid protein. Amyloid accumulation in the brain is one of the neuropathologic hallmarks of individuals dying with Alzheimer's disease, the other finding being the accumulation of neurofibrillary tangles. The other known mutations on chromosome 1 (the PS2 or presenilin 2 gene) and chromosome 14 (the PS1 or presenilin 1 gene) code for proteins for which a direct etiologic role is uncertain at this time, but indirect effects on processing the amyloid protein is one speculative mechanism. In the case of the chromosome 1 mutations, these cases have all occurred in a small group of ethnic Germans originating in the Volga valley of Russia in the 18th and

The prevalence of dementia doubles every 5 years between ages 60 and 85 years, beginning at 1 percent to 2 percent, and leveling off at approximately 50 percent in people older than age 85 years.

TABLE 21-2. GENETICS OF ALZHEIMER'S DISEASE

Causal Genes
  Chromosome 1: Early onset familial Alzheimer's disease, Volga Germans, PS2 gene mutation
  Chromosome 14: Early onset familial Alzheimer's disease, PS1 gene mutation
  Chromosome 21: Early onset familial Alzheimer's disease, amyloid precursor protein gene mutation, Downs syndrome
Established Risk Factor Genes
  Chromosome 19: Late onset Alzheimer's disease associated with apolipoprotein E4 allele
Other Risk Factor Genes (less firmly established)
  Chromosome 6: Sporadic Alzheimer's disease, association with HLA antigen A2
  Chromosome 12: Beta-2 macroglobulin
  Additional genes

19th centuries.[27] Although these genetic discoveries are of great importance to research in Alzheimer's disease, such cases are unlikely to be commonly seen among elders. All of the known gene mutations in Alzheimer's disease occur most commonly in the relatively rare instances of early-onset (before age 60), familial (two or more affected first-degree relatives) Alzheimer's disease.

Much more common is a history of affected family members in a patient age 60 or older. In these later onset cases, family history increases the risk, but the mode of inheritance and exact degree of susceptibility is difficult to determine in an individual family member. A gene locus coding for a lipid transport protein, apolipoprotein E, has been found to clearly modulate the risk of developing later onset Alzheimer disease.[27, 28] Apolipoprotein E occurs as 3 allele types: E2, E3, E4. The homozygous state, E4/E4, is reported to increase the risk of Alzheimer's disease 3 to 7 times. The variable risk is likely related to whether one is a man, in which case the risk appears to be similar whether one is homozygous or heterozygous for E4, as opposed to women, where the homozygous state for E4 increases the risk relative to being heterozygous.[29] For those with both an E4 allele and a family history of dementia, the relative risk of dementia is further increased. The majority of patients with Alzheimer's disease are in an age group (those over 80 years) in which the high risk apolipoprotein E4 allele does not seem to play as significant a role. Other factors may play an important role such as the presence of concomitant vascular disease[30] and ethnic background.[31]

WHO TO ASSESS

Principles of Case Detection and Identification

The most obvious reason to assess an individual for dementia is that a patient is complaining of cognitive impairment and requests an evaluation to understand what is happening. Since up to 25 percent of patients will have no complaints of memory impairment despite being mildly, but clearly demented.[32] Another important role of assessment is case detection when dementia is at a mild or early stage and can be missed because the patient is socially appropriate and engaging. Some health care providers do not believe there is any premium on early detection or assessment of dementia. This attitude generally stems from a concern that there is little to be gained from pursuing a work-up as the most common forms of dementia in elders have no cures. This approach ignores four important considerations. First, it implies that if the patient or family were aware of the deficits they would not wish to pursue the cause of the dementia, which could be discovered on proceeding with the evaluation.[33] Second, it prevents the possibility of uncovering the important 10 percent to 14 percent of reversible dementias, which respond increasingly less well to treatments when the dementia has been allowed to progress.[34] Third, in those cases where there is no curative therapy, it prevents the patient and family from developing a proactive management plan with the patient's full participation in what often becomes an increasingly difficult to manage chronic disease. In the latter case, the ultimate role of assessment is in determining prognosis and developing a care plan. Last, with the advent of new treatments for Alzheimer's disease (e.g., donepezil), delaying the diagnosis deprives patients of using proven therapies. Although the effect of medications on cognitive function can be modest, patients and families may chose treatment after alternatives and risks have been discussed.

When considering who should be assessed for dementia, one must take into account patient characteristics (risk factors or complaints of cognitive impairment), the stage or point of presentation, and the clinical context or setting of the assessment. There is currently little systematic information to guide the generalist health care provider as to which, or in fact whether all elders should be screened for dementia similar to routine blood pressure surveillance. There are few instances where dementia assessment should proceed in clearly asymptomatic people. These preclinical cases are currently restricted to the genetically determined dementias such as Huntington's disease or familial Alzheimer's disease, where family members may wish to have presymptomatic testing. Such evaluations should only proceed within the context of a genetic counseling, which provides education regarding the significance of positive and negative results, and psychological support.[35]

Routine screening may be indicated in the oldest old (people aged 85 years or older), given the high prevalence of cognitive impairment and dementia in this age group, and the high rate of functional impairment that dementia engenders. Table 21-3 lists triggers for assessment for dementia. The 25 percent to 30 percent of nondemented elders over age 65 who complain of memory im-

TABLE 21-3. TRIGGERS FOR ASSESSMENT FOR DEMENTIA

Triggers for assessment for dementia include problems with the following.
  Learning and retaining
  Handling complex tasks
  Reasoning
  Spatial ability and orienting
  Language
  Behavior

pairment,[32, 36, 37] may represent another group appropriate for cognitive screening. Some people with memory complaints have mild dementia, whereas others are at high risk of developing dementia, especially if they have objective evidence of memory dysfunction on formal testing.[38] Clinical assessments in cases with subjective complaints are primarily focused on mild symptoms and similar to the patient who presents for assessment with early, but definite cognitive impairment. On the other hand, dementia assessments in more advanced stages of disease focus on quite different aspects of the dementia syndrome, which tend to predominate in later disease. Often, the etiologic diagnosis may have already been established and the assessment challenge is directed at other signs and symptoms such as neurologic deficits, functional impairment, or behavioral disturbances.

Stages of Dementia

A number of staging systems can aid the health care provider in determining to what point along the clinical continuum an individual patient has progressed. To properly apply these ratings, one needs to perform a comprehensive evaluation including a cognitive and functional assessment, outlined as follows. Two systems, the Global Deterioration Scale (GDS) (see Appendix #20)[39] and the Clinical Dementia Rating Scale (CDR;) (see Chapter 3, Table 3-11),[40, 41] are widely recognized. The GDS describes seven levels of cognitive and functional change ranging from none to very severe cognitive decline. The first two stages are not accompanied by significant functional deficits and thus, encompass most patients presenting without obvious histories of impairment. For example, a GDS stage of 2 should describe a patient with concern about his or her memory without objective deficits of memory on office testing. Such systems can only be a gross guide, however, as there are no sharp demarcations between "normal" and deficient cognitive performance or, at later stages, between severe and very severe cognitive deterioration. Further, depending on age, cultural background, education, gender, or work or social situation demands, functional decline might be perceived at different points in time despite equivalent levels of memory or cognitive impairment.

The CDR has five levels of staging: normal (0), questionable (0.5), mild (1.0), moderate (2.0), and severe (3.0) dementia. Recently, two further stages termed profound (4.0) and terminal (5.0) have been added. The CDR simultaneously describes the dementia syndrome stage across six factors: memory, orientation, judgment, problem solving, community affairs, home and hobbies, and personal care. To be applied properly, it requires a semistructured interview.

Perhaps the simplest system is the three-stage system of the DSM-III-R, where once memory and at least one other area of cognitive function are impaired, the following stages are recognized: (1) mild dementia: impairment of work or social activities, but capacity for independent living remains, with relatively intact judgment and adequate personal hygiene; (2) moderate dementia: some supervision is necessary, independent living is hazardous; and (3) severe dementia: activities of daily living are so impaired that continual supervision is required (e.g., unable to maintain minimal personal hygiene, largely incoherent, or mute).

The Setting for Assessments

Aside from the ways in which the type of patient and the clinical stage of presentation will affect who has a dementia assessment, the place in which the patient resides or in which the assessment takes place can also significantly determine not only who is assessed, but how the assessment is carried out. The majority of assessments are likely to occur in the primary care outpatient clinic or office setting. These settings produce several important challenges. Not the least of these challenges is the limited time that may be available to interview not only the patient, but a collateral historian as well, and then to perform a complete mental status examination. For the specialist, the patients evaluated may be referred for a second opinion, for special documentation of clinical status such as mental competency or for research purposes. From time to time, health care providers may be asked to evaluate patients in the hospital setting. Here, patients are likely to be on multiple medications or have alterations in their level of consciousness, making some acutely confused patients appear to be demented unless proper assessment for delirium is made. Another institutional setting that is likely to engender yet another set of evaluations is the long-term care facility ranging from residential care facilities to nursing homes. Because the majority of residents in these settings are cognitively impaired, it is almost always appropriate to perform an assessment for dementia. These assessments are often focused on behavioral changes, neurologic signs, and functional abilities.

HOW TO ASSESS
Principles of the Dementia Assessment

It is frightening to confront the loss of one's mental life. When there is little insight or concern, patients with early dementia may be suspicious or paranoid about an assessment that inquires into

The key to the diagnosis of dementia is a careful history, taken from both the patient and a reliable informant, focusing on main symptoms. This is complemented by a symtematic mental status evaluation, a physical and neurologic examination, and appropriate laboratory tests.

their thinking abilities. Thus, it is important at the very outset to put patients at ease. Loss of cognitive processing speed occurs in the majority of dementias. Histories and examinations conducted at a rapid pace are unlikely to be informative. There can be a tendency to ignore the patient after it is apparent that the history they can provide will be unreliable. It is always appropriate to at least state to the patient that because there is some concern about his or her memory; many questions will be posed to his or her spouse or companion, although he or she should feel free to speak up at any time. From time to time during such interviews, the patients can be asked for their input to continue to involve them in the interview. In some instances, this is obviously disruptive, in which case it can be more appropriate to press on to the examination and to plan to obtain further history at a later point, when the collateral historian can be interviewed separately.

Perhaps no other principle is as important in the assessment of dementia as obtaining a reliable history. Since implicit in the definition of dementia is a change or decline in cognitive or functional abilities from a previous level, the examiner must be able to establish in what way and to what degree this has occurred. Impaired insight regarding deficits in early dementia will often require a collateral informant. This is usually a spouse or an adult child. With proper consent, other family members, friends and other health care providers (e.g., social workers) are often helpful.

Sometimes, obtaining the history from family members can create disagreement. A common scenario is a longtime spouse who is not aware of how much answering he or she has begun to perform for the spouse. Children who may only see their parents infrequently, on the other hand, can be struck by changes that are not as apparent to the spouse. Thus, just as one gauges the degree to which the patient can provide a reliable history, it is equally important to monitor the insight of collateral informants. This is particularly important among elders or in certain cultures where an attitude that memory loss is an acceptable or expected part of aging can lead to minimization of symptoms. Older collateral informants may themselves have memory impairment.[42] This has an important impact on both the reliability of the interview, as well as on future planning for the patient and care provider. It is also important to keep in mind that many people may not want to contradict or upset their spouse or parent during the history taking. They may minimize any deficiencies during the interview. Thus, it is important to gauge the reaction of the collateral historian during the interview, and to plan to ask them if they felt comfortable with the account as told by the patient or if they had to "hold back" for fear of upsetting the patient.

In order to obtain a reliable history, it is of value to focus on single events or activities and the way in which the patient performed during these occasions. Specific examples of memory lapses are more revealing than more general descriptions. Signal events might be forgetting prominent events or important appointments, getting lost in familiar places, consistently losing household or personal items, or an inability to solve problems or follow instructions. Reviewing the activities of a typical day from rising in the morning to going to bed at night can be highly revealing if each component step (e.g., dressing, preparing meals, driving, recalling events during the day later in the evening) is queried. This also is a useful way of establishing a baseline of function.

In addition to focusing on cognitive performance, the patient's personality and behavior should be specifically addressed. These changes are often present in early or mild dementia.[43] In patients with Alzheimer's disease, approximately half of all families will, in retrospect, recall changes other than memory as the first sign of the dementia syndrome.[44] Most often, families report a change toward being more withdrawn, less talkative, and less open to new ideas or activities.[43, 44] Alternatively, the patient may appear less mature, more suspicious, anxious, impatient, and irritable. Many families interpret these changes as a mild depression or change of life associated with the frustrations of aging. On the other hand, significant depression or major affective disorder is an important concomitant or even precursor of dementia. After a 3-year follow-up of 225 nondemented depressed elderly patients presenting to a dementia assessment clinic, 57 percent had developed a clear dementia syndrome.[45] Nonaffective, noncognitive behavioral symptoms, especially prominent delusions, hallucinations, and poor judgment, which appear early in the course of the dementia, can be important diagnostic clues to several non-Alzheimer dementias.

Approximately 10 percent of patients with Alzheimer's disease will, prior to memory failure, have more apparent disorientation to time or place, language difficulties (aphasia), or dyspraxia.[44] These nonmemory deficits at presentation can suggest other neurologic disorders ranging from vascular dementia to relatively rare neurodegenerative syndromes such as corticobasal ganglionic degeneration.[46]

Aside from the assessment of cognition and behavioral change, an important element of the history of dementia is the functional ability of the patient. Functional assessment is discussed in general in Chapter 2. Functional assessment of the demented patient is usually divided into basic and more complex or instrumented activities of daily living (IADLs). Complex tasks, such as managing finances, tracking medications, or maintaining a household, become impaired earliest in the course of dementia. Typically, the early patient will have no difficulty with basic activities such as eating, dressing, grooming and bathing, toileting and mobility. Determining these functional landmarks is critical for making recommendations and designing a comprehensive care plan. They represent highly relevant markers of progression of dementia.[47] As previously noted, one efficient means of obtaining this information is by asking the patient and family to describe a typical day. More structured or formal scales exist to test functional abilities and these are discussed in the following sections.

Past Medical and Family History

A complete review of the past medical history is essential. Whenever possible, previous medical records should be obtained for review. The examiner must be careful to independently judge the patient and not to be unduly biased by medical records, as some health care providers in the past have indiscriminately labeled cognitively impaired elders as having "senile dementia" or Alzheimer's disease without considering further evaluation. In the setting of dementia assessment, those medical conditions that are most likely to compromise brain function either in a primary or secondary role need to be reviewed. In elders, vascular disease and its risk factors (e.g., hypertension, diabetes, and cardiac arrhythmias) are often present and must be assessed for their potential role in the dementing symptoms or signs, and as comorbid conditions whose management can be affected by the presence of dementia.[48] Prior history of complex partial seizures, transient ischemic attacks, or recurrent syncope must be carefully considered. Various chronic medical conditions that may appear minor must be reviewed and include endocrine disturbances, anemia, cancer, vitamin deficiencies and, infections. Alcohol use must be carefully reviewed.

The average community-dwelling elder fills 13 prescriptions during the course of a year and takes 3 to 4 medications.[49] Many of these drugs have central nervous system side effects. Particularly important to review are medications with sedating effects, anxiolytics, and anticholinergic medications including antidepressants. Over-the-counter medications such as ibuprofen or antihistamines, and others, can cause confusion in elders and may be forgotten unless specifically queried.[50]

It is important to assess the family history for related disorders.[51] In general, for autosomal dominant disorders such as some familial Alzheimer's disease pedigrees, two or more first-degree relatives in successive generations must be clearly affected in order to establish this pattern. This can be difficult for a number of reasons. First, even though parents of the current generation of elders may have had dementia in some cases, symptoms may have been accepted as a normal accompaniment of aging. Asking if the parent exhibited persistent memory loss, difficulty recognizing family members, or died in a nursing home can be more informative than asking if a parent had Alzheimer's disease. Second, small families, or families where relatives died at a young age from illnesses unrelated to dementia, may not allow accurate assessment of risk in the current generation because too few relatives may have lived to an old enough age to have become demented. This is particularly true in late-onset dementias. In addition to some forms of Alzheimer's disease, frontotemporal dementia,[52] Huntington's disease, Gerstmann-Straussler disease, Creutzfeld-Jakob disease, and cases of vascular dementia[53] can all demonstrate strong familial aggregation.

Examination of the Patient

Although the mental status examination is the central focus of the patient assessment for dementia, the general physical examination is essential. The examination is informed by clues from the history and review of the major organ systems. Sensory deficits are very common with usual aging and a thorough assessment of hearing and vision, with appropriate intervention, has the practical potential of optimizing the function of a cognitively impaired person. The mental status examination will be significantly affected by the patient's ability to hear and see.

The neurologic examination extends the history and often indicates which brain areas or levels of the neuraxis are involved. This is particularly useful in aiding the differential diagnosis of dementia. Thus, a systematic review of the cranial nerves, motor systems, reflexes, gait and posture, and sensory function are all part of the thorough assessment of dementia. Evidence of focal signs raises the suspicion of cerebrovascular disease or other structural brain pathology. The presence of unexplained focal signs requires a neuroimaging study.[54]

The cranial nerve examination can reveal an abnormal sense of smell in the most common dementias. This has been considered to be an early sign of Alzheimer's disease, but also declines with uncomplicated aging. Decrements in smooth pursuit and saccadic eye movements are seen in Alzheimer's disease, but this is difficult to distinguish clinically from uncomplicated aging. A diminished excursion of the eyes in voluntary upward gaze is common with healthy aging. On the other hand, impairment of downward gaze (pursuit, saccades, or optokinetically induced), which can be overcome by oculocephalic maneuvers (passive head movements) can

The neurologic examination in patients with dementia can reveal typical, but exaggerated, age-related changes such as slowing, parkinsonism, gait abnormalities, or focal neurologic changes.

be somewhat more specific in pointing to the possible presence of early progressive supranuclear palsy (PSP),[55] or rarely, other disorders including cerebrovascular disease. Dementia in PSP is usually mild or absent when the eye signs first appear.[56]

Many dementias especially affect the motor systems. Examination for signs of parkinsonism includes assessment of muscle tone, speed and quality of movement, and posture. Loss of arm swing, short steps, and shuffling of the feet can characterize gait. Hydrocephalus or bilateral frontal lobe damage are characterized by a wide-based, hesitant, "magnetic" gait, with prominent difficulty initiating walking and turning. There can be increased tone, predominantly in the legs. Extensor plantar responses (Babinski sign) can be present. Both syndromes are associated with prominent dementia. Longitudinal studies have shown that extrapyramidal signs (resting tremor, rigidity, akinesia or slowing, and gait impairment)[57] and motor slowing[58] may be present in patients destined to develop Alzheimer's disease prior to the development of dementia.

Primitive reflexes or release signs such as the grasp, snout, or the palmomental sign are observed in an optimally healthy elderly.[59] When they are easy to elicit, prominent, or present in a younger person, these reflexes can indicate a pathologic disorder. When asymmetrical or unilateral, these indicate focal cerebral pathology, until proven otherwise. Abnormal involuntary movements, such as tremor and myoclonus, should also be watched for. Myoclonus is seen in about 10 percent of late-stage Alzheimer's disease patients, but if it appears early in the course of dementia, suggests Creutzfeld-Jakob disease. Aside from decreased vibratory sense in the toes, the sensory examination should not be impaired in the healthy elder. Absent vibration sense, or the loss of other sensory modalities (position sense, pinprick sensation, and light touch), suggests a neuropathy or myelopathy and can serve as a clue to a systemic disease causing the dementia such as a vitamin deficiency, collagen vascular disorder, or vasculitis.

Mental Status Examination for Dementia

It is important to ensure the patient's best possible performance during the mental status examination. A magnifying glass and a simple battery operated microphone-amplifier device are useful tools to have in the office to assist patients with vision or hearing impairment. The patients age, level of education, possible life-long weaknesses (e.g., "math-phobia," dyslexia) or strengths (e.g., professional mnemonist), primary language, and socioeconomic and cultural background can influence performance on the cognitive examination, and need to be considered in interpreting performance.

Much can be learned by simply observing the patient. It should be apparent long before the formal mental status examination whether the patient is attentive, conversant, and at ease with the examiner. Patients who are paranoid, or have poor attention, may only answer a few questions and then refuse to proceed further. Thus, careful consideration should be made as to the few key questions that might be successfully completed in such a potentially limited examination.

Behavioral or mood state can effect responses on mental status testing. These must be considered before proceeding with assessing cognitive function. A patient who complains somewhat bitterly about memory failure, and then proceeds to recall several specific instances of this failure may be depressed. The subsequent examination in depressed patients can be colored by frequent, I can't do that, or, I don't know, answers despite being able to perform some of the tasks quite well if coaxed. These patients will classically appear to have little energy, make poor eye contact, be slow to respond, and show incongruous or patchy strengths across multiple cognitive domains. Addressing the issue by asking the patients if they are depressed, sad or blue, should be done, at a minimum. Asking about anhedonia, guilt, sleep disturbance, and appetite loss can be nearly as effective as more detailed assessments in screening for depression, but more time efficient.[60, 61] More detailed assessment instruments (described later) are more sensitive, and are useful in tracking changes with treatment.

The specific setting dictates the form of the mental status examination. For screening patients with low suspicion of cognitive impairment, an abbreviated clinical mental status examination is reasonable in the context of a busy primary care setting, bearing in mind that some cases of early asymptomatic cognitive impairment will be missed. In a patient with a clear complaint, or history suggesting dementia, a more complete mental status examination is necessary. In the following description of cognitive function assessment, a relatively complete, although not exhaustive clinical mental status examination is described (Table 21-4). This examination can be modified according to the patient and the setting in which the evaluation is performed. After presenting this examination, an abbreviated approach will be presented for screening in the active primary care office or at the bedside. Finally, the use of more formal screening instruments and the role of neuropsychological consultations will be presented.

Language assessment begins during the initial conversation with the patient before any formal testing has occurred. Attention should be paid to the patients use of grammar and syntax. Does

A core mental status evaluation can include assessment of spontaneous speech, registration of four or more words, listing as many animals as possible in 1 minute, clock drawing, and testing recall without and with cueing.

Exaggerated complaints of cognitive impairment, lack of effort, and frequent "don't know" answers on the mental status examination in a patient who has a depressed affect suggests a diagnosis of depression.

TABLE 21-4. ITEMS IN A CLINICAL COGNITIVE ASSESSMENT FOR DEMENTIA	
COGNITIVE DOMAIN	TASK EXAMPLES[a]
Attention and concentration	Digit spans
Memory	Recall of old knowledge
	Immediate and delayed recall
Language	Spontaneous speech
	Verbal fluency
	Naming
	Comprehension
Visuospatial perception	Clock or figure drawing
Reasoning and abstract concept formation	Word pair association
	Solving crisis situations

[a]Many tasks tap more than one domain.

the patient speak in full sentences or is there reduced fluency? The average English speaker uses phrases that are at least 5 words in length. Are there frequent pauses for word finding and are there paraphasic errors (replacing words, sounds, and letters with erroneous ones) such as "hog" for "dog." Paraphasic errors are seen in patients with progressive aphasias, stroke, or Alzheimer's disease. Does the patient tend to be echolalic (repeat what you say) or produce intrusions of incongruous words or phrases?

Rather than beginning with the classic question, can you tell me today's date, it is less off-putting to begin to assess longer term memory along with orientation by asking questions about specific current events and important life events. The examiner can begin this by asking the patient to give autobiographic details such as their place and date of birth, education, and job history. The examiner can then begin to discuss current events. Obviously, establish the correct answers to these questions must be established.

It is useful to describe and give simple examples of what the patient is asked to do. Because memory function is prominently effected in many dementias, it should be assessed fully and early in the mental status evaluation. Since most patients will have some understanding that the reason for the assessment is related to problems with memory, many questions can be framed in these terms. Attention and concentration can be assessed by asking the patient to "recall" or repeat some numbers after he or she is told them: "so if I say 1-2-3, you say 1-2-3; listen first, then repeat". All elders should be able to repeat at least 5 digits forward. The more difficult task of reversing the number strings can logically be asked next.

Most elders can correctly reverse at least 4 digits. This reversal task taps several mental faculties including immediate recall of the forward number string, maintenance of the string in mind, and serial reversal. This task taps working memory.

The tradition of giving the patient three words to remember for later recall is not sensitive for detection of early dementia. It is better to present to the patient at least four words, which the examiner asks for immediate repetition and then later recall after distracter tasks.[62] The words should be in unrelated categories (e.g., rose, swallow, trombone, and brown) so that if, on later recall, they cannot be remembered, a superordinate cue or category prompt such as "it was a flower" can be presented. Elders should be able to immediately repeat the four words. If there is difficulty with this immediate registration, the individual should be given the words multiple times (up to five times). This is an attempt to have them learn the list; then proceed to other "distracter" tasks (see the following) before coming back to the word list later to assess delayed recall. Visual or place memory can be tested in patients who give a history of losing or misplacing items by placing four objects around the room for later identification.

Another sensitive, time efficient approach to memory assessment is adapted from a standardized test, the Rey Auditory Verbal List Learning Test.[63] The patient is sequentially presented with a list of common words (chimney, salt, harp, button, meadow, train, flower, finger, rug, and book) each on a 3 × 5 card, and at each presentation, asked to use the word in a sentence. The list is then presented again and the patient is asked to use the words in a sentence, even if the sentence is the same as the one used previously. The patient is then asked to perform two other tasks that have been shown to be useful for detection of early dementia.

The first test examines concentration as well as verbal fluency by asking the patients to name as many animals as they can "recall" in 60 seconds. Again, the test is framed as a memory test for the patient, although strictly speaking, this task tests other domains, in particular generative category thinking characteristic of frontal lobe function. Most should be able to produce a list of at least 12 animals.

Similarly, the patient can be asked to produce as many words as he or she can recall that begin with a particular letter such as the letters F, A, or S. A cutoff of 11 words (mean of three lists) at any age or education is below age-expected performance. Age and education influence this test. Thus, the cutoff for a normal 70 to 75 year old with more than high school education is 20 words. These conservative cutoffs are approximately 2 standard deviations below the average performance at this age.[64] A discrepancy between category and word fluency can suggest early dementia consistent with Alzheimer's disease. This task should take about 4 to 5 minutes.

The examiner can then ask the patient to draw a clock and set the hands to read 10 minutes to 11. Drawing a clock has gained popularity as a planning and construction or visual-perceptive task for assessing dementia. Although it is a gross screen of both left (language dominant) and right hemisphere function, it is often not affected early in dementia. Clock drawing has the advantage of requesting the patient to reproduce a familiar item, containing details, and a natural symmetry. There are many scoring systems for this task. One simple approach is to rate the drawing on 5 key features that have been shown to suggest cerebral damage when present.[65, 66] These include: (1) omission or fragmentation of elements (numbers, hands); (2) poor integration (numbers not in sequence or off to one side); (3) distortion or rotation of the figure by more than 45 degrees (twisting or unusual outline to clock face); (4) perseveration or repetition of the clock or its elements; and (5) addition of extraneous elements.

At this point, 6 to 10 minutes have passed and the patient is now asked to recall as many of the words presented previously as he or she can. Most nonimpaired elders between ages 65 and 85 years can recall 6 ± 2 words from the 10-word list. This procedure, unlike many other dementia screening tests, is designed to examine those domains most likely to be effected early in dementia. The supraspan list of words exceeds the usual immediate recall limit of 7 ± 2. The procedure constrains and standardizes the way the participant learns, enhancing the normal opportunity to learn the list. Additionally, a reasonable time delay is interspersed to truly test delayed recall. Another similar combination of tests, using a different memory test, has been shown to be useful in assessing patients for dementia.[67]

If the examiner had given the patient a 4-word list, recall can be tested at this time. If he or she cannot recall the four words, category cues or prompts should be given for each missed item. If cues do not improve performance, then a list of three choices should be given. In this way, the examiner can estimate the degree to which delayed recall is impaired. An average person over age 65 should be able to recall at least three of the four words spontaneously and should improve with cues.

Language function is further tested by repetition of phrases such as "no ifs, ands, or buts." The patient is asked to demonstrate how they follow a sequence of tasks (language comprehension), such as asking the patient to point to the pen, the floor, and your nose. The inability to name objects is frequently an early sign of dementia. Asking the patient if they recall the name of items pointed to can test this. The items should include both relatively frequently (e.g., pen, shoe, and watch) and infrequently used words, including parts of the objects presented (e.g., clip, sole, and watch crystal or winder). An alternative means of performing the assessment of naming abilities (although not entirely equivalent) is to have a set of standard pictures for naming. In this version of the naming task, the test is posed as a screen for vision ("can you see this picture?"). For agitated demented patients, this can be a less "insulting" or embarrassing task. To complete the assessment of language function, the patient is next asked to read. For example, patients can be asked to read a simple sentence and do what it says. The patient can also be asked to read a paragraph from a magazine. Comprehension and recall of elements of the paragraph can subsequently be tested. The patients should be asked to write a complete sentence. Both reading and writing can amplify deficits seen in patients with aphasia. In addition to providing the assessment of written language abilities, writing allows the health care provider to further observe the patient's motor skills, monitoring for tremor or micrographia.

The composed, cooperative patient will have persevered through earlier questions. Patients with poor impulse control and easily agitated may also have complied with this examination if the questions were posed as primarily a test of memory function, rather than as challenges of the patient's intelligence and reasoning. Judgment and reasoning skills, however, are especially important to test in this latter group of patients. Thus, it is recommended that the end of the mental status examination be reserved for testing so-called complex or higher-order mental faculties of reasoning and abstraction. An example of this is the ability to relate word pair similarities of increasing difficulty into a single class or related function. Some word pair examples to use are carrots–peas (vegetables), bicycle–train (transportation), painting–music (arts), and cat–goldfish (pets). A related higher order function is judgment, which can be tested by asking participants to provide verbal solutions to crisis or challenging situations. The patient's ability to approach the problem logically and come up with a reasonable plan is considered. The fact that the patient can give the appropriate response does not necessarily mean that in the actual situation he or she would perform according to the answer. Thus, the examiner might ask what the patient would do if they were walking in the woods and got lost or if they developed a flat tire on an abandoned road and discovered their spare tire was flat too. These situations can be made geographically and culturally appropriate.

The mental status examination takes approximately 20 to 25 minutes. This is a good investment in time. In some situations, however, such as when there is low suspicion for dementia or when the health care provider wishes to evaluate the cognitive function of a patient as part of a general health screen, an abbreviated approach can be taken. Memory function is the most important cognitive domain to tap for such a screening evaluation. It is less useful to ask about old, often over-learned information such as where the patient lives, or the name of the president, because this information will be preserved in many patients. The recall of three words with a short delay is also insensitive to early dementia.

Standardized Cognitive Tests

A large number of relatively brief screening tests are available for the assessment of dementia. These tests are reliable and useful measures of dementia.[68] They provide a numerical score that can be used to follow the patient over time, but are not a substitute for a careful history and examination.

Probably the best known of these mental status tests is the Mini-Mental State Examination (MMSE) (see Appendix #29).[69, 70] It is not a good test for detecting early or mild dementia. Although the items seem fairly straightforward, there is clear variability in the way the test is administered. The specific three words presented for recall are chosen at the examiner's discretion. Low frequency words make the recall task more difficult. The MMSE is brief, and usually takes less than 10 minutes to administer, but in some patients with motor or cognitive slowing, may take longer to complete. Because of its widespread use, however, it has to some degree become a common currency for describing the severity of dementia. Thus, when a health care provider in Tampa describes a patient with a MMSE score of 17, a provider in Portland has a good sense of that patient's gross level of cognitive function. Another advantage to the MMSE is that there are also numerous nonEnglish versions of the test.[71] Additionally, there is a wealth of research literature of its use in different clinical settings.[72] This literature has shown that, by and large, a score of 23 or less suggests cognitive impairment, although adjustments must be made for age, educational level, and ethnic or cultural background.[73, 74] In practice, scores of 0 to 10 are considered consistent with severe dementia, 11 to 20 moderate dementia, and above 21, mild dementia. The average annual rate of change on the MMSE has also been established as 2 to 5 points per year (in Alzheimer's disease patients) and can be used as a guide to the rate of progression of dementia.[75]

A number of other brief cognitive status tests are also available. These include the Blessed information–Memory–Concentration Test (IMCT),[76] Short Portable Mental Status Questionnaire (SPMSQ) (see Appendix #41),[77] and the Short Test of Mental Status.[78]

The Information–Memory–Concentration Mental Status Test (IMCT) has found wide use in North America and the United Kingdom. This 26-item test has been used frequently as a gross test of the correlation between cognitive function and the pathologic features of Alzheimer's disease. The original 26 items have been reduced to a short 6-item version (the Blessed Orientation–Memory–Concentration Test, BOMC), which contains a delayed recall item, asking the patient to remember a name and address after approximately 2 minutes delay. The test uses a weighted scoring system such that the memory item is given more significance to the total score. Thus, out of a possible total error score of 28, 10 points are added to the total if the name and address cannot be recalled. Ninety percent of nonimpaired elders (mean age, 87) have a weighted error score of 6 or less on the BOMC.[79] The average annual rate of change of the error score is 4 ± 3.6 (SD) points.[80] In severely impaired patients, the test is not sensitive to change. There is considerable overlap in the performance of patients on the BOMC and the MMSE, with a correlation of up to −0.83 between tests.[81] Telephone administration of this test (which requires no visual materials) has been shown to correlate with in-person administration results.[82]

The Short Test of Mental Status is another brief test that screens 8 cognitive domains yielding a maximum correct score of 38.[78] This screening test is a relative newcomer and has not been used as widely as the MMSE or the BOMC, but has the advantage of providing a potentially more sensitive measure of delayed recall with a list of four words for recall and a delay occurring over a 5-minute period. A cutoff of less than 31 is suggested as indicative of dementia with an age adjustment of 1 point subtracted from the 31-point cutoff for each decade over the age of 50.[83] The reported sensitivity is approximately 86 percent to patients with dementia. Not surprisingly, the STMS is well correlated with the MMSE (0.74) and the Blessed (−0.86) Scales.

The 10-item Short Portable Mental Status Questionnaire (SPMSQ) is perhaps the briefest of all formal cognitive screening scales taking only several minutes to complete in the relatively intact elder.[77] Most nondemented persons miss less than two of the ten items. On the 9-item version (deleting the question, "What is the name of this place?"), community-based elders, ages 85 to 89, made on average 4 errors.[84] More than other brief measures, the SPMSQ relies heavily on old learning and orientation and has no questions addressing new learning or recall. Similar to most short composite batteries such as the MMSE, it is not sensitive to detecting early dementia. These short tests tend to ignore cognitive abilities associated with the frontal lobes such as executive function. A recent study, using a number of tests sensitive to executive function, found that these abilities may be particularly important factors in determining the level of care needed by elders.[85]

Aside from these brief batteries, there are also what might be called intermediate length cognitive survey batteries. These include the Mattis Dementia Rating Scale (MDRS),[86] the Alzheimer Disease Assessment Scale (ADAS),[87] the Neurobehavioral Cognitive Status Examination (NCSE),[88] and expanded versions of the Mini-Mental State Examination (e.g., the 3MS).[89] These scales are all more comprehensive in the scope of cognitive domains tested than the brief scales described. In general, they take at least 15 to 20 minutes, or longer, to administer depending on the level of impairment of the demented patient. Both the MDRS and the NCSE are designed to have a screening item for each domain so that if the patient passes that item, he or she immediately proceeds to the next question. Thus, a cognitively intact individual can proceed quite quickly through these examinations. The ADAS has, in addition to a survey of the pertinent cognitive domains, an assessment of the patient's noncognitive or behavioral symptoms. The cognitive portion of the ADAS has been widely used as an outcome measure in clinical drug trials. It does not have a metric that allows a participant to pass to the next item and, therefore, can take up to 20 minutes to administer.

Finally, more in depth, detailed tests of cognitive function can be obtained through a complete neuropsychologic evaluation performed by a qualified neuropsychologist. These evaluations are especially useful in several situations: (1) to demonstrate subtle cognitive impairment in early cases or in individuals with high premorbid cognitive skills; (2) to evaluate in greater detail patients presenting with relatively isolated impairments such as in primary progressive aphasia[90] or frontotemporal dementia; (3) to distinguish depression from dementia; (4) to distinguish malingering from dementia: and (5) to document decision-making capacity. Some familiarity with the standardized tests and approaches used by the neuropsychologist allow the request for evaluation to be more focused.[91]

Behavioral Assessment of Dementia

The original case of dementia reported in 1907 by Alois Alzheimer was noteworthy for the presence of behavioral disturbances consisting of paranoia and personality change. These and other noncognitive symptoms may be present at any time in the course of most dementias, but commonly, specific types of behavioral disturbances are observed during discrete periods of the illness.[92] In Alzheimer's disease, depressive symptoms are present early and may even be a presenting sign in retrospect. Anxiety and irritability can also be present early, but increase in frequency with more advanced disease. Delusions are usually not observed initially, but are more common in mid-course of the dementia. Hallucinations, most commonly visual or auditory, are generally observed somewhat after delusions. Patients with primary visual or auditory deficits can be especially prone to hallucinations. This pattern of behavioral expression can differ in patients with dementias affecting the frontal lobes. Thus, early inappropriate social behavior, irritability, or delusions can be observed. In dementia with Lewy bodies, visual hallucinations are a prominent, early feature.[12]

It is common that the more disruptive symptoms will be brought up at the interview by the family. In some cases, however, the behaviors are considered bizarre or embarrassing, especially if of a sexual nature, and unless the clinician inquires specifically about behavioral change, these can go unreported. Rarely, patients with relatively intact insight experience hallucinations, which are troubling to them, but are not reported by them so as not to appear "crazy." Again, specific inquiry must be made.

A number of instruments have been designed to assess noncognitive symptoms in dementia. These generally address either a single symptom complex such as depressive symptoms or agitation.[93] Other scales are more inclusive, surveying multiple behavioral domains including depression, anxiety, agitation, delusions, and hallucinations. Until relatively recently, there were few scales that were designed specifically for dementia patients. Many were adapted from the general or psychiatric assessment. Among widely used depressive symptom inventories that were used in assessment and adapted for patients with dementia are the Hamilton Depression Scale[94] and the Geriatric Depression Scale[95] (see Appendix #16). The latter is a self-administered questionnaire that is valid in patients with a MMSE score above 15/30. The Cornell Scale for Depression in Dementia specifically targets dementia patients.[96] It requires a semistructured interview of the patient and a collateral informant. These single symptom domain scales are useful when there is a prominent behavioral sphere that is affected and the patient is to be followed for changes in behavioral status after institution of therapy.

A growing number of more broadly based screening instruments for noncognitive or behavioral symptoms in dementia (including depression) are available.[97] These include the behavioral portion of the Alzheimer's Disease Assessment Scale,[87] the Behavior Pathology in Alzheimer's Disease Rating Scale,[98] the CERAD Behavior Rating Scale for Dementia,[99] the Neuropsychiatric Inventory (NPI),[100] the Revised Memory and Behavior Problem (RMBPC) Checklist[101] and the Columbia Rating Scale for Psychopathology in Alzheimer's disease.[102] Although these scales are useful for assessing a broad range of behavioral changes, their major

Behavioral symptoms, including anxiety, agitation, aggression, depression, sleep disruption, delusions, hallucinations, repetitive behaviors, and wandering, occur commonly in patients with dementia. These should be addressed regularly in the follow-up of patients with dementia.

drawback is that some take up to 45 minutes to administer. The NPI and the RMBPC take approximately 20 minutes to administer.

Functional Assessment Scales

As noted earlier, the definition of dementia in some diagnostic systems, such as the DSM-IV, includes not only cognitive impairment for the diagnosis of dementia, but also functional decline. Assessing functional decline in dementia is particularly important because these abilities are key to the patient's maintenance of a relatively independent life. This element of the history is usually based on queries related to the ability to perform common basic and more complex activities of daily living. Performance based tests where the individual is observed completing the tasks may have greater face validity, but require props and more time to administer. Several brief scales have been developed to quantify the level of functional abilities. Most of these rely on the history of a caregiver or person living with the patient to provide his or perception of what the patient can or cannot do. The Katz Index of Activities of Daily Living is among the briefest scales assessing bathing, dressing, toileting, transfer, continence, and feeding[103] (see Appendix #24). Obviously, this kind of scale will only be sensitive to those with already significantly compromised function. Other scales such as the Blessed Dementia Rating Scale (IADL portion),[76] the OARS Multidimensional Functional Assessment Questionnaire (in it's abbreviated form),[104] or the Philadelphia Geriatric Center Instrumental Activities of Daily Living Scale[105] and the functional assessment questionnaire[106] additionally survey more complex tasks. These include orienting in the community, shopping, meal preparation, housework, and handling money. Recently developed instruments have attempted to address both the severity and duration of functional impairment in dementia patients.[47] Staging instruments such as the Clinical Dementia Rating Scale[41] or the Global Deterioration Scale[39] rely not only on cognitive function, but the level of functional abilities. This later approach has the advantage of combining both major domains into a global score, thus integrating both the cognitive impairment and functional disabilities. Individual function items can be recorded separately for later referral by the health care provider.

Impairment in activities of daily living (e.g., walking, dressing, bathing, and grooming) and instrumental activities of daily living (e.g., bill paying, taking medications, shopping, transportation, and telephoning) develop over the course of dementia, and should be systematically addressed during follow-up to identify care needs.

Social and Caregiver Assessment

Dementia significantly affects not just an individual patient, but an entire family. Assessment of the caregiver and family has an important place in the dementia evaluation.[107] The psychosocial interview should be considered preventative medicine. It is a means of preparing or maintaining the caregiver to most effectively cope with the demands of dementia care. In the outpatient setting, the health care provider should, at a minimum, review the caregiver's knowledge about the dementing disorder, the caregiver's capacity to provide quality care, the extent of outside support, and the degree to which advanced directives have been addressed. Depending on the stage of dementia, safety issues such as driving and the use of firearms should be frankly reviewed. After the initial assessments, or during the moderate stages of dementia, alternative care contingency plans should be addressed. In some instances, the caregiver may need referral for mental health services or a support group. All families should be aware of the resources available through the national Alzheimer's Association (**www.alz.org**).

Laboratory Tests

The use of laboratory testing in the assessment of dementia is a natural extension of the history and physical examination (Table 21-5). The blood tests may uncover previously unsuspected disorders in a cost effective fashion,[108] and are currently recommended in the United States.[2, 3]

Clinical experience teaches that certain signs or symptoms are more likely to yield a positive or "diagnostic" test result; they raise the probability that a condition is present. The impact of a diagnostic test on making a specific diagnosis depends on the prior probability of the condition (which is affected by clinical signs and symptoms), the prevalence of the condition, and how good the test is. For example, a very low vitamin B_{12} level is very specific for having a clinically relevant vitamin deficiency. It has a high likelihood ratio (the probability that a test outcome is the result of a disease entity divided by the probability that the test result would be associated with an absence of the disease). Thus, a low vitamin B_{12} level greatly increases the likelihood of having this clinical disorder. Conversely, a normal level is rarely associated with dementia related to B_{12} deficiency. The pretest probability or odds of a disease associated with an abnormality is clearly dependent on the prevalence of the disease in the population being studied. In the case of vitamin B_{12} testing, patients with anemia and a macrocytosis would have an increased likelihood of dementia related to cobalamin deficiency. The presence of a neuropathy and gait abnormalities would further increase the likelihood. If two conditions are common, it is plausible that they might coexist by chance alone.

Core laboratory investigations in patients with dementia include a complete blood count, glucose, electrolytes, including calcium, liver and renal function tests, urinalysis, vitamin B_{12} level, thyroid function tests, and a CT scan in most patients.

TABLE 21-5. TESTS USED IN THE ASSESSMENT OF DEMENTIA	
Blood	Metabolic-chemistry screen (electrolytes including calcium, liver and renal function tests)[a]
	Complete blood count[a]
	Vitamin B_{12} level[a]
	Thyroid function tests[a]
	Folate level
	Toxicology
	Syphilis serology
	Sedimentation rate
	HIV studies
Urine	Urinalysis[a]
	Culture
	Toxicology
Cerebrospinal fluid	Cell count
	Chemistry
	Special antibody tests (β-amyloid, tau, 14-3-3, etc.)
	Cytology
	Cultures
	PCR tests (Whipple's, herpes, etc.)
Cardiorespiratory	Routine
	Holter monitor
	Chest x-ray
Neuropsychologic evaluation	Psychometric testing
Electroencephalogram	Routine
	Sleep deprived
	Sleep studies
Neuroimaging	Computed tomography
	Magnetic resonance imaging
	Single photon emission computed tomography
	Positron emission tomography

[a]These tests are the most commonly used. The use of any ancillary laboratory test depends on the history and examination. An algorithm and patient information can be found on the Alzheimer's Association website (www.alz.org).

Unfortunately, for even the most relatively common conditions, estimates of the pretest odds of a particular diagnosis may not be known. Moreover, likelihood ratios for common tests are not widely available.[109] Frequently, there are gray zones such as the "low-normal" cobalamin level where a more sensitive or specific test such as a methylmalonic acid or homocysteine level may be required for diagnosis. The sensitivity and specificity of many tests are further dependent on the age of an individual. Often, there is little test performance data for the oldest old, a section of the population with the highest prevalence of dementia. Finally, many dementing disorders are relatively rare and the ability to collect true sensitivity and specificity data is practically limited by their infrequency in the population.

Given these considerations there is a series of tests that have been found to be useful in many instances for the diagnosis of dementia (Table 21-5). These include complete blood count, serum electrolytes, glucose, blood urea nitrogen, creatinine, liver function tests, thyroid function tests (thyroid stimulating hormone and free thyroid index), serum vitamin B_{12}, and syphilis serology.[110] Other tests that may be useful but clearly depend on clinical circumstance are serum folate, sedimentation rate, HIV testing, urine analysis, urine collection for heavy metals, and toxicology screens. A minimum screen that has been suggested is a complete blood count, chemistry panel, and thyroid function tests.[111]

As noted previously, determination of apolipoprotein E genotype has been found to significantly influence the risk of Alzheimer's disease.[28] The association is not absolute, however, and cannot be used to predict with certainty exactly when or if an individual will develop Alzheimer's disease.[112, 113] informed risk estimates must take into account the patient's age, gender, degree of vascular disease, family history of dementia, and ethnic background. The relatively rare genetic mutations on chromosomes 21, 14, and 1 that cause Alzheimer's disease can be identified. Genetic testing for these rare mutations which occur predominantly in early onset familial Alzheimer's disease, should be done only with the guidance of a genetic counseling program.

Among the more controversial tests to order is a neuroimaging study of the brain; either computed tomography (CT) or magnetic resonance imaging (MRI). These studies should be considered, although not necessarily ordered, in all patients evaluated for dementia. The true yield of these studies is difficult to determine in that there is little population-based data to guide the prior probability of finding the most common treatable brain lesions likely to be discovered by CT or MRI. A recent study based on retrospective record review of over 30,000 patients age 65 years or older with chart-based documentation of "clinically significant" subdural hematoma, hydrocephalus, and intracranial tumors suggested that these lesions rarely presented as isolated dementia.[114] Others have reached similar conclusions from the perspective of specialty clinics.[34, 48] The frequency with which these lesions are missed (i.e., not reported or recorded in general practice), however, is not known. A study of the cost-effectiveness of CT or MRI in the diagnosis of dementia considered several levels of "best-case" or "worse case" scenarios and concluded that given the high cost of long-term care, CT was probably cost effective despite the relative rarity of discovering occult pathology because only a few missed cases will result in the need for expensive long-term care.[115]

Another argument for performing imaging studies is often not fully expressed, but commonly practiced. This is the practice of obtaining an imaging study to support a diagnosis and give the family and patient closure on the final diagnosis of a fatal disease. Thus, the identification of large temporal horns in a 65-year-old patient with classic symptoms of Alzheimer's disease is useful confirmatory diagnostic information. Although, it will not change management, the comfort that a family takes in knowing that a stroke or mass lesion has been ruled out is not easily measured and has not been extensively studied.

In lieu of better data to guide ordering of neuroimaging studies, several pragmatic recommendations can be made. Patients less than about age 70 years should be imaged unless there is an obvious medical cause for the dementia. This is because the incidence of degenerative dementias such as Alzheimer's disease is relatively rare in this age group. Any patient with a history of transient neurologic deficit or focal signs is clearly a candidate for neuroimaging. Patients with new onset of headache, ataxia, visual field obscuration or defect, and seizures are also appropriate candidates, regardless of age. In general, patients presenting with early cognitive impairment of duration less than a year, and thus most likely to have reversible abnormalities if discovered on neuroimaging, should be studied.[116] In clinics and medical practices where cognitive screening is routinely performed, this means that most patients with dementia will have at least a CT scan of the brain.

In patients with a suspected cerebrovascular cause of dementia, evaluation should be similar to that conducted for cerebrovascular disease in general and can include, in addition to CT or MRI scan, evaluation of the extra and intracranial vessels (e.g., carotid ultrasound, magnetic resonance angiography) as well as the cardiovascular system (e.g., electrocardiogram, chest x-ray, and echocardiography).

Other studies of the nervous system are applied selectively. Lumbar puncture for evaluation of cerebrospinal fluid (CSF) is generally reserved for cases of suspected infectious disease, demyelinating disease, vasculitis, or neoplastic disease. Recently, the identification of tau protein and the β amyloid (1-42) protein in CSF has suggested potential diagnostic utility for Alzheimer's disease[117, 118] but this is not yet an established test. In Creutzfeld-Jacob disease, abnormal cerebrospinal fluid proteins have been identified, which may aid in the differential diagnosis of patients with rapidly progressive dementia.[119, 120]

The electroencephalogram (EEG) is primarily of value in differentiating seizures as either a primary cause of dementia or as a signature of an underlying disease causing dementia. The EEG is very useful in the diagnosis of spongiform encephalopathies, such as Creutzfeldt-Jakob disease, where the distinctive periodic complexes are almost pathognomonic in the setting of a rapidly progressing dementia with myoclonus. Unfortunately, many cases do not develop characteristic EEG changes.[121]

Other studies are sometimes performed as diagnostic adjuncts, but their relative expense and uncertain sensitivity and specificity in routine clinical venues make their use more commonly restricted to research studies. Thus, single photon emission computed tomography (SPECT), which has generally been used to measure cerebral blood flow (rCBF), demonstrates characteristic patterns of rCBF in several dementing conditions. Most notably, patients with Alzheimer's disease show reduced rCBF in temporal and parietal lobe regions.[122, 123] Using current technology, such findings do not predict the development of dementia in patients with memory loss alone.[124,125] Patients with frontal lobe dementias of the non-Alzheimer type show reduced rCBF in the frontal lobes. Patients with multiple infarctions show asymmetrical and patchy rCBF deficits. These asymmetries can be indistinguishable from early Alzheimer's disease. Standardized application of SPECT can be helpful in the differential diagnosis of dementia.[126] Positron emission tomography (PET) is the quantitative cousin of SPECT, which cannot only measure rCBF but also glucose metabolism. This research tool produces similar patterns as the SPECT studies.

COMMON PROBLEMS IN ASSESSMENT

Mild or Early Cognitive Impairment

Among the more difficult assessment issues is the distinction between expected age-associated changes in cognitive function and deteriorating cognition indicative of early dementia. In this context, a large number of conditions have been described, although their long-term outcome is incompletely known (e.g., age-associated memory impairment, mild cognitive impairment, late-life forgetfulness, and age-associated cognitive impairment). In general, these conditions overlap but are not the same as the clinical and psychometric criteria required for these designations, which shift somewhat arbitrarily from author to author.[37, 127] Because changes with age are associated with a loss of efficiency of cognitive function (decreased speed and intermittent, nonrepetitive errors) as opposed to actual defective task performance (consistent inability to perform to criterion levels), the guidelines presented previously under the cognitive assessment section should suggest those areas where performance is pathologic. Nevertheless, since the transition from nonimpaired to dementia is a continuous function, there will be patients where the only practical recourse is to perform careful follow-up. It is these patients where careful documentation of baseline cognitive function is critical for diagnosis. In a study of 250 men and women between the ages of 60 and 78 years with subjective complaints of memory loss, Mini-Mental State Examination Scores above 23 and psychometric test scores *below* cutoffs considered objective evidence for memory impairment, only 9 percent met criteria for dementia after a mean of 3.6 years of follow-up.[128] Interestingly, about 14 percent of individuals demonstrated performance superior to their original level or no longer had subjective memory complaints suggesting that many younger elders turn out to be "worried well." Whereas people with documented severe memory impairment may be at greater risk of progression to dementia,[38] others with mild cognitive impairment may be less likely to decline.[129]

The Oldest Old

Most patients with dementia are among the oldest old. Alzheimer's disease is the most common etiology of dementia in this age group, but vascular ischemic dementia also occurs, given the exponential increase in the incidence of cerebrovascular disease with age.

The assessment of cognitive impairment consistent with dementia in those 85 years and older is fraught with potential difficulties. At the outset, some degree of hearing and vision deficits in this population are almost universal and can significantly affect the results of the cognitive assessment. There is a very high prevalence of dementia in this age group ranging from 25 percent[130] to up to 50 percent,[19] or more at the extremes of life.[131] Thus, there is a high statistical probability of just "guessing right" and this can bend the health care provider's judgment towards dementia as a diagnosis. Because most psychometric research on dementia in elders focused on the under 85 patient group, there has been relatively little psychometric test data to guide the health care provider as to what to expect either in the average oldest old[132–134] or in those who retain excellent health (so-called maximum expected function).[135] As in the very mild cognitively impaired younger patient, the only certain means of confirming the clinical diagnosis of early dementia in the oldest old is through well-documented follow-up.[135, 136]

Delirium

In the absence of a clear sensorium, reliable testing of multiple cognitive domains is not possible.[137, 138] Thus, any patient presenting with presumptive cognitive deficits needs to be first assessed for a disturbance in level of consciousness[139-141] and followed serially for fluctuations. The acute confusional state, or delirium, is commonly thought to present with acute onset. The agitated delirium patient may talk to himself or herself incoherently, with impaired flow of thought; be difficult to redirect; or thrash about in bed. Less well-recognized are patients with a quiet "apathetic" form of delirium where there is a less obvious abrupt onset with reduced motor activity and quiet speech, muttering, or no speech at all. Diagnostic confusion can result if it is not realized that dementia patients are more susceptible to delirium because of underlying compromised brain function. The two conditions often coexist. Thus, a new seemingly minor infection or drug can disrupt the patient's already compromised cerebral function and produce an acute confusional state. Up to 40 percent of all demented hospital patients will have delirium[142] and up to 25 percent of those initially diagnosed with delirium will be found to also have dementia.[143]

> It is critical to consider delirium in any patient with a fluctuating level of consciousness, and impaired attention and thought-processes. Delirious patients can be hyperactive or withdrawn and hypoactive.

Depression and Behavioral Disturbances

As noted, many patients with cognitive deficits will appear withdrawn, less communicative, and sad. Those in whom depression is responsible for these symptoms may complain bitterly of their forgetfulness, out of proportion to the degree of memory impairment documented on examination. Such patients will characteristically pepper their efforts with a despondent "I don't know" or "I can't," but if gently coaxed, may be able to correctly complete cognitive tasks. The depressed patient generally has mild cognitive deficits in comparison to the mood disorder symptoms. Patients with depressed mood and psychotic symptoms can have hallucinations and nihilistic or paranoid delusions. These symptoms would be unusual in most typical dementias in the absence of at least moderate cognitive deficits.[92] Important exceptions are patients with frontotemporal dementia, dementia with Lewy bodies, or patients with cerebrovascular events. Additionally, patients with depression do not have cortical signs of dementia such as aphasia, apraxia, or visuospatial impairment. Psychotic features in the absence of other signs of dementia raise the possible diagnosis of paraphrenia or late-life psychosis.

Some elements of the history can also help in the diagnosis of depression. A relatively rapid onset, a prior history of depression, a family history of affective disorders, and prominent vegetative symptoms are features that suggest that the cognitive symptoms are secondary to a primary depression. As the diagnosis of these entities is purely clinical, there are always patients in whom it is not entirely clear as to whether the patient has a primary dementia or depression. An empirical trial of antidepressant therapy can be appropriately instituted. A favorable outcome in terms of depressive symptoms may be seen whether the patient has dementia with depressive symptoms or primary depression. In the latter case, with appropriate antidepressant therapy, depressed patients with mild to moderate cognitive deficits should improve more markedly than the demented patient.

The Severely Impaired

Mental status assessment instruments used in mild and moderate dementia are not as helpful in assessing severely demented patients where behavioral problems and functional impairment are the main problems. Specific instruments to assess congnitive function in severely impaired patients are becoming increasingly available.

A major clinical challenge is assessment of the severely impaired dementia patient not previously seen by the health care provider. These patients can present labeled with a diagnosis that has been carried over for many years. Most standard screening mental status tests, such as the MMSE or the SPMSQ, have significant floor effects and are, therefore, insensitive for assessment of these patients. They fail to take into account the difference between a patient who can give a month of the year, albeit incorrectly, as opposed to the patient who cannot discern what a month is. Both individuals would achieve a score of zero for these two very different responses. There are a number of assessment tools that have recently been designed to extend the cognitive examination of the more severely impaired. These include the Severe Impairment Battery[144] and the Test for Severe Impairment.[145] These tools take into account more basic cognitive abilities that may remain preserved such as the recognition of social symbols (shaking hands) and praxis ("show how you use a cup"). Their sensitivity to change over time has not been well-studied.[146]

A thorough neurologic examination can be rewarding both diagnostically and therapeutically in severely impaired patients. Clinical questions to address in such patients are: Does the patient have significant parkinsonian signs indicative of the Lewy body dementias and likely to be highly sensitive to drugs affecting the dopamine system? Are they poorly attentive and distractible suggesting that caregivers must limit instructions to single step activities? Should sedative or neuroleptic medications be discontinued because the patient appears drowsy, unsteady or parkinsonian? and Does the patient have visual neglect or a field deficit characteristic of right hemisphere infarction, mandating the need for care givers to approach visual space in a selective manner and the physician to institute specific prophylactic therapies to prevent recurrent cerebrovascular events?

Dementias Without Distinctive Neurologic Signs or Evidence of Neurologic or Medical Disease

Among the dementias presenting without prominent neurologic signs, such as disturbances of movement, focal motor, or sensory signs, Alzheimer's disease is clearly the predominant disorder. Categorizing Alzheimer's disease as presenting without focal neurologic signs is a bit misleading in that the cognitive impairment of Alzheimer's disease is not global, but selective in its presentation. Thus, the earliest signs of memory failure are most likely reflected by concentration of pathology in the hippocampi and medial temporal lobes of the brain. As the disease progresses, there is subsequent involvement of other cortical and subcortical regions. Declines in language function, visuospatial skills,[147] and executive functions (problem solving, abstract reasoning, and judgment)[148] then become apparent. In middle and latter stages, behavioral changes[92] and motor signs emerge.[149]

There are several important variations to the classic pattern just described, which are helpful diagnostically. Prominent early behavioral and personality changes (impulsivity, repetitive stereotyped behavior, and disinhibition) with little memory or visuospatial impairment suggests a frontotemporal dementia. Most of these syndromes have an earlier age of onset in the fifth or sixth decade. Speech output can be progressively affected leading to a decrease in fluency to the point of mutism. The best known frontal dementia syndrome is Pick's disease, which grossly affects the frontal and anterior temporal lobes with characteristic neuronal inclusion bodies (Pick bodies). A number of patients with a similar presentation and course, however, do not demonstrate the classic neuropathology of Pick's disease.[150] These have been termed frontotemporal dementia, or frontal lobe degeneration of the non-Alzheimer type, to distinguish them from both Pick's disease and Alzheimer's disease.

A minority of patients can present with prominent aphasia out of proportion to memory deficits.[151, 152] In some cases, this aphasia progresses to a more diffuse dementia but without marked behavioral disturbances. Nonspecific temporal lobe degeneration, Alzheimer's disease pathology, or Pick's disease may be found at autopsy. These language disorders are generically termed primary progressive aphasias in their early stages when there is relative sparing of other cognitive functions. Some cases can be familial or associated with motor neuron disease.

Other initially focal dementias can present with constructional apraxia and cortical sensory loss of the left hand, but progress to a

Acquired, progressive, impairment in behavior in the setting of preserved memory and visuospatial skills suggests the diagnosis of frontotemporal dementia and related disorders if structural causes are excluded.

syndrome clinically and pathologically like Alzheimer's disease.[153, 154] A number of patients also present with pronounced complex visual impairments preceding other characteristics of a more widespread dementia.[155] These syndromes predominantly affect posterior cortical regions. Such patients may exhibit Balint's syndrome (ocular apraxia, simultanagnosia, and cortical paralysis of fixation). Other patients can present with alexia, agraphia, acalculia, right–left disorientation, visual agnosia, or fluent aphasia.[10]

Dementias with Neurologic Signs Without Obvious Medical Disease

Many dementias will be associated with neurologic signs. These range from obvious hemiplegia or involuntary movements, such as tremor or chorea, to more subtle signs, such as increased muscle tone or reflex asymmetry. In the proper setting, these signs provide very helpful clues in the assessment and differential diagnosis of dementia.

MOVEMENT DISORDERS AND DEMENTIA

Dementia with parkinsonism (the combination of resting tremor, rigidity, akinesia, and postural and gait disturbance) occurs in Alzheimer's disease, dementia with Lewy bodies, Parkinson's disease with dementia, progressive supranuclear palsy, and vascular ischemic dementia.

Among the most striking neurologic signs associated with the dementias are movement disorders. Elements of parkinsonism (rigidity, bradykinesia, and tremor) may be found in up to a third of patients with the clinical diagnosis of Alzheimer's disease. This is often related to the postmortem observation of the co-occurrence of Alzheimer's disease pathology with varying distributions of the pathologic marker of Parkinson's disease, the Lewy body.[156] When Lewy bodies are confined to the brainstem, the disease pathologically resembles typical idiopathic Parkinson's disease. Lewy bodies may also be found more widely distributed in the basal forebrain.[157] Whether this disorder is best considered a variant of Alzheimer's disease or a separate entity (diffuse Lewy Body disease or dementia of the Lewy body type) is unsettled. Clinically, these patients do not have prominent parkinsonism early on and rest tremor is rare at any stage. Psychotic symptoms with hallucinations or delusions can be present early, before more clear cut parkinsonism emerges.[158] These patients also exhibit early visuospatial impairment. For example, they have impaired clock drawing without significant improvement on attempting to copy a well-drawn clock.[159] A diagnostic trial of levodopa is generally not as confirmatory as in classic idiopathic Parkinson's disease. The motor syndrome may respond to L-dopa, but the psychotic symptoms may be exacerbated by these drugs.[159] Similarly, such patients may be very sensitive to dopamine blocking drugs used to manage psychotic symptoms and carry a risk of causing disabling parkinsonism.

Other less common dementias are frequently diagnosed by their association with characteristic movement disorders. These include choreiform movements in patients with Huntington's disease, the axial extensor dystonia (or flexion posture in some patients) and vertical supranuclear palsy of progressive supranuclear palsy, and the ataxia associated with a number of cerebellar degeneration syndromes. Most of these disorders have their peak age at onset as young adults in the fourth through sixth decade, but later onset cases have been reported as well. Myoclonus in the setting of a rapidly progressing dementia requires the consideration of Creutzfeld-Jacob disease. Myoclonus can appear late in the course of Alzheimer's disease in about 10 percent of patients. In this setting, myoclonus is not indicative of Creutzfeld-Jakob disease. A number of patients will present with several months of mild cognitive decline with concomitant change in gait. The gait is characteristic in that it is short-stepped and narrow based, with difficulty initiating steps. When this clinical picture is accompanied by urinary incontinence, symptomatic hydrocephalus must be ruled out because it is a treatable entity.[160, 161] Motor neuron disease and dementia present in a number of degenerative dementias. The hallmark of these disorders is weakness with amyotrophy (muscle wasting) and fasciculations. The dementia is more of the frontotemporal type and is clinically indistinguishable from the frontotemporal neurodegenerations such as Pick's disease. Although, classically, amyotrophic lateral sclerosis does not usually involve a dementia, this may not always be the case.[162]

The diagnosis of dementia with Lewy bodies is suggested by dementia in the setting of two core features among fluctuations in conciousness, visual hallucinations, and parkinsonism. Supported features include falls, syncope, neuroleptic sensitivity, and delusions.

Vascular Dementias

Ironically, dementias secondary to underlying vascular disease can be the result of "silent" multiple small strokes and thus, can be categorized as dementias without distinctive neurologic signs. This perception most likely prevails when the diagnosis is made in a patient with vascular risk factors and an imaging study that shows a single unexpected small cerebral infarction or has been given the designation of "leukoaraiosis indicative of ischemic white matter disease." Many of these patients turn out to have concomitant Alzheimer's disease pathology and are then termed "mixed dementia." In fact, cerebrovascular disease may influence the onset and expression of Alzheimer's disease.[163] Recent introduction of a number of research criteria has not resolved the difficulties in categorizing ischemic vascular dementia.[164] Cerebrovascular disease can lead to dementia in a number of ways.[165, 166] These can be related to the type of vascular territories affected. Classic multi-infarct dementia is secondary to occlusion of several major branch vessels affecting cortical regions. In these cases, the patient should have evidence of amnesia, aphasia, apraxia, or agnosia. Involvement of small penetrating vessels (e.g., lenticulostriate) results in small infarcts termed lacunes in the deep white matter, and leads to a syndrome of motor and intellectual slowing. Because this ischemic damage tends to distribute preferentially in the frontal white matter, there are more commonly observed signs of frontal lobe dementia with apathy, poor insight, and judgment. A related disorder is termed Binswanger's disease, which affects the medullary arteries of the white matter and is clinically indistinguishable from multiple lacunar infarctions. Cerebral hypoperfusion due to bilateral carotid stenosis may also lead to dementia.[166]

Although vascular dementia may be less common than previously recognized, cerebrovascular disease and its risk factors may contribute to the risk of Alzheimer's disease.

All of the above vascular dementias discussed previously are secondary to multiple infarctions or relatively widespread ischemic damage. A number of single infarctions are strategically located so that they masquerade as a dementia. These strategic infarct dementias include occlusion of the left inferior parietal branch of the middle cerebral artery (angular gyrus syndrome: agraphia, alexia, anomia, left–right disorientation, constructional apraxia, and finger agnosia),[6] infarction of the genu of the internal capsule (inattention, amnesia, apathy, abulia, and psychomotor slowing),[167] and thalamic infarction (amnesia, apathy, and executive dysfunction).[168] Interestingly, these strategic infarcts are more often associated with left hemisphere vessel occlusions.

Dementias With Clinical or Laboratory Evidence of Other Disease

A number of dementias can be discovered on clinical examination or laboratory screening, either intentionally as part of a dementia assessment, or inadvertently during a health maintenance screen. They include discovery of the signs or symptoms of a particular disease entity such as the lethargy, weakness, change in voice, and depressed reflexes of a hypothyroid patient to the more common occurrence of discovering on laboratory testing, the biochemical signature of the disease, in this case, an elevated TSH and low free T_4 level. Accordingly, many of the conditions that belong to this group are those that are commonly thought of as the treatable or reversible dementias (Table 21-6). It is important to keep in mind that not only metabolic or drug-related dementias will present as general medical illnesses without classic neurologic signs, but that structural causes of dementia (cerebral tumors or subdural hematomas) can present in elders with minimal or no focal neurologic

TABLE 21-6. MAJOR CATEGORIES OF POTENTIALLY REVERSIBLE DEMENTIAS	
Drugs	Sedative-hypnotics
	Anticholinergic drugs
	Antianxiety drugs
	Antidepressants
	Cardiac drugs
	Abused drugs, alcohol
Metabolic and endocrine	Hypernatremia or hyponatremia
	Hypoglycemia
	Hyperthyroidism or hypothyroidism
	Hypercalcemia
	Hypoparathyroidsm
	Renal failure
	Hepatic failure
Nutritional	Vitamin B_{12} deficiency
	Thiamine deficiency
Infectious	Fungal meningitis or encephalitis
	Parasitic meningitis or encephalitis
	Viral meningitis or encephalitis
	Bacterial meningitis or encephalitis
	Lyme disease
	Neurosyphilis
Inflammatory disorders	CNS vasculitis
	Sjögren's syndrome
	Systemic lupus erythematosis
CNS disorders	Subdural hematoma
	Hydrocephalus
	Tumor (primary or metastatic)
	Seizure disorder

signs. These may only be uncovered with a neuroimaging study.[169] Laboratory testing in patients with dementia is generally recommended, as discussed.[107, 171, 172] Attention to clues on the history or physical and neurological examination is important in guiding the workup.

A major challenge with this group of disorders in elders is to determine the degree to which common, highly prevalent medical disorders significantly contribute to the change in cognitive function. This concept is inherent in the criteria for the clinical diagnosis of Alzheimer's disease, which requires "absence of systemic disorders or other brain disease that in and of themselves could account for the progressive deficits in memory and cognition."[172] In a review of 2889 patients evaluated for dementia in 32 separate studies, the three major scenarios for uncovering a secondary cause of dementia were drug effects, depression, and metabolic conditions (such as cobalamin deficiency or thyroid disease).[173] The frequency with which these or other disorders causing dementia will be uncovered will be modified by the profile of the population that presents to the health care provider. Ultimately, when a particular medical condition is considered suspicious for playing a role in the dementia, the disorder in question needs to be successfully treated or optimally managed before it can be said with certainty that the dementia is not caused or significantly modulated by that illness.

SUMMARY

The assessment of dementia requires a unique combination of skills involving knowledge of the wide variety of causes of dementia as well as excellent interviewing and diagnostic techniques. Unfortunately, many cases of dementia are recognized late, missing the opportunity to determine the prognosis and develop a care plan for both the elder's and his or her family's benefit. Assessment involves confirmation of the presence of dementia, arriving at a probable cause, and deciding what stage of dementia is present. Standardized tests are useful but do not supplant an in-depth cognitive evaluation. Behavioral and functional assessment are necessary components of the process in order to rule out other causes and to reduce excess disability from co-morbid conditions. Social and caregiver assessment is also needed to provide effective care planning. Finally, it is important to rule out potentially reversible dementias in every case. A comprehensive assessment of an elder with memory loss is the foundation of care of the patient with dementia.

REFERENCES

1. Agency for Health Care Policy and Research (AHCPR). *Early Identification of Alzheimer's Disease and Related Dementias.* U.S. Department of Health and Human Services; 1996:27.
2. Corey-Bloom J, Thal L, Galasko D, et al. Diagnosis and evaluation of dementia. *Neurology.* 1995;45:211–218.
3. Small G, Rabin P, Barry P, et al. Diagnosis and treatment of Alzheimer disease and related disorders. *JAMA* 1997;278:1363–1371.
4. Callahan C, Hendrie H, Tierney W. Documentation and evaluation of cognitive impairment in elderly primary care patients. *Ann Intern Med.* 1995;122:422–429.
5. American Psychiatric Association. *Diagnostic and Statistical Manual of Mental Disorders,* 4th ed. Washington, DC: American Psychiatric Association; 1995:494.
6. Cummings J, Benson D. *Dementia—A Clinical Approach,* 2nd ed. Boston: Butterworth-Heinemann; 1992.
7. Kaye J. Diagnostic challenges in dementia. *Neurology.* 1998; 51(suppl):S45–S52.

8. Neary D, Snowden J, Gustafson L, et al. Frontotemporal lobar degeneration. *Neurology.* 1998;51:1546–1554.

9. Levine D, Lee J, Fisher C. The visual variant of Alzheimer's disease. *Neurology.* 1993;43:305–313.

10. Caselli R. Asymmetric cortical degeneration syndromes. *Curr Opin Neurol.* 1996;9:276–280.

11. American Psychiatric Association. *Diagnostic and Statistical Manual of Mental Disorders,* 4th ed. Washington, DC: American Psychiatric Association; 1994:886.

12. McKeith I, Galasko D, Kosaka K, et al. Consensus guidelines for the clinical and pathologic diagnosis of dementia with Lewy bodies (DLB): report of the consortium on DLB international workshop. *Neurology.* 1996;47:1113–1124.

13. Christensen H, Henderson A, Korten A, Jorm A, Jacomb P, Mackinnon A. ICD-10 mild cognitive disorder: its outcome three years later. *Int J Geriatr Psychiatry.* 1997;12:581–586.

14. Erkinjuntti T, Steenhuis R, Hachinski V. The effect of different diagnosis criteria on the prevalence of dementia. *N Engl J Med.* 1997;337:1667–1674.

15. Schneider L, Olin J, Lynness S, Chui H. Eligibility of Alzheimer's disease clinic patients for clinical trials. *J Am Geriatr Soc.* 1997;45:923–928.

16. Barberger-Gateau P, Dartigues J, Letenneur L. Four instrumental activities of daily living score as a predictor of one-year incident dementia. *Age Aging.* 1993;22:457–463.

17. Corrada M, Brookmeyer R, Kawas C. Sources of variability in prevalence rates of Alzheimer's disease. *Int J Epidemiol.* 1995;24:1000–1005.

18. Ritchie K, and Kildea D. Is senile dementia "age-related" or "aging-related"—evidence from meta-analysis of dementia prevalence in the oldest old. *Lancet.* 1995;346:931–934.

19. Evans D, Funkenstein H, Albert M, et al. Prevalence of Alzheimer's disease in a community population of older persons higher than previously reported. *JAMA.* 1989;262:2551–2556.

20. Gao S, Hendrie H, Hall K, Hui S. The relationship between age, sex and the incidence of dementia and Alzheimer disease. *Arch Gen Psychiatry.* 1998;55:809–815.

21. Jorm A, Jolley D. The incidence of dementia. *Neurology.* 1998;51:728–733.

22. Launer L, Andersen K, Dewey M, et al. Rates and risk factors for dementia and Alzheimer's disease. *Neurology.* 1999;52:78–84.

23. Nyenhuis D, Gorelick P. Vascular dementia: a contemporary review of epidemiology, diagnosis, prevention and treatment. *J Am Geriatr Soc.* 1998;46:1437–1448.

24. Gorelick P. Status of risk factors for dementia associated with stroke. *Stroke.* 1997;28:459–463.

25. Hendrie H. Epidemiology of Alzheimer's disease. *Geriatrics.* 1997;52:S4–S8.

26. Lendory C, Ashall F, Goate A. Exploring the etiology of Alzheimer disease using molecular genetics. *JAMA.* 1997;277:825–836.

27. Levy-Lahad E, Bird T. Genetic factors in Alzheimer's disease: a review of recent advances. *Ann Neurol.* 1996;40:829–840.

28. Seshardi S, Drachman D, Lippa C. Apolipoprotein E Σ4 allele and the lifetime risk of Alzheimer's disease. What physicians know and what they should know. *Arch Neurol.* 1995;52:1074–1079.

29. Payami H, Montee K, Kaye J, et al. Alzheimer's disease, apolioprotein E4, and gender. *JAMA.* 1994;271:1316–1317.

30. Slooter A, Tang M, van Duijn C, et al. Apolipoprotein E E4 and the risk of dementia with stroke. *JAMA.* 1997;277:818–821.

31. Tang M, Stern Y, Marder K, et al. The APOE-E4 allele and the risk of Alzheimer disease among African Americans, whites and Hispanics. *JAMA.* 1998;279:751–755.

32. Grut M, Jorm A, Fratiglioni L, Forsell Y, Viitanen M, Winblad B. Memory complaints of elderly people in a population survey: variation according to dementia stage and depression. *J Am Geriatr Soc.* 1993;41:1295–1300.

33. Boise L, Morgan D, Kaye J, Camicioli R. Delays in the diagnosis of dementia: perspectives of family caregivers. *Alzheimer Dis.* 1999;(14):20–26.

34. Freter S, Bergman H, Gold S, Chertkow H, Clarifield M. Prevalence of potentially reversible dementias and actual reversibility in a memory clinic cohort. *Can Med Assoc J.* 1998;159:657–662.

35. Furtado S, Suchowesky O. Huntington's disease: recent advances in diagnosis and management. *Can J Neurol Sci.* 1995;22:5–12.

36. Koivisto K, Reinikainen K, Hanninen T, et al. Prevalence of age-associated memory impairment in a randomly selected population from eastern Finland. *Neurology.* 1995;45:741–747.

37. Larrabee G, McEntee W. Age-associated memory impairment: sorting out the controversies. *Neurology.* 1995;45:611–614.

38. Petersen R, Smith G, Waring S, Ivnik R, Tangalos E, Kokmen E. Mild cognitive impairment. *Arch Neurol.* 1999;56:303–308.

39. Reisberg B, Ferris S, de Leon M, Crook T. The global deterioration scale for the assessment of primary progressive dementia. *Am J Psychiatry.* 1982;139:1136–1139.

40. Hughes C, Berg L, Danizger W, Coben L, Martin R. A new clinical scale for the staging of dementia. *Brit J Psychiatry.* 1982;140:566–572.

41. Morris J. The clinical dementia rating (CDR): current version and scoring rules. *Neurology.* 1993;43:2412–2414.

42. Boucher L, Renwall M, Jackson J. Cognitively impaired spouses as primary caregivers for demented elderly people. *J Am Geriatr Soc.* 1996;44:828–831.

43. Wild VK, Kaye JA, Oken BS. Early noncognitive change in Alzheimer's disease and healthy aging. *J Geriatr Psychiatry Neurol.* 1994;7:199–205.

44. Oppenheim G. The earliest signs of Alzheimer's disease. *J Geriatr Psychiatry Neurol.* 1994;7:118–122.

45. Reding M, Haycox J, Blass J, et al. Depression in patients referred to a dementia clinic: a three year prospective study. *Arch Neurol.* 1985;42:894–896.

46. Litvan I, Agid Y, Goetz C, et al. Accuracy of clinical diagnosis of corticobasal degeneration. *Neurology.* 1997;48:119–125.

47. Galasko D, Bennett D, Sano M, et al. An inventory of assess activities of daily living for clincial trials in Alzheimer's disease. *Alzheimer Dis Assoc Disord.* 1997;11:S33–S39.

48. Walstra G, Teunisse S, van Gool W, van Crevel H. Reversible dementia in elderly patients referred to a memory clinic. *J Neurol.* 1997;244:17–22.

49. La Vange L, and Silverman H. Outpatient prescription drug utilization and expenditure patterns of noninstitutionalized aged medicare beneficiaries. *National Medical Care Utilization and Expenditure Survey.* Washington, DC: Health Care Financing Administration; 1987.

50. Flaherty J. Psychotherapeutic agents in older adults. Commonly prescribed and over-the-counter remedies: causes of confusion. *Clin Geriatr Med.* 1998;14:101–127.

51. Lovestone S. Early diagnosis and the clinical genetics of Alzheimer's disease. *J Neurol.* 1999;246:69–72.

52. Pasquier F, Delacourte A. Non-Alzheimer degenerative dementias. *Clin Geriatr Med.* 1998;11:417–427.

53. Joutel A, Vahedi K, Corpechot C, et al. Strong clustering and stereotyped nature of Notch3 mutations in CADASIL patients. *Lancet.* 1997;350:1511–1515.

54. Price T, Manolio T, Kronmal R, et al. Silent brain infarction on magnetic resonance imaging and neurological abnormalities in community-dwelling older adults. *Stroke.* 1997;28:1158–1164.

55. Litvan I. Progressive supranuclear pasly revisited. *Acta Neurol Scand.* 1998;98:73–98.

56. Robbins T, James M, Owen A, et al. Cognitive deficits in progressive supranuclear pasly, Parkinson's disease and multiple system atrophy in tests sensitive to frontal lobe dysfunction. *J Neurol Neurosurg Psychiatry.* 1994;57:79–88.

57. Richards M, Stem Y, Mayeux R. Subtle extrapyramidal signs and incident dementia: a follow-up analysis. *Neurology.* 1995;45:1942.

58. Camicioli R, Howieson D, Oken B, Sexton G, Kaye J. Motor slowing precedes cognitive impairment in the oldest old. *Neurology.* 50: 1496–1498.

59. Kaye J, Oken B, Howieson D, et al. Neurologic evaluation of the optimally healthy oldest old. *Arch Neurol.* 1994;51:1205–1211.

60. Lebowitz B, Pearson J, Schneider L, et al. Diagnosis and treatment of depression in late life. *JAMA.* 1997;278:1186–1190.

61. Brody D, et al. Identifying patients with depression in the primary care setting: a more efficient method. *Arch Intern Med.* 1998;22: 2469–2475.

62. Simpson N, Black F, Strub R. Memory assessment using the Strub-Black Mental Status Exam and the Wechsler Memory Scale. *J Clin Psychol.* 1986;42:147.

63. Knopman D, Ryberg S. A verbal memory test with high predictive accuracy for dementia of the Alzheimer's type. *Arch Neurol.* 1989;46:141–145.

64. Bolla K, Gray S, Resnick S, Galante R, Kawas C. Category and letter fluency in highly educated older adults. *Clin Neuropsychol.* 1998;12:330–338.

65. Tuokko H, Hadjistavropoulos T, Miller J, Beattie B. The Clock Test: a sensitive measure to differentiate normal elderly from those with Alzheimer's disease. *J Am Geriatr Soc.* 1992;40:579–584.

66. Mendez M, Ala T, Underwood K. Development of scoring criteria for the clock drawing task in Alzheimer's disease. *J Am Geriatr Soc.* 1992;40:1095–1099.

67. Solomon P, Hirschoff A, Kelly B, et al. A 7 minute neurocognitive screening battery highly sensitive to Alzheimer's disease. *Arch Neurol.* 1998;55:349–355.

68. Camicioli R, and Wild K, Assessment of the elderly with dementia. In: *Handbook of Neurologic Rating Scales.* Herndon RM, ed. New York Demos Vermande. 1997:265.

69. Folstein M, Folstein S, McHugh P. "Mini-Mental State"—a practical method for grading the cognitive state of patients for the clinician. *J Psychiatr Res.* 1975;12:189–198.

70. Tombaugh T, Mclntyre N. The Mini-Mental State Examination: a comprehensive review. *J Am Geriatr Soc.* 1992;40:922–935.

71. Mungas D, Marshall S, Weldon M, Haan M. Age and education correction of Mini-Mental State Examination for English and Spanish-speaking elderly.*Neurology.* 1996;46:700–706.

72. Crum R, Anthony J, Bassett S, Folstein M. Population-based norms for the Mini-Mental State Examination by age and education level. *J Am Med Assoc.* 1993;269:2386–2391.

73. Bohnstedt M, Fox P, Kohatsu N. Correlates of Mini-Mental Status Examination scores among elderly demented patients: the influence of race-ethnicity. *J Clin Epidemiol.* 1994;(47):1381–1387.

74. Murden R, McRae T, Kaner S, Bucknam M. Mini-Mental State Exam scores very with education in blacks and whites. *J Am Geriatr Soc.* 1991;39:149–155.

75. Galasko D, Edland S, Morris J, Clark C, Mohs R, Koss E. The consortium to establish a registry for Alzheimer's disease (CERAD). *Neurology.* 1995;45:1451–1455.

76. Blessed G, Tomlinson B, Roth M. The association between quantitative measures of dementia and of senile change in the cerebral gray matter of elderly subjects. *Br J Psychiatry.* 1968;114:797–811.

77. Pfeiffer E. A Short Portable Mental Status Questionnaire for the assessment of organic brain deficit in elderly patients. *J Am Geriatr Soc.* 1975;23:433–441.

78. Kokmen E, Naessens J, Offord K. A short test of mental status: description and preliminary results. *Mayo Clin Proc.* 1987;62: 281–288.

79. Katzman R, Brown T, Guld P, Peck A. Validation of a short orientation-memory-concentration test of cognitive impairment. *Am J Psychiatry.* 1983;140:734–739.

80. Katzman R, Brown T, Thal L, et al. Comparison of rate of annual change of mental status score in four independent studies of patients with Alzheimer's disease. *Ann Neurol.* 1988;24:384–389.

81. Thal L, Grundman M, Golden R. Alzheimer's disease: a correlational analysis of the Blessed Memory Concentration Test and the Mini-Mental State Exam. *Neurology.* 1986;36:262–264.

82. Kawas C, Karagiozis H, Resau L, Gorrada M, Brookmeyer R. Reliability of the Blessed Telephone Information-Memory-Concentration Test. *J Geriatr Psychiatry Neurol.* 1995;8:238–242.

83. Kokmen E, Smith G, Peterson R, Tangalos E, lvnik R. The Short Test of Mental Status: correlations with standardized psychometric testing. *Arch Neurol.* 1991;48:725–728.

84. Scherr P, Albert M, Fundenstien H, et al. Correlates of cognitive function in an elderly community population. *Am J Epidemiol.* 1988;128:1084–1101.

85. Royall DR, Cabello M, Polk MJ. Executive dyscontrol: an important factor affecting the level of care received by older retirees. *J Am Geriatr Soc.* 1998;46:1519–1524.

86. Mattis S. Dementia Rating Scale: Professional Manual. Odessa FL: Psychological Assessment Resources, 1988.

87. Rosen W, Mohs R, Davis K. A new rating scale for Alzheimer's disease. *Am J Psychiatry.* 1984;141:1356–1364.

88. Kiernan R, Mueller J, Langston J, Van Dyke C. The Neurobehavioral Cognitive Status Examination: a brief but differentiated approach to cognitive assessment. *Ann Intern Med.* 1987;107:734–739.

89. Teng E, Chui H. The modified Mini-Mental State (3MS) Examination. *J Clin Psychiatry.* 1987;48:314–318.

90. Westbury C, Bub D. Primary progressive aphasia: a review of 112 cases. *Brain Lang.* 1997;60:381–406.

91. Lezak M. *Neuropsychological Assessment,* 3rd ed. New York: Oxford University Press; 1995.

92. Mega M, Cummings J, Fiorello T, Gornbein J. The spectrum of behavioral changes in Alzheimer's disease. *Neurology.* 1996;46:130–135.

93. Cohen-Mansfield J. Agitated behaviors in the elderly II. *J Am Geriatr Soc.* 1986;34:722–727.

94. Williams J. A structured interview for the Hamilton depression scale. *Arch Gen Psychiatry.* 1988;45:742–747.

95. Yesavage J. Geriatric depression scale. *Psychopharmacol Bull.* 1988;24:709–713.

96. Alexopoulos G, Abrams R, Young R, Shamoian C. Cornell scale for depression in dementia. *Biol Psychiatry.* 1988;23:271–284.

97. Weiner M, Wild K, Folks D, Tariot P, Luszczynska H, Whitehouse P. Measures of psychiatric symptoms in Alzheimer patients: a review. *Alzheimer Dis Assoc Disord.* 1996;10:20–30.

98. Reisberg B, Borenstein J, Franssen E, Salob S. BEHAVE-AD: A Clinical Rating Scale for the Assessment of Pharmacologically Remedial Behavioral Symptomatology in Alzheimer's Disease, ed. H Altman. New York: Plenum; 1987.

99. Tariot P, Mack J, Patterson M, et al. The Behavior Rating Scale for Dementia of the Consortium to Establish a Registry for Alzheimer's disease. *Am J Psychiatry.* 1995;152:1349–1357.

100. Cummings J, Meda M, Gray K, Rosenberg-Thompson S, Carusi D, Gornbein J. The Neuropsychiatric Inventory: an efficient tool for comprehensively assessing psychopathology in dementia. *Neurology.* 1994;44:2308–2314.

101. Teri L, Truax P, Logsdon R, Uamoto J, Zarit S, Vitaliano P. The Revised Memory and Behavior Problems Checklist. *Psychol Aging.* 1992;7:627–631.

102. Devanand D, Miller L, Richards M, et al. The Columbia University Scale for Psychopathology in Alzheimer's disease. *Arch Neurol.* 1992;49:371–376.

103. Katz S. Assessing self-maintenance: activities of daily living, mobility and instrumental activities of daily living. *J Am Geriatr Soc.* 1983; 31:721–727.

104. Fillenbaum G. Multidimentional functional assessment of older adults: The Duke Older Americans Resources and Services Procedures. Hillsdale, NJ: Lawrence Erlbaum Associates; 1988.

105. Kuriansky J, Gurland B. The performance test of activities of daily living. *Intl Aging Hum Develop.* 1976;7:343–352.

106. Pfeffer R, Kurosaki T, Harrah C, Chance J, Filos S. Measurement of functional activities in older adults in the community. *J Gerontol.* 1982;37:323–329.

107. Dunkin J, Anderson-Hanley C. Dementia caregiver burden. *Neurology.* 1998;51(suppl):S53–S60.

108. van Creve H, van Gool W, Waslstra G. Early diagnosis of dementia which tests are indicated? What are their costs? *J Neurol.* 1999; 246:73–78.

109. Siu A. Screening for dementia and investigating its causes. *Ann Intern Med.* 1991;115:122–132.

110. American Academy of Neurology. Practice parameter for the diagnosis and evaluation of dementia (summary statement). *Neurology.* 1994;44:2203–2206.

111. Larson E, Reifler B, Sumi A, Canfield C, Chinn N. Diagnostic tests in the evaluation of dementia: a prospective study of 200 elderly outpatients. *Arch Intern Med.* 1986;146:1917–1922.

112. Relkin NR, et al. Apolipoprotein E genotype in Alzheimer's disease. *Lancet.* 1996;347:1091–1095.

113. Farrer L, Cupples L, Haines JL, et al., Effects of Age, Sex, and Ethnicity on the Association between Apolipoprotein E Genotype and Alzheimer Disease. JAMA, 1997;278:1349–1356.

114. Alexander E, Wagner E, Buchner D, Cain K, Larson E. Do surgical brain lesions present as isolated dementia? A population-based study. *J Am Geriatr Soc.* 1995;43:138–143.

115. Simon D, Lubin M. Cost-effectiveness of computerized tomography and magnetic resonance imaging in dementia. *Med Decisi Making.* 1985;5:335–354.

116. Mohr E, Feldman H, Gauthier S. Canadian guidelines for the development of antidementia therapies: a conceptual summary. *Can J Neurol Sci.* 1995;22:62–71.

117. Motter R, Vigo-Pelfrey C, Kholodenko K, et al. Reduction of β amyloid peptide 42 in the cerebrospinal fluid of patients with Alzheimer's disease. *Ann Neurol.* 1995;38:643–648.

118. Galasko D, Chang L, Motter R, et al. High cerebropsinal fluid tau and low amyloid $\beta42$ levels in the clinical diagnosis of Alzheimer disease and relation to Apolipoprotein E genotype. *Arch Neurol.* 1998;55:937–945.

119. Harrington M, Merril C, Ahser D, Gajdusek D. Abnormal proteins in the cerebrospinal fluid of patients with Creutzfeldt-Jakob disease. *N Engl J Med.* 1986:315:279–283.

120. Zerr I, Bodemer M, Gefeller O, et al. Detection of 14-3-3 protein in the cerebrospinal fluid supports the diagnosis of Creutzfeldt-Jakob disease. *Ann Neurol.* 1998;43:32–40.

121. Brown P, Gibbs J, Rodger-Johnson P, et al. Human spongiform encephalopathy: The National Institutes of Health series of 300 cases of experimentally transmitted disease. *Ann Neurol.* 1994;35: 513–529.

122. Bergman H, Chertkow H, Wolfson C, et al. HM-PAO (CERETEC) SPECT brain scanning in the diagnosis of Alzheimer's disease. *J Am Geriatr Soc.* 1997;45:15–20.

123. Masterman D, Mendez M, Fairbanks L, Cummings J. Sensitivity, specificity and positive predictive value of technetium 99-HMPAO SPECT in discriminating Alzheimer's disease from other dementias. *J Geriatr Psychiatry Neurol.* 1997;10:15–21.

124. McKelvey R, Bergman H, Stem J, Rush C, Zahirney G, Chertkow H. Lack of prognostic significance of SPECT abnormalities in non-demented elderly subjects with memory loss. *Can J Neurol Sci.* 1999;26:23–28.

125. Black S. Can SPECT predict the future for mild cognitive impairment? *Can J Neurol Sci.* 1999;26:4–6.

126. Talbot P, Lloyd J, Snowden J, Neary D, Testa H. A clinical role for ^{99}cmTc-HMPAO SPECT for the investigation of dementia? *J Neurol Neurosurg Psychiatry.* 1998;64:306–313.

127. Ebly E, Hogan D, Parhac I. Cognitive impairment in the non-demented elderly: results from the Canadian study of health and aging. *Arch Neurol.* 1995;52:612–619.

128. Hanninen T, Hallikainen M, Koivisto K, et al. A follow-up study of age-associated memory impairment: neuropsychological predictors of dementia. *J Am Geriatr Soc.* 1995;43:1007–1015.

129. Helkala E, Koivisto K, Hanninen T, et al. Stability of age-associated memory impairment during a longitudinal population-based study. *J Am Geriatr Soc.* 1997;45:120–121.

130. Graham J, Rockwood K, Beattie B, et al. Prevalence and severity of cognitive impairment with and without dementia in an elderly population. *Lancet.* 1997;349:1793–1796.

131. Thomassen R, van Schaick W, Blansjaar BA, Prevalence of dementia at 100. *Neurology.* 1998;50:283–286.

132. Ivnik R, Malec J, Smith G, et al. Mayo's older Americans normative studies: WMS-R norms for ages 56 to 94. *Clin Neuropsychologist.* 1992;6(suppl)49–82.

133. Ivnik R, Malec J, Smith G, et al. Mayo's older Americans normative studies: WAIS-R norms for ages 56 to 97. *Clin Neuropsychologist.* 1992;6(suppl):1–30.

134. Johansson B, Zarit S, Berg S. Changes in cognitive functioning of the oldest old. *J Gerontol.* 1992;47:75–80.

135. Howieson D, Dame A, Camicioli R, Sexton G, Payami H, Kaye J. Cognitive markers preceding Alzheimer's dementia in the healthy oldest old. *J Am Geriatr Soc.* 1997;45:584–589.

136. Johansson B, Allen-Burge R, Zarit S. Self-reports on memory functioning in a longitudinal study of the oldest old: relation to current prospective and retrospective performance. *J Gerontol.* 1997; 52B:139–146.

137. Rummans T, Evans J, Krahn L, Fleming K. Delirium in elderly patients: evaluation and management. *Mayo Clin Proc.* 1995;70: 989–998.

138. Jacobson S. Delirium in the elderly. *Geriatr Psychiatry.* 1997; 20:91–110.

139. Inouye S, Van Dyck C, Alessi C, Balkin S, Siegal A, Horwitz R. Clarifying confusion: the Confusion Assessment Method. *Ann Intern. Med.* 1990;113:941–948.

140. Rockwood K, Goodman J, Flynn M, Stolee P. Cross-validation of the Delirium Rating Scale in older patients. *J Am Geriatr Soc.* 1996;44:839–842.

141. O'Keeffe S, Gosney M. Assessing attentiveness in older hospital patients: global assessment versus tests of attention. *J Am Geriatr Soc.* 1997;45:470–473.

142. Levkoff S. Delirium: the occurrence and persistence of symptoms among hospitalized elderly patients. *Arch Intern Med.* 1992; 152:334–340.

143. Erkinjuntti T. Dementia among medical inpatients, evaluation of 2000 consecutive admissions. *Arch Intern Med.* 1986;146:1923–1926.

144. Saxton J, McGonigle-Gibson K, Swihart A, Miller V, Boller F. Assessment of the severely impaired patient: description and validation of a new neuropsychological test battery. *Psychol Assess J Consult Clin Psychol.* 1990;2:298–303.

145. Albert M, Coher C. The test for severe impairment: an instrument for the assessment of patients with severe cognitive dysfunction. *J Am Geriatr Soc.* 1992;40:449–453.

146. Wild K, Kaye J. The rate of progression of Alzheimer's disease in the later stages: evidence from the Severe Impairment Battery. *J Intl Neuropsychol Soc.* 1998;4:512–516.

147. Locascio J, Growdon J, Corkin S. Cognitive test performance in detecting, staging, and tracking Alzheimer's disease. *Arch Neurol.* 1995;52:1087–1099.

148. Perry R, Hodges J. Attention and executive deficits in Alzheimer's disease. *Brain.* 1999;122.

149. Ellis R, Caligiuri M, Galasko D, Thal L. Extrapyramidal motor signs in clinically diagnosed Alzheimer's disease. *Alzheimer Dis Assoc Disord.* 1996;10:103–114.

150. Mann D, Snowden J. Dementia of frontal lobe type: neuropathology and immunohistochemistry. *J Neurol Neurosurg Psychiatry.* 1993; 56:605–614.

151. Weintraub S, Rubin N, Mesulam M,-M. Primary progressive aphasia: longitudinal course, neuropsychological profile and language features. *Arch Neurol.* 1990;47:1329–1335.

152. Hodges J, Patterson K. Nonfluent progressive aphasia and semantic dementia: a comparative neuropsychological study. *J Intl Neuropsychol Soc.* 1996;2:511–524.

153. Crystal H, Horoupian D, Katzman R, Jotdowitz S. Biopsy-proved Alzheimer disease presenting as a right parietal syndrome. *Ann Neurol*. 1982;12:186–188.

154. Ross S, Graham N, Stuart-Green L, et al. Progressive biparietal atrophy: an atypical presentation of Alzheimer's disease. *J Neurol Neurosurg Psychiatry*. 1996;61:388–395.

155. Benson D, Davis R, Snyder B. Posterior corical atrophy. *Arch Neurol*. 1988;45:789–793.

156. Hulette C, Mirra S, Wilkinson W, Heyman A, Fillenbaum G, Clark C. The consortium to establish a registry for Alzheimer's disease (CERAD). *Neurology*. 1995;45:1991–1995.

157. Gomez-Tortosa E, Ingraham A, Irizarry M, Hyman B. Dementia with Lewy bodies. *J Am Geriatr Soc*. 1998;46:1449–1458.

158. Burkhardt C, Filley C, Kleinschmidt-DeMasters B, et al. Diffuse Lewy body disease and progressive dementia. *Neurology*. 1988: 1520–1528.

159. Gnanalingham K, Byrne E, Thornton A, Sambrook M, Bannister P. Motor and cognitive function in Lewy body dementia: comparison with Alzheimer's and Parkinson's disease. *J Neurol Neurosurg Psychiatry*. 1997;62:243–252.

160. Vanneste J. Three decades of normal pressure hydrocephalus: are we wiser now? *J Neurol Neurosurg Psychiatry*. 1994;57:1021–1025.

161. Krauss J, Droste D, Vach W, et al. Cerebrospinal fluid shunting in idiopathic normal-pressure hydrocephalus of the elderly: effect of periventricular and deep white matter lesions. *Neurosurgery*. 1996;39:292–300.

162. Massman P, Sim J, Cooke N, Haverkamp L, Appel V, Appel S. Prevalence and correlates of neuropsychological deficits in amyotrophic lateral sclerosis. *J Neurol Neurosurg Psychiatry*. 1996;61: 450–455.

163. Snowdon D, Greiner L, Mortimer J, Riley K, Greiner P, Markesbery W. Brain infarction and the clinical expression of Alzheimer disease. *JAMA*. 1997;277:813–817.

164. Wetterling T, Kanitz R, Borgis K. Comparison of different diagnostic criteria for vascular dementia (ADDTC, DSM-IV, ICD-10, NINDS-AIREN). *Stroke*. 1996;27:30–36.

165. Amar K, Wilcock G. Vascular dementia. *BMJ*. 1996;312:227–231.

166. Pasquier F, Leys K. Why are stroke patients prone to develop dementia? *J Neurol*. 1997;244:135–142.

167. Tatemichi T, Desmond D, Prohovnik I, Eidelberg D. Dementia associated with bilateral carotid occulusions: neuropsychological and haemodynamic course after extracranial to intracranial bypass surgery. *J Neurol Neurosurg Psychiatry*. 1995;58:633–636.

168. Tatemichi T, Desmond D, Prohovnik I, et al. Confusion and memory loss from capsular genu infarction: a thalamocortical disconnection syndrome? *Neurology*. 1992;42:1966–1979.

169. Steinke W, Sacco R, Mohr J, et al. Presentation and prognosis of infarcts and hemorrhages. *Arch Neurol*. 1992;49:703–710.

170. Chui H, Zhang Q. Evaluation of dementia: a systematic study of the usefulness of the American Academy of Neurology's practice parameters. *Neurology*. 1997;49:925–935.

171. Piccini C, Bracco L, Amaducci L. Treatable and reversible dementias: an update. *J Neurol Sci.* 1998;153:172–181.
172. McKhann G, Drachman D, Folstein M, et al. Clinical diagnosis of Alzheimer's disease: Report of the NINCDS-ADRDA Work Group under the auspices of Department of Health and Human Services Task Force on Alzheimer's disease. Neurology 1984;34(7):939–44.
173. Clarfield A. The reversible dementias: do they reverse? *Ann Intern Med.* 1988;109:476–486.

CHAPTER 22

URINARY INCONTINENCE

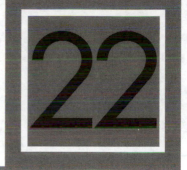

JOSEPH G. OUSLANDER

Urinary incontinence is a classic geriatric condition. Prevalent, morbid, and costly, incontinence is often hidden by elders and shunned by health care providers. The pathophysiology of incontinence is multifactorial, and the basic underlying anatomic and neurourologic mechanisms of continence remain poorly understood. Despite the availability of a variety of efficacious treatments, they remain underutilized.

Urinary incontinence can have adverse effects on physical health, psychological well-being, and the costs of health care. Urinary incontinence is uncomfortable, can result in skin irritations and contribute to pressure ulcers; lead to urinary tract infections if managed improperly; and irritative symptoms, especially nocturia; and contribute to sleep disruption and falls. Urinary incontinence is also embarrassing, frustrating, and can predispose to social isolation and depression. The costs of managing urinary incontinence and its complications are now estimated to exceed $20 billion annually in the United States.

Recently developed guidelines, including those promulgated by the Agency for Health Care Policy and Research (AHCPR),[1] the Health Care Financing Administration (HCFA) in its minimum data set (MDS) and resident assessment protocols (RAPs),[2] and the American Medical Directors Association (AMDA)[3] provide

The Agency for Health Care Policy and Research (AHCPR) was renamed in December 1999.
This agency is now known as the Agency for Healthcare Research and Quality (AHRQ).

specific recommendations about the diagnostic assessment of incontinent elders.

The purpose of this chapter is to present a brief overview of the problem, its clinical manifestations and underlying causes; and to provide health care providers with the tools necessary for the optimal assessment of incontinent people.

DESCRIPTION OF THE PROBLEM

Definition

Urinary incontinence is defined as the involuntary loss of urine sufficient in severity to be a problem for the affected individual and/or a caregiver. Although this may seem to be a straightforward definition, several factors make it more complicated. Since many elders are embarrassed by their incontinence, and also believe it is an inevitable consequence of aging, they do not report their symptoms to a health care provider. In addition, many frail incontinent elders try to hide their incontinence from their families, especially since residential care facilities frequently exclude individuals who are incontinent. Finally, what constitutes a "problem" for elders or their caregivers varies considerably. Some are very bothered by even infrequent losses of small amounts of urine, whereas others consider more frequent larger volume losses only a minor annoyance.

Prevalence

About one third of community-dwelling older women admit to some degree of urinary incontinence. The prevalence in men is about half of this rate. Of community-dwelling elders, 5 percent to 10 percent have severe incontinence, requiring the use of protective pads or undergarments.

Approximately one third of community-dwelling women older than 60 years have some degree of urinary incontinence, and close to 75 percent of men older than 50 years have symptoms referable to the urinary tract.[4] Between 5 percent and 10 percent of community-dwelling people older than 60 years have "severe" urinary incontinence, which occurs more than once per week and/or requires the use of a pad. Among the frail and cognitively impaired community-dwelling elders, the prevalence of urinary incontinence is 30 percent to 50 percent. In acute care hospitals the prevalence of urinary incontinence is just over one third, and 50 percent to 70 percent of residents of U.S. nursing homes have severe urinary incontinence.

Risk Factors

There are two predominant risk factors for the development or presence of urinary incontinence: cognitive impairment and mobility problems.[5] Other risk factors have been variably identified in several studies, however, impaired cognitive function and/or mobility appear to be the most important in elders. Clearly, the use of rapid acting diuretics, most commonly furosemide, is an important risk factor for incontinence, especially among the frail elders with mobility problems. A past history of multiple vaginal deliveries or genitourinary surgery (such as a previous cystocele repair or bladder suspension) can also be important risk factors among older women.

Clinical Manifestations

Table 22-1 illustrates a classification of the basic types of urinary incontinence.[6] Many elders have mixtures of these types of incontinence. Among women younger than 75 years, stress incontinence symptoms, either alone or in combination with urge symptoms, are common. The predominant abnormality of lower urinary tract functioning found among older and frail individuals is detrusor hyperactivity (involuntary bladder contractions found on cystometry; also termed detrusor instability, unstable bladder, and detrusor hyperreflexia, the latter in the presence of a neurologic disorder). Although most often associated with urge-type urinary incontinence, detrusor hyperactivity is commonly seen in conjunction with sphincter weakness and stress urinary incontinence among women, and with obstruction in men with benign or malignant prostatic enlargement. Patients with detrusor hyperactivity can also have incontinence without urgency, or, on the other hand, urgency and other irritative symptoms without incontinence. In frail older patients, detrusor hyperactivity is commonly associated with impaired bladder contractility resulting in incomplete bladder emptying (termed detrusor hyperactivity with impaired contractility, or DHIC).[7] People with DHIC can have symptoms that mimic stress or overflow, as well as urge incontinence. Functional-type urinary incontinence should be a diagnosis of exclusion because many elders, especially in nursing homes, have impairments of cognitive and/or physical functioning that can interfere with their ability to toilet. These people can also have other potentially treatable conditions contributing to their urinary incontinence. Thus, a search for reversible factors and other types of urinary incontinence should be completed before labeling a person's incontinence as "functional".

WHO TO ASSESS

It is important to screen all elders for urinary incontinence and related symptoms for several reasons. First, urinary symptoms,

TABLE 22-1. BASIC TYPES AND CAUSES OF URINARY INCONTINENCE		
TYPE	SYMPTOMS	COMMON CAUSES
Stress	Involuntary loss of urine (usually small amounts) simultaneous with increases in intra-abdominal pressure (such as those caused by coughing, sneezing, laughing, etc); patients with sphincter deficiency may have constant wetting	Weakness and laxity of pelvic floor musculature resulting in hypermobility of the bladder base and proximal urethra Bladder outlet or urethral sphincter weakness (intrinsic sphincter deficiency) related to prior surgery or trauma
Urge	Leakage of urine (usually larger, but variable volumes) because of inability to delay voiding after sensation of bladder fullness is perceived	Detrusor hyperactivity isolated or associated with one or more of the following: Local genitourinary condition such as cystitis, urethritis, tumors, stones, diverticula, and outflow obstruction Central nervous system disorders such as stroke, dementia, parkinsonism, spinal cord injury, or disease
Overflow	Leakage of urine (usually small amounts) resulting from mechanical forces on an over-distended bladder	Anatomic obstruction by prostate, large cystocele Acontractile bladder associated with diabetes mellitus or spinal cord injury
Functional	Urinary leakage associated with inability to toilet because of impairment of cognitive and/or physical functioning, psychological unwillingness, or environmental barriers	Severe dementia Immobility Physical restraints Inaccessible toilets Unavailability of regular toileting assistance Depression

Note: Functioning incontinence should be a diagnosis of exclusion. Most elders have functional factors that can contribute to incontinence, but may also have reversible and specifically treatable conditions underlying the incontinence.

especially incontinence, are frequently under-reported by patients. This may in part be due to embarrassment, and in part because of ageist attitudes on the part of patients, families, and health care providers. Second, there are substantial changes over time in the reporting of urinary incontinence symptoms in both community-dwelling elders and nursing home residents. Third, urinary symptoms are almost always treatable with substantial cure and improvement rates. Finally, urinary incontinence may be the manifestation of a potentially serious and curable disorder, either outside or within the lower urinary tract, such as obstruction and malignancy.

Among community-dwelling cognitively intact elders, general screening questions can be helpful, such as "Do you have any trouble with your bladder?", "Do you ever lose urine when you don't want to?", "Do you often have to rush to the bathroom?", and "Do you ever wear pads or other protection to prevent your getting wet?" For frail and cognitively impaired community-dwelling elders, family members are often helpful in identifying urinary symptoms because of experiences or in finding soiled laundry.

In acute hospitals and nursing homes, urinary incontinence can be directly identified by observing voiding behavior and detecting wetness. A systematic record, such as the one depicted in Figure 22-1, can be helpful. Reports of incontinence by aides in nursing homes are generally reliable and valid. Federal regulations for nursing home care in the United States require a comprehensive assessment (the minimum data set, or MDS) at the time of admission and periodically thereafter.[2] One component of the MDS assesses continence status (Table 22-2). Because many nursing home residents are admitted from acute hospitals, they frequently arrive at the nursing home with an indwelling bladder catheter. In this situation, it is essential to determine why the catheter was placed (i.e., to monitor urinary output versus urinary retention versus management of urinary incontinence) and to consider the resident for a bladder retraining program after the catheter has been removed. If a catheter is to remain in place, the resident should have an appropriate indication for its chronic use because of the morbidity associated with chronic indwelling catheters.[4] Residents with chronic indwelling bladder catheters should have an appropriate indication documented (Table 22-3).

HOW TO ASSESS

Overview

The United States federal government, through the AHCPR, published a clinical practice guideline on urinary incontinence in adults,[1] and the Health Care Financing Administration (HCFA) provided a basic strategy for assessing urinary incontinence among nursing home residents as one of eighteen resident assessment protocols or RAPs.[2] The American Medical Directors Association (AMDA) also published guidelines specifically for long-term care settings.[3] The recommendations presented herein are basically consistent with those contained in the cited sources.

Half or more of older people who suffer from incontinence do not consult a health professional about it.

The basic objectives of assessing urinary incontinence and related symptoms are:
Identification of potentially reversible factors (Table 22-4).
Identification of potentially serious underlying conditions, and/or conditions that may require further urologic, gynecologic, and/or urodynamic evaluation (Table 22-5).
Determination of the cause of the symptoms and an appropriate management plan.

INCONTINENCE MONITORING RECORD

INSTRUCTIONS EACH TIME THE PATIENT IS CHECKED
1) Mark one of the circles in the BLADDER section at the hour closest to the time the patient is checked.
2) Make an X in the BOWEL section if the patient has had an incontinent or normal bowel movement.

| ◗ = Incontinent, small amount | ∅ = Dry | X = Incontinent BOWEL |
| ● = Incontinent, large amount | △ = Voided correctly | x = Normal BOWEL |

PATIENT NAME _____ ROOM # _____ DATE _____

| | BLADDER | | | BOWEL | | | |
	INCONTINENT OF URINE	DRY	VOIDED CORRECTLY	INCONTINENT X	NORMAL x	INITIALS	COMMENTS
12 am	● ●	○	△ cc ___				
1	● ●	○	△ cc ___				
2	● ●	○	△ cc ___				
3	● ●	○	△ cc ___				
4	● ●	○	△ cc ___				
5	● ●	○	△ cc ___				
6	● ●	○	△ cc ___				
7	● ●	○	△ cc ___				
8	● ●	○	△ cc ___				
9	● ●	○	△ cc ___				
10	● ●	○	△ cc ___				
11	● ●	○	△ cc ___				
12 pm	● ●	○	△ cc ___				
1	● ●	○	△ cc ___				
2	● ●	○	△ cc ___				
3	● ●	○	△ cc ___				
4	● ●	○	△ cc ___				
5	● ●	○	△ cc ___				
6	● ●	○	△ cc ___				
7	● ●	○	△ cc ___				
8	● ●	○	△ cc ___				
9	● ●	○	△ cc ___				
10	● ●	○	△ cc ___				
11	● ●	○	△ cc ___				

TOTALS:

FIGURE 22-1 Example of a bladder record for institutional settings. (Reprinted, with permission, from The Regents of the University of California.)

TABLE 22-2. CONTINENCE STATUS SECTION FROM THE MINIMUM DATA SET[a]

1. Continence self-control categories
   (Code for resident performance over all shifts)
     Continent: Complete control
     Usually continent, bladder: incontinent episodes once a week or less; bowel: less than weekly
     Occasionally incontinent, bladder: 2+ times a week but not daily; bowel: once a week
     Frequently incontinent, bladder: tended to be incontinent daily, but some control present (e.g., on day shift); bowel, 2–3 times a week
     Incontinent, Had inadequate control. Bladder, multiple daily episodes; bowel, all (or almost all) of the time.

   a. Bowel continence   Control of bowel movement, with appliance or bowel continence programs, if employed
   b. Bladder continence   Control of urinary bladder function (if dribbles, volume insufficient to soil through underpants), with appliances (e.g., Foley) or continence programs, if employed

2. Bowel elimination pattern	Bowel elimination pattern regular (at least one movement every 3 days) ☐	Diarrhea ☐
	Constipation ☐	Fecal impaction ☐
		NONE OF ABOVE ☐

3. Appliances and programs	Any scheduled toileting plan ☐	Did not use toilet room/
	Bladder retraining program ☐	commode/urinal ☐
	External (condom) catheter ☐	Pads/briefs used ☐
	Indwelling catheter ☐	Enemas/irrigation ☐
	Intermittent ☐	Ostomy present ☐
		NONE OF ABOVE ☐

4. Change in urinary continence   Change in urinary continence has changed as compared to status of 90 days ago (or since last assessment if less than **90 days**)
   0. No change   1. Improved   2. Deteriorated

[a]Continence status is assessed over the past 14 days at the time of nursing home admission and quarterly thereafter.

TABLE 22-3. DOCUMENTATION OF APPROPRIATE INDICATIONS FOR CHRONIC INDWELLING BLADDER CATHETER USE

Urinary retention that:
  Causes persistent overflow incontinence, symptomatic infections, or renal dysfunction
  Cannot be corrected surgically or medically
  Cannot be managed practically with intermittent catheterization
Skin wounds, pressure ulcers, or irritations that are being contaminated by urine
Care of terminally ill or severely impaired patients for whom bed and clothing changes are uncomfortable or disruptive
Preference of patient or caregiver when patient has failed to respond to more specific treatments

TABLE 22-4. POTENTIALLY REVERSIBLE CONDITIONS THAT CAN CAUSE OR CONTRIBUTE TO URINARY INCONTINENCE	
CONDITION	MANAGEMENT
Irritation or inflammation in or around the lower urinary tract	
Urinary tract infection (symptomatic with frequency, urgency, sudden onset, or worsening of incontinence, unexplained fever or functional decline)	Antimicrobial therapy
Atrophic vaginitis and urethritis	Oral or topical estrogen
Stool impaction	Disimpaction Appropriate use of stool softeners, and laxatives if necessary Adequate mobility and fluid intake
Increased urine production	
Metabolic (hyperglycemia, hypercalcemia)	Better control of diabetes mellitus Therapy for hypercalcemia depends on underlying cause
Excess fluid intake	Reduction in intake of diuretic fluids (e.g., caffeinated beverages)
Volume overload	
Venous insufficiency with edema	Support stockings Leg evaluation Sodium restriction Diuretic therapy
Congestive heart failure	Medical therapy
Drug side effects	
Rapid acting diuretics causing frequency and urgency	Discontinuation of the offending medication if possible Dosage reduction or modification (e.g., flexible scheduling of rapid acting diuretics)
Anticholinergics, narcotics, calcium channel blockers, alpha adrenergic agonists (in men) causing urinary retention Alpha adrenergic antagonists causing urethral relaxation and stress incontinence Psychotropic drugs with sedative or extrapyramidal effects causing sedation and immobility that interfere with toileting	
Impaired ability or willingness to reach a toilet	
Delirium	Diagnosis and treatment of underlying cause(s) of acute confusional state
Illness, injury, or restraint that interferes with mobility	Regular toileting assistance Use of toilet substitutes Environmental alterations (e.g., bedside commode)
Depression	Appropriate pharmacologic and/or nonpharmacologic treatment

TABLE 22-5. EXAMPLES OF CONDITIONS THAT MAY REQUIRE FURTHER UROLOGIC, GYNECOLOGIC, AND/OR URODYNAMIC EVALUATION	
CONDITION	COMMENTS
History	
Recurrent symptomatic urinary tract infections in addition to the incontinence	A structural abnormality or pathologic condition in the urinary tract predisposing to symptomatic infection should be excluded
Physical examination	
Marked pelvic prolapse protruding through the vaginal introitus	Consideration should be given to surgical repair or pessary management to prevent discomfort and tissue erosion, as well as to treat the incontinence
Suspicion of prostate cancer	Although surgical intervention to cure the cancer would not be appropriate for most elders, diagnosis of the cancer may be important in managing the incontinence and other complications
Urinalysis	
Hematuria (sterile)	Urologic evaluation should be considered to identify urinary tract pathology
Post-void residual determination	
Residual volumes > 200 mL	Although no precise cutoff point can be recommended, residual volumes > 200 mL are abnormal, and should lead to consideration of further evaluation of the urinary tract to identify complications (e.g., hydronephrosis, renal function impairment) and to determine the cause of the retention (obstruction, impaired bladder contractility, or both)

Although there remains some controversy about the appropriate extent and the cost effectiveness of various diagnostic strategies, two fundamental principles should be kept in mind.

1. Diagnostic tests should be performed only if the results will change the patient's management.
2. The consequences of misdiagnosis should be considered. For example, missing a bladder cancer or an obstruction in a patient to be treated with bladder relaxant medication can cause considerable morbidity.

Identification of Potentially Reversible Factors

Because the pathogenesis of urinary incontinence among elders is often multifactorial, involving urologic and gynecologic conditions, neurologic disorders, behavioral and psychological factors, and functional impairments, the approach to assessment as well as treatment must be comprehensive and consider all of these potential factors. The most important factors to consider are those that are *reversible* (Table 22-4).[5] Identification and management of these reversible factors may not cure the incontinence, however, the severity can be reduced. In addition, identification and management of these conditions can have important benefits for the patient's overall functioning and quality of life. The potentially reversible factors that can cause or contribute to urinary incontinence (Table 22-4) can be remembered by the acronym, DRIP: *D*elirium; *R*estricted mobility, retention; *I*nfection, inflammation, impaction; *P*olyuria, pharmaceuticals. The basic elements of an evaluation of an incontinent person are seen in Table 22-6.

History

Table 22-7 illustrates the key aspects of the history. A bladder record, such as the one depicted in Figure 22-2, can be helpful for elders who can keep them. In nursing homes, facility staff members can be very helpful in identifying many of these symptoms among residents who cannot reliably report them, as well as in assessing the timing and nature of fluid intake and monitoring voiding activity using a record such as the one shown in Figure 22-1.

Several studies have shown a poor correlation between symptoms and urodynamic findings (especially urge symptoms and detrusor hyperactivity), however, the history is important for several reasons. First, a careful history can assist in diagnosis and treatment planning. Specific symptoms, such as clearly described stress incontinence in the absence of any irritative complaints, is reasonably sensitive and specific for the diagnosis of stress incontinence associated with urethral hypermobility. Second, the pattern of symptoms (either related verbally or via a bladder record) can be helpful in making a diagnosis. For example, frequency, urgency, and inconti-

TABLE 22-6. BASIC EVALUATION OF INCONTINENCE
Focused history
Targeted physical examination
Urinalysis
Estimation of post-void residual volume

TABLE 22-7. KEY ASPECTS OF AN INCONTINENT PATIENT'S HISTORY

Active medical conditions, especially
  Neurologic disorders, diabetes mellitus, congestive heart failure, and
    venous insufficieny
Medications
Fluid intake pattern
  Type and amount of fluid (especially before bedtime)
Past genitourinary history, especially
  Childbirth, surgery, dilatations, urinary retention, radiation, and recur-
    rent urinary tract infections
Symptoms of incontinence
  Onset and duration
  Type—stress versus urge versus mixed versus other
  Frequency, timing, and amount of incontinence episodes and of conti-
    nent voids
Other lower urinary tract symptoms
  Irritative—dysuria, frequency, urgency, and nocturia
  Voiding difficulty—hesitancy, slow or interrupted stream, straining,
    and incomplete emptying
  Other—hematuria, suprapubic discomfort
Other symptoms
  Neurologic (indicative of stroke, dementia, parkinsonism, or spinal
    cord disorder)
  Psychological (depression)
  Bowel (constipation, stool incontinence)
  Symptoms suggestive of volume-expanded state (e.g., leg edema, short-
    ness of breath while horizontal or with exertion)
Perceptions of incontinence
  Patient's concerns or ideas about underlying cause(s)
  Interference with daily life, sexual activity
  Severity (e.g., Is it enough of a problem to consider surgery)
  Most bothersome symptom(s)
Environmental factors
  Location and structure of bathrooms
  Availability of toilet substitutes

nence in the morning in an elder on furosemide probably represents diuretic-induced incontinence; nocturia and nocturnal incontinence can be the manifestation of congestive heart failure, excessive fluid intake, or prostatic enlargement in men. Third, since elders often have multiple symptoms, it is important to get a sense of what their most bothersome symptom is, and how bothersome it is. For example, many women have symptoms of both urge and stress incontinence, but one is often more bothersome than the other. If behavioral therapy is planned, the distinction may not be critical because bladder training, pelvic muscle exercises, and related techniques are effective for urge, stress, and mixed types of urinary

Bladder Record

_____   Date: _____/_____
                                              month   day

INSTRUCTIONS:

In the 1st column make a mark every time during the 2-hour period you
urinate into the toilet

Use the 2nd column to record the amount you urinate (if you are measuring amounts)

In the 3rd or 4th column, make a mark every time you accidentally
leak urine

Time Interval	Urinated in Toilet	Amount	Leaking Accident	*or*	Large Accident	Reason for Accident*
8 am						
10 am						
4 pm						
6 pm						
8 pm						
10 pm						
2 pm						
Midnight						

Number of pads used today: _____

*For example, if you coughed and have a leaking accident, write "cough."
If you had a large accident after a strong urge to urinate, write "urge."

FIGURE 22-2 Example of a bladder record for ambulatory clinic
settings. (Reprinted, with permission, from Kane RL, Ouslander
JG, Abrass IB, ed. *Essentials of Clinical Geriatrics,* 2nd ed. New
York: McGraw-Hill; 1989:156.)

incontinence. If pharmacologic or surgical intervention is being
considered, however, the distinction is essential in targeting
therapy.

The key components of the physical examination are listed in
Table 22-8. Because impairments of cognitive and physical function
are commonly associated with incontinence among frail elders, the
physical examination should include an assessment of these areas
specifically related to the patient's ability to use the toilet, and
manage his/her clothing and hygiene.[8]

The general physical examination should exclude volume overload (i.e., venous insufficiency, congestive heart failure) and previously undiagnosed neurologic conditions that might contribute

Physical and occupational
therapists can be helpful in assessing toileting and hygiene
skills among incontinent
elders.

TABLE 22-8.   KEY ASPECTS OF AN INCONTINENT PATIENT'S PHYSICAL EXAMINATION

Mobility and dexterity
 Functional status compatible with ability to self-toilet
 Gait disturbance (parkinsonism, normal pressure hydrocephalus)
Mental status
 Cognitive function compatible with ability to self-toilet
 Motivation
 Mood and affect
Neurologic
 Focal signs (especially in lower extremities)
 Signs of parkinsonism
 Sacral arc reflexes
Abdominal
 Bladder distension
 Suprapubic tenderness
 Lower abdominal mass
Rectal
 Perianal sensation
 Sphincter tone (resting and active)
 Impaction
 Masses
 Size and contour of prostate
Pelvic
 Perineal skin condition
 Perineal sensation
 Atrophic vaginitis (friability, inflammation, and bleeding)
 Cystourethrocele and pelvic prolapse
 Pelvic mass
 Other anatomic abnormality
Other
 Lower extremity edema or signs of congestive heart failure (if nocturia
  is a prominent complaint)

to the incontinence (e.g., signs of parkinsonism, spinal cord compression). Rectal examination is done to assess resting and active sphincter tone, exclude fecal impaction, and assess the prostate in men. The size of the prostate on physical examination, however, can neither diagnose nor exclude the presence of urethral obstruction. In women, the pelvic examination should assess perineal and vulvar skin condition, exclude pelvic masses and marked pelvic prolapse (i.e., a cystocele that protrudes through the vaginal introitus), and evaluate the vaginal epithelium for signs of inflammation (erythema, friability, and bleeding) that suggest atrophic vaginitis. Pelvic muscle strength can also be assessed by having the patient attempt to squeeze on the examiner's fingers during the vaginal exam. A cough test to detect stress incontinence can also be done at the time of the pelvic examination. This test is best performed in the standing position with a comfortably full bladder. Small bladder volumes and severe urgency at the time of the test can result in a false negative test. A positive cough test while the patient is supine with a relatively empty bladder is suggestive of intrinsic sphincter deficiency.

The primary purposes of the urinalysis are to exclude sterile hematuria, which may be a sign of bladder or upper urinary tract pathology, and to exclude significant bacteriuria in patients who have symptoms (other than chronic, stable incontinence) suggestive of a urinary tract infection (dysuria, recent onset or worsening of their incontinence or other irritative symptoms, and unexplained fever or functional decline). There is no evidence that treating bacteriuria among patients with stable incontinence symptoms affects the severity of the incontinence. Among nursing home residents, this is true whether or not pyuria is present.[9] Evidence is also lacking for a beneficial effect of treatment for asymptomatic bacteriuria on morbidity and mortality.[10, 11] In addition, bacteriuria is known to spontaneously resolve in a substantial proportion of elders. Thus, unless an incontinent elder has symptoms other than stable incontinence (such as those listed earlier), it is reasonable to leave the bacteriuria untreated. Neither symptoms nor physical examination signs (suprapubic palpation, bimanual examination) are highly sensitive or specific in detecting significant residual volume. A portable ultrasound device is now available (Bladder Scan, Diagnostic Ultrasound, Redmond, WA) that can noninvasively measure residual urine with reasonably good accuracy among incontinent elders. Post-void residual volume can have substantial intra-individual variability. The timing of the determination in relation to a void, the degree to which the void was natural for the patient, the nature of instructions given to the patient, the amount of straining, and body position can all influence the post-void volume obtained. Thus, when moderately elevated volumes are detected (e.g., 150 to 300 mL), repeated determinations may be appropriate. In these situations, the ultrasound can be especially valuable in avoiding the need for repeated catheterizations. Repeated residual volumes of more than 200 mL should prompt consideration of whether the patient should be referred for further evaluation (Table 22-5).

Further Assessments

In determining the need for further evaluation, the most important consideration is whether the results will change the way the patient's incontinence will be managed.

Some incontinent people benefit from further diagnostic tests and, urologic, gynecologic, and/or urodynamic evaluation (Table 22-5). Urodynamic evaluation is essential for a patient in whom surgery is being considered (e.g., a woman with symptoms and signs of severe stress incontinence, or a man with symptoms and signs suggestive of obstruction).

A person with urinary retention who is not a candidate for surgical intervention is unlikely to benefit from a urodynamic evaluation to diagnose the cause of the retention; they should be managed by intermittent or chronic catheterization. Table 22-9 lists various diagnostic tests and procedures and examples of indications for each. The role of urodynamic testing in the evaluation of incontinence and related symptoms remains controversial. Complex urodynamic tests [including cystometry, with simultaneous measurement of bladder and abdominal pressure; voiding pressure-flow study; measurement of urethral pressure at the time of leakage with straining (leak point pressure); sphincter electromyography; and videourodynamic studies] have been shown to be safe and feasible even among frail elders.[6] This type of testing is essential to accurately diagnose obstruction, DHIC, and the type of stress incontinence (i.e., primarily due to urethral hypermobility versus intrinsic sphincter deficiency). Because the testing procedures are relatively costly, involve some discomfort, and require specialized equipment and trained personnel, they should only be performed

TABLE 22-9. EXAMPLES OF INDICATIONS FOR DIAGNOSTIC TESTS IN THE ASSESSMENT OF AN INCONTINENT ELDER

TESTS	INDICATIONS
Urine culture and sensitivity	Patients with the new onset or worsening of incontinence, or symptoms or signs of a urinary tract infection (other than stable incontinence)
Blood urea nitrogen, serum creatinine	Urinary retention
Renal ultrasound	Urinary retention
Blood glucose, calcium	Polyuria
Urine cytology	Hematuria
	Recent onset of irritative symptoms
	Risk factors for bladder cancer (smoking history, exposure to industrial carcinogens, e.g., aromatic amines contained in aniline dyes)
Prostate specific antigen	Suspected cancer on examination in patients for whom diagnosis will influence management
Urodynamic tests	Diagnosis will determine therapy
	Suspected obstruction
	Urinary retention

in patients for whom the results are necessary to determine an appropriate treatment plan.[12] Simple urodynamic tests, including a pad test for stress incontinence and bedside cystometry, have been described that do not require specialized equipment. The stress test is performed by having the patient cough forcefully, preferably in the standing position, when their bladder is relatively full (but not in the presence of a strong urge to void). The test is positive if there is immediate leakage similar to the volume and circumstance of the resident's usual incontinence. If the test is negative and the total bladder volume (voided volume plus residual volume) is less than 200 mL, the test should be repeated. If the post-void residual determination has been done by catheterization, the bladder can be filled with sterile water (by gravity) to a volume of 200 mL for the stress test. Simple cystometry can also be performed immediately after catheterization for a post-void residual determination. This test can be helpful for identifying involuntary bladder contractions, but low pressure involuntary contractions (such as those seen in many patients with DHIC) are easily missed. In addition, straining can be difficult to detect and is easily misinterpreted as an involuntary contraction, especially in cognitively impaired elders. Among incontinent nursing home residents, stress tests and simple cystometry have not been found to be helpful in identifying those who respond well to daytime prompted voiding.[13] Urodynamic diagnosis also does not predict responsiveness to bladder training in community-dwelling older women.[14] Thus, if behavioral interventions such as bladder training and prompted voiding are to be used as the initial therapy, urodynamic testing is not necessary before a therapeutic trial. Urodynamic testing to help differentiate stress from urge and mixed (stress and urge) incontinence should be considered for patients who do not respond well to the behavioral intervention and for whom more specific therapy (e.g., pharmacologic or surgical treatment) is planned.

Urodynamic tests can be helpful for making a specific diagnosis for the incontinence, but should only be performed if the findings will help determine a treatment plan.

HOW TO USE THE ASSESSMENT DATA

The first step in managing the incontinent elder is to treat any potentially reversible conditions detected during the basic assessment. If the incontinence resolves, or if the incontinence is ameliorated to the patient and/or caregiver's satisfaction, then periodic follow-up is all that is necessary to ensure that the symptoms do not recur.

The vast majority of older women will have either urge, stress, or mixed (urge and stress) incontinence based on the basic assessment. For women with pure stress incontinence, there are four basic options: behavioral therapy, drug therapy (an alpha agonist to which estrogen can be added), a combination of behavioral and drug therapy, or surgery. Surgery for stress incontinence has good short term results (e.g., 90 percent cure rates) in young and middle-aged women, however, long-term outcomes (longer than 5 years) are much less impressive. Periurethral injection of collagen is also an option, and may be appropriate for many older women with stress incontinence associated with urethral sphincter weakness. For urge and mixed incontinence, behavioral therapy or drug therapy (a bladder relaxant such as tolterodine or oxybutynin, or imipramine in patients with mixed incontinence) or a combination can be used. Drug therapy for urge and mixed incontinence should be initiated at low doses because elders frequently develop an intolerable dry mouth from standard doses.

Behavioral therapies are very effective in functional and motivated patients.[13] These include various bladder training techniques, pelvic muscle exercises, and biofeedback. The latter is used to enhance patients' abilities to learn pelvic muscle exercises and strategies to manage urgency. For functionally impaired incontinent patients, prompted voiding can be helpful if caregivers are available and motivated to assist the patient in maintaining dryness.[12]

The management of incontinence in older men is more complicated because of the possibility of the presence of obstruction, and the possibility of precipitating urinary retention by bladder relaxant treatment of urge symptoms (by far the most common and bothersome in this population). If behavioral therapies are ineffective, not feasible, or not wanted, a decision must be made between a trial of a bladder relaxant, an alpha blocker, or consideration of surgery. This decision must be based on the patient's overall health status, preferences, and, if appropriate, the results of further urodynamic and/or urologic evaluation.

SUMMARY

Urinary incontinence is an embarrassing problem that frequently is inadequately assessed. Health care providers caring for elders should routinely inquire about urinary incontinence. Those with incontinence should be assessed for the type and cause of incontinence. The primary care provider can usually conduct such an assessment. Many strategies exist to help the patient with incontinence including behavioral, pharmacologic, and surgical interventions. On occasion, patients will require a referral for more complicated diagnostic testing or management. Older persons should never have their incontinence labeled as due to "old age."

REFERENCES

1. Fantl JA, Newman DK, Colling J, et al. Urinary incontinence in adults: acute and chronic management. *Clinical Practice Guideline, no. 2. Update.* U.S. Department of Health and Human Services, Public Health Service, Agency for Health Care Policy and Research. AHCPR Publication No. 96-0682, Rockville, MD: USDHHS; 1996.

2. Health Care Financing Administration. U.S. Department of Health and Human Services. *Resident Assessment Instrument MDS,* version 2.0. Washington DC: Heaton Publications; 1995.

3. American Medical Directors Association. *Urinary Incontinence: Clinical Practice Guideline.* Columbia, MD: AMDA; 1996.

4. Thomas DH, Brown JS. Reproductive and hormonal risk factors for urinary incontinence in later life: a review of the clinical and epidemiologic literature. *J Am Geriatr Soc.* 1998;46:1411–1417.

5. Ouslander JG, Schnelle J. Incontinence in the nursing home. *Ann Int Med.* 1995;122:438–449.

6. Kane RL, Ouslander JG, Abrass IB. *Essentials of Clinical Geriatrics,* 4th ed. New York: McGraw-Hill; 1999.

7. Resnick NM, Yalla SV, Laurino E. The pathophysiology of urinary incontinence among institutionalized elderly persons. *N Engl J Med.* 1989;320: 1–7.

8. Williams ME, Gaylord SA. Role of functional assessment in the evaluation of urinary incontinence. *J Am Geriatr Soc.* 1990;38: 296–299.

9. Ouslander J, Schapira M, Schnelle, J, et al. Does eradicating bacteriuria affect the severity of chronic urinary incontinence among nursing home residents? *Ann Int Med.* 1995;122:749–954.

10. Nicolle LE, Bjornson J, Harding GMK, et al: Bacteriuria in elderly institutionalized men. *N Engl J Med.* 1983;309:1420–1425.

11. Nicolle LE, Henderson E, Bjornson J, McIntrye M, Harding GK, MacDonell JAA. The association of bacteriuria with resident characteristics and survival in elderly institutionalized men. *Ann Intern Med.* 1987;106:682–686.

12. Ouslander JG, Leach G, Staskin D, et al. Prospective evaluation of an assessment strategy for geriatric urinary incontinence. *J Am Geriatr Soc.* 1989;37:715–724.

13. Ouslander J, Schnelle J, Nigam J, Uman G, Fingold S, Tuico E. Predictors of Successful prompted voiding among incontinent nursing home residents. *JAMA.* 1995;273:1366–1370.

14. Fantl JA, Wyman FJ, McClish DK, et al. Efficacy of bladder training in older women with urinary incontinence. *JAMA.* 1991;265:609–613.

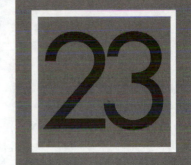

CHAPTER

23

FALLS AND GAIT DISORDERS

LAURENCE Z. RUBENSTEIN

Difficulties with ambulation and the related phenomenon of falling are among the most common and serious problems facing elders— causing considerable mortality, morbidity, reduced functioning, and premature nursing home admissions. Impaired gait and balance rank among the most important causes for falls, and are also common consequences of falls. These disorders are generally the result of multiple and diverse etiologies, and health care providers must use careful and thorough diagnostic approaches to identify the most likely causes, contributing factors, and associated comorbidity—many of which conditions respond successfully to treatment.

DESCRIPTION OF THE PROBLEM

Epidemiologic Considerations

Both the incidence of falls and the severity of fall-related complications rise steadily after entering the sixth decade. Accidents are the fifth leading cause of death in elders, and falls constitute two thirds of these accidental deaths. About three fourths of deaths due to falls in the United States occur in the 13 percent of the population age 65 years and over.[1]

Fall incidence varies among settings and populations. The lowest rates are reported among community-living, generally healthy elders, about a third of whom will fall each year, with an overall rate of about 0.6 falls per person annually. Most of these falls result

Falls constitute two thirds of accidental deaths of elders.

573

in no serious injury, but in a given year, about 5 percent of these community fallers experience a fracture or need hospitalization, a proportion much higher than among younger fallers. Incidence rates in nursing homes and hospitals are almost three times the community rates (1.5 falls per bed annually), and complication rates are also considerably higher (10 percent to 25 percent of institutional falls result in fracture, laceration, or need for hospital care).[1] Thus, an important issue concerning falls in elders is not simply the high incidence, because children and athletes have even higher fall incidences, but rather a combination of a high incidence together with a high susceptibility to injury.

This injury susceptibility in elders results from a high prevalence of comorbid diseases (e.g., osteoporosis) and age-related decline (e.g., slowed reflexes), which make even a relatively mild fall particularly dangerous. Fear of falling and the post-fall anxiety syndrome result in loss of self-confidence and self-imposed functional limitations among both community-dwelling and nursing home residents who fall. Falls and instability are a leading precipitating cause of nursing home admissions. Recent national data indicate that falls were the largest single cause of restricted activity days among elders. Other national data indicate that fall-related injuries recently accounted for 6 percent of all medical expenditures for persons age 65 years and older.

Injury susceptibility in elders makes even a relatively mild fall dangerous.

The related problems of gait and balance disorders are also extremely prevalent among elders and can have similarly profound impacts on physical health, quality of life, and capacity for independent living. Detectable gait abnormalities affect 20 percent to 40 percent of people age 65 years and older, and about half of these people have a grossly abnormal gait.[2] Gait problems are even more common in older subgroups, affecting 40 percent to 50 percent of those over age 85 years. In a large study of community-dwelling persons age 75 and older, 10 percent needed assistance to walk across a room, 20 percent were unable to climb a flight of stairs without help, and 40 percent were unable to walk half a mile.[3] As will be shown, gait and balance disorders are among the most highly predictive risk factors for falling.

Causes of Falls and Disordered Gait

A number of predictable changes of normal aging adversely affect gait and balance. These include stiffening of connective tissue, loss of muscle mass, slowing of nerve conduction, decreasing visual acuity, and impaired proprioception. These directly result in decreased joint range of motion, reduced muscle strength, prolonged reaction time, impaired depth perception, and increased postural sway. Consequently, with aging, gait becomes slower, with a shortened step length, decreased cadence, and a wider base of support. Feet are not picked up as high and are more prone to tripping. Slowed reaction time makes it less likely for an elder to stop a fall once a trip, slip, or other sudden displacement has occurred.[2, 3]

In addition to these age-related changes, specific conditions and disease processes contribute to pathologic gait. These factors are outlined in Table 23-1 and include pain, joint immobility, muscle weakness, spasticity, sensory deficits, and impaired central processing. For example, arthritis, present in over half of all elders, interferes with normal joint mobility through both pain and deformity of the joint. Muscle weakness, often the result of disuse, is also endemic in elders and results in decreases in step height, stride length, gait speed, and stability. Disorders of the central nervous system, such as stroke and parkinsonism, cause a variety of abnormalities affecting gait, including weakness, sensory impairment, decreased proprioception, spasticity, and tremor. It has also been shown that mobility deteriorates as the number of chronic conditions increase. Other risk factors associated with declines in mobility in large studies include increasing age, low income, smoking, obesity, and low physical activity levels.[4] A careful assessment outlined as follows, should enable the health care provider to establish the existence of a mobility problem, identify the major age-related or disease process(es) involved, and detect other associated risk factors, which will enable formulation of a comprehensive therapeutic plan.

TABLE 23-1. MAJOR CAUSES OF PATHOLOGIC GAIT

Pain
  Arthritis
  Injury
Weakness
  Deconditioning
  Myopathy and neuropathy
  Pulmonary and cardiovascular
    problems
  Loss of muscle mass
Sensory impairment
  Stroke
  Spinal cord lesion
  Peripheral neuropathy
  Proprioceptive impairment
  Visual impairment

Bone and joint abnormalities
  Arthritis
  Contractures
  Leg injury or shortening
  Connective tissue stiffening
Impaired central processing
  Dementia
  Stroke
  Normal pressure hydrocephalus
  Parkinson's disease
  Age-related slowing
Spasticity
  Stroke
  Spinal cord lesion

TABLE 23-2. CAUSES OF FALLS IN ELDERS: SUMMARY OF 12 LARGE STUDIES		
CAUSE	MEAN (PERCENT)[a]	RANGE[b]
Accident and environment-related	31	1–53
Gait and balance disorders or weakness	17	4–39
Dizziness and vertigo	13	0–30
Drop attack	9	0–52
Confusion	5	0–14
Postural hypotension	3	0–24
Visual disorder	2	0–5
Syncope	0.3	0–3
Other specified causes[c]	15	2–39
Unknown	5	0–21

[a]Mean percent calculated from the 3,628 reported falls.

[b]Ranges indicate the percentage reported in each of the 12 studies.

[c]This category includes: arthritis, acute illness, drugs, alcohol, pain, epilepsy, and falling from bed.

(Adapted, with permission, from Rubenstein LZ. Falls. In: Yoshikawa TT, Cobbs EL, Brummel-Smith K, eds. *Ambulatory Geriatric Care.* St. Louis: Mosby-Year Book, Inc.; 1993:296–304.)

Table 23-2 lists the major precipitating causes of falls and their relative frequencies based on published studies.[1, 5] The relative importance of causes differs depending on the population studied. For example, frail, high-risk populations have increased rates of medical-related falls and also a higher incidence of falls of all types than do healthier populations. Overall, "accidents," gait and balance disorders, and the nonspecific symptom of dizziness are the three most frequent causes of falls.

Accidents, generally involving some environmental hazard, are usually reported as the most common cause of falls and account for 30 percent to 50 percent in most studies. In reality, however, most of the falls attributed to accidents stem from the interaction between an environmental hazard (e.g., an irregular floor, a wet surface) and increased susceptibility to these hazards because of the effects of aging or disease. Age-associated changes in gait and posture control, along with impairments in vision, hearing, and memory tend to impair an elder's ability to avoid hazards and recover from a trip or stumble. Unfortunately, the homes of such susceptible elders are commonly filled with avoidable environmental hazards, such as throw rugs, dim lighting, trailing electrical cords, unsafe stairs, and accumulated clutter (see Chapters 9, 14, 15, 21).

The second most common cause of falls is the broad category of gait problems and weakness. As described earlier, gait problems are common and can be caused by many factors. Muscle weakness is also extremely common among elders, much of it stemming from disease and inactivity rather than aging *per se.* Studies report the prevalence of easily detected leg weakness ranging from about 50 percent among community-dwelling elders to over 80 percent among nursing home residents. Common causes of weakness include deconditioning, stroke, parkinsonism, skeletal abnormalities, arthritis, myopathies, neuropathies, and cardiorespiratory disorders, in addition to age-related muscle loss.[2, 3, 6, 7]

The sensation of dizziness is a very common complaint of elders who fall. Because the symptom is subjective and can reflect a number of different causes and mechanisms, a careful history is required. True vertigo, a sensation of rotational movement, can indicate a disorder of the vestibular apparatus (e.g., benign positional vertigo, acute labyrinthitis, or Meniere's disease). Symptoms described as imbalance on walking often reflect a gait disorder. Many patients describe a vague light-headedness that can reflect cardiovascular problems, hyperventilation, orthostatic hypotension, drug side effects, anxiety, or depression. Another common cause of dizziness or unsteadiness is a combination of visual loss and peripheral neuropathy, which must be sought on physical examination.

Drop attacks are sudden falls associated with abrupt leg weakness without loss of consciousness or dizziness, sometimes precipitated by sudden change in head position. This syndrome has been attributed to transient vertebrobasilar insufficiency, although it is probably caused by more diverse pathophysiologic mechanisms. The leg weakness is usually transient but can persist for hours. Recent studies, employing stricter diagnostic criteria, are finding this to be a much less common cause for falls than earlier reported.[5]

Confusion and cognitive impairment are often associated with falls and can reflect an underlying systemic or metabolic process causing both the confusion and the fall (e.g., electrolyte imbalance, fever). Dementia can cause an increase in falls by impairing judgment, visuospatial perception, and ability to orient oneself geographically. Dementia-related wandering activities are also often associated with falls.

Orthostatic hypotension, most often defined as a consistent drop of 20 mm Hg or greater in systolic blood pressure after standing from a supine position, has a 5 percent to 25 percent prevalence among normal elders living at home. It is even more common among persons with certain predisposing factors, such as autonomic dysfunction (often related to age, diabetes, or central nervous system damage), hypovolemia, low cardiac output, parkinsonism, metabolic and endocrine disorders, and medications (particularly sedatives, antihypertensives, and antidepressants). The orthostatic drop may be more pronounced on arising in the morning, since the baroreceptor response is diminished after prolonged recumbency, as well as after meals (post-prandial hypotension). Fortunately, most people with orthostatic hypotension adjust to the phenomenon and are able to avoid falling, which is why it is a less common cause of falls than its high prevalence might suggest.

Syncope is a serious but less commonly reported cause of falls. It is, however, much more common than the mean figure listed in Table 23-2 because several of the falls studies specifically excluded patients with syncope. Syncope, defined as a sudden loss of consciousness with spontaneous recovery, usually results from decreased cerebral blood flow or occasionally, from metabolic causes such as hypoglycemia or hypoxia. Among elders, its most frequent causes are cardiac arrhythmias (especially ventricular tachycardia and sick sinus syndrome), orthostatic hypotension, situational reflex syndromes (e.g., micturition syncope, Valsalva maneuver), and the very common "syncope of unclear etiology." Less common causes of syncope are vasodepressor–vasovagal reactions, transient ischemic attacks, and seizures. A history of syncope can be difficult to obtain because many elders do not remember exactly what occurred during the fall, and they may confuse drop attacks or dizziness for syncope.

Other specific causes of falls include visual problems, disorders of the central nervous system, drug side effects, and alcohol intake. Diseases of the central nervous system (e.g., cerebrovascular disease, normal pressure hydrocephalus, and parkinsonism) often result in falls by causing dizziness, orthostatic hypotension, and gait disorders. Drugs frequently have side effects that result in impairment of mentation, circulatory integrity, body stability, and gait. Especially strong relationships between falls and drugs have been noted for psychotropic agents (e.g., sedatives, hypnotics, anxiolytics, and antidepressants) as well as with total number of medications taken. Similar, but less consistent, risks have been associated with antihypertensives, diuretics, vasodilators, and beta blockers. Alcohol use is an under-reported but common problem among the elderly population. Elders should be specifically questioned about this, since alcohol can be an occult cause of instability, falls, and serious injury. Other less common causes of falls include seizures, anemia, hypothyroidism, unstable joints, foot problems, and severe osteoporosis with spontaneous fracture.[1, 5, 8]

Risk Factors

In many cases, because a single specific cause for falling cannot be identified, and because falls are usually multifactorial in etiology, many epidemiologic case-control studies have been conducted to identify risk factors that increase the likelihood of falling. Taken

TABLE 23-3. IMPORTANT RISK FACTORS FOR FALLS: SUMMARY OF 17 CONTROLLED STUDIES			
RISK FACTOR	SIGNIFICANT/TOTAL[a]	MEAN RR-OR[b]	RANGE
Weakness	12/12	4.9 (8)	1.9–10.3
Balance deficit	10/10	3.2 (5)	1.6–5.4
Gait deficit	8/9	3.0 (5)	1.7–4.8
Visual deficit	5/9	2.8 (9)	1.1–7.4
Mobility limitation	9/9	2.5 (8)	1.0–5.3
Cognitive impairment	4/8	2.4 (5)	2.0–4.7
Impaired activity of daily living	5/6	2.0 (4)	1.0–3.1
Postural hypotension	2/7	1.9 (5)	1.0–3.4

[a]Number of studies with significant association/total number of studies examining the possible risk factor.

[b]Relative risks (prospective studies) and odds ratios (retrospective studies). Number in parentheses indicate the number of studies that reported RR or OR for each factor.

(Adapted, with permission, from Rubenstein LZ. Falls. In: Yoshikawa TT, Cobbs EL, Brummel-Smith K, eds. *Ambulatory Geriatric Care*. St. Louis: Mosby-Year Book, Inc.; 1993:296–304.)

together, these studies indicate that leg weakness, gait and balance disorders, functional impairment, visual deficits, cognitive impairment, and polypharmacy (defined as taking five or more prescription medications) are the most important risk factors for falls. Table 23-3 summarizes the data from 17 studies that determined fall risk factors. For example, from the risk factor column it can be seen that people with leg weakness have about a five-fold increase in fall risk, whereas those with impaired gait or balance have about a three-fold increase. Visual deficit, mobility limitation, cognitive impairment, postural hypotension, and impaired function have also been identified as risk factors in several studies, although these associations are somewhat weaker.

Risk factors specifically for injurious falls have been identified in seven additional studies, and by and large, the factors are the same as those for falls in general, with the addition of factors associated with osteoporosis (e.g., female gender, being underweight, and decreased bone density) as well as the use of physical restraints. Recent studies confirm earlier suspected relationships between the type of fall and whether a wrist or hip fracture is sustained. Wrist fractures are associated with falls forward or backward onto the hands, older age, and taller stature. Hip fractures are associated with falls on the side and also taller stature. People falling directly onto the buttocks have the lowest rate of fractures.[8]

Perhaps as important as identifying individual risk factors is appreciating the interaction and probable synergism between multiple risk factors. Several studies have shown that risk of falling increases dramatically as number of risk factors increases. For example, three studies have reported that 65 percent to 100 percent of individuals with three or more risk factors fell in a 12-month observation period compared to 8 percent to 12 percent of persons with no risk factors.[4, 8]

It is possible to identify those at substantially increased risk of sustaining a fall or fall-related injury. Once identified, such individuals will need a personalized and comprehensive approach to their evaluation and therapy. Similarly, those identified with gait and balance abnormalities deserve a focused diagnostic assessment and structured therapeutic plan to optimize their functioning and long-term outcomes.

WHO TO ASSESS AND HOW TO ASSESS

Because of the importance of falls and impaired gait and balance in elders, and the fact that these problems are relatively easy to detect and effectively intervene with once the health care provider is sensitized to them, it is probably worthwhile to regulary screen all elders for mobility impairments and fall risk factors noted in Table 23-3. This could readily be accomplished in the course of the periodic history and physical examination or could be performed via focused screening programs in the community center or managed care program. Such a screening would include, at a minimum, inquiring about recent falls or near falls, observing a person getting up and walking, and checking for orthostatic hypotension, avoidable medications, and visual disorders (including checking visual fields and perhaps depth perception, in addition to simple acuity). In addition, the person should be specifically questioned about mobility, inquiring about ability to get out of the house, go shopping, use transportation, and climb stairs, as well as estimating walking distance (e.g., number of blocks). For those individuals identified by screening, questioning, or via a referral to have a mobility impairment or significant fall risk factors, a more detailed assessment is warranted. The extent and direction of the assessment should depend on the nature and severity of the suspected problem.

Another important time for a comprehensive falls assessment is after a fall has occurred. A number of practice guidelines and clinical recommendations for the post-fall assessment have been proposed and vary somewhat depending on the purpose and clinical setting (e.g., emergency department, nursing home, home, and hospital).[1, 9-11] These usually include recommendations for a focused history (inquiring about recent falls, mobility, medications, vision, hearing, and comorbid conditions) and physical examination (including postural vital signs, neurologic examination, cardiovascular assessment, and careful observation of gait and balance). Studies have shown that the post-fall assessment can identify treatable causes for the fall as well as additional risk factors and can ultimately lead to improved outcomes. Of course, outcome improvement depends upon the specific treatment prescribed, a discussion of which is beyond the scope of this chapter. But treatments that have been shown promising in fall prevention trials include exercises (specifically those geared to improving strength, balance, and endurance), multiple risk-factor abatement programs, and environmental inspection and modification.[12]

Assessing Gait and Balance

A number of techniques are available to assess the nature and severity of a suspected problem of gait and/or balance. These range from simple screening maneuvers (e.g., the Get Up and Go Test),[13] to more detailed gait observation, to quantitative observational scales (e.g., the Tinetti POMA, see Appendix 36; or the Berg Balance Scale),[14, 15] to formal high-technology tests in a gait laboratory. The choice of test depends on the purpose of the assessment, the degree of impairment, the availability of the technology, and the potential for benefit.

Like other aspects of geriatric assessment, the purposes of mobility assessment can be multiple and include: screening for unsuspected abnormalities, characterizing the abnormalities, facilitating diagnosis, quantifying severity, predicting outcomes (e.g., falls, mortality), assisting treatment planning, and establishing baseline data for future comparison. Tests useful for screening should be brief, sensitive, and easy to administer. Tests useful for specific diagnosis or treatment planning need to be more precise and detailed and ordinarily require more time and knowledge to administer. Tests used for assessing elders with more substantial impairments prior to beginning a rehabilitative or research program also need to be of the more precise, quantitative variety.

Many tests have been designed to measure specific mobility parameters, such as gait speed, flexibility, or balance stability. These are especially helpful in research settings or in rehabilitative programs working on single areas of improvement. Many other tests have been designed to measure multiple mobility tasks and to produce a summary mobility score. These latter multitask tests have been more useful in screening and clinical settings, such as comprehensive assessment programs or general rehabilitation centers.

Among the simplest of the multi-task screening tests is the Get Up and Go test.[13] This test asks the participant to stand up from a chair, walk 3 meters, turn around, walk back, and sit down.

A single overall judgement score is given: 1 = normal, 2 = slightly abnormal, 3 = mildly abnormal, 4 = moderately abnormal, 5 = very abnormal. Although clearly simple, the subjectivity of the scoring has limited this test's usefulness. In response, a more quantitative version, the Timed Get Up and Go test, has been devised, in which the time taken to perform the test is measured and used as a score (> 15 seconds is abnormal).[16] This simple time measurement has been reported to have high reliability, to give a useful clinical index, and to be very easy to obtain during a routine examination.

A slightly more involved protocol, and perhaps the most widely used mobility screening test, is the Tinetti Performance Oriented Mobility Assessment Scale (POMA).[14] Several slightly different versions of this have been described, none clearly superior. In the POMA, the participant is asked to stand up from a chair without using the arms (if possible), step forward, put the feet as close together as possible, receive a mild nudge to the sternum from the examiner (who also gives standby support), with eyes open and shut, then turn around 360 degrees, walk about 25 feet at normal speed, turn around and walk back to the chair at a faster speed, and sit down. This routine is scored according to the protocol, which gives a total score of 0 to 28, with both gait and balance subscores. After a very few practice sessions, the examiner becomes proficient in observing and scoring the participants. The test has been shown to be very reproducible, and is quite sensitive in detecting clinically important gait or balance problems. It also seems to provide a fairly sensitive index of improvement over time. Moreover, it has been shown to be a good predictor of fall likelihood; for example, scores under 20 (out of 28) are associated with a fivefold increased risk of falling.

Somewhat more involved than the POMA is the Gait Abnormality Rating Scale (GARS),[6] which also produces an index summating qualitative judgments of specific aspects of gait. It adds several items on upper extremity motion during gait. Each item is rated on a 4-point scale (1 = normal, 4 = severely impaired). The GARS is less practical in the clinical setting, however, as it requires videotaping of gait, and takes longer than the POMA. Moreover, it has not been shown to be clinically superior.

Developed for use in mobility-impaired and hospitalized elderly patients, the Physical Performance and Mobility Examination (PPME)[17] has been recently described and validated. Included are six tasks: bed mobility, transferring, rising from chair, standing stability, stepping up, and walking. Two scoring options for each item are offered: a pass–fail screening score (each item 0 or 1, total score 0 to 6), and a more quantitative score (each item 0 to 2, total score 0 to 12), which is better suited to measuring change over time. This measure may well turn out to be the mobility measure of choice for very frail persons, but as yet, its use has been limited.

Among the most detailed of the performance-based mobility scales is the Berg Balance Scale.[15] This rates performance on 14 balance tasks, each on 0 to 4 point scale, with a total score of from 0 to 56. As implied by the name, this scale emphasizes balance over gait activities. A disadvantage is that it can take 10 to 15 minutes to administer by including fairly long tests of sitting balance, comfortable stance, and parallel stance. Its strength seems to be its ability to discriminate when balance is poor, which makes it another potentially very good test among very frail persons. Its predictive value relative to the POMA and other scales has yet to tested, although its length and detail decrease its usefulness as a screening test.

One benefit of learning to administer any of the quantitative tests is that they sensitize the examiner to detection of abnormal mobility. Even if a formal test is not used routinely in the clinical practice setting, simply having learned how to perform any of the tests can be of value in improving the examiner's assessment skills. Assessment of gait and mobility is usually omitted from the standard history and physical examination, but once a health care provider has learned how to observe gait—a task greatly facilitated by use of these instruments—its assessment will likely be included as a matter of habit.

Once a gait or balance problem has been detected on screening and characterized by detailed observation or use of a more detailed quantitative protocol, further testing can be warranted. Formal testing of gait and balance in a gait laboratory is sometimes helpful in quantifying the deficit, planning rehabilitative strategies, and following progress over time. Similarly, formal tests of vestibular function, vision, muscle function, and joint mobility can sometimes be helpful in selected cases with problems suspected in these areas. Formal testing is usually not necessary, however, when evaluating a detected mobility problem. In most cases, careful observation is all that is needed to identify the abnormality and the pathologic processes involved, which can usually be classified into the six major types listed in Table 23-1.

Astute observation of gait generally requires an understanding of the normal gait cycle and what to look for at each phase (Figure 23-1). The *gait cycle* is usually defined as beginning when the right heel contacts the ground and ending when the same heel strikes the ground again after having moved forward a step. Each foot undergoes two phases in the gait cycle, stance and swing. *Stance phase* is the interval when the foot in in contact with the ground, generally about 60 percent of the normal gait cycle, and *swing phase* is the interval when the foot is not contacting the ground

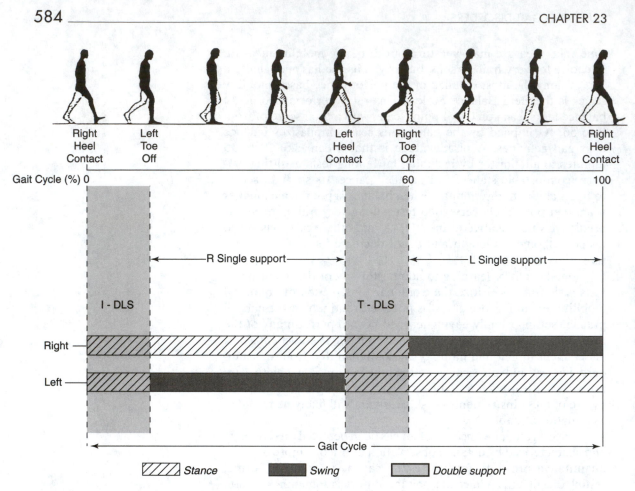

FIGURE 23-1   The Normal Gait Cycle. I-DLS, initial double limb support; T-DLS, terminal double limb support. (Adapted, with permission, from Rubenstein LZ. Falls. In: Yoshikawa TT, Cobbs EL, Brummel-Smith K, eds. *Ambulatory Geriatric Care.* St. Louis: Mosby-Year Book, Inc.; 1993:296–304.)

(i.e., swinging forward), generally about 40 percent of the cycle. *Double limb support* time is the interval, occurring twice during the gait cycle, when both feet are on the ground and weight is being transferred from one foot to the other. *Stride length* is the distance of the full gait cycle, measured as the distance between consecutive heel strikes of the right (or left) foot, and usually averages about 1.5 meters in normal participants. With aging, there is predictable shortening of the stride length and increase in the double support time.

Gait should be observed from both the side and the back. While viewing from the side, several things should be looked for, as summarized in Figure 23-2. At *initial contact* (the first segment

Normal Gait

	Stance (60%)					Swing (40%)		
	Initial Contact	Loading Response	Mid-stance	Terminal stance	Pre-swing	Initial swing	Mid-swing	Terminal swing
Hip	30° flexion	Extending to 5° flexion	Extending to neutral	10° of hyper extension	Neutral extension	20° Flexion liopsoas	30° Flexion	30° Flexion
Knee	Full extension	15° Flexion	Extending to neutral	Full extension	35° Flexion	60° Flexion	From 60° to 30° flexion	Extension to 0°
Ankle	Neutral heel first	15° Plantar flexion	From plantar flexion to 10° Dorsi flexion	Neutral with tibia stable and heel off prior to initial contact of opposite foot	20° Plantar flexion	10° Plantar flexion	Neutral	Neutral

FIGURE 23-2   Normal angular rotations and critical events at the hip, knee, and ankle joints during each portion of stance and swing phase of the normal gait cycle. (Adapted, with permission, from Trueblood P, Rubenstein LZ. Assessment of instability and gait in elderly persons. *Comp Therapy.* 1991;17(8):20–29.)

of stance phase), does the heel touch the ground first (normal), or does the whole foot touch together, or worse, does the forefoot touch first (both of which indicate weak dorsiflexors)? During *mid-stance,* are the hip and knee in neutral position while the ankle moves into slight dorsiflexion? During *terminal stance,* does the heel leave the ground as it should before the opposite foot makes contact? In the *pre-swing* segment of stance phase, does the knee move from neutral to a normal 30 to 40 degrees of flexion in preparation for swing phase, in which it should achieve 60 degrees of flexion? In swing phase, is the limb propelled forward normally and far enough before contacting the ground? Observing from the back, is there lateral trunk or limb deviation? Is there asymmetry between the right and left? Does the pelvis raise normally during swing phase or does it sag with each step (*Trendelenburg gait*)? With practice, this observational gait analysis will lead to recognition of all the major gait deviations. In combination with the rest of the evaluation (including joint range-of-motion testing, manual muscle testing, sensory examination, and balance screening), the most likely cause(s) can be identified and an appropriate treatment plan devised without the need for a formal gait laboratory.

Common Problems in Assessment

The major problems in assessment of falls and gait disorders concern underdiagnosis and misdiagnosis. Both are potentially very serious and can result in occurrence of avoidable falls, reduced function, as well as inappropriate treatment.

Underdiagnosis is the failure to identify in an elder the presence of a mobility problem or a high-risk situation for falls. This can result from a failure to look for the problem, a failure to report the problem by the patient or family, or a masking of the problem by the presence of multiple other disorders or comorbidities. Similarly, misdiagnosis can stem from incomplete evaluation of a reported problem or misreporting of the problem, both of which can lead to wrong conclusions, unnecessary evaluations, or inappropriate therapies. All of these situations can be minimized if the health care provider makes a systematic effort to inquire about, screen for, and evaluate fall risk factors, as outlined in the chapter.

SUMMARY

Falls and gait disorders are among the most common and disabling conditions of elders. A systematic approach to their assessment should lead to the development of an effective treatment plan that improves mobility and minimizes fall risk. As described in this chapter, this assessment involves identification of the problem in the face of an often-incomplete history, detection of treatable underlying causes and risk factors, and diagnosing the specific mobility abnormality through careful observational and functional testing using one or more validated measures. A logical and effective treatment approach should emerge that involves a combination of medical, rehabilitative, environmental, and psychosocial interventions.

REFERENCES

1. Rubenstein LZ, Josephson KR, Robbins AS. Falls in the nursing home. *Ann Intern Med.* 1994;121:442–451.
2. Trueblood P, Rubenstein LZ. Assessment of instability and gait in elderly persons. *Comp Therapy.* 1991;17(8):20–29.

3. Alexander NB. Gait disorders in older adults. *J Am Geriatr Soc.* 1996;44:434–451.

4. Robbins AS, Rubenstein LZ, Josephson KR, et al. Predictors of falls among elderly people: results of two population-based studies. *Arch Int Med.* 1989;37:562–569.

5. Rubenstein LZ. Falls. In: Yoshikawa TT, Cobbs EL, Brummel-Smith K, eds. *Ambulatory Geriatric Care.* St. Louis: Mosby-Year Book, Inc.; 1993:296–304.

6. Wolfson L, Whipple R, Amerman P, Tobin JN. Gait assessment in the elderly: a gait abnormality rating scale and its relation to falls. *J Gerontol A Biol Sci Med Sci.* 1994;45:M12–M19.

7. Wolfson L, Judge J, Whipple R, King M. Strength is a major factor in balance, gait, and falls. *J Gerontol A Biol Sci Med Sci.* 1995;50(A):64–67.

8. King MB, Tinetti ME. Falls in community-dwelling older persons. *J Am Geriatr Soc.* 1995;43:1207–1213.

9. Baraff LJ, Della-Penna R, Williams N, Sanders A. Practice guidelines for the ED management of falls in community dwelling elderly persons. *Ann Emerg Med.* 1997;30:480–489.

10. Josephson KR, Fabacher DA, Rubenstein LZ. Home safety and fall prevention. *Clin Geriatr Med.* 1991;7:707–731.

11. American Medical Directors Association and the American HealthCare Association. Falls and fall risk. *Clinical Practice Guideline.* Author; 1998.

12. Wolter LL, Studenski SA. A clinical synthesis of fall intervention trials. *Top Geriatr Rehabil.* 1996;11(3):9–19. Gaithersburg, MD.

13. Mathias S, Nayak USL, Isaacs B. Balance in elderly patients: the "Get Up and Go" test. *Arch Phys Med Rehabil.* 1986;67:387–389.

14. Tinetti ME, Ginter SF. Identifying mobility dysfunctions in elderly patients. *JAMA.* 1988;259:1190–1193.

15. Berg KO, Maki BE, Williams JL, et al. Clinical and laboratory measures of postural balance in an elderly population. *Arch Phys Med Rehabil.* 1992;73:1073–1080.

16. Posiadlo D, Richardson S. The timed "Up and Go": a test of basic functional mobility for frail elderly persons. *J Am Geriatr Soc.* 1991;38:142–148.

17. Winograd CH, Lemsky CM, Nevitt MC, et al. Development of a physical performance and mobility examination. *J Am Geriar Soc.* 1994;42:743–749.

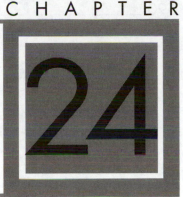

DECISION MAKING

MARSHALL KAPP / TOM FINUCANE

> *Case Vignette: A frail elderly man develops colon cancer with likely metastasis. He has mild dementia. There is a small chance that aggressive treatment might cure him, and a slightly better chance that such treatment would prolong his life. Most likely, it would do neither. The treatment would certainly cause some combination of pain, indignity, disability, disfigurement and expense.*

In this case, the health care provider is forced to do one of two things: give treatment, and cause suffering to a person who is most likely dying, or withhold treatment, and forgo a potentially life-saving intervention for an ill, vulnerable person. Although decisions about life-sustaining treatment receive great attention, day-to-day decisions about frail elders are much more common and, often, as problematic. The purpose of this chapter is to outline how decisions like this are made.

In the United States, the value of autonomy has achieved preeminence in the canon of modern medical ethics. To know what to do for someone, ask him or her. The word *autonomy,* from the Greek for "self rule," was first applied to Greek city-states. It has now come to refer to a general concept that a person should be free to "rule" the course of his or her life. Autonomy is valued so highly because it is seen in the dominant American culture as the optimal way to show respect for another person. Respect for the person is thus seen to require that someone who is able to guide the course of his or her own medical care should do so. As we see in this chapter, other cultures find different ways to show respect for a person. Advance directives are intended for a person who has lost the ability to make decisions to allow the exercise of autonomy more or less *in absentia*. Advance directives are discussed in Chapter 25. If the person is incapable of making a decision and has not established advance directives, decision making by substitutes becomes necessary. Substitutes make decisions on behalf of elders because (1) the individual has previously formally designated them to do so; (2) a legal proceeding has named them to do so, as in a guardianship; or (3) because they seem like the logical people to do so.

This chapter begins with a discussion of informed consent, and the limits imposed by cultural context. Next, we discuss the central question of competence. How do we know if this person is capable of making a meaningful and valid decision? For that matter, what do "meaningful" and "valid" mean? The remainder of the chapter concerns substitute decision makers. What are the rights and responsibilities of the various categories of substitute? When is a court proceeding advisable? What standards should be used when substitutes act on behalf of others and must make these difficult decisions?

INFORMED CONSENT

Informed consent is more than having the patient sign a form before surgery is performed. It involves ensuring that the patient has all the information he or she needs to make an informed decision.

A fundamental principle of American society is that each person has the right to determine what shall be done with/to his or her person. There are few exceptions to this rule. A person should provide autonomous authorization for any medical procedures that are proposed. In order to achieve informed consent, several elements must be present (Table 24-1). There must be *disclosure* of all relevant risks and alternative approaches. The elder must *comprehend* the essential material. The decision must be *voluntary* and free from coercion. The person must be *competent* to make decisions. Finally, the individual must *express a decision*. Each of these elements can be extremely difficult to clearly define. It is

TABLE 24-1. ELEMENTS NECESSARY TO PROVIDE INFORMED CONSENT
A patient with the capacity to make decisions
Adequate disclosure of all information
Comprehension by the patient of the information
An expression of a decision
Assurance that the decision is voluntary

also important to keep separate the roles of informed consent in research and in clinical care. In the former case, higher standards are often required.[1]

Most health care providers struggle with how much to disclose during the informed consent process. The ideal information to be provided for informed consent is shown in Table 24-2. Two competing standards regarding disclosure have been used in many court cases. With the older standard, that of "professional practice," what a health care provider must disclose is determined by the prevailing practices in his or her professional community. More recently, several courts have embraced the "reasonable person" standard. Here, the provider is required to disclose any information that a reasonable person would want to know in order to make the decision in question.

In general, physicians often underestimate how much information the patient desires. Patients almost always want more information provided in order to make the most educated decision.

> *Case Vignette: A 65-year-old man develops atrial fibrillation. The physician offers him coumadin anticoagulation. In doing so, she warns him about necrosis of the penis and possible amputation, a complication that occurs in less than one in a thousand male patients. After she shows him relevant photographs, he chooses to take aspirin only.*

At one extreme, adequate disclosure would suggest that health care providers should act like waiters who are simply showing elders the "menu" of choices. This is clearly an inadequate formulation. On the other hand, providers cannot act by pure paternalistic authoritarianism. This area of uncertainty in ethics, law, and clinical practice is difficult to answer. Deciding how much information to provide based solely on the desire to protect oneself from liability is generally a fruitless endeavor. In the previous case, if the fully informed patient were to have a stroke, a lawsuit could certainly follow. If the patient were to take coumadin without being warned of the possibility of skin necrosis, then a lawsuit could just as easily follow. Some form of middle ground must be sought.

One well-established exception to the rule of autonomy is emergency treatment. If emergency treatment for a critically ill and incapacitated patient is likely to produce substantial benefit,

TABLE 24-2. COMPONENTS OF INFORMED CONSENT

The recommended treatment
The benefits and risks of the recommended treatment
Any alternative treatments available, with attendant benefits and risks
What is likely to occur if no treatment is chosen

and if delaying treatment is likely to lead to irreversible harm, emergency treatment without consent is widely accepted. This exception is limited, however, when a patient has previously expressed a desire not to undergo the proposed emergency treatment. A do-not-resuscitate (DNR) order is acceptable when there has been a clearly stated wish in advance to avoid this intervention. The exact meaning and role of DNR orders remain extremely controversial. To some observers, attempting resuscitation on an elder who is almost certainly dying is barbaric, while to others, withholding this treatment from an emergently ill, highly vulnerable elder is criminally neglectful. In many cases, the patient has not made a decision in advance. The use of DNR orders has increased markedly in the last 10 years, especially in long-term care settings. In acute care settings, however, health care providers and health care institutions tend strongly to preserve life.

The second major exception to the rule of autonomous authorization is called therapeutic privilege. In this case, the physician may believe that fully informing a patient about his or her medical situation would clearly be more harmful than beneficial. The role of therapeutic privilege is highly suspect in the United States, but is widely accepted in most other cultures in the world.

Therapeutic privilege, the act of a physician withholding information in the patient's best interest, is highly suspect in the United States. But many other cultures still see it as a valuable tool for the physician.

> *Case Vignette: An 88-year-old nursing home resident is unable to speak following resection of laryngeal cancer. Hemiparetic, bedfast, and indifferent from a previous stroke, he responds appropriately to simple questions. He will not cooperate with mental status testing. He is hard of hearing, and has poor vision and chronic stable angina. A chest x-ray done because of suspected pneumonia shows a malignant-appearing lung mass with enlarged mediastinal nodes.*

Caring for this resident under the strict doctrine of autonomy, the physician should, in principle, make a determined attempt to inform him about his situation, the possible diagnostic interventions and treatments, and the likely consequences of the various choices. In practice, this would require shouting in the man's ear to inform him that he was almost certainly mortally ill, and repeating this until he acknowledged that he understood. Some ethicists, and many fewer health care providers, believe that the value of autonomy is so great that such a conversation must follow. In many other societies, such an approach would seem cruel and primitive. In Japan, for example, it is likely that during the long terminal illness of the late Emperor Hirohito, he was never informed of his diagnosis.[2] In that society, individual autonomy does not have the same overpowering value that it does in the United States.[3] In an ethnographic study, Carrese and Rhodes[4] have shown that in Navajo culture, thinking or speaking of possible bad events in the future is believed to increase the likelihood that those events will occur and that, therefore, establishing advance directives creates unnecessary risk. In some parts of western Europe until recently, it was a criminal act to inform a patient of the diagnosis of terminal cancer. In the United States, holding a person in "the glare of autonomy," requiring him or her to understand his or her situation and all the possible ways it could go wrong, may be unnecessarily cruel.

Capacity to Make Decisions

Several factors can interfere with a person's ability to make sound decisions about medical treatment, or about other decisions regarding self-care, such as the proper use of financial resources. Dementia and psychiatric illness are well-recognized conditions that affect reasoned decision making. The terms *competence* and *capacity* are often used interchangeably, although the former has a more specific legal connotation: in guardianship proceedings a court may often find a person incompetent. Decision-making capacity is task- or decision-specific. A person may be capable of making medical decisions but not to manage finances, or to refuse amputation but not nursing home placement. When a health care provider is asked to determine if a person has the capacity to make a decision, the reply should be a question: What decision?

In deciding whether a person has decisional capacity, objective testing is of limited value. If a person is conscious, communicative, and willing to express a decision, there is almost no level of cognitive impairment and no score on a mental status test that, by itself, resolves the question of competence. For people who are unable to express a decision, incompetence is present by definition, although the health care provider must be certain of the person's inability to communicate. For an individual who can express a decision, a general clinical rule is that he or she should be able to demonstrate an understanding of the proposed alternatives and the consequences of the various options, then explain reasonably why he or she has chosen the option that he or she has. What constitutes reasonable explanation is often a matter of opinion, however, and a determination of decision-making capacity almost invariably contains some subjective elements.

A health care providers's assessment of an elder's capacity to make the decision at hand is further influenced by what is at stake. If a person declines a risky or uncomfortable procedure that is proposed for a condition where the benefits of treatment are small,

Competence and *capacity* are often used interchangeably. But health care providers deal mostly with issues of whether a patient has the capacity to make a particular decision.

the health care provider will generally not question the person's competence or attempt to force the issue. If a very demented woman declines mammography, even in barely coherent terms, few physicians would mount a serious challenge to her decision. On the other hand, if risks are low and treatment is likely to be successful, physicians might seriously question a patient's decision to forgo treatment. A patient with appendicitis who refuses surgery is likely to undergo much more careful scrutiny.

At times, decisions about capacity are like a Rorschach inkblot test. The physician's judgment tells more about the physician than about the patient. Some physicians are avid to respect patient autonomy, or at least to avoid acting coercively. Others wish to avoid preventable harm to persons who are ill and impaired in their ability to make decisions. The relative weighting of these values will inevitably influence a physician's decisions.

In geriatrics, the border between social and medical problems can be obscure and questions about competency often arise in patients with cognitive impairment who live in unsafe living conditions. Whereas a competent person is free to take calculated risks, people who behave in very risky ways should be able to understand the dangers. An extremely difficult situation arises when progressive dementia develops in people who live alone and who have long, consistent records of saying that they would never want to leave their homes, and that they would rather die than live somewhere else. As the dementia progresses, the risk to the elder rises, and the ability to recognize and understand the risk diminishes. A common approach to this situation is to optimize supportive services in an attempt to reduce the risk. But often, efforts at persuasion fail and guardianship is sought only after elders have sustained an injury.

In summary, assessment of an elder's decision-making capacity begins with a clear statement of the decision that the person is facing. Cognitive testing is not definitive. A person's ability to think about options and their consequences and to make uncoerced, reasonable choices among them is the central feature of capacity. Over 20 years ago, Roth, Meisel, and Lidz formulated the situation succinctly.[5]

> The search for a single test of competence is a search for the Holy Grail. Unless it is realized that there is no magical definition of competency to make decisions about treatment, the search for an acceptable test will never end. . . Judgments (about competence) reflect social considerations and societal biases as much as they reflect matters of law and medicine.

Whereas neuropsychiatric impairment ranges along a continuum, a decision about legal competence is all-or-nothing. Judging

Determining a patient's capacity to make a particular decision is not based solely upon a cognitive test or psychiatrist's evaluation.

a person to be incompetent should be difficult. Once that decision is made, the patient loses a wide spectrum of civil and human rights, from involuntary residential placement to unwanted medical treatment. Fortunately, the legal determination of competence is not necessary in most cases seen in geriatric health care. Surrogate decision makers, usually the patient's spouse or adult children, can provide proxy decisions in the clinical situation.

STANDARDS FOR SURROGATE DECISION MAKING

Substituted Judgment

Current ethical and legal consensus promotes the concept that proxies and surrogates should make decisions for incapacitated patients. Furthermore, they should base such decisions on the principle of *substituted judgment*.[6] This view has been endorsed by the President's Commission for the Study of Ethical Problems in Medicine and Biomedical and Behavioral Research,[7] the New York State Task Force on Life and the Law,[8] the Uniform Health Care Decisions Act adopted by the National Conference of Commissioners on Uniform State Laws,[9] and a host of judicial decisions and state statutes.

Using substituted judgement, a proxy attempts to infer from an individual's earlier statements and actions what choices that person would make now if he or she were able to express an autonomous decision. Because it attempts to account for the individual's unique, even idiosyncratic characteristics and beliefs, substituted judgment is thought of as a subjective approach to decision making. Substituted judgment is the most authentic when the individual has stated treatment preferences before the capacity to decide was lost. Ideally, such preferences would have been stated straightforwardly, unambiguously, and repeatedly. Because such clear statements are unusual, most states permit and indeed encourage proxy (surrogate) decision making on the basis of whatever reasonable inferences about the person's preferences can be drawn by piecing together the individual's informal statements and actions. Since each state is idiosyncratic about its use of the terms "proxy" and "surrogate," this chapter will treat them as equivalent. The reader should refer to his or her own state statute for specific terminology.

> A surrogate decision maker should attempt to decide what the patient would have wanted in this circumstance, not what the surrogate wants.

Some commentators have criticized the concept of substituted judgment as an artificial "legal fiction" or "invented consent," and too speculative a foundation on which to predicate the withdrawal or withholding of medical treatment, especially if it is life-sustaining.[10] One charge is that there are inherent uncertainties in trying to determine the true present wishes of a person incapacitated to make decisions. Many currently competent people might have difficulty articulating precisely some of their own values and preferences. Further, even when the person has left clear instructions concerning his or her feelings about a particular treatment in the future, it can be difficult to draw from that statement meaningful conclusions about the individual's attitude toward another treatment, which had not been previously contemplated. Even if the person previously made a precise statement about the medical intervention now at issue, there is no assurance that the person's preferences in that matter have remained firm and stable over time.

This inevitable uncertainty leads in many cases to proxies or surrogates guessing wrongly about specific treatment preferences of the person for whom they are purporting to exercise substituted judgment. This discordance between patients and their chosen proxies who become decision makers by default, has been well-documented empirically.[11]

Best Interests

Application of the substituted judgment test to a particular situation is sometimes impossible without undue speculation. Where a credible prediction of the incapacitated patient's current preference cannot be made, health care providers are obligated by the principles of beneficence and nonmaleficence (i.e., the duty not to cause harm) and the fiduciary or trust nature of the provider–patient relationship to act in the patient's best interests. This standard is purportedly an objective one; it holds that proxy or surrogate decisions ought to benefit the patient according to the socially shared values of a theoretical reasonable person.

Determining what course of action (or deliberate inaction) would serve a person's best interests in a particular set of circumstances can be problematic. Proper analysis involves weighing the likely benefits versus the predictable burdens (e.g., pain and suffering and loss of independence, privacy, and dignity) of specific alternatives for that person, from the perspective of that person. Reasonable people may disagree about how to strike the balance, when what is really at stake is a judgment about the ambiguous but vital concept of the individual's present and future quality of life.

Conflicts of Interest

In reality, proxies and surrogates commonly make decisions for incapacitated patients based on neither a careful substituted judgment nor a best interests analysis, but instead based on a history of family relationships, religious convictions, and a personal sense of love or guilt. Family members may stand to gain financially from the medical decisions they make for their loved ones. The physician must remain in the role of the patient advocate to ensure that the surrogate decision maker is truly attending to the patient's best interests.

Conflicts of interest, both real and in appearance, can also exist between an incapacitated patient and the health care providers. To guard against such potential conflicts affecting medical decision making, many commentators have urged that health care providers, especially physicians, should never assume the formal function of decision-making proxy or surrogate for their own incapacitated patients. In this view, the conflicts are irreconcilable. Theory aside, in practice, the health care provider sometimes functions *de facto* as the surrogate and this pragmatic accommodation goes on without adverse legal consequences to the provider or negative consequences to the patient.

Even when a surrogate decision maker is available to assist an incapacitated patient, the physician must remain in the role of the patient advocate to ensure that the surrogate is truly attending to the patient's best interests.

SURROGATE DECISION MAKING BY DEFAULT

Devolution of Authority to the Family

The topic of advance planning, including the execution of advance medical directives, is discussed in Chapter 25. In situations where the patient is incapable of making a decision and has executed a valid advance medical directive, decision-making authority may devolve or pass from the patient to someone else by operation of a statute, regulation, or judicial precedent. Family consent statutes in 30 states set forth legal authority empowering specifically designated relatives to make particular kinds of medical decisions on behalf of incapacitated persons who have not executed a living will or durable power of attorney (Table 24-3).[12] Health care providers ought to familiarize themselves with the normal legal progression of medical decision-making authority applicable in their own state. They should also educate patients to make sure that this default progression comports with their wishes and to encourage them to take prospective action if it does not.

In addition to family consent statutes and implementing regulations, courts in an increasing number of states are formally recognizing in test cases the authority of the family to exercise an incompetent person's decision-making rights for him or her. Just as notably, most of these judicial decisions explicitly establish legal precedent for families to act in future cases without the need for

		TABLE 24-3. SURROGATE CONSENT IN THE ABSENCE OF AN ADVANCE DIRECTIVE		
STATE AND CITATION	GENERAL TYPE OF STATUTE	PRIORITY OF SURROGATES (IN ABSENCE OF APPOINTED PROXY OR GUARDIAN WITH HEALTH POWERS)	LIMITATIONS ON TYPES OF DECISIONS	DISAGREEMENT PROCESS AMONG PRIORITY SURROGATES
1. Alabama Ala. Code 1975 §22-8A-11 and –6 (1997), enacted 1997	Comprehensive Health Decisions Act	Spouse Adult child Parent Sibling Nearest relative Attending physician and ethics committee	Patient must be in terminal condition of permanently unconscious	Consensus required
2. Arizona Ariz. Rev. Stat. Ann. §36-3231 (West 1998), enacted 1992	Comprehensive Health Decisions Act	Spouse Adult child Parent Domestic partner Sibling Close friend	N/A to decisions to withdraw nutrition or hydration	Majority rule
3. Arkansas Ark. Code Ann. §20-17-214 (1997)	Living Will Statute	Parents of unmarried minor Spouse Adult child Parents Sibling Persons in loco patients Adult heirs	Patient must be in terminal condition or permanently unconscious N/A if pregnant	Majority rule
4. Colorado Colo. Rev. Stat. Ann. §15-18.5-103 (West 1999)	Separate Surrogate Consent Act	The following "interested persons" must decide who among them shall be surrogate decision-maker: Spouse Either parent Adult child Sibling Grandchild Close friend	N/A to withholding or withdrawal of artificial nourishment and hydration unless specified conditions are met	Consensus required
5. Connecticut Conn. Gen. Stat. Ann. §19a-571 (West 1998)	Comprehensive Health Care Decisions Act	Physician authorized in consultation with next of kin	Limited to the removal or withholding of life-support systems, and patient is in terminal condition or permanently unconscious N/A if pregnant	None listed
6. Delaware Del. Code Ann. tit. 16, §2507 (1998)	Comprehensive Health Care Decisions Act	An individual orally designated as surrogate Spouse Adult child Parent Sibling Grandchild Close friend	Patient must be in terminal condition or permanently unconscious N/A if pregnant	If in health care institution, refer to appropriate committee for a recommendation
7. District of Columbia D.C. Code 1981 §21-2210 (1998)	Durable Power of Attorney for Health Care Act	Spouse Adult child Parent Sibling Religious superior if patient is member of a religious order or a diocesan priest Nearest living relative	N/A to abortion, sterilization, orpsycho-surgery, convulsive therapy, or behavior modification programs involving aversive stimuli	None listed

TABLE 24-3.   SURROGATE CONSENT IN THE ABSENCE OF AN ADVANCE DIRECTIVE (*Continued*)

STATE AND CITATION	GENERAL TYPE OF STATUTE	PRIORITY OF SURROGATES (IN ABSENCE OF APPOINTED PROXY OR GUARDIAN WITH HEALTH POWERS)	LIMITATIONS ON TYPES OF DECISIONS	DISAGREEMENT PROCESS AMONG PRIORITY SURROGATES
8. Florida Fla. Stat Ann. §765.401 (West 1998)	Comprehensive Health Care Decisions Act	Spouse Adult child Parent Sibling Close adult relative Close friend	N/A to abortion, sterilization, electroshock therapy, psychosurgery, experimental treatment, or voluntary admission to a mental health facility Applies to withholding or withdrawal of life-prolonging procedures only if patient is in terminal condition and will not regain decision-making capacity N/A if pregnant	Majority rule
9. Georgia Ga. Code Ann. §31-9-2 (1998)	Informed Consent Statute	Spouse Adult child Parent Sibling Grandparent	Not explicitly applicable to refusals of treatment	None listed
10. Hawaii Haw. Rev. Stat. Ann. §327D-21 (Lexis 1998)	Living Will Statute	Attending physician and family under "ordinary standards of current medical practice" (interpreted by court decision)	Limited to the withdrawal or withholding of life-sustaining procedures	None listed
11. Idaho Idaho Code §39-4303 (Lexis 1998)	Informed Consent Statute	Either: Parent Spouse If none, then any relative or . . . any other person representing himself or herself responsible for the health care of such person	None listed	None listed
12. Illinois 755 ILCS 40/25 (Smith-Hurd 1998)	Separate Surrogate Consent Act	Spouse Adult child Either parent Sibling Adult grandchild Close friend Guardian of the estate	N/A to admission to mental health facility, psychotropic medication, or electroconvulsive therapy (see 405 ILCS 5/1-121.5; 5/2-102; 5/3-601.2, amended 1997) If decision concerns forgoing life-sustaining treatment, patient must be in terminal condition, permanently unconscious, or incurable or irreversible condition	Majority rule
13. Indiana Ind. Code Ann. §16-36-1-1 to –14 (West 1998)	Health Care Agency and Surrogate Consent Act	Any of the following: Spouse Parent Adult child Sibling Religious superior if the individual is a member of a religious order	None listed	None listed

		TABLE 24-3. SURROGATE CONSENT IN THE ABSENCE OF AN ADVANCE DIRECTIVE (Continued)		
STATE AND CITATION	GENERAL TYPE OF STATUTE	PRIORITY OF SURROGATES (IN ABSENCE OF APPOINTED PROXY OR GUARDIAN WITH HEALTH POWERS)	LIMITATIONS ON TYPES OF DECISIONS	DISAGREEMENT PROCESS AMONG PRIORITY SURROGATES
14. Iowa Iowa Code Ann. §144A.7 (West 1998)	Living Will Statute	Spouse Adult child Parent or both parents, if reasonably available Adult sibling	Limited to the withholding or withdrawal of life-sustaining procedures, and patient is in terminal condition or comatose N/A if pregnant	Majority rule
15. Kentucky Ky. Rev. Stat. §311.631 (Baldwin 1999)	Living Will Statute	Spouse Adult child Parents Nearest relative	N/A to withholding or withdrawal artificial nutrition and hydration unless specified conditions are met	Majority rule
16. Louisiana La. Rev. Stat. Ann. §40:1299.58. 1 to 10 (West 1999)	Living Will Statute	Spouse Adult child Parents Sibling Other relatives	Limited to patient in terminal and irreversible condition and comatose	Consensus required
17. Maine Me. Rev. Stat. Ann tit. 18-A, §5-801 to §5-817 (West 1998)	Comprehensive Health Care Decisions Act	Spouse Adult child Parent Sibling Adult grandchild Adult niece or nephew Adult relative familiar with patient's values Close friend	Limited to withdrawal or withholding of life-sustaining treatment, and patient is in terminal condition or persistent vegetative state	Majority rule, although referral to dispute resolution assistance is mentioned as option
18. Maryland Md. Health-Gen. Code Ann., §5-605 (Lexis 1998)	Comprehensive Health Care Decisions Act	Spouse Adult child Parent Sibling Friend or relative who has maintained regular contact with the patient	N/A to sterilization or treatment for mental disorder Applicable to life-sustaining procedure only if the patient as been certified to be in a terminal condition, persistent vegetative state, or end-stage condition Applicable to DNR order only under certain conditions	If in hospital or nursing home, refer to ethics committee If elsewhere, consensus required
19. Mississippi Miss. Code 1972 Ann. §41-41-211 (1998)	Comprehensive Health Care Decisions Act	Individual orally designated by patient Spouse Adult child Parent Sibling Close friend	None listed	Majority rule
20. Montana Mont. Code Ann. §50-9-106 (1997)	Living Will Statute	Spouse Adult child Parents Sibling Nearest adult relative	Limited to withholding or withdrawal of life-sustaining treatment, and patient is in terminal condition N/A if pregnant	Majority rule

| | | PRIORITY OF SURROGATES (IN | | DISAGREEMENT |
| | GENERAL TYPE OF | ABSENCE OF APPOINTED PROXY OR | LIMITATIONS ON TYPES | PROCESS AMONG |
STATE AND CITATION	STATUTE	GUARDIAN WITH HEALTH POWERS)	OF DECISIONS	PRIORITY SURROGATES
21. Nevada Nev. Rev. Stat. §449.626 (1997)	Living Will Statute	Spouse Adult child Parents Sibling Nearest adult relative	Limited to withholding or withdrawal of life-sustaining treatment, and patient is in terminal condition N/A if pregnant	Majority rule
22. New Mexico N.M. Stat. Ann. 1978 §24-7A-5 (1998)	Comprehensive Health Care Decisions Act	An individual designated as surrogate Spouse Individual in long-term spouse-like relationship Adult child Parent Sibling Grandparent Close friend	None listed	Majority rule
23. New York N.Y. Pub. Health Law §2965 (McKinney 1999)	Specialized Surrogate Consent Statute (applicable only to DNR orders)	Spouse Adult child Parent Sibling Close friend	Limited to consent to a DNR order, and patient is in terminal condition, or permanently unconscious, or where resuscitation is futile or extraordinarily burdensome	Refer to dispute mediation system
24. North Carolina N.C. Gen. Stat. §90-322 (Michie 1997)	Living Will Statute	Spouse Majority of relatives of the first degree	Limited to the withholding or discontinuance of extraordinary means or artificial nutrition or hydration, and patient is in terminal condition, or persistent vegetative state, and meets other conditions	Majority rule
25. North Dakota N.D. Cent. Code §23-12-13 (Michie 1997)	Informed Consent Statute	Spouse Adult children Parents Siblings Grandparents Adult grandchildren Close adult relative or friend	Not explicitly applicable to refusals of treatment N/A to sterilization, abortion, psychosurgery, and some admissions to a state mental facility	None listed
26. Ohio Ohio Rev. Code Ann. §2133.08 (Baldwin 1999)	Living Will Statute	Spouse Adult child Parents Sibling Nearest adult relative	Limited to consent for withdrawal or withholding of life-sustaining treatment, and patient is in terminal condition or permanently unconscious Nutrition and hydration may be withheld only upon the issuance of an order of the probate court N/A if pregnant	Majority rule
27. Oklahoma Okla. Stat. Ann. tit. 63 §3102A (West 1999)	Specialized provision (applicable only to experimental treatments)	Spouse Adult child Parent Sibling Relative	Limited to experimental treatment, test, or drug approved by a local institutional review board	None listed

TABLE 24-3. SURROGATE CONSENT IN THE ABSENCE OF AN ADVANCE DIRECTIVE (Continued)

TABLE 24-3. SURROGATE CONSENT IN THE ABSENCE OF AN ADVANCE DIRECTIVE (Continued)				
STATE AND CITATION	GENERAL TYPE OF STATUTE	PRIORITY OF SURROGATES (IN ABSENCE OF APPOINTED PROXY OR GUARDIAN WITH HEALTH POWERS)	LIMITATIONS ON TYPES OF DECISIONS	DISAGREEMENT PROCESS AMONG PRIORITY SURROGATES
28. Oregon Or. Rev. Stat. §127.635 (1998)	Comprehensive Health Care Decisions Act	Spouse Adult designated by others on this list, without objection by anyone on list Majority of adult children Either parent Majority of siblings Adult relative or adult friend Attending physician	Limited to withdrawal or withholding of life-sustaining procedures, and patient is in terminal condition, or permanently unconscious, or meets other conditions	Majority rule
30. South Carolina S.C. Code 1976 Ann. §44-66-30 (1998)	Separate Surrogate Consent Act	Person given priority to make healthcare decisions for the patient by another statute Spouse Parent or adult child Sibling, grandparent, or adult grandchild Other close relative Person given authority to make healthcare decisions for the patient by another statutory provision	N/A if patient's inability to consent is temporary and delay of treatment will not result in significant detriment to the patient's health	None listed
31. South Dakota S.D. Codified Laws Ann. §34-12C-1 to -8 (1998)	Separate Surrogate Consent Act	Spouse Adult child Parent Sibling Grandparent or adult grandchild Aunt or uncle or adult niece or nephew	None listed	None listed

32. Texas
Tex. [Health & Safety] Code Ann. §672.009 (West 1997)
	Living Will Statute	At least two persons, if available, in the following priority:
		  Spouse
		  Majority of reasonably available adult children
		  Parents
		  Nearest relative
			N/A if pregnant	Majority rule

Tex. [Health & Safety] Code Ann. §674.001 to .024, specifically §674.008(b) (West 1997)	Specialised provision (applicable to **DNR** orders)	Same as above. Incorporates the terms of §672.009	Same as above	Same as above

33. Utah
Utah Code Ann. 1953 §75-2-1105, -1105.5, -1107 (Lexis 1998)
	Comprehensive Health Care Decisions Act	Spouse
		Parents or surviving parent
		Adult child
		Nearest reasonably available relative
		When patient is terminal or in a permanent vegetative state:
		  Spouse
		  Parent
		  Adult children
			N/A if pregnant	Majority rule

STATE AND CITATION	GENERAL TYPE OF STATUTE	PRIORITY OF SURROGATES (IN ABSENCE OF APPOINTED PROXY OR GUARDIAN WITH HEALTH POWERS)	LIMITATIONS ON TYPES OF DECISIONS	DISAGREEMENT PROCESS AMONG PRIORITY SURROGATES
34. Virginia Va. Code 1950 §54.1-2986 (Michie 1997)	Comprehensive Health Care Decisions Act	Spouse Adult child Parent Sibling Other relative in the descending order of blood relationship	N/A to nontherapeutic sterilization, abortion, psychosurgery, or admission to a mental retardation facility or psychiatric hospital	Majority rule
35. Washington Wash. Rev. Code Ann. §7.70.065 (West 1998)	Informed Consent Statute	Spouse Adult children Parents Siblings	Not explicitly applicable to refusals of treatment	Consensus required
36. West Virginia W. Va. Code 1966 §16-30B-1 to –16 (Lexis 1998)	Separate Surrogate Consent Statute	Spouse Adult child Parent Sibling Adult grandchild Close friend Any other person or entity according to DHHR rules If there are multiple surrogates at the same priority level, provider must choose one who appears best qualified according to statutory criteria; may also choose lower level surrogate if deemed best qualified	None listed	Others on the permissible surrogate list have a 72-hour window to seek court challenge of a decision made by selected surrogate
37. Wyoming Wyo. Stat. 1997 §3-5-209 and §35-22-105(b) (1998)	Durable Power of Attorney Statute and Living Will Statute (Identical provisions)	All family members who can be contacted through reasonable diligence	Limited to withholding or withdrawal of life-sustaining procedures, and patient is in terminal condition or irreversible coma	Consensus required
Uniform Health-Care Decisions Act	Comprehensive Health Care Decisions Act	Individual orally designated by patient Spouse Adult child Parent Sibling Close friend	None listed	Majority rule

Source: ABA Commission on Legal Problems of the Elderly, 1999.

obtaining prior court authorization.[13] Information regarding state-specific advance directives and regulations can be found on the web site of the organization Choice in Dying (**www.choices.org**).

In the absence of an advance directive or any specific statute, regulation, or court order delegating authority to a substitute decision maker for an incapacitated patient, neither the family as a whole nor any of its individual members (nor any nonrelatives) possess any special legal authority to make decisions on behalf of

Check state regulations regarding advanced directives and whether there is a specified order of whom to consult as surrogates in the absence of a formal advance directive.

a patient who cannot speak for himself or herself. Nonetheless, it has long been a widely known and implicitly accepted medical custom for families to be relied on by health care providers as the empowered decision maker, even in the absence of express legal authority. The courts, in turn, have been very careful not to second-guess health professional deference to family decisions made on behalf of incapacitated patients, except under the most extreme and compelling circumstances.

This devolution of authority is predicated on the family's position as the basic moral unit in society. Family members are presumed to best know the basic values and preferences of their relatives, thereby facilitating accurate substituted judgment. Family members are also often expected to act as zealous advocates for the patient's best interests. Individuals who believe their family members will not carry out their personal wishes have the opportunity, as well as the obligation, to engage in timely advance medical planning to make alternative proxy arrangements. Studies have shown, however, that the overwhelming proportion of elders prefer that their family members serve as proxies or surrogates if necessary, and that elders assume that this will occur even in the absence of any affirmative direction on their part.[14]

Practical Considerations and Conflicts in Family Involvement

Whatever the formal or informal source of family decision-making authority, most family decisions sooner or later are reached as a matter of consensus through a process of communication, negotiation, and sometimes compromise. Major, irresolvable conflicts among family members or between the family and the health care team are very much the exceptional circumstance.

Nevertheless, in some cases, substitute decision making by family members may not work well. Problems are especially likely when the family's authority is informal and the elder's family cannot agree as to the patient's prior wishes. Family members may so fundamentally disagree among themselves that voluntary consensus becomes unattainable. Most of the time, there is an implicitly understood hierarchy of family surrogates (i.e., spouse to adult children to siblings to other relatives), and states with family consent statutes have specified this sort of hierarchy legislatively. When conflicts develop, it is desirable to include in discussions all family members who wish to be part of the decision-making process. Generally, one particular family member will ultimately be relied on as the authorized agent to accept or refuse medical recommendations, but achieving broad family consensus on important issues to the greatest degree feasible is an ideal to be pursued.

Family members may make decisions that seem to be at odds with the earlier expressed or understood preferences of the elder or that clearly appear not to be in the individual's best interests. The possibility of actual or apparent financial and/or emotional conflicts of interest was mentioned previously. Conflicts of interest are potentially more troublesome when decision making devolves to a family surrogate by default, as opposed to the frequent situations in which the elder knew of the conflict but nonetheless consciously chose to name the relative as formal proxy decision maker anyway.

Factual misunderstandings, a family member's idiosyncratic religious beliefs, and the surrogate's own emotional or cognitive impairments can skew substitute decision making seriously away from the ideal. Even when none of the foregoing factors is present and the family knows (or thinks it knows) what treatment choice its incapacitated loved one would currently make, the family may consciously disregard the elder's wishes because the relatives simply think they "know better." In other words, the family thinks it knows what's "best" for the person more than he or she does. In addition, the family may request a course of conduct that seriously contradicts the personal sense of ethical integrity held by the physician, other members of the care team, or the health care facility.

When any of these situations happen, the various interested parties can resort to petitioning a court to appoint a guardian or conservator with the power to make decisions on behalf of the incompetent person. The guardianship option is discussed in the following section. Other external arbitrators or mediators also may be drawn into trying to resolve decision-making situations gone awry, for example, institutional ethics committees and long-term care ombudsmen may help to resolve disputes.

Timely, thoughtful family discussions can assist the elder to reduce the possibility that acrimonious scenarios will unfold in his or her own life. These discussions need to commence well in advance of medical crises, at a time when the individual is able to fully participate in, indeed, to direct their content.

GUARDIANSHIP AND CONSERVATORSHIP

Definitions and Rationales

When other, more private and less intrusive forms of proxy or surrogate decision making for a cognitively or emotionally incapable patient have failed, guardianship or conservatorship may be needed. Guardianship is a legal relationship, created by a state court (in most states in the probate division), between a ward (the

Guardianship usually refers to control over the person's medical decisions, whereas conservatorship often refers to control over the person's finances.

person whom the court has adjudicated as incompetent to make particular kinds of decisions) and a guardian (whom the court appoints as the proxy decision maker for the ward). Conservatorship is usually applied to management of the person's estate or finances, though precise terminology regarding this legal relationship varies somewhat among jurisdictions. For instance, a court-appointed proxy with total authority over both the ward's personal and financial matters is called a plenary guardian. One given authority only over financial issues is a guardian of the estate or conservator, and a proxy decision maker regarding personal (including medical and residential) choices is a guardian of the person. Because the terminology is not standard, readers should familiarize themselves with the terms used in their own respective states.

Two fundamental ethical principles form the justification for judicial imposition of a proxy decision maker for an incapacitated person regarding personal and/or financial questions. The principle of nonmaleficence guides health care providers to "do no harm" to others (*primum non-nocere*). The related precept of beneficence tells health care providers to assist others who need help, to positively "do good." These ethical principles have been translated into the legal doctrine of *parens patriae,* the inherent authority and obligation of a benevolent society to intervene, even over objection, to protect people who cannot properly take care of themselves and their own interests. It is the power of government to protect incapacitated individuals from themselves, if necessary.

Reasons Guardianship Is Sought

Guardianship is generally sought for one of two reasons. First, there is altruism, a sincere wish to benevolently protect a vulnerable human being. Thus, guardianship petitions often are generated by members of the helping professions, social agencies, and private citizens (relatives and friends) who seek an effective legal mechanism for assuming necessary control over the personal or financial affairs of a cognitively or emotionally compromised person.

The second sort of motivation for guardianship petition initiation is more pragmatic; guardianship may be sought for the primary purpose of benefiting a service provider, for example, a physician or other health care professional, nursing facility, or hospital. These providers, out of anxiety about their own liability exposure, may resort to the guardianship system to definitively establish a party who is responsible for paying for services used by the ward and who is legally empowered to provide binding informed consent for medical treatment. Guardianship petitions can be made as a result of mandated provider compliance with state elder abuse and neglect reporting requirements. These motivations often are quite legitimate, but they illustrate the point that, much of the time, guardianships are created more to protect a third party than to benefit the proposed ward directly.

Powers and Limits of Guardians

Judicial appointment of a guardian means that the ward no longer retains the power to exercise decisional rights that have been assigned to the guardian. Historically, the legal system has treated guardianship as an all-or-nothing proposition, with global findings of incompetence being accompanied by virtually complete loss of rights on the part of the ward. Recently, the trend has been toward statutory and judicial recognition of the concept of limited or partial guardianship, which takes into consideration the decision-specific nature of mental capacity and the ability of some people to rationally make certain kinds of decisions, but not others. Under this arrangement, a guardian is given power to make only those limited kinds of decisions that the court finds the ward unable to make personally. The right to make decisions on other matters is retained by the ward.

Courts also have the authority to appoint a guardian on a temporary basis when the ward is expected to regain capacity in the foreseeable future. Most states now require periodic review of guardianship orders, although the burden of proof regarding decisional capacity ordinarily shifts at that point to the ward to provide evidence that capacity has been restored. States provide an array of procedural due process protections against unwanted intrusions for the proposed ward prior to the imposition of a guardianship, and the appointing court maintains oversight jurisdiction as long as the guardianship remains in effect. Realistically, the extent and quality of continuing judicial monitoring of guardians after their appointment frequently is quite weak, in light of constrained court budgets and resources.

THE INCAPACITATED ELDER WITHOUT FAMILY AND FRIENDS

For a growing number of elders whose cognitive or emotional impairments are severe enough to technically qualify them for guardianship, whether plenary or limited, the most pressing practical problem is the unavailability of family members or close friends who are willing and able to accept guardianship duties. Some states have legislation creating public guardianship systems, under which a government agency itself acts as guardian of last resort or contracts out those services.[15] Further information regarding legal issues can be found on the web site of the American Bar Association's Commission on Legal Problems of the Elderly (**www.abanet.org/ elderly**). In a few localities, religious or other private community organizations have formed volunteer guardianship programs to help meet temporary needs. When the proposed ward has adequate financial assets, the services of a growing number of private, for-profit professional guardians can be purchased through the probate courts.

When these alternatives are not available, the incapacitated person with no family or friends often is in severe jeopardy of literally "falling between the cracks" of the service delivery system. Significant decisions, including those pertaining to medical treatment, by default go without being made until an emergency has developed and the doctrine of presumed consent applies to justify intervention without formal permission. Consultation with institutional ethics committees or consultants, as well as institutional legal counsel, can be especially useful in these circumstances.

Alternatives to Guardianship

Guardianship usually is an expensive, time-consuming, and emotionally draining experience for everyone involved, often without producing satisfactory offsetting benefits. A number of less restrictive and intrusive alternatives exist for assisting elders with cognitive or emotional impairments to navigate through the challenges of daily life and, ideally, to keep private decisions within the private, nonjudicial sphere. Some of these alternatives to guardianship are planned by the competent individual in anticipation of incapacity at some future time.

Planned alternatives for financial purposes include such strategies as joint bank accounts, various forms of living trusts, direct deposit of checks, and personal money management services. Living wills and durable powers of attorney are potentially useful medical advance planning options. For financial matters, federal law has established various representative payee programs to handle government benefit checks on behalf of incapacitated beneficiaries who have not previously made alternative arrangements.[16] Another important means of surrogate decision making is Adult Protective Services (APS). These agencies, located in every state, provide a constellation of social, legal, medical, and basic maintenance services to community-dwelling elders in need. Ordinarily, services are accepted voluntarily by the beneficiary, and the most

Local adult protective services agencies can often provide assistance is managing incapacitated elders who have no family or friends to act as surrogates.

pressing issue is how to obtain enough resources to satisfy the individual's needs and desires. State APS statutes usually contain provisions authorizing involuntary imposition of services, over the elder's objections, in emergency circumstances based on an abbreviated application and hearing. APS is not really a complete alternative to guardianship because, once an immediate emergency has abated, the APS agency must go through the entire formal guardianship process before proceeding with further intervention over the individual's objection.

SUMMARY

Autonomy has become the centerpiece of medical decision making in contemporary American medical ethics. At the same time, powerful technology has developed that can prolong life, although often simultaneously imposing serious burden on the patient. Making decisions for frail elders, who are often cognitively impaired and near death, is a difficult problem that will likely grow more frequent. In general, if a person has the capacity to make decisions, the best way to know what is good for him or her is to ask. In particular, health care providers should recognize explicitly the right of every competent individual to say, "I do not want this treatment."

Good medical decision making requires informed consent. Enough information must be provided to the person in a manner that it will be understood so that an educated decision can be made. Emergency treatment and therapeutic privilege are the two most well-accepted exceptions to this rule. Health care providers must act benevolently and offer their best advice, but the patient will have the final decision.

Determination of decision-making capacity depends on the nature of the decision. It cannot be determined on the basis of a mental status score or a psychiatrist's consultation. Such determinations require in-depth discussions with patients or their surrogates. There is no objective finding that provides a definitive answer.

For incapacitated elders who lack advance directives, substitute decision making becomes necessary. The roles and authority of substitutes designated by the individual, those designated by the courts, and those who are acting by default are variable from jurisdiction to jurisdiction, as is the terminology used to identify these roles. In general, patient-designated substitutes (e.g., health care agents or proxies) have wide authority to make decisions. Substitutes acting by default, often-close family members, are viewed in some states as trustworthy allies, and in other states, their authority is sharply circumscribed. The trend in guardianship proceedings is to name guardians for very specific tasks, rather than assigning them broad authority over the person. Alternatives to guardianship are being developed.

REFERENCES

1. Faden RR, Beauchamp TL. *A History and Theory of Informed Consent.* New York: Oxford University Press; 1986.
2. Harfield P. Tokyo perspective: informed consent *Lancet.* 1993;341: 1141.
3. Long SO, Long BD. Curable cancers and fatal ulcers: attitudes toward cancer in Japan. *Soc Sci Med.* 1982;16:2101–2108.
4. Carrese JA, Rhodes LA. Western bioethics on the Navajo reservation: benefit or harm? *JAMA.* 1995;274:826–829.
5. Roth LH, Meisel A, Lidz CW. Tests of competency to consent to treatment. *Am J Psych* 1977;134:279–284.
6. Welch DD. Walking in their shoes: paying respect to incompetent patients. *Vanderbilt Law Rev.* 1989;42:1617.
7. Helm A. Summary of the President's Commission for the Study of Ethical Problems and Biomedical and Behavioral Research. *Mil Med.* 1987;152:425–430.
8. Daly RW. When others must choose: deciding for patients without capacity. The New York State Task Force on Life and the Law. *HEC Forum.* 1993;5:100–107.
9. Galambos CM. Preserving end-of-life autonomy: the Patient Self-Determination Act and the Uniform Health Care Decisions Act. *Health Soc Work.* 1998;23(4):275–281.
10. Suhl J, Simons P, Reedy T, Garrick T. Myth of substituted judgement: surrogate decision making regarding life support is unreliable. *Arch Intern Med.* 1994;154:90–96.
11. Sulmasy DP, Terry PB, Weisman CS, et al. The accuracy of substituted judgements in patients with terminal illness. *Ann Intern Med.* 1998;128:621–629.
12. Areen J. The legal status of consent obtained from families of adult patients to withhold or withdraw treatment. *JAMA.* 1987;258: 229–235.
13. Schmidt W. *Guardianship: The Court of Last Resort for the Elderly and Disabled.* Durham, NC: Carolina Academic Press; 1995.
14. High DM. Surrogate decision making: who will make decisions for me when I can't? *Clin Geriatr Med.* 1994;10:445–462.
15. Kapp MB. Ethical aspects of guardianship. *Clin Geriatr Med.* 1994;10(3):501–512.
16. Veterans Affairs 38 C.F.R. Sec. 13.1-13.111. Department of Defense 37 U.S.C. Sec. 601-604, Railroad Retirement Board 20 C.F.R. Sec. 266-11-266.13, Office of Personnel Management 5 U.S.C. Sec. 8345(e), Social Security Programs (Old Age, Survivors, and Disability Insurance 20 C.F.R. Sec. 404.2001-404.2065).

ADVANCE DIRECTIVES

ROBERT A. PEARLMAN

The principal goal of advance care planning (ACP) is to promote good medical decisions for patients who become decisionally incapacitated. Advance care planning aims to achieve this either by having the patient's autonomous wishes, expressed during a period of prior decisional capacity, serve as an action guide, or by having the specified proxy decision maker or the next-of-kin make decisions.[1]

In the chapter, advance care planning and the role of advance directives are described. After presenting limitations inherent in ACP and the use of advance directives, a framework to help health care providers facilitate ACP discussions with patients is provided. Several case examples are given throughout the chapter to highlight important clinical complexities. Explanatory considerations for approaching these difficult issues are also offered. The chapter concludes with a call for education and research to improve the process of ACP.

UNDERSTANDING ACP AND THE USE OF ADVANCE DIRECTIVES

ACP is a two-step process. The first step is a cognitive process in which people formulate preferences for future medical care in the event of decisional incapacity. In this process, a person may consider many issues, such as quality of life, outcomes of treatment, and personal values. In this first step, a person may identify the individual he wants to speak on his or her behalf in medical care decisions. Ideally, a person should clarify his or her personal threshold for acceptability of the benefits and burdens of medical treatment under plausible future conditions of decisional incapacity. The second step of ACP is a communicative process. Communication should make sure that the identified potential proxy decision maker is willing to assume this responsibility. Moreover, communication should ensure that the elder's health care providers and institutions are familiar with his or her preferences for future medical care. Communication also should provide an accurate and useful description of these preferences.

Where should ACP take place? Although the Joint Commission for the Accreditation of Health Care Organizations (JCAHO) requires that patients be made aware of their right to have an advance directive on admission to health care institutions, this may not be the ideal time.[2] Thoughtful ACP can occur more readily in the home and outpatient settings without the stress of acute illness. It is recommended, however, that a person's previously stated preferences be reviewed on admission to a hospital, nursing home, home care program, or hospice to ensure that there has not been a change.

Advance directives are the means to communicate and/or document ACP. Advance directives can be written or verbal, formal or informal, and legally approved or unofficial. Written directives have the advantage of providing evidence of prior wishes. The validity of directives is maximized by thoughtful reflection, authentic preferences, and unambiguous communication. Advance directives are generally of two types: instructional (e.g., living wills) and proxy [e.g., durable power of attorney for health care (DPAHC)]. Instructional directives allow the patient to specify care preferences about treatments in terminal conditions (living wills) and nonterminal conditions, as well (other types of written advance directives). Physicians and others, however, often have trouble interpreting these written directives as the instructions are often too vague or too constrained, and may, in any case, not correspond to the situation at hand.[3]

Proxy directives officially appoint spokespersons for decision making if the person becomes decisionally incapacitated. Simply appointing a proxy, however, does not necessarily increase the proxy's understanding of the individual's values or wishes.[4] The following case illustrates paradigmatic issues that arise with regard

Instructional directives allow the patient to specify care preferences about treatments in terminal conditions (living wills) and nonterminal conditions (other types of advance directives).

Proxy directives officially appoint spokespersons for decision making if the patient becomes decisionally incapacitated.

to understanding ACP communication and interpreting advance directives.

Case Vignette: Family Conflict and Ambiguous Communication

HISTORY. *A 65-year-old woman asked that her sister be her proxy decision maker in the event that she became decisionally incapacitated. She told her sister that she would not want to receive life-sustaining treatment, including the artificial provision of hydration and nutrition, if she "lost her mental faculties and was suffering." She recently developed pneumonia and confusion. Over a prolonged hospital course, she has remained confused and become malnourished. In order to manage the infection properly, the doctors want to use a feeding tube. The sister thinks that this is not appropriate because of what she was told by her sister. A brother has visited, however, and disagrees with his sister.*

CONSIDERATIONS. *This case demonstrates the importance of clear communication and shared understanding in ACP communication. It is difficult to know whether the patient's wishes were intended to apply to potentially reversible situations. Moreover, the suffering is an ambiguous term. Patients need to clarify what they mean by suffering. Similar problems arise with terms such as independence, dignity, pain, burden, and hope(less).*

The conflict between family members is troublesome. Although the designation of proxies is supposed to reduce family conflict, this may not always be the case. Similarly, although the designated proxy is authorized legally to make the decision, family dynamics and social roles make this authority less clear. Health care providers often attempt to achieve consensus among family members before acting for a person who is decisionally incapacitated. It is advisable for health care providers to ask the family members to try to represent the patient's interests and wishes, rather than their own values. It also is advisable to inform nondesignated family members that the patient chose one family member for a reason and that honoring that selection shows respect for the patient. Persistent family conflicts can interfere with timely medical decision making. In these circumstances, appeal to an ethics committee or suggesting that the nondesignated family member go to court for determination of the most appropriate decision maker are options to consider.

DIFFERENT APPROACHES TO ADVANCE DIRECTIVES

Instructional Directives

Starting in the 1970s, California passed a living will statute, referred to as the Natural Death Act.[5] Briefly, this Act specified that terminally ill patients could issue directives to their physicians to withhold or withdraw life-sustaining treatment that merely prolonged the moment of death. It serves as a model for many other states. Currently, many living will statutes include permanent vegetative state as a condition under which life-sustaining treatment is to be withheld or withdrawn, and some statutes specify the inclusion or exclusion of medical hydration and nutrition from the definition of life-sustaining treatment. In addition, some natural death acts offer space for patients to indicate other wishes pertinent to decision making at the end of life. When completed according to state specifications (e.g. witnessing or notarization), natural death acts and living will statutes serve as state-approved directives for withholding and withdrawing life-sustaining treatment in the event of terminal illness and decisional incapacity. The Department of Veteran Affairs (VA) has developed an advance directive form for use in VA health care institutions throughout the United States (see Appendix #44).

A popular, unofficial instructional directive is the Medical Directive. A major section of this document presents brief clinical scenarios, such as coma, terminal illness, dementia, and one's current state of health, and requests that patients express their preferences for numerous life-sustaining treatments under those conditions.[6] Patients can indicate whether they want, do not want, want a therapeutic trial (if feasible), or are undecided about each of the listed treatments. (A sample page from the Medical Directive is on Appendix #28)

Value statements are alternative forms of expression that serve as instructional directives. Many patients use them as a means to communicate their ACP preferences. Value statements often pertain to issues concerning dignity, independence, burden, and suffering. For example, the Values History form contains questions for patients to answer, such as, "Do you consider yourself an independent person?" "What goals do you have for the future?" "Are prayer and worship important to you?[7]" Another set of values questions/statements includes issues such as, I want to feel safe and secure, and, I want to be treated with respect. These types of value statements, however, have limited relevance to decisions about using or forgoing life-sustaining treatments. For this reason, value statements from an ACP workbook entitled, *Your Life, Your Choices,* are included in the appendix to this chapter.[8]

Proxy Directives

In every state in the United States, statutes exist sanctioning the appointment of a proxy decision maker for medical decisions (health care agent) if a person were to become decisionally incapacitated. These documents, called durable power of attorney for health care (DPAHC), usually do not allow an involved health care provider to become the health care agent. When completed according to state specifications, these documents empower a specified decision maker, who may be a family member or not. Use of this form of directive (proxy-type) is particularly suited for patients who do not have a nuclear family or for situations in which family conflict is anticipated. The Durable Power of Attorney for Health Care form utilized in the VA health care system is Part 1 of the VA Advance Directive on Appendix #44.

Combination Directives

Combination directives appoint a proxy decision maker and provide instructions, preferences, or relevant value statements. These instructions are intended to provide guidance for health care agents so that medical decisions are framed by this kind of expression of patient values. The Medical Directive is a combination directive. Combination directives may be the most useful form of directive. They help ensure that the proxy decision maker knows the relevant, health-related values and preferences of the patient.

LIMITATIONS OF ADVANCE DIRECTIVES

Many of the current limitations in formulating and executing advance directives exist as a result of insufficient knowledge about successful alternative approaches. Examples of limitations are organized by category and presented as follows.

Theoretical Issues

Advance directives raise at least three distinct theoretical concerns that health care providers need to be aware of. First, advance

Written instructional directives usually are framed in the direction of foregoing life-sustaining treatment.

Many patients are not interested in executing advance directives for legitimate reasons.

The interests and resulting preferences that are expressed in a directive may not be relevant to the future situation.

directives are intended to foster patient self-determination in medical decision-making, yet written instructional directives are usually framed in the direction of foregoing life-sustaining treatment. In part, this reflects an underlying professional norm and a societal goal. The professional norm in medicine is to support life. The societal goal of advance directives is to curtail excessive treatment by the medical profession and promote death with dignity. The negative slant to advance directives however raises the dual risk of inhibiting patient expression of countervailing attitudes and creating health care provider expectations that it is not as acceptable to want life-sustaining treatments as it is to forego them.

A second concern is that many people are not interested in executing advance directives for legitimate reasons. Some think that directives reflect an attempt to cut health care costs at their expense. Others fear that health care providers will misinterpret their preferences in the same way that a "no-cardiopulmonary resuscitation (CPR)" policy sometimes slips into a "no intensive care" or "no curative treatment" policy. Although people have the autonomous right to not be burdened with advance directives and can opt for informed refusal, they need to understand the implications of not having an advance directive. For example, they need to know who the health care provider will turn to for help with decision making.

A third theoretical concern is that a person's interests and preferences that are expressed in a directive may not be relevant to a future situation.[9] An active businessman who says that he would prefer to die from a life-threatening illness than live with brain damage or severe cognitive deficits may not retain the same perspective after becoming demented. Although most patients would argue that their current (precognitive impairment) preferences should be determinative, returning to this case example can demonstrate the weakness of this position. If this hypothetical business person develops severe dementia and lives in a nursing home, but enjoys the attention from the nursing staff and the affection of the institution's pet cat, it is legitimate to question whether the previous statement of preferences should outweigh the man's positive elements of quality of life and apparent contemporaneous best interests. This case example shows how this theoretical concern has practical implications. Another similar case is presented as follows.

Case Vignette: Substituted Judgment Versus Best Interests

HISTORY. *After reading a poignant article in The New Yorker, a 66-year-old widow told her daughter that if she ever* *became demented, she would not want to live like that. Some years later, she developed dementia and was placed in a nursing home. Recently, she stopped eating and the nursing home staff wants her to have a PEG tube placed for provision of hydration and nutrition. Her daughter wants to respect her earlier wishes, but she has second thoughts. Her mother seems to enjoy herself in the nursing home, obtaining pleasure in watching television and appreciating her monthly visits (although she does not recognize her).*

CONSIDERATIONS. *According to many sources, substituted judgment is the highest standard of surrogate decision making. Yet, sometimes contemporaneous best interests conflict with prior expression of preferences. In this case, the ACP conversation did not identify the mother's rationale for stating that she would not want life-sustaining treatment. The conversation also did not address what the mother envisioned when she talked about dementia. She may have thought about screaming, wandering, paranoid patients who do not interact meaningfully with and derive pleasure from their environment. Without more information, it is impossible to know what is the most likely right thing to do. When patients are asked about this potential, many want their prior wishes honored. Others recognize that good judgment needs to be included in the actual decision making. Thus, this issue is an important element of ACP discussions. This case also emphasizes the importance of quality ACP discussions before the need for implementing a directive. Health care provider involvement in the formulation of preferences can serve as a quality assurance safeguard for ambiguous preferences.*

Logistical Issues: Who, When, and How Often

Advance directives have been described as interventions in preventive ethics. Prevention strategies in health care always raise questions about who should be targeted, when should the screening occur, and how often should it be repeated. Similarly, these questions should be asked about the formulation of advance directives from patients.[10]

Although advance directives are recommended for everyone, this lack of specificity reduces the cost-effectiveness of this activity and can undermine quality ACP discussions between people and

Knowledge is lacking about who should be targeted, when should the screening occur, and how often should it be repeated.

their health care providers. A target population might include those at risk for needing life-sustaining treatment under conditions of decisional incapacity. This target population is not easily identifiable, but it might include those who are dying, at risk for strokes, those with early dementia, and those who engage in risky behavior, such as riding motorcycles or not wearing seat belts in moving automobiles.

People can change the content of their advance directives. If they change their preferences without changing their directives, they put themselves at risk for treatment that does not match their wishes. Because health care providers have an interest in promoting the patients' well being, they have an interest in avoiding this occurrence. It is unclear under which circumstances people change their preferences, so it is recommended that whenever there is a significant change in health or social situation, the general content of advance directives should be reviewed. This would argue for reviewing advance directives prior to discharge from a health care facility, upon follow-up in an outpatient setting, and as needed.

Physicians and other health care providers often report that the value of advance directives is limited by the fact that elders can change their preferences. By repeatedly reviewing an elder's advance directive, it is possible to gain a greater understanding about the stability of preferences and what kinds of considerations lead to the changes. This information can be very informative and helpful if and when advance directives are utilized. For example, if a person often changes his or her preferences, the health care provider should encourage the individual to appoint a proxy decision maker. The health care provider also should encourage the person to have the proxy use his or her judgment of the person's best interests as the guide for future decisions. A statement about this "interpretive leeway" can be incorporated into the directive.

Another logistical aspect of advance directives pertains to the determination of when they should go into effect. Advance directives are intended to go into effect when people become decisionally incapacitated. Unfortunately, criteria for this are imprecise and a person can become incapacitated temporarily. This is especially worrisome with elders who are at risk for transient incapacity due to medications and acute illness. Thus, it is recommended that the profession develop practice guidelines for the determination of decisional incapacity that balance the competing interests of respect for patient self-determination and well being. It might also be reasonable for involvement by ethics committees when conflicts exist over health care provider judgments of a patient's decisional incapacity. The following cases illustrate several of these challenges to ACP.

Patients who change their thinking and preferences without changing their directives put themselves at risk for treatment that does not match their wishes.

Under nonemergency situations, causes for the temporary loss of decisional capacity should be investigated before invoking an advance directive.

Case Vignette: Fluctuating Mental Status

HISTORY. *A physician enters a 74-year-old female patient's room before morning rounds to obtain informed consent for mediastinoscopy to evaluate adenopathy and an abnormal chest x-ray. The physician finds the patient to be confused and conducts a Mini-Mental State Examination, which reveals a score of 22. It is unclear whether this is a new finding. The patient has a durable power of attorney for health care. Should the physician meet with the health care agent to obtain consent for the mediastinoscopy?*

CONSIDERATIONS. *Mini-Mental State scores are insensitive measures of decisional capacity. An interview is required to ascertain whether the patient lacks decisional capacity for consenting to the procedure. The acute onset of altered mental status suggests the need to review medications and investigate other causes of the change, such as the onset of an infection. If the patient is deemed to be decisionally incapacitated at this time, deferring the nonemergency procedure is appropriate. It would be premature at this time to proceed by obtaining proxy consent.*

Case Vignette: Decisional Capacity for Executing an Advance Directive

HISTORY. *An elder with early dementia desires an advance directive. Another physician previously communicated to this patient that the purpose of a directive is to avoid over-treatment and abuses by the health care "system" near the end of life. The patient states that he wants a directive specifically to avoid any unnecessary life-sustaining treatment.*

CONSIDERATIONS. *Decisional capacity to choose a medical treatment is not the same as capacity to complete an advance directive. Choosing treatment(s) in a directive is more complicated than choosing to receive or forego a recommended treatment due to a contemporaneous problem. Formulating preferences for a directive requires a patient to consider a future time and hypothetical circumstances involving interactions between treatments and health states.*

Decisional capacity to execute an advance directive presupposes meaningful, comprehensive communication between the health care provider and the individual. Health care providers should try to ensure that the person understands and appreciates that the choices articulated in a directive will be used in the future when he or she is no longer capable of participating in the decision-making process. Moreover, the health care provider should ensure that the person understands that choices can involve medical treatments and the designation of a proxy, and the relative strengths and weaknesses of alternative approaches to advance directives. The person should be able to understand that his or her choices can change over time, and if they do, he or she should change the directive.

Early dementia does not necessarily preclude decision-making capacity to formulate an advance directive; however, physician language may need to be simplified. In addition, the steps involved in discussing ACP may need to be broken down into understandable pieces.[11]

Case Vignette: Depression and Treatment Refusals

HISTORY. *An 80-year-old male patient involved in a home care program has long-standing depression. Several treatment trials have not provided appreciable benefit over the preceding 2 years. He wants to execute an advance directive stating his wish to refuse all life-sustaining treatments, including hospitalization.*

CONSIDERATIONS. *The blanket use of a psychiatric diagnosis to connote decisional incapacity is not appropriate. In general, psychiatric diagnoses are too nonspecific to use as measures of decisional incapacity. The lack of decisional capacity has to be discerned by determining whether the depression is directly affecting the decision to execute an advance directive. For example, many patients with mild depression are able to formulate valid advance directives.[12] If a patient does not have any hope, feels worthless, or cannot envision a better future, however, then this might modify his ability to rationally weigh the benefits and burdens of a treatment and be grounds for considering the patient to be decisionally incapacitated and incompetent to execute an advance directive.*

The elder's reasons for refusing all life-sustaining treatment should provide insight into the person's capacity to execute an advance directive. The health care provider needs to listen carefully to appreciate the difference between an elder's legitimate difference in values and priorities versus not being able to appreciate the ramifications of the decision due to the psychiatric disease.

These can be difficult cases to manage and psychiatry consultation and ethics consultations can be of assistance.

Questions of Interpretation

ARE WE SPEAKING THE SAME LANGUAGE?

People and their health care providers often formulate advance directives using short-hand terms that decrease the likelihood of shared understanding. Patients often use expressions such as, "I wouldn't want to live like a vegetable," "I want to die with dignity," and "I do not want to be a burden on my family." Health care providers often use terms such as coma and dementia. All of these examples of patients' expressions and clinical terms lack sufficient description to characterize with precision the level or intensity of these issues. "Burden" is an example: how much burden is unacceptable? Does the patient mean his or her own subjective sense of burden on the family or the actual burden felt by the family? Dementia may conjure up an image of a person with mild forgetfulness or an image of a patient in an institution with severe dementia and a complete lack of awareness of his or her surroundings.

Patient and health care provider language is often imprecise and difficult to interpret reliably.

DO THE EXPRESSED PREFERENCES PERTAIN TO THIS SITUATION?

After a patient has executed an advance directive interpretive issues often arise. Do the statements in the directive pertain to this situation? Many patients complete living wills with the intention that they will serve as directives for nonterminally ill situations of decisional incapacity (e.g., dementia, coma, or stroke) and for circumstances in which the life-sustaining treatment might be successful in prolonging a life with unacceptable quality. Unfortunately, living wills usually require that two physicians agree about the patient's terminal diagnosis, and thus, living wills are not relevant to these nonterminal situations. This characterizes one limitation in the interpretation of a directive. Another limitation occurs when patients communicate their values with simplified, blanket statements such as, "As long as there is hope, I want treatment." Rarely in clinical medicine are circumstances completely binary. With prognosis, likelihood of successful treatment can range from near zero to near 100 percent, but there will always be a lack of certainty for the individual. In addition, hope is subjective and influenced by affect. Thus, hope may often be at variance with prognosis. Another example of interpretive difficulty occurs when the particularities of the current situation do not match the specifics in the advance directive. Advance directives will never overcome this limitation. Some information is probably better than no information, however, and the challenge to developing good advance directives is having them elicit enough information to infer an accurate profile of preferences and values.

Another major interpretive area concerns whether a person's advance directive is to be interpreted as a set of instructions or as a general guide. Without explicit communication (in the directive itself or in additional conversation), the degree of interpretive leeway is not addressed. Excessive leeway, especially occurring without previous knowledge, can undermine a person's intent and decision-making authority. Lack of leeway can expose the individual to insensitive treatment that does not seem to fit the clinical reality. The following case provides another illustration of potential interpretive difficulties in ACP.

Whether advance directives should be interpreted as a set of instructions or as a general guide usually is not clarified.

Case Vignette: Directive Requesting CPR Despite Terminal Illness

HISTORY. *An older patient with disseminated breast cancer failed the previous course of chemotherapy, and due to hypercalcemia became decisionally incapacitated. The physicians decide that it would be a good idea for her to have a "no-CPR" or "Do Not Resuscitate" order on the chart, but learn that in her advance directive she stated that she wanted CPR if decisionally incapacitated, even if her life expectancy was short.*

CONSIDERATIONS. *ACP discussions should be documented in progress notes and described in sufficient detail for health care providers and proxy decision makers to glean the patient's understanding of CPR, the anticipated indications for its use, and the rationale for her stated preference. Without written documentation or personal recall of the discussion, it is possible that stated preferences do not apply to the current situation. This patient may have wanted CPR because she thought it was as successful as it usually is presented on television. In addition, this patient's advance directive raised the issue of an abbreviated life expectancy. This may not have meant terminal illness. Thus, ACP discussions need to be recorded in sufficient detail so that the meaning and values that underlie the preferences are understood and can be applied if appropriate.*

If the advance directive asks health care providers to engage in medical practice that is outside the standards of the profession, this is a good reason for obtaining an ethics consultation. If CPR in this situation is clearly futile (i.e., the patient is dying of metastatic cancer), this can be legitimate grounds for overriding the directive.

Again, it is wise to have ethics committee input as the subjectivity of medical futility judgments opens the door to capricious expressions of medical paternalism.

Engaging in Advance Care Planning

It is unknown whether the quality of ACP is enhanced by having one professional versus another conduct the discussions. It is known that ACP discussions can range in specificity from a general statement of values or the naming of a proxy decision maker to the articulation of preferences based on the likelihood of success for treatment given a patient's underlying condition and medical prognosis. Properly trained members of the geriatric assessment team, such as nurses, social workers, and chaplains, can introduce the topic, elicit preferences and values, and answer many of the patient's questions. Physicians, however, need to be involved for several reasons. First, they have a key role in quality assurance in terms of determining whether the patient's preferences make medical sense and have internal consistency. Second, they have the ultimate responsibility for implementing decisions and are more likely to respect patient wishes if they have discussed them ahead of time. Finally, other physicians are presumably more likely to accept preferences that have been signed off by another health care provider in their discipline.

Developing advance directives with patients requires additional time during outpatient visits and is contrary to the managed health care trend toward shorter and more standardized patient visits. In addition, patients may ask questions such as the acceptability outside the state, the difference between withholding treatment and euthanasia, and the legal weight of informal directives, which physicians are unprepared to answer. Questions such as these may fall outside the expertise of the physician. Thus, additional resources from the geriatric assessment team, such as social work and legal and pastoral information, need to be readily available.

Advance directives are intended to help guide medical decisions when people have lost decisional capacity, and therefore, are essential parts of medical records at all levels of care. One frequent limitation is that directives are not incorporated into the medical record in a way that permits easy availability. A second limitation occurs when medical or nursing staff are confused about the difference between an advance directive and an order for "no-CPR." This requires repeated staff education articulating that directives go into effect in circumstances of decisional incapacity, whereas "no-CPR" orders are orders, and are applicable regardless of mental status. A third operational limitation pertains to portability outside the institution or between institutions.[13] To reduce this

Other members of the geriatric assessment team can help patients and their physicians in their ACP discussions.

occurrence, health care providers in one health care setting need to communicate with those in another. In addition, patients need to assume partial responsibility by communicating and/or transferring documents to the appropriate parties and institutions before the need arises.

WHY ADVANCE CARE PLANNING RATHER THAN ADVANCE DIRECTIVES

ACP embraces the entire process from deciding to formulate an advance directive to selecting what should be communicated in one. ACP is analogous to informed consent; informed consent requires effective transfer of information to a patient, comprehension of relevant information, and weighing of alternatives in order to make a decision. The consent form, a document that does not ensure any of the aforementioned prerequisites, is comparable to the directive. Thus, the heart and soul of this endeavor to extend autonomy into circumstances of decisional incapacity rests in the ACP process of becoming informed and then communicating effectively to ensure shared understanding.

Advance directives represent the communicative output of ACP, and as a result, can be limited by both the prior communication and deliberative aspects of ACP. Without high quality ACP, advance directives can be fraught with problems. For example, preferences can be internally inconsistent (e.g., "I want to receive CPR, but do not want to be hospitalized"). Moreover, the anticipated role of the person's family can be inconsistent with the family's previous relationships, and the proxy decision maker and the health care provider may not have a shared understanding of the individual's wishes and values.

The quality of advance directives rests on the quality of prior ACP.

Advance directives that are formulated without communication between a person and health care providers can be influenced by misperceptions or misunderstandings, and be incompatible with the standards of the medical profession. Thus, ACP requires a core discussion in which relevant issues are laid out so that a full engagement with, refining of, and balancing of issues can occur. The field of ACP struggled for years when trying to determine whether values or concrete treatment preferences were more important. Ultimately, it has become clear that both are needed, since people think in terms of both.

Validated advance directive instruments can be used not only as an accurate recording of wishes but also as a worksheet that can help people raise, consider, and articulate views on all major relevant issues. In this latter application, advance directives serve as worksheets for ACP. Well-designed instruments help people, in practical ways, identify their personal thresholds for treatment, acknowledge relevant experiences in their life, and articulate relevant beliefs, values, and primary concerns. Four examples of worksheets are illustrated in Appendix #28: the sample page from the Medical Directive (previously discussed as an unofficial, instructional directive), the values statements from *Your Life, Your Choices,* a quality of life exercise, and a sample page of health state and treatment preferences from *Your Life, Your Choices.*

FACILITATING THE DELIBERATIVE PROCESS OF ACP

People are at different stages of readiness with regard to engaging in ACP. Stages of behavioral change is a concept that is employed frequently in health promotion strategies and it offers guidance to ACP. Five basic stages of change have been identified: precontemplation (not aware of need for ACP, not yet interested in getting involved in ACP), contemplation (considering ACP, intending to engage in ACP), preparation (gathering information, getting ready to talk about preferences), action (documenting and/or communicating ACP preferences), and maintenance (reviewing and revising ACP preferences, repeat ACP discussions). This organizing model of behavior change is important for ACP discussions because it explicitly recognizes that change is an extended, complex process, and that individuals are at different points in thinking about and engaging in ACP

Figure 25-1 presents a diagram of stages of behavioral change. Associated with each stage is a health care provider's goal for the ACP discussion and an example of what the person might be

Precontemplation
Health care provider's role:
Increase awareness of ACP

Patient's response:
"I might be in an accident tomorrow"

Maintenance
Provide new knowledge
and encourage review

"How often do I revise?"
"Who needs to know ?"

Contemplation
Motivate and educate

"What do I need to know
to do this well?"

Action
Provide scripts and prompts

"What are my preferences?"
"How do I document them?"
"Who do I tell?"

Preparation
Facilitate identification
and integration of factors

"What is most important to me?"

FIGURE 25-1   Stages of Behavioral change

anticipated to think as a result of effective communication. As characterized, this representation of stages of change presupposes an individualistic decision-making model. If a person comes from a different cultural tradition, it should be modified or even abandoned if necessary. For example, an individual may come from a tradition in which important decisions are made jointly by the family. The model would have to be expanded to incorporate the family unit. If the person was Navajo, ACP would have to be modified as described in the following case.[14]

Case Vignette: Cultural Objections to ACP

HISTORY. *An older Navajo man is admitted to a Western hospital for a complication of diabetes mellitus. The health care providers in the hospital want to follow the Patient Self-Determination Act (PSDA) and JCAHO guidelines and discuss ACP with the patient. Navajo beliefs and culture are such that discussing negative outcomes "witches" the outcome.*

CONSIDERATIONS. *ACP is intended to promote well being and show respect for patient self-determination. The manner is which ACP is approached in this chapter reflects Western dominant culture. With a traditional Navajo patient, ACP may conflict with deeply held values. Furthermore, forcing an ACP discussion can cause harm to the patient. In this type of situation, it might be worthwhile to ask how important decisions are made in this patient's life, and who knows the person the best. Having a general conversation about important values without discussing life-sustaining treatments in hypothetical situations of decisional incapacity also would be useful.*

Within the stages of change organizing concepts, the health belief model helps to analyze and promote behavior change. Behavior change comes about by addressing (1) perceived threats (susceptibility or risk if one does not have an advance directive and severity or seriousness of the outcome, i.e., wishes will not be followed; (2) perceived benefits (e.g., increase in patient autonomy, help family members speak on one's behalf); and (3) perceived barriers (e.g., disagreement among family members, time and effort required). These elements are important to incorporate in ACP discussions to provide motivation and remove some of the barriers that interfere with ACP.[15]

The concept of self-efficacy complements the health belief model by clarifying efficacy expectations and outcome expectations. Efficacy expectations are the person's own beliefs about whether he or she can actually take some action—in this case thinking through ACP or completing an advance directive. Outcome expectations are expectations about whether taking such action would have any meaningful effect, for example, forecasting what the impact ACP communication would have on future treatments. A person might not feel capable of thinking through the issues involved or completing all the required paperwork correctly (poor efficacy expectation). Alternatively, the person might believe that regardless of having advance directives on record, health care decisions will not follow the wishes expressed in the forms (poor outcome expectation). An ACP discussion that fails to change such expectations probably will not motivate or change behavior.

In addition to the behavioral change and efficacy concepts, human information processing needs to be considered in ACP. An important goal of an ACP discussion is to lead a person to well thought out decisions, such as, "Do I want an advance directive and, if so, which one best suits me?" and "Do I want life-sustaining treatment if I'm in Z state of health?" As such, the process must meet three cognitive challenges. It must effectively bring essential considerations or factors to light, help the individual to think clearly about each factor in turn, and help the patient to think about how the factors interact or combine.

When a person thinks through a complex problem, it is difficult to bring to mind all relevant aspects of the problem. It is often hard to exhaustively search for all possibly relevant factors. In addition, thinking about one factor makes it that much harder to think of another. For example, if a person is considering what it would be like to have suffered a stroke, he or she might think about no longer being able to walk, but not think about his or her abilities to still get around in the community, think clearly, and appreciate the love of others. The first challenge for the health care provider in an ACP discussion is to help a person identify the essential factors within an ACP decision policy.

The second challenge for the health care provider is to help the person to think clearly or accurately about the relevant factors involved in formulating any ACP preference or decision. For example, the person may have no way of judging whether cardiopulmonary resuscitation is painful. In addition, the person may incorrectly assume that the use of a mechanical ventilator would not affect the ability to speak. What comes to mind when a factor is brought up depends on the way new information is explained, the context within which it is framed, and the patient's past experiences. If a health care provider discusses CPR as a means to restart the heart, most elders consider this desirable. After learning that CPR is usually unsuccessful, however, many elders express a desire to forego this particular life-sustaining treatment. If a person has witnessed use of a feeding tube in a patient who is not eating due to complications of cancer and chemotherapy, he or she may attribute pain and suffering to the feeding tube rather than the underlying disease and other therapies. The challenge for the health care provider in this last example is to identify and correct the misattribution.

Even if all factors bearing on a decision are well known and at hand, it can still be very difficult to know how to combine them. A person thinking through treatment decisions may have to think about many factors that interrelate. For example, a person who is considering his or her preferences for CPR should take into account (1) adequate information about what is involved in receiving CPR; (2) the probabilities of different outcomes; (3) preferences for each of the possible outcomes; and (4) other personal factors, such as religious beliefs or worries about being a burden. The third challenge in an ACP discussion is whether the health care provider can help the person find a way to represent these factors as interrelating, rather than in isolation.

The anticipated value and approach to ACP are influenced by cultural factors. To facilitate deliberation about ACP, health care providers need to consider communication in multi-ethnic settings. Affirming different explanatory models, negotiating potential and real conflicts in models, and using experience-near, culturally-informed idioms and metaphors create the circumstances for providing culturally appropriate approaches to illness and clinical practice.[16] The explanatory models approach is now widely used to improve clinical communication across cultural and ethnic lines and has applicability to ACP. With regard to etiology and treatment of illness, it involves asking a standard set of questions about the meaning of the illness experience, the level of functioning, the treatment regimen and its effects, and what is most feared about the future direction of the illness course and outcome. With regard to ACP, a culturally sensitive approach involves asking questions about the meaning of the illness and life, the relationship between the present and the future, and the preferred process and participants in medical decision making.

FACILITATING ACP COMMUNICATION

ACP can involve several periods of communication. In Figure 25-2, a model of interactions and communication episodes is presented. Introductory communication needs to motivate and inform. Subsequent conversations between health care providers and patients need to continue to inform by answering questions and clarifying ambiguities, facilitate communication between the person and next-

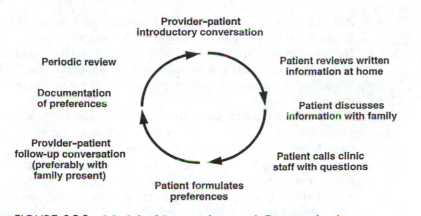

FIGURE 25-2   Model of Interactions and Communication

of-kin or designated proxy, and facilitate written documentation if the patient is so inclined.[17]

Clarification of a person's preferences about future health care can be thought of as involving three activities: (1) individual clarification of values about health care by the person; (2) double-checking and fine-tuning of these values and preferences with the family or proxy; and (3) doing the same with the doctor.

An initial issue for a person to consider in the first set of activities is how the goals of medical care change in different situations. For example, a person initially can consider his or her current state of health. Most people would want all treatments, including life-sustaining ones, if there was a reasonable likelihood of returning to the usual state of health. When someone is dying or suffering, however, he or she might not want treatments that put off the time of death or prolong the suffering.

ACP Questions

There are several questions that people can be asked that complement this line of inquiry and that should help them clarify their preferences about future medical care.*

- Who should speak on your behalf if you are so sick that you cannot speak for yourself?
- If you became seriously ill today with a life-threatening problem, what should be the goals of your medical care, cure or comfort? Why?

*Source: Pearlman RA, Back AL. Ethical Issues in geriatric care. In: Hazzard WR, Blass JP, Ettinger WH, et al, eds, *Principles of Geriatric Medicine and Gerontology,* 4th ed. New York: McGraw-Hill, 1999:564.

- Are there any circumstances where you would prefer to die rather than receive life-sustaining treatment. Why?
- Have you ever heard about a situation where you have said to yourself, "I would not want to be kept alive like that."
- What is it about these circumstances that make you feel as you do?
- Are there any life-sustaining treatments that you know you would always want or never want regardless of the situation? Why? (Sometimes a person will say that a mechanical ventilator or being fed through tubes is not desired. Additional questions about the difference between permanent use of these life-sustaining treatments versus short-term "therapeutic trials" should be asked.)
- Where do you want to receive your medical care in the event you are dying? Why?
- Should your current preferences be strictly applied to future situations or serve as a guide for your proxy decision makers? Why?

The more explicit people are in explaining their preferences and values, the greater will be their and others' understanding of what is best for them. People and health care providers need to remember that there are no right or wrong answers to these questions.

These questions and the answers should serve to guide the person's thinking about the use of life-sustaining treatment. The next step is for the person to sit down with his or her family and the person(s) he or she would want to be the proxy, and discuss these questions and responses. The individual might find that family members or the person he or she designates to be a surrogate decision maker challenge some of his or her assumptions. This can be helpful because the person may have some misunderstandings. These areas of doubt and confusion are important topics to discuss with the health care provider. The person may find in these conversations with health care providers that both he or she and the family were off the mark in terms of an expectation. If so, they all have the opportunity to revise their values with additional information. After these three steps, the clarified values about health care and preferences can serve to help him or her plan the advance directive.

OVERCOMING BARRIERS TO ACP

Many policy recommendations and initiatives promote the use of advance directives. A few illustrative examples include Supreme

Court Justice O'Connor's opinion pertaining to the case of Nancy Cruzan.[2, 18–20] Despite these initiatives and people's preferences to be involved in life-sustaining treatment decisions, however, a minority of Americans have ACP discussions with health care providers, and even fewer (estimated between 9 percent and 23 percent) have executed formal, written advance directives.[21–23]

ACP and the use of advance directives create challenges to some health care providers because it forces them to share uncertainty and authority with a person.[24] ACP and advance directives place the person or his or her proxy decision maker in the driver's seat. Shared medical decision making is the recommended model for the patient–provider relationship, and advance directives obligate the use of this model. In order for people to engage fully in ACP, health care providers need to talk to them about topics not commonly addressed in the clinical encounter: goals of medicine, patient values, hypothetical future situations, treatments neither currently under consideration nor indicated, uncertainty, and quality of dying. Perhaps most challenging, ACP discussions have the potential to be overly simplified as well as excruciatingly detailed and burdensome. The providers' general lack of experience in having these discussions and peoples' variability in conceptualizing ACP issues often result in awkward discussions.[25]

Even when ACP communication occurs, there are flaws in the process, as the goal of shared understanding is not realized. Several studies have shown that physicians who engage in ACP discussions do not appear to understand what their patients would want under circumstances of decisional incapacity. Similarly, there is limited understanding between people and their proxies, as demonstrated by poor concordance of preferences.[4] Of course, the quality of these discussions has been dubious. Barriers exist beyond the aforementioned. The barriers identified in Table 25-1 serve as a reminder of issues deserving consideration in ACP.

FURTHER CONSIDERATIONS ABOUT ACP

Sociocultural Considerations

ACP discussions need to relate to people about the issues that are relevant to them, with respect to health, culture, stage of personal maturity, driving psychological or religious issues, and so forth. This requires that health care providers be flexible in their approach to the discussions. Health care providers need to create a milieu that signals the person that it is acceptable to raise issues that may not fit in the dominant culture's perspective.

TABLE 25-1. BARRIERS TO EFFECTIVE ADVANCE CARE PLANNING	
DOMAINS	POSSSIBLE RESPONSES
Patient, family, and health care provider difficulty with thinking and talking about death and dying	Professional and public education Marketing strategies to encourage a cultural shift Practice
Directives often focus on treatment preferences rather than the interests and concerns of patients and their families	Explore concerns of patients and families first Explore patients' health state preferences, then check for consistency of treatment preferences
Limited health care provider training in conducting ACP discussions	Education and skills training Role modeling by experts
Differential knowledge and experience with life-sustaining treatments	Communication aimed at shared understanding Help patients and families separate disease-related effects from the treatment(s) Help patients and families appreciate differences between past experiences and the present situation
Limited opportunities for clear, in-depth discussions	Encourage system changes in scheduling (outpatient setting) and reimbursement Stage discussions over time

Health care providers need to allow sufficient air time in ACP discussions to hear what people might want to say. This opening can permit a person to indicate that his or her primary desire is to know that a family member will serve as a proxy decision maker. Another person, such as a Navajo patient, may let the physician know if it is acceptable to talk about tragic scenarios. Similarly, an older person may decline to formulate preferences about future hypothetical decisions and draw attention to the desire to die without becoming a burden on family members.

Decision Support

For people who want to express preferences for life-sustaining treatment, the use of a visual aid is sometimes quite helpful. Figure 25-3 presents a decision-making "treatment board." This ori-

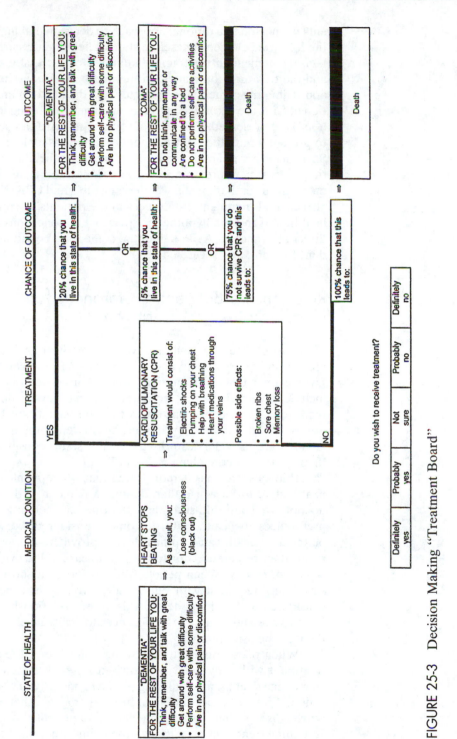

FIGURE 25-3 Decision Making "Treatment Board"

ents the person to a rational approach to decision making involving the following elements: baseline state of health, intercurrent problem, recommended treatment, likelihood of successful treatment, and the treatment outcomes. In the figure, a baseline health state approximating dementia is characterized, the need for and description of CPR are described, and the outcomes (including their likelihood) are presented. This kind of treatment board can be modified to present a multitude of treatment descriptions and health states. Such an aid in research was successfully used to facilitate the elicitation of treatment preferences for antibiotics, short- and long-term mechanical ventilation, dialysis, feeding tube, and CPR.[26] This study also elicited treatment preferences in the patients' current state of health, and in four hypothetical permanent conditions that have direct relevance to ACP: dementia, coma, bed bound and dependent for care, and severe pain.

Relationship Between Preferences for Health States and Treatments

Many people seem to want an advance directive to avoid receiving life-sustaining treatment under circumstances considered to be "worse than death." Common circumstances described as such include severe dementia, permanent coma, severe unrelievable pain, total dependence on others for care, significant burden on others, and dependence on a mechanical ventilator until death.[27] Health care providers can discuss health states considered worse than death as a core element in ACP.

Prior research has demonstrated that when people consider a health state to be worse than death, 85 percent of the time they do not want any life-sustaining treatment.[26] Relating treatment preferences to health state outcomes considered worse than or better than death can help health care providers talk with people about their preferences for future health care in the event of decisional incapacity. When people want to forego a short-term life-sustaining treatment with only mild morbidity in a health state considered worse than death, this direct relationship between health state and treatment preferences logically gives credence to the treatment preference.

When people indicate they want a short-term life-sustaining treatment with only mild morbidity in a health state considered worse than death, this should trigger the need for further communication. Either the person is confused or has another value that outweighs this relationship. For example, a person may want a life-sustaining treatment even though the living situation is considered worse than death if (1) the refusal of treatment is considered morally unacceptable; (2) the dying process is feared to be worse than the situation described as worse than death; (3) the person merely describes the health state as worse than death to indicate that it was rather awful, but not necessarily to communicate that death is preferable to living; and (4) the family wants the person to continue living and the person places more weight on this desire than his or her own. Probing apparent inconsistencies between health state and treatment preferences facilitates the identification of personal values that enrich ACP discussions.

Probing apparent inconsistencies between health state and treatment preferences facilitates the identification of personal values that enrich ACP discussions.

FUTURE NEEDS

Health care providers are expected to facilitate ACP and the majority of people report that they want them to. Providers usually are not trained, however, and there is a paucity of role modeling that occurs in the clinical setting. If ACP is to become a part of clinical practice, it needs to be formally incorporated into traditional clinical education, similar to taking a history and conducting a physical examination, and become part of the professional culture.

As is true of any endeavor in its infancy, research needs to answer a multitude of questions to improve the quality of ACP. As a start, research should determine what approaches to ACP work well with certain types of people in certain settings. Research should evaluate the effectiveness of different approaches to promoting shared understanding of values and preferences that would inform future situations of medical decision making if decisionally incapacitated. For example, does communication with simple expressions of preferences, such as, "I don't want to live like a vegetable," as opposed to more specific expressions of treatment preferences, impair the proxy's ability to represent the person. It would be helpful to know whether one discipline of health care providers does a better job than another (given the same training), and how ACP can occur most cost effectively. Thus, to help guide clinical practice, research needs to characterize the effectiveness of different approaches to ACP.

The author wishes to acknowledge that many of the issues presented in this chapter are the result of a long-standing collaboration with the following scholars at the University of Washington and the VA Puget Sound Health Care System: Kevin C. Cain, William G. Cole, Donald L. Patrick, and Helene E. Starks. He is deeply grateful for their interdisciplinary insights.

REFERENCES

1. Buchanan AE, Brock DW. *Deciding for Others: The Ethics of Surrogate Decision Making*. Cambridge, England: Cambridge University Press; 1989.

2. Joint Commission on the Accreditation of Health Care Organizations. *Accreditation Manual for Hospitals*. Vol. R1.1.1.3.2.1. Oak Brook Terrace, IL: Joint Commission on the Accreditation of Health Care Organizations; 1993:106.

3. Schneiderman LJ, Pearlman RA, Kaplan RM, Anderson JP. Relationship of general advance directive instructions to specific life sustaining treatments. *Arch Int Med*. 1992;152:2114–2122.

4. Uhlmann RF, Pearlman RA, Cain KC. Physician's and spouse's predictions of elderly patients' resuscitation preferences. *J Gerontol*. 1988;43(5):M115–M121.

5. California's Natural Death Act. *West J Med*. 1978;128(4):318–328.

6. Emanuel LL, Emanuel EJ. The medical directive: a new comprehensive advance care document. *JAMA*. 1989;261:3288–3293.

7. Gibson, JM. National values history project. *Generations*. 1990; (suppl.)51–64.

8. Pearlman R, Starks H, Cain K, Rosengren D, Patrick D. *Your Life, Your Choices—Planning for Future Medical Decisions: How to Prepare a Personalized Living Will*. Springfield, Virginia: U.S. Department of Commerce, National Technical Information Service. PB #98159437. 1998.

9. Dresser R. Advance directives: implications for policy. *Hastings Center Rep*. 1994;24:S2–S5.

10. Pearlman RA. Advance directives research: are we asking the right questions of the right people in the right circumstances? *Hastings Center Rep*. 1994;24:S24–S26.

11. Finucane TE, Beamer BA, Roca RP, Kawas CH. Establishing advance medical directives with demented patients: a pilot study. *J Clin Ethics*. 1993;4(1):41–44.

12. Lee MA, Ganzini L. Depression in the elderly: effect on patient attitudes toward life-sustaining therapy. *J Am Geriatr Soc*. 1992; 40(10):983–988.

13. Danis M, Southerland LI, Garrett JM, et al. A prospective study of advance directives for life-sustaining care. *N Engl J Med*. 1991; 324:882–888.

14. Carrese JA, Rhodes LA. Western bioethics on the Navajo reservation: benefit or harm? *JAMA*. 1995;274(10):826–829.

15. Pearlman RA, Cole WG, Patrick DL, Starks HE, Cain KC. Advance care planning: eliciting patient preferences for life-sustaining treatment. *Patient Edu Couns*. 1995;26:353–361.

16. Kleinman A. *The Illness Narratives: Suffering, Healing, and the Human Condition*. New York: Basic Books, Inc., 1988.

17. Emanuel LL, Danis M, Pearlman RA, Singer PA. Advance care planning as a process. *J Am Ger Soc*. 1995;43;440–446.

18. Pearlman RA. Clinical fallout from the Supreme Court decision on Nancy Cruzan: Chernobyl or three Mile Island? *J Am Geriatr Soc*. 1991;39(1):92–97.

19. *Omnibus Budget Reconciliation Act of 1990* (Western Supplement 1991). Vol. Pub. L. No. 101-508, 4206, 4751. codified in scattered sections of 42 USC, especially 1395cc, 1396a. 1990.

20. Department of Veterans Affairs. *Veterans Health Administration Manual* M-2, Clinical Affairs, Part 1, General Vol. November 18. Washington, DC: 1991; Chapter 31.

21. Teno JM, Licks S, Lynn J, Wenger N, et al, for the SUPPORT Investigators. Do advance directives provide instructions that direct care. *J Am Ger Soc.* 1997;45(4):508–512

22. Emanuel LL, Barry MJ, Stoeckle JD, Ettelson LM, Emanuel EJ. Advance directives for medical care: a case for greater use. *N Engl J Med.* 1991;324(13):889–895.

23. Emanuel EJ, Weinberg DS, Gonin R, Hummel LR, Emanuel LL. How well is the Patient Self-Determination Act working? An early assessment. *Am J Med.* 1993;95:619–628.

24. Katz J. *The Silent World of Doctor and Patient.* New York: Free Press; 1984.

25. Tulsky JA, Fisher GS, Rose MR, Arnold RM. Opening the black box: how do physicians communicate about advance directives? *Ann Intern Med.* 1998;129:441–449.

26. Patrick DL, Pearlman RA, Starks HE, Cain KC, Cole WG, Uhlmann RF. Validation of life-sustaining treatment preferences: implications for advance care planning. *Ann Intern Med.* 1997;127(7):509–517.

27. Pearlman RA, Cain KC, Patrick DL, et al. Insights pertaining to patient assessments of states worse than death. *J Clin Ethics.* 1993A;4(1):33–41.

FAMILY AND COMMUNITY-BASED CARE: THE SUPPORTS FOR CARE PLAN IMPLEMENTATION

JOANN DAMRON-RODRIGUEZ

FAMILY AS THE KEY INFORMAL SUPPORT

A comprehensive geriatric assessment produces a care plan aimed to optimize functioning of an elder. Successful care plan implementation necessitates consideration of the elder within the context of his or her social environment. Without the consideration of environmental support, after a comprehensive assessment, the older adult may, in one elder's words, "be all assessed up with no place to go." The required ecological perspective views elders and their supports, both formal and informal, as interactively adaptive.[1] The aim is to achieve a goodness-of-fit between the elder and his or her social environment to maximize functioning and the quality of late life.[2] Informal and formal supports make major and distinct contributions to care plan implementation.[3]

This chapter examines the social environment in terms of the informal supports of family, friends, and neighbors, and the formal delivery system of health and social services. It provides a theoretical framework as well as practical referral information. The first two sections describe major issues in the contemporary family and service delivery system that relate to achieving care plan goals. The final section presents a social care framework for facilitating the optimal use of the elder's support system and community resources.

It is singularly important to understand the importance of the family as the major support system for elders.[4,5] Research results

Healthcare providers must examine myths regarding the contemporary family to develop realistic expectations of caregiver roles.

estimate that the family provides the majority, up to 85 percent of care to elders.[6] Despite the fact that family care is the most researched area in gerontology, health care providers often hold the belief that elders are abandoned by their families[1] (see Chapter 4).

Eldercare Past and Present

FAMILY SIZE SMALLER AND MORE GENERATIONAL TIERS

The dramatic aging of the population added to other social and demographic factors have transformed the contemporary family.[6, 7] Using the previous turn of the century as the point of comparison, the following major contrasts in the family past and present become apparent (Table 26-1). In 1900, the average life expectancy was 47 years, today that number has almost doubled. Only 21 percent of adults had a living grandparent; currently, 76 percent do.[8] Since 1900, the chance of having at least one parent still living for adults age 60 years increased from 8 percent to 44 percent.[8] Today, families have multiple elders, parents, parent's in-law, step parents, aunts and uncles, to whom they may have some level of responsibility. Overall, families are smaller today but have more generations represented. This is referred to as the verticalization of the family system and is described as the bean pole family structure. Increasingly, families have as many as five living generations.[9] Furthermore, at the turn of the past century, only 10 percent of marriages ended in divorce compared to a current divorce rate of 50 percent.[10] This greatly adds to the complexity of intergenerational family roles and responsibilities.

TABLE 26-1. CONTRASTS IN FAMILY ELDERCARE: PAST AND PRESENT

In the "Good Old Days" (1900)
  Fewer elderly
  Larger families, living closer together
  Connected family economics
  Higher mortality
  Less prolonged needs for care
Today
  Dramatically increased number of elders with more than one eldercare responsibility per family
  Decreased family size with more generations
  Urbanization—less geographic proximity
  Increase in women working, 60% age 45–54
Increase in elders living with chronic illness with a longer time period of need for assistance

FAMILIES ARE MORE GEOGRAPHICALLY DISBURSED

Professional ties can move families far from their parents in contrast to family economic ties of the past (i.e., the family farm, that kept relatives in close proximity).[9] The site of many of the major life transitions, death and birth, for the majority no longer take place within the home, ritualized by traditional beliefs.[4]

WOMEN IN THE WORKFORCE

Women's roles have concomitantly changed. Caregiving is frequently an "add on" to multiple other roles such as grandparent, parent, spouse, community-member, and worker. The composite description of the elder caregiver is a wife or daughter in her late 50s.[11, 12] Women increasingly work outside the home, frequently in order to ensure the economic survival of the family.[4, 3] Yet, they maintain the major role of caregiver to dependent persons, sometimes through the management of paid providers.[14]

ACUTE VERSUS CHRONIC ILLNESS

The tremendous progress of medicine in this century, including the introduction of antibiotics, allows people to survive infectious diseases and other acute illnesses. People now live much longer but may live longer with one or more chronic illnesses (60 percent over age 65 and with increasing levels of disability).[15] Though age, chronic illness, and disability are not synonymous, they are associated. An estimated 5.6 million elders lived in the community in 1990 and required assistance with two or more activities of daily living (ADLs). This is more than the number of people living in nursing homes (1.6 million).[16] Further, the number of elders with functional limitations living in the community is projected to increase to 6.7 million by 2001.[17] The time committed to caregiving for functionally impaired elders is frequently lengthy and intermittently intense. Primary caregivers spend 5 to 7 years, more than the average person spends getting a college degree, and some caregivers may have as many as 17 years of varying levels of elder care responsibility.[18]

Thus, the eldercare of the past cannot be compared with contemporary family responsibilities. It is a myth to romanticize the family of the past as one that provided elder care within the warm embrace of an intergenerational family, and contrast the families of today as abandoning their elders. The fact is that the majority of elders have family, interact with them frequently, and when necessary, receive their primary support from family.[1, 4] Approximately half of the elders have spouses and about 80 percent have children.[19] Forty percent to fifty percent of elders see adult children weekly.[20] Interaction within the intergenerational family is an active

Each care plan should identify interacting family members as a key element in the
support of the elder. Interdisciplinary team members must
specifically note the following
characteristics of caregivers.

- Multiple caregiving respon-
  sibilities
- Number of potential family
  supports
- Geographic distance
- Employment conflicts
- Time commitment to care-
  giver roles

Health care providers can
work to encourage the contributions of elders within the intergenerational family.

process that links the majority of elders to other family members.[21] Only 7 percent of people over 65 years of age enter a nursing home from the community in any 2-year period, and the family is the single most explanatory variable in differentiating those who are placed in an extended care facility from those who are not.[22, 23] Elders without family should be targeted for assistance that can provide alternative supports.

Cost of Elder Care to Families

ELDERS GIVING AND RECEIVING

It is difficult to conduct a cost–benefit analysis of so complex a human experience as family caregiving. Research has focused on the debits of family caregiving but less is known about the rewards of eldercare. In considering the impact of eldercare, it must first be recognized that elders in general give as much they receive from the family. Elder assistance to younger family members can be monetary, instrumental (grandparent roles), or emotional, as well as the transfer of history and culture. This balance of interdependency tips when the elder reaches advanced old age, when they may require more assistance than they can give.[24] Elder interdependence should always be respected and avenues for contributing to the family strengthened.

DEFINITIONS OF CAREGIVER COST

Research describes the cost of care as stress, strain, and caregiver burden.[25] Caregiver costs can be measured in terms of monetary expenditures, time and energy taken from other family roles, economic and professional opportunity losses to the caregiver, and impact on caregiver's physical and mental health.[26] Caregiving, particularly for those whose family member is demented, is associated with increased levels of depression, anxiety, higher use of psychotropic medicines, poorer self-reported health, and compromised immune functioning.[27–29]

The impact of elder care must be individually assessed. Lustbader and Hooeyman suggest professionals ask the following types of questions: How much rest are caregivers getting? Are caregivers neglecting their own health? Have caregivers turned to alcohol or drug abuse in their distress? Has substance abuse been lifelong? Are caregivers receiving verbal or physical abuse from the person in their care?[30] Zarit developed a widely used, standardized instrument for assessing caregiver burden (see Appendix #47).[31] Indeed, institutionalization of older persons is more predicated on the perception of the burden of the caregiver than the major care variable of the elder, such as incontinence.[23] Isolation and restricted activity for the caregiver is a major factor in the perception of the burden.[32] Abuse of the care recipient can be one of the most severe outcomes of caregiver stress and requires mandatory reporting and intervention.[33] Caregiver support groups and counseling can relieve stress.[25, 34]

> Caregiver burden must be assessed and considered in ongoing care planning and implementation. Respite care and support groups should be considered proactively.

DIVERSITY OF CAREGIVER POPULATION

Though the elder caregiver is typified as female and older, the caregiver population is actually very heterogeneous. Gender, age, ethnicity, relationship to the individual, living arrangement, and environmental resources must all be considered in assessing caregiver burdens.[35–37] Men and women manage the caregiver responsibility differently.[35] Men typically assume more of a management style to caregiving involving more supplemental informal and formal support.[38] Gay and lesbian couples require special considerations in relationship to family systems and supports. Women are more likely to be serial caregivers and provide care until the level of burden is overwhelming and then require a substitute caregiver or institution.

> A coordinated care plan must consider a range of differences in the caregiver population, utilize appropriately all available family supports, and avoid placing all responsibility on a single primary caregiver.

Ethnic Dimensions in Eldercare

VALUES AND BELIEFS VERSUS DEMANDS

Values and beliefs regarding filial piety or family responsibilities to elders are strongly based in culture and must be individually ascertained.[39, 40] Health care providers must recognize they also may hold preconceptions of family responsibility based on their own cultural beliefs.[41] Ethnicity is a particularly important element considering that the minority older population, particularly Latino, is growing at a faster pace than the white elder population.[42] Ethnic families are also faced with the increasing participation of women in the workforce and multitiered generational responsibilities. Though ethnic families may hold strong values and beliefs regarding family care responsibilities, they may be challenged economically and have other pressures that make caregiving without formal supports difficult.[43]

DIVERSITY OF ETHNIC POPULATIONS

The tremendous diversity of the minority population must be taken into account as a foundation for understanding ethnicity and aging in planning long-term care.[44] The four major ethnic groups, Asian-American and Pacific Islanders, Hispanic-American, African-

American, and American Indian, display tremendous heterogeneity between and within groupings. Culture, language, national origin, immigration status, and religions vary within groups as well as health practices and beliefs.[45] Ethnic identity is also important in understanding the white elder who in the current cohort of old-old is more likely to be an immigrant. A few of the major considerations in implementing care plans for ethnic families will be highlighted.

VARYING DEFINITIONS OF FAMILY SYSTEM

First, cultural differences are marked in the prescription of the primary caregiver. In the Asian traditions, the eldest son and concurrently, his wife, are frequently called to take the main caregiving reponsibilities.[13] In most other cultures, daughters are more likely to be designated as the primary caregivers. In African-American families, fictive kin, persons with longstanding family relationships, may play key roles in eldercare.[46]

Another significant difference between majority and minority families is the increased likelihood of minority families to care for elders in an intergenerational household.[43] Unmarried, older African-Americans are twice as likely to live with family as whites and Latinos are three times more likely to live with family than whites even when income, health status, and other characteristics are controlled.[47, 48] Much of the co-residence can be ascribed to economic need and shared family resources.[49]

Based on these issues, health care providers must be cautious of the tendency to develop care plans based on the adage that minorities "take care of their own" solely within the family. The multiple responsibilities of minority families can make traditional eldercare overwhelming without appropriate community supports.[43, 49]

Informal Roles: Affection and Affiliation

SPECIFIC CHARACTERISTICS OF INFORMAL ROLES

Families in all their diversity, then, are the foundation of the support system for elders.[50] Litwak provided a useful conceptual framework for understanding the nature of family support as it relates to care plan implementation.[51] Family or informal roles are defined by face-to-face interaction or as naturally occurring systems. Informal roles are further defined by their continuity over time and affectional ties. The knowledge base and tasks of informal support are nontechnical. A family's knowledge is not of disease states or

---

Important care plan considerations for ethnic elder care include the following:

• Clarification of beliefs and values about eldercare
• Assessing family challenges to meeting traditional expectations
• Distinguishing the primary caregiver
• Understanding the importance of intergenerational households
• Recognizing higher rates of poverty

intervention methodologies but rather on the knowledge of the elder's coping over time.

Time is an important element in the differentiation of informal and formal support. Informal caregivers are not "on the clock" as formal caregivers are. Time commitment of informal caregivers requires that they respond to unpredictable demands at all hours of the day or night, as in managing incontinence. Additionally, the commitment can be extensive over time. The last feature of the nature of informal supports is that the tasks are often not discrete or easily divided, as in comforting an elder with Alzheimer's disease who may become agitated.

> Informal support is based on nontechnical knowledge and tasks are characterized by: unpredictability, continuity and time intensity.

ROLES OF FRIENDS AND NEIGHBORS

Friends and neighbors are another form of informal support. Friends are more likely to be able to provide peer influence regarding health practices and are often the best source of emotional support.[50] Elders' positive affective state is most associated with friends rather than family support.[52]

Neighbors are often the closest geographically and can be the best source of emergency support. Professionals and family can strengthen the roles of friends and neighbors by sharing information, affirming their contribution, helping them set limits, and coordinating their efforts with the other sources of support. Daily check-ins are one of the most useful functions a neighbor can do and require a minimal commitment of time. As an element in treatment planning this "just checking in" provides an important function of monitoring the elder's overall health status or knowing when he or she is "going down hill."

CARE PLAN TASKS BEST PERFORMED BY INFORMAL SUPPORTS

Informal supports include attention to socialization and life satisfaction as well as assistance in activities of daily living and personal care needs arising from disabilities.[3] Thus, informal supports are vital to quality of life in ways hired help and professionals cannot be. Hiring a companion for an elder may be necessary but must be recognized as a poor substitute for a lifelong friend. Shared holidays and religious ceremonies are essential to integrity in the life cycle. Community organizations, churches, synagogues, as well as family and friends, help with this important area. Care planning must consider not only the medical needs but the social and interpersonal nature of the elder's well-being, as well as the caregiver.[34]

People who have known the elder over time are important sources of history as well as current functioning. Interviewing family

> Friends and neighbors play important roles in emotional support and emergency response but rarely can be counted on for long-term, time-intensive service.

Care plan implementation includes attention to informal supports for:

- Socialization
- Emotional support
- Monitoring health status
- Emergency response
- Assistance with daily functioning
- Linking with formal services

caregivers is an important adjunct to the individual assessment process. If the elder and caregiver are interviewed together, the older adult should be addressed first and respectfully. The caregiver interview is supplemental or ancillary to the interview of the elder. The degree of additional or confirming information will vary based on the competence of the elder. The caregiver's perspective of functioning and assistance needs, however, provides an invaluable perspective for all elders. Requesting the permission of the older adult to speak with or ask questions of the caregiver is essential. If the elder is seated closer to the interviewer and the family member slightly behind the elder, the provider can assess nonverbal cues signifying differences of opinion. As an example, the elder may communicate a high degree of independence and the family member may respond with a look of astonishment. This requires further questioning. Guidelines from interviews with families are summarized in Table 26-2. The frequency of family contact should be noted in the assessment. Other family members may be long-distance caregivers relying on telephones for their interaction and monitoring.

The concept of a trajectory is helpful to understand this dynamic. A trajectory is the unfolding of a disease or condition in relation to the total organization of care aiming to control it. Rather than focusing on an episode of care, the trajectory views the course of the illness. Many elders' chronic illness could benefit from a better orchestration of their support systems in order to impact its trajectory.

Families should be encouraged to view eldercare over "the long haul" and not prematurely develop dependency. Though the trajectory of an illness can require sudden increases in assistance, the majority of eldercare must be more incrementally responsive to small declines.

TABLE 26-2. GUIDELINES FOR INTERVIEWS WITH FAMILIES
Set ground rules (i.e., no interrupting, want to hear from everybody)
Clarify the purpose of interview
Maintain neutrality and empathy
Be aware of power and decision making
Be aware of alliances; who sides with whom
Summarize what has been accomplished
Include educational materials and information about condition and/or services

Source: Bumagin VE, Hirn KF. *Helping the Aging Family.* New York: Springer-Verlag; 1990.

FORMAL SERVICES IN THE COMMUNITY

Social Care Model

Together informal and formal services from the social care framework. Social care, as defined by Cantor, is the entire spectrum of helping that supports elders in their environment.[47] Social care is functionally based and operates from the principle that services augment individual competency and mastery of the environment rather than increasing dependency.[53] Social care incorporates quality of life and life satisfaction as key variables relating to the interfacing of formal and informal support.

COMPLEMENTARY ROLES

The concentric circle presentation of informal and formal supports can illustrate the complementary levels of support (Figure 26-1). Social care is depicted as a series of concentric circles with the elder in the center. Ripples of change at any level of support have ramifications for the other levels of support. This model, rather

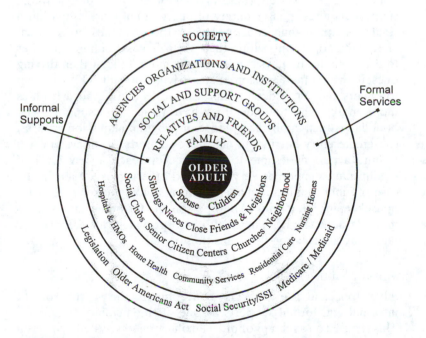

FIGURE 26-1 Social care for older adults: informal and formal supports.

The elder and/or caregiver must play an active role in care planning and contracting for care plan implementation.

than substituting informal supports for formal or providing formal supports only when family caregiving options are exhausted, advocates for the best use of both informal and formal supports in an interactive process.[54] A key role of family is in decision making in concert with the elder regarding the selection of community services and medical care.[39, 55]

Elders must be questioned at each step of care planning and a contract of support drawn for implementation. If the elder is not competent and/or family is actively involved in care, a family member or surrogate should be an active part of the team planning process. If this does not take place, a well-laid treatment plan can be sabotaged or destroyed because the values and preferences of the informal support system are not considered.[55]

TRANSITIONS BETWEEN LEVELS OF SUPPORT

Independence is particularly important for current cohorts of elders. Moving from relying completely on oneself to relying even on the closest family member can be very difficult, though ethnic differences in the value of independence and interdependence vary. Each of the circles in Figure 26-1 represents a different system level. Each system has boundaries. For the elder to move past a boundary of one system (family), to another system for help and support requires greater outlay of energy than working within a single system. Moving from one level to the next takes more system energy than operating within the system. To ask a family member to drive one to the physician's office is more difficult than driving oneself, even if failing vision makes driving difficult. This can help to understand why elders do not ask for needed support. It takes more energy than the elder may have to seek out support. The boundaries (i.e., family acceptance or program admission criteria) can create entry barriers to accessing supports. Each system will require a period of time to rebalance or reach a new level of equilibrium, sometimes very short and other times longer, in the case of more significant changes. Hiring a homemaker helps with housekeeping but it brings a new person into the home and requires multiple adjustments. The health care provider can prepare the family by anticipating this transition period.

Health care providers can assist elders and their families by anticipating the reluctance to ask for help and the time needed to adjust to new care arrangements.

AUXILIARY FUNCTIONS

Silverstone and Burack-Weiss conceptualize the shared role of informal and formal supports as one of the auxiliary functions.[2] This is based on a metaphor of an auxiliary energy system triggered into action by failure of the permanent system. The auxiliary system adds to, fills in for, and bolsters that which is depleted in the elder's support system. The auxiliary system aims to meet not only the temporary needs but to restore the sytem to its previous level of functioning as soon as possible.

The elder's energy can be depleted slowly with advanced age or suddenly through loss of functioning because of a stroke or a fall. The depletions affect physical, mental, as well as social resources. Further, this model distinguishes between primary and secondary depletions. A medical problem can quickly lead to a loss of functioning mentally and/or socially. Hearing loss leading to social isolation leading to depression is an example of primary loss leading to secondary loss.

This model requires using family and formal services only to the degree required and withdrawing the additional supports as soon as they are no longer needed. Short-stay nursing home placement for rehabilitation is an example. Home health services post hospitalization can end abruptly. This can require homemaker or home health services to "titrate" supports and not continue to add one on top of the other or contrastingly, to stop all of them inappropriately. Care planning is an ongoing process for elders with long-term needs and requires monitoring at specific points in time.

> Monitoring of care plan implementation is required to achieve the appropriate level of assistance at each stage of recovery. Too many supports can create excess disability. Abrupt interruption of support can precipitate a crisis.

Issues of Access

Formal services founded in social policy form a comprehensive and complex web that provides a safety net for elders in need of assistance.[56] These programs are the outer circle of Figure 26-1. Post-World War II categorical funding has resulted in numerous agencies with specific social service functions to supplement health care services. Though this provides a rich array of programs, it is indeed a fragmented or a "many splintered thing," creating problems for accessing services.[56] Health and social services are often dichotomized and are not parts of an integrated system of care.[57]

Varying Eligibility Requirements

Further, the doors to community health and social services open under different locks and keys. Access can be based on type of health care coverage: Medicare or Medicaid or private insurance. There can be geographical restrictions to service. Specific diseases may be targeted, such as cancer, heart disease, or stroke. Services are provided under federal, state, county, and city auspices. Formal assistance can be public, nonprofit, or proprietary. It is difficult for elders to know what key opens what service door or what information they need to give to get help. Social workers, as part of the interdisciplinary team, can decipher this complex system.

Mobilizing community-based services requires confronting access barriers to help:

- Give service recommendations in writing
- Provide service directions and information
- Link patients to the social worker and care manager

It has been estimated that it takes the average elder five telephone calls to locate one service that they need. This assumes that the elder perseveres in calling after the first unsuccessful contact. An Oregon example describes it as taking a care manager 35 hours and 41 agencies to obtain the needed services for a client with multiple needs.[58] If it were an elder calling with hearing loss, speech problems, a language difference, or other cognitive or communication problem, imagine the time and energy involved with less success anticipated. Service directories for area agencies in aging should be made available at all program sites for the care of elders. One knowledgeable team member or staff should be "in charge" of accessing services.

ETHNIC ELDERS' UNDERUTILIZATION OF FORMAL SERVICES

Minority elders have a higher need for health and social services yet use community-based care and nursing homes less.[40, 44] Emergency room use, however, is higher for ethnic elders.[59] Thus, service utilization by ethnic elders is not appropriate to the level of need.

BARRIERS TO LONG-TERM CARE SERVICES

Barriers to formal service use by ethnic elders are classified into cultural and structural barriers.[60] Cultural barriers relate to the characteristics of the ethnic group that influence service preference including: language, level of acculturation, education, family support system, and religion. Structural barriers are defined in terms of service delivery system characteristics: affordability, availability, and outreach to the ethnic population. A major structural barrier is economic, particularly for recent immigrant elders, who may have no healthcare coverage. Elderly immigrants must wait for 5 years after legal entry as permanent residents to receive Medicare coverage. Other long-term residents may have worked in jobs outside the Social Security system and have no benefits. Both cultural and structural barriers must be considered in care plan implementation for ethnic elders. For care planning implementation for ethnic elders refer to Table 26-3.

Formal Roles: Expertise and Reimbursement

CHARACTERISTICS OF FORMAL SUPPORTS

The medical and technologic revolution of the 20th century mandates that certain functions are best performed by people with specialized knowledge and skill. Professionals and paraprofession-

TABLE 26-3. CARE PLANNING IMPLEMENTATION FOR ETHNIC ELDERS
Language differences between elder and service providers
Bilingual staff
Translated materials
Family interpreters
Cultural differences through outreach
Use of community volunteers from different cultures
Community access
Services in the neighborhoods where ethnic elders live
Transportation when needed
Affordability
Based on type of coverage ethnic elders have

als bring to geriatric service knowledge of disease, conditions, and/or interventions, which the elder and his or her family do not possess.

CARE PLAN TASKS BEST PERFORMED BY FORMAL SUPPORTS

Skilled medical care in the home is an area best performed by health care providers. Advanced decubiti care is an example of an area of need that in the institutionalized setting would be the responsibility of staff members as part of formal hospital services. When patients are discharged home requiring higher levels of care than in the past, families are often given responsibility of care that requires technical knowledge and skill. Though home care providers teach family members these new tasks, informal support members, by nature, are not suited to provide this skilled level of care. An elderly wife may respond that she is happy to be by her husband's bedside at all hours, provide nourishment, change the bed, and give medicine, but feel inadequate to changing dressings or tube feeding. This is an example of substituting informal support for formal care that is problematic. It can and is done in implementing care plans but the difficulties that families experience in this change of roles must be respected.

ACCESSING THE SUPPORTS FOR IMPLEMENTING THE CARE PLAN

Assessment and Referral

Appropriate community-based care referrals are founded in geriatric assessment in collaboration with family caregivers. Figure 26-2 presents a model for assessment and referral that integrates infor-

Formal support roles are characterized by:

- Professional knowledge of disease, problem, and/or interventions
- Technical tasks that are time specific

Formal services are needed for the following.

- Assessment and monitoring of disease states and functioning
- Interventions performed by health care providers
- Technical tasks and teaching related to use of medical equipment

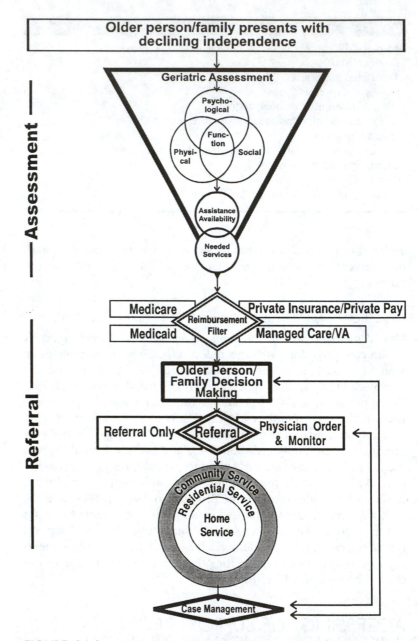

FIGURE 26-2 Community-based elder care: assessment and referral.

mal and formal supports. For elders presenting with problems of declining independence in functioning, a comprehensive geriatric assessment (CGA) may be required. This section presents the referral process, which follows assessment. The primary care physician may need to refer to a geriatrician or an interdisciplinary geriatric team for consultation in interviewing family and accessing community services (see Chapter 6, 7, and 27). The major components of the CGA are physical examination, history, review of medications, determination of acuity and complexity, psychological assessment, cognition, and social status evaluation, including family support, culture, finances, and living arrangement. Standardized instruments for the CGA have been presented in previous chapters. The link between the CGA and the referral process, as pictured in Figure 26-2, is the interlocking circles at the base of the assessment triangle. These are the assessment of assistance available to meet the need for services arising from functional deficits. Functioning in terms of activities of daily living (ADLs) and instrumental activities of daily living (IADLs) are central to assessment. The needs that arise from functional deficits, such as assistance with toileting, are addressed in the care plan. The need can be met by either informal or formal assistance. The key is recognition of the skills and deficiencies of the elder that then must be matched with available external resources.

The Assessment of Living Skills and Resources (ALSAR) is an assessment tool that systematically evaluates the accomplishment of 11 tasks and matches these with available supports.[61] This tool is consistent with the auxiliary function framework in which elders are seen as at risk based on interplay of deficits and supports (see Appendix #2).

Increasingly, resources to meet these needs consist of assistive devices and technology. Durable medical equipment, emergency response systems, and home modification may alone, or in consort with family and community resources, meet a functional challenge.

The degree of deficit must be matched with the strength of the resource. An elderly disabled caregiver may be available for assistance with toileting but require bathroom modifications and respite from community services. In addition to care plan implementation based on functional assessment, diagnoses for medical conditions may necessitate certain referrals to community-based services. For example, exercise programs for elders with arthritis can be important and are available through recreation programs or the YMCA. Addressing depression or grief reactions can be identified in the care plan and the individual referred to a community mental health service for counseling or hospice grief support groups.

Figure 26-2 delineates the process of referral in interplay with elder and family decision making. Each element is described as it is shown on the diagram; first consideration of the reimbursement filter and second, special considerations for elders with decision-making deficits. Third, the circular referral continuum based in home, residential, or community services is described. Finally, care management and monitoring of care plan implementation is discussed.

REIMBURSEMENT FILTER: HEALTH CARE BENEFITS BY PAYER SOURCE

The most critical access issues relate to health care financing and individual health care coverage.[62] Income maintenance forms the safety net of social care. The major income maintenance programs are Social Security Assistance (SSA) and Supplemental Security Income (SSI). Both are federally established by the Social Security Act. Health care coverage relates to income maintenance programs: Medicare to SSA and Medicaid to SSI coverage. SSA and Medicare are entitlement programs based on earnings contributions. Approximately 95 percent of the occupations in the United States are covered by Social Security, and thus, Medicare. SSI and Medicaid coverage is based on income eligibility. SSI is based on the individual's current income and assets, weighed against his or her ability to meet "standard living expenses" in his or her state. SSI and Medicaid are state-administered programs for low income elderly and disabled persons and are subject to variations and fluctuations in state support. Over half of elders eligible for SSI/Medicaid do not apply. Major differences in Medicare and Medicaid that are important considerations in care plan implementation are the benefits for nursing home care, home health, and medications.

Appropriate referral to community-based services must be filtered through the reimbursement or payer source in order to determine options for care (Figure 26-2). The reimbursement mechanisms are briefly described in Table 26-4. The accompanying reimbursement code is used in Appendix 11 to delineate coverage for specific services.

ELDERS AND IMPAIRED DECISION MAKING

Elders and their families are most interested in what the service does (function) and what needs it addresses (problem).[54] Time is a major factor in care planning and deciding if informal or formal supports are most appropriate. Time-related questions that must be asked to utilize informal and formal supports effectively are: "How long has this problem/need existed?"; "Why do you feel additional help is needed now?"; "What did you or your family

Table 26-4. Healthcare Reimbursement Mechanisms

Code	Program	Eligibility	Benefits
M/SS	Medicare Federal, linked to Social Security	A person 62 years of age or older is eligible to begin receiving Social Security benefits (based on 40 quarters employment). All persons eligible for Social Security benefits plus Civil Service and Railroad retirees. Social Security Disability recipients including end-stage renal disease patients. Requires a monthly co-payment for Part B	Part A covers 80% of approved hospital expenses and skilled nursing care/rehabilitation services at home or in a nursing home. Covers skilled nursing care, which includes a nursing or rehabilitation therapy service that requires the special skills of technical or professional health care providers. For nursing homes when skilled care is required, the beneficiary pays Days 1–20 → nothing Days 21–100 → share of cost Days ≥101 → all costs. Part B covers 80% of approved ambulatory care medical visits, durable medical equipment, and some prosthetic devices.
MDC/SSI	Medicaid State and Federal, linked to Supplemental Security Insurance (SSI)	Low income (SSI eligible) 65+, blinded or disabled or medically needy. Individuals who do not qualify for SSI but have extraordinarily high medical expenses pay a share of cost. In Home Supportive Services (INSS) recipients	Covers custodial nursing care including assistance with activities of daily living, medication, and meals. Also pays for pharmaceuticals, durable medical equipment, and restorative care. Once qualified, long-term nursing care is covered with only a share of cost, if any.
VA	VA Benefits Federal, Veterans Health Administration	Any honorably discharged veteran. Percent of service-connected disability	Combination health and long-term care, prescriptions, assistive devices. Includes Service Connected Compensation, Non-Service Connected Pension, and Aid and Attendance.
MC	Managed care Not for profit or for profit corporations, health maintenance organizations (HMO), preferred provider organizations (PPO)	Medicare assignment. Employment related coverage. Individual enrollment	Consumers should be provided with a list of covered services.
PI/PP	Private insurance (including MediGap) Private pay	Purchased services	As determined by providers. Private insurance may require physician order and use ancillary Medicare. Medigap may provide long nursing home stay and nursing service in home.
SL	Sliding scale		Sliding scale based on income: family service and community services often SL or NC.
NC	No cost		

Care plan implementation must relate to the elder's definition and history of the problem.

do in the past?"; "How long do you anticipate needing help?" "What times of the day do you need help the most?"

The elder is the primary decision maker for care options and, as has been described, is the center of care plan implementation considerations. The following are important alternatives to assist in decision making when the elder is significantly impaired.

OPTIONS WHEN AN ELDER NEEDS HELP IN MANAGING AFFAIRS

An elder with physical, functional, or cognitive impairment is not able to adequately manage his or her own, financial and personal affairs. It can be necessary to mobilize additional support. The following list outlines some options from least restrictive to total control of an individual's affairs.

- Direct deposit: checks deposited directly to an elder's bank account.
- Joint tenancy: two or more people have equal control over property such as a bank account.
- Durable power of attorney: a legal document that gives another person the authority to act on behalf of another only when the elder lacks the capacity for decision making.
- Advance directives for health: written instructions used only in the event that the person is incapacitated and unable to make his or her wishes known to the health care providers. Advance directives include living wills, durable power of attorney for health care, and health care proxy (see Chapter 25).
- Representative payee money management: a service to manage the person's finances. A representative payee is a person who has the authority to receive, sign, and cash another person's public benefit check.
- Conservatorship/guardianship: A conservator/guardian has the authority over the elder's living arrangements, property/finances, and/or health care decision making, depending on powers granted by the court (see Chapter 24).

Referral: Community-Based Elder Care Continuum

The formal service network has been conceptualized in various ways. Traditionally, various levels of care have been differentiated ranging from the least to the most restrictive. These levels have been presented as a linear continuum from home care to nursing home.

The inadequacy of the linear model is exemplified by understanding that home hospice care for a terminally ill patient is not at a lower level of care than a short rehabilitation stay in a nursing home for an elder with a recent hip fracture. A circular rather than a linear framework for long-term care is presented in both Figure 26-2 and again in Figure 26-3. Both medical and social services are included and listed according to the site of care.

Figure 26-2 illustrates three locations of service: the community, the home, and in residential care. Services can be combined

Home Services

- Emergency response systems
- ✓ Home-delivered meals
- ✓ Home health care
- ✓ Home Health Aide
- Homemaker/Companion
- Telephone Reassurance Friendly Visitor
- ✓ Hospice
- Home repair

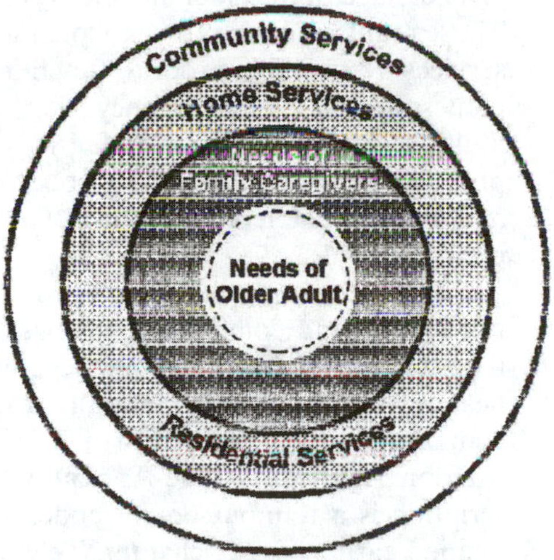

Residential Services

- ✓ Assisted living
- Continuing care retirement community
- ✓ Nursing Home
- ✓ Residential care (Board & Care)
- Senior Citizen Apartments
- Shared Housing

All of these services may provide a needed service.
- Most need only a referral.
- ✓ These services may require a physician order and

Community Services

- Adult day care
- ✓ Adult day health care
- Congregate meals
- Exercise programs
- Information and referral
- Legal
- Money management
- ✓ Outpatient mental health
- Protective Services
- Public Guardian
- Recreation
- Respite care
- Senior Center
- Support Groups
- Transportation

FIGURE 26-3 Community-based elder care referrals. A dynamic model of long-term care allows for varying levels of intensity of care provided in home and residential settings supplemented by community services. (Modified from Damron-Rodriguez J, Frank J, Heck E, et al. Physician knowledge of community-based care: what's the score? *Ann Long-Term Care* 1998;6(4):112–121).

The appropriate "package" of social and health services must combine resources to create the appropriate level of care in home, residential care, and nursing home setting.

Formal services must be combined to create an *appropriate* type and level of care that is *accessible* to the older adult and *acceptable* to him or her and the family.

from various sites to meet specific needs and movement between sites will be more rapid than in the past. Elders residing in residential care facilities can benefit from linkage to community services as much as elders living at home. Increasingly, services will be noninstitutional and of shorter duration based on assessed, documented need and careful care planning with the informal support network.

The major settings of care relate to care plan recommendations in the following ways. All formal services, regardless of setting, must meet three standards to successfully meet the needs of elders and their families. They must be appropriate, accessible, and acceptable.[60] Appropriateness requires a match between the type, level of need of the elder and family and the intensity of the service. Those requiring long-term care planning have the need for multiple services over time in order to function. An example of inappropriateness is the use of emergency rooms for assessment of elders with multiple chronic problems.[59] Meeting these standards is particularly problematic for minority elders because of the potential structural and cultural barriers inherent in the development of private and public services.

Figure 26–3 provides a listing of the services provided in home, residential, and community settings. Further, the diagram designates those services that require a physician order or medical verification. Physicians are generally less familiar with their role in community-based care.[63] For a brief description of each service listed in Figure 26–3 (see Appendix #11); accompanying each description is a reimbursement code, for example, M = Medicare, defined earlier in this chapter. Telephone references for community-based services are provided in Appendix #10.

Home Service

Home care is the fastest-growing segment of health care today.[64] A range of levels of assistance for people with functional limitations are available within their home for varying periods of time. Home care has options for both health and social services, from home repair and domestic help to skilled services that provide sophisticated medical technology. Succinct referral information is provided in Appendix #11. Older adults living at home with high levels of disability require high levels of informal support as well as home care, and require a primary caregiver.

Home health services at the skilled level provided by a Medicare certified home health agency include nursing, occupational therapy, physical therapy, social work, speech therapy, and the services of a nutritionist. Home health care services require a physician's order and ongoing physician consultation for the home health nurse. Home care assistance supplements home health care and is provided by a continuum of providers each with specific functions: companion, homemaker, and home health aide. A home health aide will be covered in addition during the period skilled nursing or rehabilitation therapy is approved. Medicare reimbursed services are for medically necessary care that is for a limited period of time or sickness episode. Each visit by a health care provider is for the time required to accomplish the interventions. Family must be prepared not to expect a nurse who will stay with them for a certain number of hours.

Private insurance or private pay services can provide homemakers, home health aid, and nursing care on an hourly or shift basis. Community services through social clubs, churches, and synagogues can provide volunteer companion services. Medicaid covers a smaller range of professional home health services for shorter periods of time. Medicaid is compatible with Title XX support for In Home Supportive Services (IHSS), which provides homemaker services for low-income elders.

In implementing a care plan that includes home care, particularly assistance at the lower levels of provider skill, the elder or the family must be prepared to become an employer. This is frequently an unanticipated role. Homemaker assistance can be arranged through domestic services and the family may wish to hire a live-in assistant. This requires that the elder and/or family be prepared to become an employer and adjust to the transition of supervising an assistant. Several helpful guides provide guidelines for this role (see, for example Lustbader and Hooyman).[30] Tips include making a list of tasks, avoiding over surveillance, praising extra effort, and correcting major errors with information rather than criticism.

RESIDENTIAL SERVICE

For elders, who maintain a significant level of independence but would be aided by congregate living supports, (i.e., three meals provided, socialization, and emergency responses) residential care should be considered. However, elders who require 24 hours a day care and intensive rehabilitation may require nursing home or post-acute care. Institutional care need not be long-term but can be needed for an episode of disability.

If an elder is substantially independent in activities of daily living, the following residential care facilities should be considered before a nursing home. Brief descriptions, including payment sources and references for referral information are listed in Appendix 11. The residential options are listed by approximate level of care.

Senior Apartments (subsidized and unsubsidized).

Retirement housing for elders provides a safe environment but limited or no supportive services. Recreational activities are usually available. Most of the buildings are disabled accessible, have emergency bells, building security, and are near shopping and other services. Some buildings have a van for medical appointments and weekly shopping. The subsidized units for elders and disabled persons, subsidized senior apartments (Title VIII), have rent schedules that are income adjusted. This type of living arrangement meets a real need for many elders and the subsidized housing units may have waiting times of many years.

Shared Housing.

This option is available in some communities. In this arrangement, an elder with a home can provide housing in exchange for assistance.

Residential Care Facilities For the Elderly (RCFE) (Retirement homes/board and care homes).

A wide variety of facilities fall into the residential care category of housing including retirement homes and board and care homes. RCFEs range from small family-owned facilities to large facilities with more than 100 residents. Sleeping quarters are separate, but the dining room and recreational area are shared. Services in residential care include: meals, weekly housekeeping, and socialization activities. Assistance with medications is usually available. Personal care can be arranged, but for additional cost.

Continuing Care Retirement Community (CCRC).

Lifelong living arrangements are offered in continuing care retirement communities, which provide a continuum of options including: retirement homes, senior apartments, assisted living, and nursing home care. Elders can move in at higher levels of functioning and, over time, move to a setting with high levels of assistance. Frequently, this continuum of care is provided for retirees of religious orders but is also now offered under proprietary auspices. Substantial life-time savings investment can be required.

Assisted Living.

Assisted living facilities are newer, enhanced types of residential living and are a rapidly growing form of care. The primary distinction is that in addition to standard services, assisted living provides personalized care (dressing, grooming, bathing, and feeding) based on individual needs. The personal cost of assisted living care is frequently high.

Post-acute Care.   "Sub-acute" care is comprehensive inpatient care for a person following an acute illness or exacerbation of a condition. It is often housed in a skilled nursing facility or in a separate section of an acute care hospital. Skilled nursing facility care is Medicare reimbursable if it requires skilled professional services for the purpose of rehabilitation. If the forms of residential care are inadequate to meet the needs of the elder and family, nursing home placement may need to be considered for maintenance care. Maintaining elders at their current level is not Medicare reimbursable. For this, Medicaid or private pay for nursing home care will be required. Risk factors for nursing home placement include not only the need for 24-hour care but problems that are particularly burdensome to families (see Chapters 1 and 9). Lustbader and Hooyman describe the following risk factors for placement: incontinence, need for heavy lifting, and frequent nighttime awakening. Others describe combative behavior as a major problem for caregivers in anticipating placement. Nursing home placement is frequently considered after an increasingly short acute care stay. The family may want to have a trial home stay before making this decision.[30]

COMMUNITY SERVICE

The Older Americans Act created a network of social services for elders. Services ranging from preventive to custodial care are provided in community agencies for limited periods of time each day. To participate, elders need to be ambulatory and have transportation. Two key sources for families to learn more about the appropriateness and availability of community services are: the Office on Aging and Hospital Social Service Departments. Office on Aging is the primary source of support for the development of senior citizen centers. Senior centers provide information and referral (I&R) services. I&R is basically a question and answer process and does not involve the evaluation of patient needs. Hospital discharge planners have the potential for providing information and referral based on individual and family need.

Increasingly, self-care and mutual help groups play an important role in social care for elders. Care plans may call for these supports for health promotion, rehabilitation, and tertiary level support to maintain current functioning. Mutual help groups share a common concern or condition. These serve an important function for elders and caregivers. Caregiver support groups have been extensively used.[34] Bereavement groups and Alzheimer's support groups are two supports that should frequently be considered in care planning. Socialization activities are essentially recreational, but for many elders are also buffers against isolation and thus, are therapeutic.

Care plan implementation should thoughtfully address the need for mental health services for elders and/or family members. Depression is a frequent companion to medical illness in late life. Without addressing this condition, other areas of the care plan may not be implemented due to symptoms of depressive illness. Elders underutilize community-based mental health services. Mental health services specifically designed for older adults are generally more acceptable to elders. Elders' response to psychotherapy is generally comparable to adults of any age.[65]

Adult Day Care.   This can provide an option for respite during the day for the caregiver and for socialization and/or rehabilitation for the elder living at home. These services fall into two major categories. The social day care model provides a caring environment for frail elders who require supervision but not skilled nursing or rehabilitation therapies. The programs are usually affordable. This level of support has been particularly helpful for persons with Alzheimer's disease and many programs are particularly developed for this population. The second model is adult day health care and is Medicaid reimbursable. The physician must order this level of care: A multidisciplinary team provides a range of rehabilitation services. Adult day health care is based on the particular medical condition of the elder and is time limited. Both of these are underutilized resources.

Care Management

Care management: A person-to-person method of managing care of people with, or at-risk for, catastrophic or complex long-term medical/psychiatric conditions so as to improve both continuity and quality of care while controlling cost.[66]

As Figure 26–2 illustrates, elders whose decision-making capacity is impaired and without adequate family decision makers can require ongoing assistance in coordinating supports. Additionally, elders with complex medical and psychological problems need ongoing monitoring, which may require a care manager. The care manager must have a direct relationship with the patient to coordinate informal and formal supports. The components of care management are: case finding; functional assessment; care planning; implementation monitoring; and formal reassessment at regular intervals.

PEOPLE IN NEED OF CARE MANAGEMENT

First, elders' needs are of an intensity that without additional supports they are unable to meet basic living demands as measured by the assessment of ADLs and IADLs. Second, targeted older adults require multiple services based on both multiple functional impairments and the lack of adequate family supports. Third, vulnerable elders require services over time not only subsequent to acute care, usually for at least 6 months but frequently, indefinitely. The needs for support can vary markedly over time in the mix and intensity of need. If an elder's needs meet these criteria, care management should be considered to address the coordination issues and assure the appropriate level of care.

> Care management is important for elders whose needs are marked by: intensity, multiplicity, and longevity.

Social workers and nurses within the interdisciplinary geriatric team may perform care-management functions. Managed care organizations or other health care systems can have designated care managers for targeted populations. Clinical care managers should be distinguished from individuals who monitor fiscal resources through chart review only. County and state programs have care managers, as in the California Multipurpose Senior Services Program (MSSP).

SUMMARY

Developing a treatment plan for elders with multiple medical problems and significant limitations in functioning requires comprehensive assessment, frequently by an interdisciplinary geriatric team. Equally complex is the utilization of family and community-based supports, in consort with the medical care team, to implement the care plan.

Care plan recommendations entail addressing personal care and daily routines, thus inevitably contributing to the elder's quality of life.[39] Understanding the essential nature of family and community-based services assists the health care providers in the effective matching of resources. Further, appreciating both the strengths and weaknesses of these supports enable the most beneficial contribution to the care plan. Primary care providers must increasingly become familiar with the array of services available for their patients and their families, to create a supportive environment.[63] Care plan implementation is a dynamic process requiring the elders, the health care team, and the family to be interactively adaptive to provide good care over time.

REFERENCES

1. Damron-Rodriguez J. Linkage of formal and informal supports for the elderly: a research synthesis for practice. In: Stopp GH, ed. *International Perspectives on Healthcare for the Elderly.* New York: Peter Lang; 1994:chap XVII.
2. Silverstone B, Burack-Weiss A. *Social Work Practice With the Frail Elderly and Their Families.* Springfield, IL: Charles C. Thomas; 1983.

3. Silverstein M, Litwak, E. A task-specific typology of intergenerational family structure in later life. *Gerontologist.* 1993;33:258–264.

4. Burton L. Families and the aged: issues of complexity and diversity. In: Burton L. ed. *Families and Aging.* San Francisco, CA: Baywood Press; 1993:1–6.

5. Robinson KM. Family caregiving: who provides the care, and at what cost? *Nurs Econ.* 15:243(5);1997.

6. Penrod J, Kane R, Kane R, Finch M. Who cares? The size, scope, and composition of the caregiver support system. *Gerontologist* 1995;35:489–497.

7. Pearlin L, Aneshenel JM, Whitlatch, C. Caregiving and its social support. In: Binstock R., George L, eds. *Handbook of Aging and the Social Sciences.* San Diego, CA: Academic Press; 1996:283–302.

8. Quadagno J. *Aging and the Life Course.* Boston: McGraw-Hill College; 1999.

9. Bengston V, Rosenthal C, Burton L. Paradoxes of families and aging. In: Binstock R, George L, eds. *Handbook of Aging and the Social Sciences.* San Diego, CA: Academic Press; 1996:253–282.

10. Uhlenberg Peter. Demographic change and kin relationships in later life. *Ann Rev Gerontol Geriatr.* 1993;13:219–238.

11. Stone R, Cafferata GL, Sangl J. *Caregivers of the Frail Elderly: a National Profile.* Washington, DC.: U.S. Department of Health and Human Services, 1987.

12. Coon DW, Schulz R, Ory MG, the Reach Study Group. Innovative intervention approaches for Alzheimer's disease caregivers. In: Biegel DE, Blum A, eds. *Innovations in Practice and Service Delivery Across the Lifespan.* New York: Oxford University Press; 1999:295–325.

13. Boyd S, Treas S. Family care of the frail elderly: a new look at women in the middle. *Women's Studies Quarterly.* 1989;112:66–73.

14. Scharlach A. Caregiving and employment: competing or complementary roles. *Gerontologist.* 1994;34:378–385.

15. Jette, A. Disability trends and transitions. In: Binstock R, George L, eds. *Handbook of Aging and the Social Sciences.* San Diego, CA: Academic Press; 1996:94–117.

16. Maloney, SK, Finn J, Bloom, DL, Andresen J. Personal decisionmaking styles and long-term care choices. *Health Care Financing Rev.* 1996;18(1):141–155.

17. Pousada L. High-tech home care for elderly persons: what, why and how much? In: Arras JD, Porterfield HW, Porterfield L, eds. *Bringing the Hospital Home: Ethical and Social Implications of High-Tech Home Care.* Baltimore, MD: Johns Hopkins University Press; 1995: 107–128.

18. Azarnoff R, Scharlach A. Can employees carry the eldercare burden? *Personnel.* 1988;67:67–69.

19. Morioka K. Generational relations and their changes as they affect the status of older people in Japan. In: Hareven T, ed. *Aging and Generational Relations Over the Life Course.* Berlin: Aldine de Gruyter; 1996:511–525.

20. Rossi A, Rossi P. *Of Human Bonding: Parent-Child Relations Across the Life Course.* New York: Aldine de Gruyter: 1990.

21. Umberson D. Relationships between adult children and their parents: psychological consequences for both generations. *Marriage Family.* 1992;54:664–674.

22. Cowart M, Quadagno J. *Crucial Decisions in Long-Term Care.* Tallahassee, FL: Mildred and Claude Pepper Foundation; 1995.

23. Hardwick S, Pack SP, Donohoe EA, Aleksa K. *Across the States 1994: Profiles of Long-Term Care Systems.* Washington, DC: American Association of Retired Persons; 1994.

24. Spitze G, Logan J. Helping as a component of parent-adult child relations. *Res Aging.* 1992;14:291–312.

25. Whitlach C, Zarit S, von Eye A. Efficacy of interventions with caregivers. *Gerontologist.* 1991;31:9–14.

26. Gold DP, Cohen C, Shulman K, Zucchero C, Andres D, Etezad J. Caregiving and dementia: predicting negative and positive outcomes for caregivers. *Intl J Aging Hum Develop.* 1995;41:183-201.

27. 1999 MetLife Juggling Act Study, MetLife Market Institute, Westport, CT, Dec, 1999.

28. Vitaliano PP, Russo J, Young HM, Teri L, and Maiuro RD. Predictors of burden in spouse caregivers of individuals with Alzheimer's disease. *Psychol Aging.* 1991;6:392–302.

29. Wright L, Clipp E, George L. Health consequences of caregiver stress. *Med, Exercise, Nutr, Health.* 1993;2:181–195.

30. Lustbader W, Hooyman NR. *Taking Care of Aging Family Members: A Practical Guide.* New York: The Free Press; 1994.

31. Zarit SH, Reever KE, Bach-Peterson J. Relatives of the impaired elderly: correlates of "feelings of burden." *Gerontologist.* 1980; 20(6):649–655.

32. Stoller EP, Pugliesi K. Other roles of caregivers: competing responsibilities or supportive resources? *J Gerontol.* 1989;44:S231–S238.

33. Vinton L. Services planned in abusive elder care situations. *J Elder Abuse Neglect.* 1992;4(3):85–99.

34. Gallagher-Thompson, D. Direct services and interventions for caregivers: a review of extant programs and a look to the future. In: Center MH, ed. *Family Caregiving: Agenda for the Future.* San Francisco, CA: American Society on Aging; 1994:102–122.

35. Allen S. Gender differences in spousal caregiving and unmet need for care. *J Gerontol.* 1994;49:S187–S195.

36. Antonucci TC, Cantor MH. Strengthening the family support system for older minority persons. In: *Minority Elders: Longevity, Economics and Health,* 2nd ed. Gerontological Society of America; 1994,40.

37. Mui A. Caregiver strain among black and white daughter caregivers: a role theory perspective. *Gerontologist.* 1992;32:203–212.

38. Chang C, White-Means S. The men who care: an analysis of male primary caregivers who care for frail elderly at home. *J Appl Gerontol.* 1991;10:343–358.

39. Degenholtz H, Kane RA, and Kivnick HQ. Care-related preferences and values of elderly community-based LTC consumers: can case managers learn what's important to clients? *Gerontol.* 1997;37(6):767–776.

40. Wallace SP, Snyder JC, Walker GK, Ingman SR. Racial differences among users of long-term care. *Rese Aging.* 1992;14(4):471–495.

41. Grant RW, Finocchio LJ. *The California Primary Care Consortium on Interdisciplinary Collaboration: A Model Curriculum and Resource Guide.* San Francisco, CA: Pew Health Professions Commission; 1995.

42. U.S. Select Committee on Aging, House of Representatives. Demographic characteristics of the older Hispanic populatioon. Comm. Pub. No. 100–696. Washington, DC: U.S. Government Printing Office; 1990.

43. Aranda MP, and Knight BG. The influence of ethnicity and culture on the caregiver stress and the coping process: a sociocultural review and analysis. *Gerontologist.* 1997;37(1):342–354.

44. Mui A, Choi NG, Mong A. *Long-term care and ethnicity.* Westport, T: Auburn House; 1998.

45. Damron-Rodriguez JA. Multicultural aspects of aging in the U.S.: implications for health and human services. *J Cross-Cult Gerontol.* 1991;6(2):135–145.

46. Stoller EP, Gibson RC. *Worlds of Difference: Inequality in the Aging Experience.* Thousand Oaks, CA: Pine Forge Press; 1997.

47. Cantor M. Family caregiving: social care. In: Cantor M, ed. *Family Caregiving: Agenda for the Future.* San Francisco, CA: American Society on Aging; 1994:1–9.

48. Worobey JL, Angel RI. Poverty and health: older minority women and the rise of the female-headed household. *J Health Soc Beha.* 1990;31(4):370–383.

49. Tennstedt S, Chang, B-H. The relative contribution of ethnicity versus socioeconomic status in explaining differences in disability and receipt of informal care. *J f Gerontol soc Sci.* 1998;53B(2):561–570.

50. Antonucci TC. Convoys of social relations: family and friendships within a life span context. In: Blieszner R, Hilkevitch Bedford V, eds. *Handbook of Aging and the Family.* Westport, CT: Greenwood Press; 1995:355–371.

51. Litwak E. *Helping the Elderly.* New York: The Guilford Press; 1985.

52. Armstrong MJ, Goldsteen K. Friendship support patterns of older American women. *J of Aging Studies.* 1990;4:391–404.

53. Bumagin VE, Hirn KF. *Helping the Aging Family.* New York: Springer Verlag; 1990.

54. Kropf NP. Home health and community services In: Schneider RL, Kropf NP, eds. *Gerontological Social Work.* Chicago: Nelson-Hall Publishers; 1992:173–201.

55. Degenholtz H, Kane RA, Kivnick HQ. Care-related preferences and values of elderly community-based LTC consumers: Can case managers learn what's important to clients? *Gerontologist* 37(6)767–76.

56. Gelfand DE. *The Aging Network: Programs and Services,* 5th ed. Springer Publishing Company; 1999, NY.

57. Greene VL, Lovely ME, Ondrich JI. The cost-effectiveness of community services in a frail elderly population. *Gerontologist.* 1993;33(2):177–189.

58. Levinson R. Information and referral services. Washington, DC: U.S. General Accounting Office, 1978:12. *Comptroller General Report to Congress.* HRD-70–134.

59. Brokaw M, Zaraa, AS. A biopsychosocial profile of the geriatric population who frequently visit the emergency department. *Ohio Med.* 1991;87(7):347–350.

60. Damron-Rodriguez J, Wallace S, Kington R. Service utilization and minority elderly: appropriateness, accessibility and acceptability. *J Gerontol Geriatr Educ.* 1994;15(1):45–63.

61. Williams JH, Drinka TJ, Greenberg JR, Farrell-Holtan J, Euhardy R, Schram M. Development and testing of the assessment of living skills and resources (ALSAR) in elderly community-dwelling veterans. *Gerontologist.* 1991;31:84–91.

62. Wiener J. The financing and organization of health care for older Americans. In: Binstock R, George L, eds. *Handbook of Aging and the Social Sciences.* San Diego, CA: Academic Press, 1996:427–445.

63. Damron-Rodriguez JA, Frank J, Heck E, et al. Physician knowledge of community-based care: what's the score? *Ann Long-Term Care.* 1998;6(4):112–121.

64. Rowland D, Lyons B. The elderly Population in need of home care. In: Rowland D, Lyons B, eds. *Financing Home Care: Improving Protection for Disabled Elderly People.* Baltimore, MD: Johns Hopkins University Press; 1991.

65. Knight BG. *Psychotherapy for the Aged.* Newbury Park, CA: Sage Publications; 1996.

66. Rothman J. *Practice with Highly Vulnerable Clients: Case Management and Community-Based Service.* Englewood Cliffs. NJ: Prentice Hall; 1994.

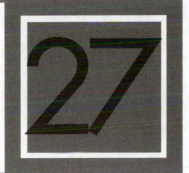

C H A P T E R

27

COMMUNICATING ASSESSMENT RECOMMENDATIONS

JANET C. FRANK / MARCIA ORY

With comprehensive geriatric assessment (CGA), a considerable amount of time and effort is invested in identifying the elder's problems and recommending potential solutions. Obviously, the goal is to act upon these treatment recommendations and assure their accomplishment. To this end, effective communication to the "partners" in care, other service providers and the elder, is essential.[1, 2]

A number of factors must be considered when deciding the best way to communicate multidimensional assessment recommendations. The communication process is at least two-directional, and is often three-directional within the assessment process. Communicating assessment recommendations can involve two or more health care providers, and most assuredly, the primary provider and the person. Since many elders bring family members with them to medical appointments, communication often involves others.[3]

One major factor in geriatric assessment that can influence the communication of recommendations is the relationship of the assessor to the health care provider(s) carrying out the recommendations. The communication process will be different for the solo practitioner versus a care team, and will be uniquely influenced by the amount of control the assessor has over the implementation

The Agency for Health Care Policy and Research (AHCPR) was renamed in December 1999.
This agency is now known as the Agency for Healthcare Research and Quality (AHRQ).

process. In many care settings, the comprehensive geriatric assessment is completed by a health care team comprised of members representing different disciplines. The multidimensional nature of the elder's condition is thought to be optimally addressed from a variety of disciplinary perspectives. Geriatric assessment teams typically include physicians, nurses, social workers, and often, allied health professionals.[4] For simplification in this chapter, the term health care provider will be used to represent any one of the disciplines involved in comprehensive geriatric assessment, although most research has focused on the physician's role in the process.

Just as importantly, the health care organizational setting in which the recommendations are being implemented has potential influence over the communication of assessment recommendations. In addition, the type(s) of recommendations provided and important characteristics of the elder often impact effective communication of assessment recommendations.

ROLE OF ASSESSOR IN PROVIDER–PROVIDER COMMUNICATION

Communication among health care providers occurs in all three types of assessment relationships: (1) when the same practitioner who does the assessment also completes the implementation (solo); (2) when a team does the assessment and one member completes the implementation (team); or (3) when a provider or team does the assessment and a separate provider completes the implementation (consultative). These three types of assessor–implementor relationships can create significant differences in the communication process. In general, the more health care providers involved in the assessment and implementation, the more complex the communication process becomes.

Solo Provider Implementation

If the provider who has completed the assessment is also responsible for managing the implementation, some recommendations can be accomplished directly with the person. Often, recommendations require the involvement of other providers, however, with the oversight of the primary provider. In this scenario, the solo provider communicates with others who have a role in the implementation process. For example, if one of the recommendations is for physical therapy, the health care provider must communicate with the physical therapist to assure that the recommendation is initiated and carried out appropriately. This communication process is the most direct between health care providers and is commonplace in medical referrals. Many of the same communication principles are applicable when making referrals as when providing consultative recommendations. The primary difference is the provider making the referral retains control over assuring that the recommendations are implemented. He or she is "ordering" services or therapies, and can expect the person's data or outcome to be reported by the secondary provider upon completion. This type of reporting back, through telephone calls or written reports, is customary between health care providers requesting and providing referred patient care services.

Assessment Team Implementation

If the team who has done the assessment is also responsible for implementing assessment recommendations, the communication process is greatly simplified. As with the solo provider, the recommendations are "owned" by team members and there is a commitment to seeing them implemented.

Communication about the implementation phase of the assessment centers on issues of team members' roles, responsibilities, and timing of recommendation implementation. In an ideal world, a detailed care plan developed in team meetings clarifies the sequencing of assessment recommendations and identifies who will be responsible for carrying out the recommendation(s) with the elder. In reality, there are often mishaps in team member communication. Misunderstandings can occur regarding the sequencing of care activities or who was responsible for following through on particular recommendations. In addition, depending on the composition of the team, follow-up patient care activities will be referred outside the team to other secondary providers for completion. In this scenario, one team member must take the lead on behalf of the elder to assure appropriate implementation of recommendation(s) and be the designated person for feedback from the other health care providers. Without such a designee, the team cannot be assured that referral recommendations are ordered or executed appropriately.

Consultative Assessment

Frequently, the health care provider who completes the assessment is serving as a geriatric consultant and must provide his or her findings to the referring provider. When the provider who has completed the assessment must relay the recommendation(s) to a different person for accomplishment, effective communication of recommendations is critical.[5]

If the assessment has been invited, and the primary provider is expecting the information, it will more likely be utilized than if the consultation is not invited. Since most health care providers currently in practice have had little or no exposure to concepts of geriatric medicine or geriatric assessment, the value of the assessment recommendations may not be immediately appreciated.[6]

Critical issues in the acceptance of consultative geriatric assessment recommendations include the clarity of the message, the perceived benefit of the treatment recommendation, the availability of resources to provide the recommended treatment, perceived patient acceptance, legal concerns, and relationship and prestige of the medical consultant.[7, 8]

In addition to face to face encounters, communication among health care providers can be accomplished using many vehicles: telephone, facsimile (fax) machine, electronic mail, and written letter reports. In-person meetings and telephone calls are more personal and provide the opportunity for interchange between the consultant and the referrer. Questions can be answered and discussion can occur. In-person meetings can be difficult to accomplish, unless the health care providers' offices are within close proximity. Calls can take more personal time, since many attempts can be required to accomplish the call. Written reports can be transmitted by fax or e-mail for expediency, or via the regular mail, but lack the opportunity for discussion.[9–11]

MEDICAL CARE ORGANIZATIONAL INFLUENCES ON COMMUNICATION

The organizational context of health care can create barriers to implementation of assessment recommendations. There is a great deal of variety among types of organizations, and within organizations, which can be similarly classified. For example, managed care organizations are quite diverse, some may have many types of care and resources, with multiple medical centers. Others may be more limited in service availability and organizational resources. The policies and procedures in place for assessment and referral, the organizational philosophy, the staff configurations, and the expertise of the professional staff all play a role in the organizational context of care.[12] For example, some managed care organizations and primary care tiered care plans may have disincentives for implementing recommendations that require costly subspecialty referrals, diagnostic tests, or treatments. Access to recommended services or tests can be limited by health plan review boards. Some services may not be available at all locations or within their particular care plan. These types of contextual constraints must be considered when making recommendations that may not be feasible to implement because of insurance coverage or organizational constraints. It is critical to find out whether the resources are available and the insurance or organizational policy allows the accomplishment of actions generated during the geriatric assessment.

Organizational structure can also influence the way comprehensive geriatric assessment recommendations are communicated to elders. As mentioned previously, assessment can be accomplished by a solo provider or a team comprised of different disciplines. In general, recommendations are provided on a one-to-one basis with the elder, although some new models of care can accomplish this in groups.[13]

Practice styles within organizations or private practice settings can also impede implementation of geriatric assessment recommendations. Principles of geriatric care may not be embraced by the health care providers receiving the referral.[7] They may be unaware of the potential benefits or scientific support for the recommendation. They may limit service based on their own beliefs of age-appropriate care.

Having noted potential organizational and practice style constraints on communication of geriatric assessment recommendations, we now turn to a key player in the communication process—the elder.

UNIQUE ASPECTS OF PROVIDER–ELDER COMMUNICATION

Although elders comprise roughly 12 percent of the population, they make up the majority of patients seen by health care providers, with an average of over 10 doctor visits per year.[14, 15] Today's elders are distinguished by several key factors that impact the elder–provider communication process. One factor is the types of health problems that bring them to the provider. A second factor is the cohort, or generation, within which they live, which shapes their psychosocial attitudes. Third is the historical context that patterns the distinct cultural experiences and social status of today's elders. As we address each of these factors relative to today's older population, it is important to keep in mind that future generations of elders may likely be quite different from the current generation.

Health Concerns as Barriers to Effective Communication

Interference to effective communication created by health problems is not unique to elders, as compared to younger persons. Health problems can hinder effective communication in any provider–person encounter. The unique aspect of health concerns for elders is the number of problems that may be present, and the fact that aspects of aging-related disorders, such as cognitive impairment or hearing loss, directly impact the capacity for effective communication.[16]

FRAILTY

Older adults, especially the very old (85 years and older), are less robust, have less reserve, and often experience limitations in activities of daily living (ADLs) due to illness.[16] Frailty is a generic concept that encompasses limitations in function, several of which are described in more detail in the following sections. A frail elder can experience high levels of fatigue from just getting dressed and getting to the doctor's office. Fatigue can interfere with the ability to listen when being given recommendations by the health care provider. Frailty can also limit the person's ability to do what is being asked.

HEARING LOSS

A substantial portion of elders have some degree of hearing loss.[16] Hearing loss is particularly prevalent in older men. Hearing aids are not always effective in correcting such loss. All elders who may benefit from a hearing aid do not own and use one. Elders may be reluctant to admit the need for one and may be skilled in convincing those around them to believe that their hearing is better than it is. If the elder does not hear well, she or he will not be able to follow instructions given by the health care provider (see Chapter 10).

COGNITIVE IMPAIRMENT

Alzheimer's disease (AD) and related dementias increase with age, with estimates of up to 50 percent of people over age 85 years having moderate to severe cognitive impairment.[16] Clinical diagnostic criteria for probable AD emphasize memory impairments and deficits in orientation, judgement, and problem solving (see Chapter 21). Language impairments are common and include disruption of verbal fluency, word finding, and object naming difficulty, and comprehension lapses.[17] These language difficulties appear as early indicators and worsen as the disease progresses.

Early stage AD patients and patients with less severe cognitive problems have a number of lucid days and assessment of communication capacity during medical visits is a critical step prior to providing information and instruction. Companions often accompany people with dementia to health care provider visits, especially after the disease progresses. Communication issues involving third persons in the encounter are discussed later.

Depression

Affective disorders in late life often go unrecognized even though these conditions are treatable.[18] Identification of depressive symptoms is difficult because elders can manifest depression differently than younger people (see Chapter 19).[19] Depression appears to hinder effective communication in the provider–elder relationship by the elder's decreasing attention, increasing fatigue, or by simply not being engaged with the provider. In addition, several simple techniques and interview approaches can address and lessen the impact of the disruption to effective communication of these health concerns, as outlined in Table 27-1.

TABLE 27-1. COMMON HEALTH PROBLEMS IMPACT ON COMMUNICATION		
HEALTH CONCERNS	IMPACT ON COMMUNICATION	TECHNIQUES TO IMPROVE COMMUNICATION
Frailty	Fatigue may decrease attention span	Limit instructions; simplify message; write down information
Hearing loss	Not able to hear or may misunderstand message	Speak slowly and clearly; create quiet environment; ask individual to repeat message to you; write down information
Cognitive impairment	May misunderstand message; may not retain information	Provide information to surrogate; simplify message; write down information; link instructions to common cues
Depression	May exhibit fatigue and short attention span; may not retain information	Treat depression; ask patient to repeat message back to you; write down information; arrange follow-up call

Psychosocial Issues as Barriers to Effective Communication

In addition to health problems that create barriers to communication, psychosocial factors also must be considered.[20] Today's generation of elders bring unique psychological and social considerations to the provider–elder relationship, which must be understood to maximize effective communication.

SELF-ASSESSMENTS OF HEALTH

How elders rate their own health can effect the provider–elder communication process. Studies show that when elders rate their health, in general, they tend to overestimate their health status, relative to an objective evaluation.[21] This may be the case because many of the chronic disabling conditions associated with age begin slowly and develop over years. This may allow people to gradually adjust to the limitations that illnesses create. Elders may also report their health in relation to others, judging themselves to be in better health than people around them.

How does this optimistic health self-assessment impact communication? First, it can limit the problems and symptoms that the elder reports. He or she may have "normalized" an ailment in that he or she no longer recognizes it as a problem in need of reporting.[22] Second, when a problem and subsequent treatment plan is identified, the elder may discount this and not agree. If he or she believes what has been identified is a "nonproblem," he or she is unlikely to agree to follow the suggested treatment regimen.[23]

Elders can feel that their health problems are "normal for their age," and therefore, believe that their problems are due to age and not treatable. When the health care provider is confronted with this scenario, he or she has a marvelous opportunity for educating the person on the issues of normal aging and disease, and exactly what kind of benefit can be expected from the treatment. For example, urinary incontinence is a common problem of older women. It is often seen as an inevitable and "normal" consequence of aging. Research has shown, however, that there are several categories of urinary incontinence that respond to behavioral, pharmacologic, or surgical intervention (see Chapter 22). Often by a combination of behavioral techniques (e.g. Kegel exercises) and medication, urinary incontinence is managed effectively. Women are relieved to find that this embarrassing and socially limiting condition can be effectively treated.

EXPECTATIONS FROM HEALTH CARE

Similar to health attitudes, expectations the elder brings to the medical encounter can impact effective communication. Since most elders have one or more chronic conditions, an expectation of cure is not realistic. The treatment approaches in these cases involve symptom management, avoidance of exacerbations, environmental adjustments, and routines of self-care. The very fact that the provider cannot "fix" the problem, but takes a problem management approach, can create discordance to expectations of some elders.

ELDERS' ATTITUDES TOWARD PROVIDERS

Compared to younger adults, the current generation of elders tends to revere physicians and health care providers. Physicians are seen as omnipotent and elders are less likely to question their wisdom or instructions.[24,25] This is true in general, with variations depending on several factors, such as the elder's educational level, acculturation status, and country of origin.

Elders' attitudes toward health care providers are changing for several reasons. First, the consumer movement has educated people to question authority figures and assure themselves that they are receiving high quality services for reasonable costs.[26] Consumerism has infiltrated medical care and has been fueled by medical care reorganization into managed care systems. The idea of getting a "second opinion" underscores the attitude of not taking the provider's word for something, but double-checking his or her finding and recommendation.

Second, medical care reorganization has changed the nature of provider–elder relationships.[27] In previous decades, people may have had more direct access and a longer relationship with their providers.[28] Today, although most people retain a primary care physician, organizational constraints often limit the autonomy of both person and provider. Due to pressures to reduce medical care costs, care decisions can be decided by a third party, such as a utilization review or insurance payer. For example, the ability to see a specialist can be routed through the primary care service, removing the sense of free choice and replacing it with a need for prior approval. The bureaucracy of the medical care organization or the insurance plan itself is often daunting, with many procedures and check-points that effectively limit access to costly services.[12] The changes in medical care organization are directly linked to elder–provider communication issues, such as how many minutes a physician is "given" for a patient appointment.[18,29] Organizational issues can also be indirectly linked to communication, for example how many people does the patient have to speak with to leave the physician a message, and how long does the elder have to sit "on hold" during this process?

Third, the nature of illness of elders requires that a treatment partnership be established to care for long-term, chronic illnesses.[30-32] As described previously, chronic illness requires self-monitoring and self-management. The health care provider makes the recommendations, but it is the individual elder, or his or her caregiver, who must carry them out. The creation of the treatment partnership shifts the power in the relationship to a more equitable basis between the person and the provider. However, some elders are not comfortable with the responsibilities which the treatment partnership invokes, they would prefer to have the provider retain his or her power and thus responsibility for care.[24, 33, 34]

Providers' Attitudes Toward Elders

Attitudes toward the care of elders are shaped by at least three factors. First, is the provider's own attitude toward elders in general and his or her own aging process. The second is the sense of capability in providing appropriate care. Third is the knowledge and skill in managing elders' medical problems. These factors are not unrelated, they often are interwoven threads that comprise the fabric of care provided to elders.

Many people hold negative attitudes towards elders, including some health care providers. The youth-oriented society has many ageist views, which devalue older members of society.[35] Providers are not exempt from holding these views, and they can interfere with the health care provider's ability to provide appropriate care. For example, medical problems may be attributed to age *per se*, so that a curable condition goes untreated.

Health care providers may feel ill-equipped to manage the myriad of chronic illnesses that elders have. Medical education does not usually provide adequate training in geriatrics or in methods of communication with elders and other providers.[36] They may feel frustrated in not being able to cure chronic health problems and this frustration can be directed to the elder.

Providers may be simply overwhelmed by the complexity of the problems that are presented by the elder. This can be exacerbated by a lack of time being made available to the health care provider in certain medical care organizations or practices. Elders have more problems, and these problems are more complex and require more time. However, physicians tend to spend less time with older, compared to younger, persons.[29] Either longer appointments or more frequent appointments are required to provide the appropriate care.

Third Party in Medical Encounter

Elders are more likely than other adults to be accompanied to provider visits by a companion, most frequently a family member, usually a spouse or adult child.[37, 38] Companions can play three basic roles in the medical encounter.[39] First, they can verify information to both person and provider. Second, they function as significant other by providing information and feedback. Third, they can assume the role of surrogate patient, answering questions for the patient. In each of these roles, they can serve either as patient advocate or antagonist.

The health care provider is challenged to manage communication well in the triadic relationship.[3, 40] The barriers to effective communication inherent in a two-way relationship are affected by the addition of the third party. It is the job of the health care provider to enlist the help of the companion, yet maintain the primary relationship with the patient. The companion's role can be useful in assuring that clear information is given to the person. With two sets of ears hearing what is being said, and with either the person, companion or both, requesting clarification, chances are likely that post-visit instructions will be understood.

> When a companion accompanies the patient, maintain the primary relationship with the patient, but enlist the help of the companion.

If the companion is functioning inappropriately, the health care provider should thank the companion for his or her insights, and redirect the discussion to the patient. In most cases, the companion should not subsume the patient role and answer for the person. The health care provider should firmly ask the companion to allow the person to answer for himself or herself, and let the companion know that he or she will have an opportunity to add insights after the person has completed the answer.

What is occurring in the provider's office can be an example of a lifetime communication pattern, where the person expects the companion to speak for him or her. The provider will need to assess whether or not the communication pattern being witnessed is typical for the person and companion. If it is, the health care provider may be helpless to intervene in such an ingrained pattern of communication.

Companions accompanying people in advanced stages of dementia may be required to assume the surrogate patient role during medical encounters.[41] If the health care provider has an established relationship with the patient, he or she will be able to assess changes in communication ability over time. If the person is a new patient, the health care provider should first address questions to the person, and only after the lack of communication ability is established, should the health care provider rely primarily on the companion. Even with severe stages of cognitive impairment, there are often still questions that the person can answer for himself or herself.

> When communicating with people with dementia, give them and their families information about the natural progression of the disease and anticipated future needs. Discuss advance directives and future care options, and assist them in setting limits when judgment becomes impaired.

When working with triads when dementia is present, it is important to integrate care for both patient and family caregiver, yet maintain the autonomy of each.[42] The health care provider must be sensitive to the negative consequences of dementia, both for person and the caregiver, and may be the first to identify caregiver stress or depression.

SOCIOECONOMIC ISSUES

The health care provider must recognize financial limitations, living conditions, access to services, or other socioeconomic concerns of the person and family when making assessment recommendations. If such limitations are not realized, recommendations may be made which are totally unrealistic for the elder. During the communication process, it may be that the elder would not bring up the concern but would listen politely with absolutely no intention of following through on the recommendation.[43] The health care provider must ask, or otherwise discern, the financial appropriateness of the recommendation. He or she may want to enlist the help of the elder in reviewing options, and have the person select the one which is the best for him or her.

Cross-Cultural Issues in Communication Between Older Persons and Providers

LANGUAGE AND CULTURAL VALUES

Differences in language are most obvious when exploring the impact of cultural diversity on communication. What is less apparent are the concerns about cultural values, traditions, beliefs, family structure, and nonverbal cues.[43-45] The major concern is improving quality of care by understanding and being responsive within the provider–elder relationship to cultural differences.

Providers regularly see people who speak different languages and hold different health beliefs, practices, and expectations from their own. In many metropolitan areas in the United States, the population may speak any of over 100 different languages. Hospitals and medical care organizations have a variety of options to bridge language differences as described in Table 27-2.

TABLE 27-2.   APPROACHES TO BRIDGING LANGUAGE BARRIERS

Extended visiting hours for family and friends
Using free interpreter services from community-based ethnic agencies, neighborhood hospitals, and courts or professional interpreter services
Matching staff and patients with the same ethnic background
Matching patients with similar ethnic background, at least one of whom speaks English
Using techniques such as diagrams, photographs, or other means for communication, such as telephone company translators

TABLE 27-3.   TIPS FOR COMMUNICATING ACROSS CULTURAL BOUNDARIES

- Demonstrate caring
  Be friendly, helpful, build rapport; develop a repertoire of knowledge: learn about special holidays, general principles of traditional medicine, a few key phrases from their native language
- Ask patients what they did before the visit
  Learn about home remedies, use of lay health consultants, and traditional or alternative healers
- Find out what patients think and do
  Ask what they think is the cause of their illness
- Involve the patient's family
  In many cultures, families are cohesive and powerful and can be sources of information to provide a better understanding of the patient's behavior; families can also be enlisted to bring group influence on the patient; understand the collective value of many cultures
- Recognize common themes in cross-cultural medicine
  Fear of blood loss
  Fear of cold
  Tradition of male dominance
  Conservatism in sexual matters
  Lack of a preventive health orientation
  Intolerance of side effects and expectations of immediate wellness
  Somatization of depression

During the medical appointment, health care providers can begin to understand the person's concept of health and disease and learn more about the person's culture by following the approaches outlined in Table 27-3. Through demonstrating a genuine interest in the person and altering the usual clinical approaches, barriers to cross-cultural communication can be opened.

THIRD PARTIES AS INTERPRETERS

As noted, family members who speak English often accompany the non-English speaking person and serve as an informal interpreter during the medical visit. When this occurs, the situation is even more complicated than the usual three-party medical visit discussed earlier.[46] The provider is arbitrarily distanced from the patient by having to communicate through a third party. The family member "cum translator" can serve any one of the companion roles. It will be more difficult for the health care provider to recognize the role, because he or she will not be able to tell how accurately the family member is translating what the person is saying.

The use of a professional translator can improve the validity of the message, however, this is not always feasible or problem-free. If family members are accompanying the elder, they may not be willing to have a "stranger" step in to translate on behalf of the person. The family member may see this as his or her valid and expected role and resent the intrusion. A second issue is the actual availability of a translator. The care organization simply may not have a person available to serve as translator, depending on the language needed. Even when a professional translator is available and welcome, biased translation can still occur. Professional translators have varied skill levels and are not without the potential of skewing translation in one direction or another during the medical encounter.

AVAILABLE, ACCESSIBLE, AND APPROPRIATE CARE

Recommended treatments must also be available, accessible, and acceptable.[47] If follow-up treatments, diagnostic tests, or recommended services are not available or affordable to the person, they are of very little use. If the location or hours are not convenient, or there is no staff member available who speaks the person's language, the recommended service probably will not be completed. It is up to the health care provider to make sure to provide all the information that is needed for the person to complete the recommendation.

EFFECTIVE ELDER–PROVIDER COMMUNICATION

Recognition of Communication Barriers

In addition to the barriers discussed, which are more frequent in relationships with elders, other types of barriers also exist.[48] Some of these barriers are clear and can be easily resolved. Other barriers are implicit and require some analysis to recognize. The provider may note indirect signs during the medical visit which indicate that an implicit barrier is present.

A verbal-nonverbal mismatch is present when the answer given is belied by nonverbal body language or an emotional response. For example, a fall assessment may include a series of questions about alcohol use, since alcohol is sometimes a factor in falls. The person may be embarrassed and not want to admit to a drinking problem. The person boldly states that he or she does not drink "much," but cannot look the provider in the eye, and begins fidgeting in discomfort. It is imperative that the health care provider be nonjudgmental and nonthreatening to try to break through the barrier and get truthful responses.

The psychological term, cognitive dissonance, refers to the holding of incompatible beliefs that creates a tension for the person to modify one of the beliefs to create compatibility. This concept is applied to provider–elder communication when the information being provided just does not "fit" the clinical picture presented. For example, the health care provider may suspect the person is withholding abuse by his or her spouse after treatment for broken bones and bruises from frequent "accidents."

In an attempt to expose the suspected abusive relationship, the health care provider may suggest that many people find it difficult to talk about abusive relationships. He or she may find unexpected resistance to this suggestion, with an emotional or angry response that may be masking fear and embarrassment.

Providers should also be vigilant to recognize how their own feelings can be triggered by information from the person. Provider discomfort can stem from his or her own personal experiences or from a previous experience with a similar personal situation. He or she also may be sensing what the person is feeling.

If the treatment is not working, the health care provider must consider that a communication barrier exists. Nonadherence to medical recommendations is common. Although nonadherence can result from a misunderstanding of instructions, it often represents a barrier that must be addressed within the provider–elder relationship. In the case of a worsening chronic illness, both the provider and elder may assume that it represents a change in the underlying disease. A thorough review of the treatment regimen is required, along with a discussion of any new situation or stressor in the person's life.

Basic Tenets of Providing Assessment Information to Elders

General communication among providers, between providers and elders, special issues of geriatric conditions, and barriers that must be recognized and addressed have been discussed. We now turn to the application of communication strategies and avoidance of pitfalls in the special case of providing assessment recommendations.

Assessment recommendations can be divided into two basic categories: those which a health care provider must first implement to enable the person to complete (provider-initiated) and those which the person can do without a provider's order (self-care).[49] Provider-initiated recommendations also differ in who will be implementing the order. As discussed in the introductory provider to provider communication section, if the follow-through is com-

TABLE 27-4. BASIC TENETS OF PROVIDING ASSESSMENT INFORMATION TO ELDERS
Simplify information
Discuss "emotional charge" issues
Limit number of recommendations or prioritize
Provide written summary of recommendations
Provide the needed resources and information to accomplish recommendations
Speak to the importance of following through on recommendation
Seek information about intentions, concerns, and potential perceived barriers
Answer questions
Treat person with respect

pleted by the same provider or team member who completed the assessment and generated the recommendation (solo or team assessment model), the communication process is greatly simplified. If the recommendation was generated as a consultation and a different health care provider is expected to do the implementation (consultative assessment model), there is an added dimension to the communication process.

Effective communication of geriatric assessment recommendations will ensure that the elder knows what he or she needs to do and has the necessary information and resources to accomplish it. In the following sections, and in Table 27-4, practical communication tips are suggested to maximize implementation of recommendations.

SIMPLIFY INFORMATION

The information relayed by a health care provider must be provided using the simplest language possible, by avoiding jargon and explaining medical terms if they must be used. For example, rather than saying that a medication for hypertension is being prescribed, a health care provider can explain that a medicine is being given to lower blood pressure. Providers relay information with the expectation that the person will understand, remember, and act upon their requests. They should ask if the person understands what has been requested. It is helpful to have the person repeat back the request when there is any suspicion that the request was not clearly understood.

DISCUSS "EMOTIONAL CHARGE" ISSUES

Some medical information provided to the person will create an emotional reaction, such as the news of a serious or life-threatening illness. A provider should anticipate this and not plan on giving detailed treatment instructions after delivering such news. People often report reactions such as, "After he told me I might have cancer, I didn't hear another word he said".

The best way a health care provider can handle this situation is, if the person has come alone to the appointment, schedule a follow-up appointment soon thereafter. The provider may also want to do a follow-up telephone call to the person a day or two after the visit to answer questions, provide additional information, or reinforce information that was given.

If the elder is accompanied to the appointment, the health care provider may want to bring in the companion and go over the information with him or her, with the person's permission.[50] The companion can be in as great a state of shock as the patient, and further instructions or comments must be gauged based on how the companion appears to be managing.

Certain types of recommendations can also elicit strong emotional reactions, even when they do not address a serious illness. For example, psychosocial problems can be difficult for the person to face. A recommendation for counseling may be extremely threatening to elders because they may equate this with the idea that they are "going crazy."

Health care providers must be aware that what may appear to them to be a very innocuous recommendation can elicit a strong emotional reaction in the patient. Vigilance about recognizing such a reaction, whether it is expressed verbally or nonverbally, is necessary. Such reactions can take the form of tears or angry outbursts. Health care providers need to acknowledge such reactions, making the individuals feel as comfortable about their concerns as possible, and let them know through words and deeds that their feelings are understood.

LIMIT NUMBER OF RECOMMENDATIONS OR PRIORITIZE

If the examiner is not the person's regular provider, but serving in a consultative manner, a number of recommendations for the person can be generated. The regular health care provider can share these over several visits. In any case, if a number of recommendations are given, they must be prioritized, if possible. Limit recommendations to no more than three or four, unless the follow-through is very simple, so that the person does not become confused. A good plan is to provide an overview of everything, and then fully explain the three most important, saving the remaining for implementation at the next visit.

PROVIDE WRITTEN SUMMARY OF RECOMMENDATIONS

A summary of exactly what the patient is expected to do should be written. A standardized "memo" form on which to write these

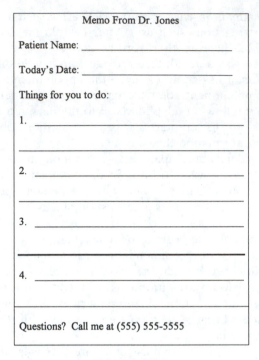

Memo From Dr. Jones

Patient Name: _____

Today's Date: _____

Things for you to do:

1. _____

_____

2. _____

_____

3. _____

_____

4. _____

Questions? Call me at (555) 555-5555

FIGURE 27-1

is shown in Figure 27-1. In writing down instructions, it is better to be specific. Thus, the directions should be "take one tablet three times each day before a meal" or "walk on flat ground for up to 15 minutes once a day."

PROVIDE THE NEEDED RESOURCES AND INFORMATION TO ACCOMPLISH RECOMMENDATIONS

The elder should be given the tools that may be needed to accomplish the requests. A recommendation that the person does not know how to complete is useless. For example, prescribing a water exercise class is not helpful if there is no pool or class available to the person (or if it is too expensive). Recommendations should be "do-able" from the person's perspective.

If the recommendation is a referral to another health care provider or the recommendations are consultative and being implemented by another provider, communicate directly to other providers as required on behalf of the person. The patient should be told that the other health care provider is expecting a call. The other provider should receive a written document with a copy sent to the elder.

SPEAK TO THE IMPORTANCE OF FOLLOWING THROUGH WITH THE RECOMMENDATION

The person needs to understand why the recommendation(s) have been made and what the expected benefit is. The examiner must be certain that these important facts are communicated clearly. As indicated in the discussion of barriers earlier in the chapter, if the person does not believe that the recommendation is addressing an important problem or will be beneficial, it likely will never be done. The person needs to know that he or she is expected to follow through with the request.

SEEK INFORMATION ABOUT INTENTIONS, CONCERNS, AND POTENTIAL PERCEIVED BARRIERS

In providing information to the patient about the potential benefits and the expectations, one can ask about his or her reactions to the recommendation. "Does he or she plan to follow the recommendation?" "Does he or she have concerns or identified reasons that would make the recommendation difficult to complete?" By posing these questions additional information can be given or problem solving can take place about what appears to be a barrier to implementation.

Patients may be reluctant to voice objections to what the health care provider has requested. Elders can be particularly reticent to share concerns or disagree that the recommendation is a good one. To elicit such information, the health care provider needs to make it "okay" to disagree. Statements such as "many elders think this is kind of a waste of time" or "some people question whether this really works" may open up communication channels. The partnership aspect of the provider–elder relationship may also need to be openly discussed.

ANSWER QUESTIONS

The well-prepared patient (or companion) may arrive with a written list of questions. Others may ask questions openly during the appointment. Many people however, are very reluctant to ask questions, or may not think of their questions until after they have left the appointment. It is up to the health care provider to anticipate the questions that may or may not be asked. If they are not asked, the examiner must ask them. Statements such as "patients often ask me," or "people often wonder about," to open the questions may be used. This is an ingenuous technique that makes it easy to provide answers to the unanswered questions of the reluctant person, or to trigger questions that will only be remembered later by others. Patients should be encouraged to write down questions as they occur between visits.

TREAT PERSON WITH RESPECT

Even the most challenging person deserves to be treated with the utmost respect. This is demonstrated in many ways: a knock on the door before entering, addressing the person by their surname, and listening intently to what the person has to say. It can be very difficult to respect a person's decision when it disagrees with the providers recommendations.

PATIENT ADHERENCE AND PROVIDER IMPLEMENTATION OF CGA RECOMMENDATIONS

We have discussed communication barriers and strategies to address these in providing geriatric assessment recommendations. We now focus on decisions to follow recommendations and other health care providers' decisions to implement consultative recommendations.

The terms adherence and compliance have both been used to portray the phenomenon of people following health care providers' recommendations. The term compliance has fallen into disfavor in behavioral health circles because of the power differential and victim-blaming application.[51]

The term adherence, meaning to stick to or stay attached to something, connotes a more accurate picture of decisions to complete or continue with a recommended course of action. Compliance, on the other hand, is defined as acquiescence or giving in to others[52] and suggests a passive person role. Adherence promotes a more involved collaborative and mutually defined effort between the health care provider and elder. There are as many types of adherence behavior as there are health care recommendations. The major reasons for patient adherence and provider implementation are presented as follows (Table 27-5). These factors are drawn from the vast body of research on health behavior and use of health services.[23, 53–60]

TABLE 27-5. WHY PEOPLE FOLLOW HEALTH CARE PROVIDER RECOMMENDATIONS

Agreement with importance of recommendation
Agreement with potential for benefit
Understanding of recommendation and access to accomplish it
Social influence
Sense of empowerment (self-efficacy) to accomplish recommendation
Recommendation(s) do not contradict basic values or interfere with lifestyle

Why Peoples Follow Health Care Provider Directions

AGREEMENT WITH THE IMPORTANCE OF THE RECOMMENDATION

People follow recommendations that they believe address important health concerns. People may define "important" differently than health care providers.[23, 61] To many people, the things that are important have immediate impact on their lives. These medical concerns may be issues that limit their ability to do the things they want. For example, foot problems can not only create pain but also limit the ability to get around to do the things that people like to do or need to do to remain independent.

If assessment recommendations identify concerns that people think are not important in their world view, they may not be followed.[23] It is crucial when providing recommendations to others to make sure that they believe that a particular recommendation is relevant as well as whether they plan to complete the recommendations since it is ultimately their decision.

AGREEMENT WITH POTENTIAL FOR BENEFIT

In addition to the belief in the importance of a recommendation, the person must also believe that it will be beneficial. He or she may have tried something like it before without success. He or she is, therefore skeptical. The more difficult the recommendation is, the more clear the benefit needs to be to the person, or he or she may decide it is not worth it. This concept is called utility, and it has been shown to be an important determinant to patient adherence.[23, 59] It makes perfect sense from the elder's viewpoint that if a recommendation is a considerable amount of trouble, with unclear potential benefit, it may not be worth doing (Figure 27-2).

There are several things that a health care provider can do to encourage an elder to complete or at least begin the recommendation. The potential benefit should be clear and tied to something important from the person's viewpoint. In addition, it is advisable to "stage in" the recommendation, by beginning with an easy aspect of the recommendation. Once that step is mastered and integrated into the person's routine, the next step can be added. A person's progress should be praised and benefits seen should be acknowledged.

Another technique that can be useful is to tailor the recommendation to the stage of readiness of the person (see Chapter 25).[62] For example, if the recommendation is for the person to lose weight, but he or she has said they do not wish to go on a diet, perhaps he or she would be willing to begin a walking program.

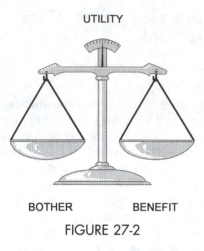

FIGURE 27-2

By slowly increasing his or her activity level, even without cutting back on calories, weight will gradually be lost.

UNDERSTANDING THE RECOMMENDATION AND ACCESS TO ACCOMPLISH IT

Of course, before the person can complete any recommendation, he or she must first understand what it is and have the means to accomplish it. Cognitive impairment, sensory disorders, frailty, and multiple chronic illnesses associated with aging, present additional barriers to communication. These barriers must be addressed to maximize effective communication, so the health care provider can be assured that the person leaves his or her office with the information and the tools to accomplish the recommendation.

SOCIAL INFLUENCE

Health care providers have a great deal of influence over patient behavior. The following communication tips assist in maximizing effectiveness. Other people can also influence the completion of assessment recommendations.[63] Elders often come to health care provider visits with a companion, therefore there may be the opportunity to discuss the recommendations with him or her directly.[45] If the recommendation must involve the companion's support or assistance, a point must be made to speak with him or her, either by telephone or in person. For example, diet modifications that impact the household or rely on someone other than the person for the shopping and/or cooking should be discussed with all the people they impact.

Social support can be either positive or negative. All health care providers have had a situation where a companion undermines the recommendation that the person was willing to do. Potential concerns or anticipated difficulties from the companion's perspective regarding the person's adherence can be elicited. Just as with the person, these insights offer clarification and problem-solving opportunities. This type of communication may not stop another's undermining behavior, but it is a step in the right direction.

SENSE OF EMPOWERMENT (SELF-EFFICACY) TO ACCOMPLISH THE RECOMMENDATION

When speaking of providing the tools necessary to accomplish the recommendation, some people need to be given a critical tool: the belief that they can do it. The concept is called self-efficacy and it means the belief of being capable of doing something.[64]

If a person does not believe that he or she is capable of doing the activities required by the recommendation, this belief must be instilled. The examiner starts by telling the person that he or she believes that the patient is capable and reviews similar accomplishments. The health care provider may also need to "step in" the recommendation, so that the person accomplishes it progressively. Previous successes will fuel future accomplishments. If these two techniques do not work, offer the person several options to accomplish the recommendation (if possible), so that they can choose the one that they feel most capable of accomplishing.

RECOMMENDATION DOES NOT CONTRADICT BASIC VALUES OR INTERFERE WITH LIFESTYLE

In making recommendations, the examiner must assess whether what is suggested is going to oppose the basic values of the person or be disruptive to their preferred lifestyle. Sometimes, this cannot be avoided, but it always needs to be recognized. People will tell the health care provider if the recommendation violates a traditional value which is nonnegotiable. They often do not tell however, if it conflicts with a value preference.[48] For example, many elders do not like taking medication. Yet, when the prescription is given, they never mention this. They may fill the prescription, but only take the medication "when they have to" and not follow the directions. After treatment failure, it is determined that the pills were not taken appropriately. When asked why they did not take the medicines, they report "Oh, I don't like taking pills."

Recommendations relating to lifestyle changes are particularly challenging.[22] These types of recommendations (lose weight, start walking) can be difficult to do.[65] The benefit is not assured, so from the person's perspective, they have low utility. There may also be an addictive component to many of these types of recommendations and a long history of doing the unwanted behaviors (e.g., smoking).

Elders can and do make such difficult lifestyle changes. Research has shown that for many behaviors, such as smoking, there are benefits in risk reduction in old age. Lifestyle behavior change is very complicated and it appears that new behaviors are easier to initiate than the termination of old behaviors. The concepts of self-efficacy, utility, staging, and tailoring of recommendations are key when addressing lifestyle behavior change. The person needs to be given the power to change, needs to understand the potential benefit, and the behavior change must be approached slowly and incrementally, to create mini-success stories to build upon. Slippage and reversals may occur; therefore providing continuous support and help ensures success.

Maximizing Successful Implementation by Other Providers

Patients are not the only set of people who, for a variety of reasons, do not follow recommendations. In consultative CGA, primary providers receive the CGA recommendation and are required to implement the recommendation in order for the participant to begin the recommendation. Health care providers receiving consultative information about patients often do not implement these recommendations.[7, 66–68] As with patient adherence, provider adherence varies by the "required" behavior, (e.g., changing a medication dosage or ordering diagnostic tests).

AGREEMENT WITH IMPORTANCE OF THE RECOMMENDATION

As with elders, other providers will be less likely to implement recommendations that are not believed to be related to an important health concern.[69] This is especially true if there are multiple recommendations for a given person. The health care provider may select the most important from his or her viewpoint, ignoring those judged to be of lesser importance.

Since many health care providers are not well trained in geriatric medicine, they may miss or be unaware of the importance of a certain recommendation. The importance of the recommendation must be conveyed in a convincing manner to the provider who will implement it, with scientific evidence to bolster the request. In a community-based consultative assessment program[69] recommendations were first discussed with the primary care physician over the telephone, followed up in writing, and mailed to them with medical journal articles that supported the recommendation. In this way, the recommendations were first suggested and discussion was possible with the primary care physician over the telephone. The mailing of the consultation summary and articles provided an opportunity for further education about the geriatric problem and the proposed recommendation.

AGREEMENT WITH POTENTIAL FOR BENEFIT

Linked to the issue of importance is the potential for benefit from the recommendation. Again, as discussed, many community physicians and other health care providers simply do not know the beneficial results attainable for certain geriatric problems or syndromes. Some of these may be functional benefits, rather than the curative focus of much medical training. The consultative interchange can be used to deliver an educational message, which providers can apply to their other older patients.

The issue is not simply the potential benefit, but the relative benefit, given the time and trouble some recommendations require.[23] The simpler the recommendation, the more often it is implemented. It makes sense then, to communicate recommendations in the most "user-friendly" manner. For example, when recommending physical therapy, provide a "prescription" for the exact recommendation, which the provider simply needs to sign, (see example in Figure 27-3). It is also helpful to provide the billing code information regarding how to charge for such an order and the names and telephone numbers of physical therapists or programs.

UNDERSTANDING OF THE RECOMMENDATION AND ACCESS TO ACCOMPLISH IT

As with patients, health care providers need a clear understanding of exactly what is recommended. Many physicians are unaware of community long-term care resources and services.[70] Informational materials available, such as a community resource directory, may need to be provided for ease of referral and contact information (see Chapter 26). The recommendation must be specific and clearly written, e.g., name specific drug rather than a medication group or category. In discussing the recommendation one needs to inquire if implementation would be difficult because of access issues. Not all services are available in certain communities or within medical care plans, so it is useful to ask whether the recommended service is available. The next best substitute to solve the problem should be sought if the service is unavailable.

CONSUMER DEMAND

Patients may enter the primary care provider's office with the list that was given to them during the assessment (Figure 27-1). They may ask for these things to be done, and probably will want to

PT/OT PRESCRIPTION

Patient Name: _____   DOB: _____

*Dx _____   Onset: _____

Condition:_____

_____

*Precautions: _____

Recommendation(s)

Physical Therapy Assessment and Treatment:

_____

_____

_____

_____

Occupational Therapy Assessment and Treatment:

_____

_____

Frequency: _____   Duration: _____

Print Name: _____   Lic. # _____

Signature: _____   Date: _____

FIGURE 27-3

know what the provider thinks of the recommendations. Although this was rare in the past, the consumer movement has spawned new assertive behaviors in the current older population group and this will likely increase in the future.[26] In a recent study of physician implementation of CGA recommendations, patient request was the major reason for the physician's action.[7] Today, the provider is caught between wanting to give the person what he or she wants, deciding if it is the best thing, and whether it is cost-effective.[71]

DEFUSE TERRITORIALITY OR "STEALING" PATIENT ISSUES

It is important at the outset in communication with the primary care provider to make sure that he or she knows that the service is consultative, and that ongoing patient care will not be provided (if this is true). Defuse any threat of taking away the patient and establish a collaborative treatment partnership in discussions with colleagues.

SUMMARY

Communication of comprehensive geriatric assessment recommendations to other health care providers, elders and their families to assure their accomplishment is a complex process. This chapter addresses the organizational, provider, and individual issues that facilitate or impede communication to accomplish recommendations and offers tips to overcome these issues and maximize effective communication. A great deal of time and effort is involved in comprehensive geriatric assessments and if the recommendations are not communicated and acted upon, the potential benefits of CGA will not be realized.[1, 68]

REFERENCES

1. Reuben DB, Frank J, Hirsch S, McGuigan K, Maly R. A randomized clinical trial of outpatient comprehensive geriatric assessment couples with an intervention to increase adherence to recommendations *J Am Geriatr Soc.* 1999;47:269–276.
2. McCormick W, Inui T, Roter D. Interventions in physician-elderly patient interactions. *Res On Aging.* 1996;18:103–136.
3. Greene M, Majerovitz G, Deborah S, Adelman R, Rizzo C. The effects of the presence of a third person on the physician-older patient medical interview. *J Am Geriatr Soc.* 1994;42:413–419.
4. Zeiss AM, and Steffen AM. Interdisciplinary health care teams: the basic unit of geriatric care. In: Carstensen LL, Edelstein BA, Dornbrand L, eds. *The Practical Handbook of Clinical Gerontology.* Thousand Oaks, CA: Sage; 1996;423–450.
5. Reuben DB, Maly R, Hirsch S. Improving physician implementation of, and patient adherence to recommendations from a comprehensive geriatric assessment. *Am J Med.* 1996;100:444–451.
6. U.S. Health Services and Resources Administration *A National Agenda for Geriatric Education: White Papers.* Washington, DC: Author; 1995.
7. Maly R, Abrahamse A, Hirsch S, Frank J, Reuben DB. What influences physician practice behavior? *Arch Fam Med.* 1996;5:448–456.
8. Shah, P.N, Maly R, Frank J.C, Hirsch, S, Reuben, D. Managing geriatric syndromes: what geriatric assessment teams recommend, what primary care physicians implement, what patients adhere to. *J Am Geriatr Soc.* 1997;45:413–419.
9. Ouslander JG, Osterweil D, Morley JE, eds. *Medical Care in the Nursing Home.* New York: McGraw-Hill; 1997:492–500, 515.

10. Fowkes W, Christenson D, McKay, D An analysis of the use of the telephone in the management of patients in skilled nursing facilities. *J Am Geriatr Soc.* 1997;45:67–70.

11. Cadogan, MP, Franzi C, Osterweil D, Hill TJ. Barriers to effective communication in skilled nursing facilities: differences in perception between nurses and physicians. *J Am Geriatr Soc.* 1999;47:71–75.

12. Ory MG, Cooper J, Siu A, eds. Aging and primary care: organizational issues in the delivery of health care services to older Americans. Health Services Research, (special supplement) 1998;33 June.

13. Beck A, Scott J, Williams P, Robertson B, Jackson D, Gade G, Cowan P. A randomized trial of group outpatient visits for chronically ill older HMO members: the cooperative health care clinic. *J Am Geriatr Soc.* 1997;5:543–549.

14. U.S. Bureau of the Census. *Current Population Reports, Special Studies: 65+ in the United States.* Washington, DC: U.S. Government Printing Office; 1996:23–190.

15. U.S. Department of Health and Human Services. *Health and Aging Chartbook.* Washington, DC: U.S. Government Printing Office; 1999.

16. Kassner E, and Bechtel R. *Midlife and Older Americans with Disabilities: Who Gets Help? A Chartbook.* Washington. DC. AARP; 1998.

17. Kemper, Anagnopoulos SC, Lyons K Heberlein W. Speech accommodations to dementia. *J of Gerontol Psychol Sci Soi Sci.* 1994; 49:P223–229.

18. Glasser M, and Gravdal J. Assessment and treatment of geriatric depression in primary care settings. *Arch Fam Med.* 1997;6:433–438.

19. Agency for Health Care Policy and Research. Clinical Practice Guidelines #5 Vol. 1. Depression in Primary Care Detection and Diagnoses. US Dept of Health & Human Services 4/93 pp 40–41. Washington, DC.

20. Greene M, Hoffman S, Charon R, Adelman R. Psychosocial concerns in the medical encounter: a comparison of the interactions of doctors with their old and young patients. *Gerontologist.* 1987;27:164–168.

21. Ory MG, Cox DM. Forging ahead: linking health and behavior to improve quality of life in older people. *Soc Indicator Res.* 1994; 33:89–120.

22. Ory, MG, and DeFriese GH, eds. *Self Care in Later Life.* New York: Springer Publishing Co.; 1998.

23. Frank JC, Hirsch S, Chernoff J, et al. Determinants of patient adherence to consultative comprehensive geriatric assessment recommendations, *J Gerontol. A Biol Sci. Med Sci.* 1997;52A:M44–51.

24. Smith R, Woodward N, Wallston B, Wallston K. Health care implications of desire and expectancy for control in elderly adults. *J Gerontol.* 1998;43:P1–7.

25. Haug M, Ory MG. Issues in elderly patient–provider interactions. *Res Aging.* 1987;3:3–44.

26. Counte M. The emerging role of the client in the delivery of primary care to older Americans. Ory MG, Cooper J, Siu A, eds. *Organizational Issues in the Delivery of Primary Care to Older Americans.* special supplement to HSR, 1998;33(2):402–423.

27. Emanuel E, Dubler N. Preserving the physician–patient relationship in the era of managed care. *JAMA*. 1995;273:323–329.

28. Health Care Financing Administration. *Medicare Managed Care Contract Report*. 1998.

29. Keeler E, Solomon D, Beck J. et al. Effect of patient age on duration of medical encounters with physicians. *Med Care*. 1982;20:1101–1108.

30. Kassebaum G, Baumann B. Dimensions of the sick role in chronic illness. *J Health Hum Behav*. 1965;6:16–27.

31. Lorig KR, Sobel DS, Stewart AL, et al. Evidence suggesting that a chronic disease self-management program can improve health status while reducing hospitalization. A randomized trial. *Med Care*. 1999;37:5–14.

32. Wagner EH. The promise and performance of HMOS in improving outcomes in older adults. *J Am Geriatr Soc*. 1996;44:1251–1257.

33. Blanchard CG, Labrecque MS, Ruckdeschel JC, Blanchard EB. Information and decision-making preferences of hospitalized adult cancer patients. *Soc Sci Med*. 1988;27:1139–1145.

34. Kaplan SH, Gandeck B, Greenfield S, Rogers W, Ware J. Patient and visit characteristics related to physician' participatory decision-making style: results from the medical outcomes study. *Med Care*. 1995;33:1176–1187.

35. Butler R. Ageism: another form of bigotry. *Gerontologist*. 1969; 9:243–246.

36. McBride C, Shugars D, DiMatteo M, Lepper H, O'Neil E, Damush T. The physician' role. Views of the public and the profession on seven aspects of patent care. *Arch Fam Med*. 1994;3:948–953.

37. Silliman R. Caring for the frail older patient: the doctor–patient–family caregiver relationship. *J Gen Intern Med*. 1989;4:237–241.

38. Silliman R, Bhatti S, Khan A, Dukes K, Sullivan L. The care of older persons with diabetes mellitus: families and primary care physicians. *J Am Geriatr Soc*. 1996;44:1314–1321.

39. Adelman RD, Greene MG, Charon R. The physician-elderly patient–companion triad in the medical encounter: the development of a conceptual framework and research agenda. *Gerontologist*. 1987; 27:729–734.

40. Beisecker AE. The influence of a companion on the doctor–elderly patient interaction. *Health Commun*. 1989;1:55–70.

41. Haley W, Clair J, Saulsberry K. Family caregiver satisfaction with medical care of their demented relatives. *Gerontologists*. 1992;32: 219–226.

42. Haug M. Elderly patients, caregivers, and physicians: theory and research on health care triads. *J Health Soc Behav*. 1994;35:1–12.

43. Rost K. Frankel R. The introduction of the older patient's problems in the medical visit. *J Aging Health*. 1993;3:387–401.

44. Saldov M, Chow P. The ethnic elderly in metro Toronto hospitals, nursing homes and homes for the aged: communication and health care. *Intl J Aging Hum Develop*. 1994;38(2):117–135.

45. Mull JD. Cross-cultural communication in the physician's office. *WJM*. 1993;159:609–613.

46. Prohaska, TR, Glasser M. Patients views of family involvement in medical care decisions and encounters. *Res Aging.* 1996;18:52–69.

47. Damron-Rodriguez, J, Wallace S, Kington R. Service utilization and minority elderly: appropriateness, accessibility and acceptability. *Gerontol Geriatr Educ.* 1994;15:45–63.

48. Haug M. Elements in physicians patient interactions in late life. *Res Aging.* 1996;18:32–50.

49. Reuben DB, Hirsch SH, Chernoff JC, et al. Project Safety Net: A health screening outreach and assessment program. *Gerontologist.* 1993;33(4):557–560.

50. Labrecque M, Blanchard C, Ruckdeschel J, Blanchard E. The impact of family presence on the physician–cancer patient interaction. *Soc Sci Med,* 1991;33:1253–1261.

51. Trostle JA. Medical compliance as an ideology. *Soc Sci Med.* 1988;27:1299–3308.

52. Guralnik D. *Webster's New World Dictionary,* 2nd ed. New York: Simon & Schuster, Inc; 1986.

53. Becker MH. The health belief model and sick role behavior. *Health Educ Monograph.* 1974;2(4):82–91.

54. DiMatteo MR. Enhancing patient adherence to medical recommendations. *JAMA.* 1994;271:79–83.

55. Kravitz R, Hays R, Sherbourne C, et al. Recall of recommendations and adherence to advice among patients with chronic medical conditions. *Arch Intern Med.* 1993;153:1869–1878.

56. DiMatteo MR, Hays RD, Gritz ER, et al. Patient adherence to cancer control regimens: scale development and initial validation *Psychol Assess* 1993;5(1):1–11.

57. Beisecker AE. Patient power in doctor–patient communciation: what do we know? *Health Commun.* 1990;2:105–122.

58. Meichenbaum D, Turk D, eds. *Facilitating Treatment Adherence, A Practitioner's Guidebook.* New York: Plenum Press; 1987.

59. Hulka B, Cassel J, Kupper L, Burdette J. Communication, compliance and concordance between physicians and patients with prescribed medications. *Am J Public Health.* 1976;66:847–853.

60. Svarstad B. Physician–patient communication and patient conformity with medical advice. In Mechanic D. ed. *The Growth of Bureaucratic Medicine.* New York: Wiley and Sons, 1971;220–238.

61. Greene M, Adelman R, Charon R. Friedmann EL. Concordance between physicians and their older and younger patients in the primary care medical encounter. *Gerontologist.* 1989;29:808–813.

62. Prochaska JO, Velicer WF, Rossi JS, et al. Stages of change and decisional balance for 12 problem behaviors. *Health Psychol.* 1994; 13:39–46.

63. Glasser M, Prohaska T, Roska J. The role of the family in medical care-seeking decisions of older adults. *Fam Commun Health.* 1992; 15:59–70.

64. Bandura A. Self-efficacy: toward a unifying theory of behavioral change. *Psych Rev.* 1977;84(2):191–215.

65. Baric L. Recognition of the at-risk role: a means to influence behavior. *Intl J Health Educ.* 1969;12:24–34.

66. Kroenke K, Pinholt EM. Reducing polypharmacy in the elderly: a controlled trial of physician feedback. *J Am Geriatr Soc.* 1990; 38:31–36.

67. Grilli R, Apolone G, Marsoni S, Nicolucci A, Zola P, Liberati A. The impact of patient management guidelines on the care of breast, colorectal, and ovarian cancer patients in Italy. *Med Care.* 1991; 29:50–62.

68. Stuck AE, Siu AL, Wieland GD, et al. Comprehensive geriatric assessment: a meta-analysis of controlled trials. *Lancet.* 1993; 342:1032–1036.

69. Cefalu CA, Kaslow LD, Mims B, Simpson S. Follow-up of comprehensive geriatric assessment in a family medicine residency clinic. *J Am Board Fam Pract.* 1995;8:263–269.

70. Damron-Rodriguez J, Frank JC, Osterweil D. Physician knowledge of community-based care: what's the score? *Ann of Long-Term Care.* 1998;6,(4),112–121.

71. Council on Graduate Medical Education. *Resource Paper: Preparing Learners for Practice in a Managed Care Environment,* Washington, DC: USDHHS; 1997.

ROLE OF THE ASSESSMENT PROCESS IN IMPROVING QUALITY OF CARE

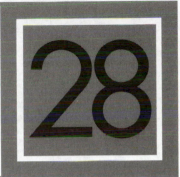

MARY JANE KOREN / MINDEL SPIEGEL

The purpose of this chapter, and the book as a whole, is to emphasize the importance of assessment in caring for elders. Assessment gives health care providers and treatment teams useful information about an elder's physical, functional, mental, and psychosocial status. In addition, assessment data can be aggregated and analyzed to improve understanding of the health care system—its effectiveness, its shortcomings, and its costs. This chapter discusses these broader uses of assessments.

How are individual assessments linked to what appear to be remote abstractions such as statutes, regulations, reimbursement methodologies, and the epidemiology of quality care? The relationship between micro- and macro-issues is sometimes difficult to ascertain. One example, however, can illustrate how such linkages occur and how they affect the lives of patients and health care providers.

In the late 1960s to the 1980s, studies of nursing home care found that the overall quality of care provided was poor, despite numerous regulations governing care provision and a well-developed process for monitoring that care. Concerned that public monies were being spent on unsatisfactory care, Congress commissioned the Institute of Medicine (IOM) to conduct a comprehensive evaluation of nursing home care. One of the many findings of the investi-

The Agency for Health Care Policy and Research (AHCPR) was renamed in December 1999.
This agency is now known as the Agency for Healthcare Research and Quality (AHRQ).

gation was that assessments of residents, if performed at all, were rarely comprehensive. Furthermore, assessments tended to be informal or used "home grown" rather than standardized instruments so that results were not reproducible and could not be used to compare residents in different facilities.[1]

Noting that high quality care begins with a thorough assessment of a patient's health, functional status, and risk factors, the IOM investigators recommended that assessment information be collected on every nursing home resident using a standardized instrument. This information would serve a dual purpose. First, and most obviously, it would identify patient problems in need of attention and, thus, provide the basis for each resident's care plan. Second, the aggregate findings of all the individual assessments could be analyzed as a means of evaluating the quality of care provided at a particular facility as well as comparing quality of care between facilities. This relationship illustrates the importance of standardized assessment as a necessary input to achieve an improvement in the mainstream of care.[2]

The IOM recommendation found its way into The Nursing Home Reform Law, a section of The Omnibus Budget Reconciliation Act of 1987 (OBRA '87), and was then carried forward in the new federal regulations issued to implement OBRA '87. Specifically, it was mandated that each resident have a comprehensive, standardized, reproducible assessment upon admission, to be reviewed quarterly, and that the assessment be repeated in its entirety either annually or whenever the health or well-being of the resident underwent a significant clinical change. This requirement led to the development of the Resident Assessment Instrument (RAI), which consists of two parts. The first part, the Minimum Data Set (MDS), elicits a variety of assessment information across several domains and is also designed to detect the presence of significant underlying problems. The second part contains 18 Resident Assessment Protocols, or RAPs, which are used to conduct more in-depth, follow-up assessments whenever MDS results indicate potentially serious problems such as delirium, incontinence, or falls. Information from both parts of the RAI provides the basis for the resident's care plan (see Chapter 9).

Gathering information for the RAI entails careful observation on the part of nursing home staff members as they examine and care for each resident. Many of the data elements seek information that goes beyond physical or clinical attributes into affective and psychosocial domains. For the staff members of most long-term care facilities, recording the results of this assessment represented a quantum leap in the amount of documentation required.

This example, then, illustrates from a public policy perspective the strong causal relationship between an initial study, the writing of statutes, issuance of regulations, creation of an assessment instrument and, finally, the instrument's promulgation and actual use. One important output of this progression is the documentation that records the assessment findings.

DOCUMENTATION

Purpose

Documented information about an individual's health and the care that person receives serves several important functions. On an individual level, this information becomes part of the patient's historical record, an account of what has been learned about the person by those who have provided care. This record also tracks results of all patient assessments and interventions, and in this way, serves as an intradisciplinary communication tool. On a macro-level, documented information about individuals can be aggregated and transformed into data used for determining reimbursement levels as well as for assessing and evaluating institutional providers and the health care system. Data profiling and pattern analyses provide a descriptive picture of the processes of care as well as the outcomes of care. The ability to analyze how effective care is and to compare common treatments in the hands of different health care providers is becoming a powerful force in improving care.

Overall, well written, thoughtful notes and the careful recording of test results can measurably enhance the quality of care provided on both a patient level and a systems level. Unfortunately, competing pressures on health care providers' time have hindered development of the art of taking good notes about patients. Despite efforts to teach health care providers how to maintain a problem-oriented medical record, poor documentation is still prevalent.

Historical Record

Health care providers for elders recognize that the complexity of each patient's condition requires comprehensive assessment in order to understand the person's problems. Assessments produce information, but if findings are not recorded, the health care provider may forget them over time and others may never know the results. The consequences can be serious.

Consider an 85-year-old woman, a widow living alone at home. She receives health care at a nearby family practice center, where staff monitor her for dietary-controlled diabetes, arteriosclerotic heart disease (ASHD), mild chronic obstructive pulmonary disease

(COPD), and hyperthyroidism. One day she falls and fractures her hip. She is rushed to the local emergency room, evaluated and admitted for surgery. Although she does well, she is quite deconditioned, requires further rehabilitation, and is transferred to a rehabilitation facility several towns away. While there, she has trouble sleeping and is given a benzodiazepine. Gradually, she becomes confused and lethargic until she is no longer considered a good candidate for rehabilitation. She is transferred to a nursing home across the street. Several weeks later she develops pneumonia and is taken to the nearest hospital. Later she is admitted to a nursing home, closer to her family.

In imagining the role of a facility staff member responsible for admission, would the information one wished to have be available? Elders who frequently travel from one care setting to another, have complicated clinical histories that they may be unable to recount and that no one else knows. The information contained in the medical record is one of their least appreciated safeguards. Avedis Donabedian, an acknowledged leader of quality measurement, notes that "the quality of recording is worthy of assessment in its own right because the record, besides being an educational and research tool, is a necessary vehicle for ensuring continuity and coordination of care, and the legal protection of patient and practitioner."[3]

Among the benefits of good record keeping is that it saves time and money because tests and procedures need not be repeated simply because no one knows whether they were done or what the results were. For the individual, it also eliminates the stress and inconvenience of repeating entire work-ups. In addition, good documentation may, literally, save patients' lives or prevent serious consequences that can result when health care providers do not know a patient's clinical history, for example, his or her allergies, previous side effects from treatments or medications, and so on. It must be kept in mind, though, that geriatric assessment is a diagnostic, not a therapeutic intervention, and by itself cannot cure chronic disease or reverse disability.[4]

Communication

The information in the medical record is not only useful as a historical record but it also provides a crucial communication link among members of the health care team. To function effectively and efficiently, teams must share information. Communication via documentation is particularly important with respect to care for chronically ill patients, who receive care over many years, often at several different health care sites. For example, a patient who needs occupational therapy may receive help at an outpatient rehabilitation center as well as at home from an aide or nurse. Communication between the therapist and the home health aide or nurse is important for coordinating the patient's care. Although verbal communication can be needed to initiate immediate action, written notes assure that all team members are kept abreast of changes, thus enabling each member to monitor the patient's progress and work in concert with other team colleagues (see Chapter 27).

Aggregating Information and Reimbursement

Over time, information about patients can be aggregated and analyzed for several purposes. For example, documentation of services provided can be obtained from the clinical record and used to authorize payment under a retrospective reimbursement system. The clinical record can be used to profile the relative complexity of the patients being cared for in order to adjust payments up or down.

In recent years, several initiatives have sought to more closely associate care provision, based on the patient's needs, with the amount that will be paid for that care. With respect to chronic or long-term care, this type of assessment, called case-mix reimbursement, has most often been applied in nursing homes. One example is the implementation of a case-mix reimbursement system that uses Resource Utilization Groups (RUGs),[5] that illustrates how individual patient assessments, when analyzed together, have a utility beyond patient care.

Case-Mix Reimbursement

Case-mix reimbursement ties payment to a system that uses a standardized assessment to group or stratify residents according to a predetermined set of characteristics such as functional level, behavior, or clinical complexity. Measurements of physical and cognitive impairments as well as social characteristics are used to predict the types and intensity or amount of services required to meet the individual's needs. The research used to develop these systems is quite complex and uses cluster analysis as well as other research designs.[6] The present prospective payment system, enacted in July 1998, is the outgrowth of the case-mix reimbursement system described as follows. The next section describes the historic evolution of this system.

The best known case-mix reimbursement system used in long-term care is the Resource Utilization Groups or RUGs. To develop this system, nursing home residents were categorized into one of five hierarchical levels, which were further subdivided according to the level of functional impairment, giving a total of 16 groups. Starting with the most resource-intensive level to the least, the five levels are rehabilitation, clinically complex, special care, behavioral, and physically disabled. Each level is further stratified according to the degree of impairment in the resident's ability to independently perform such activities of daily living (ADLs) as ambulating, toileting, and eating. A time-motion study was conducted to determine the amount of staff time or "resources" required to provide necessary care for each resident. The groups were then defined as being comprised of residents with comparable care needs, which makes it possible to predict resource utilization for each group.

One advantage of a case-mix reimbursement system is that it requires the use of a standardized assessment instrument for data collection. Although this information is collected for rate setting, it also can be used to measure the results of care. As researchers in the early 1970s demonstrated, this is possible because the data used to determine payment rates also captures changes in functional status. In 1974, Kane further refined the case-mix system by adding a "prognostic adjustment factor," which reflects the extent to which the actual outcome of care exceeds or falls short of the expected or predicted outcome.[7]

The implementation of RUGs gave rise to concerns that tying payment to patient functional level would create incentives for nursing home operators to allow their residents' health to deteriorate. In one instance, New York State wanted to use case-mix payment for nursing home residents on Medicaid, with higher payments going to facilities with a higher case-mix index, a statistic used to indicate the level of resource utilization. The federal Health Care Financing Administration (HCFA) required that the state first link such a reimbursement system to a resident-centered, outcome-oriented quality monitoring system. This system, the New York Quality Assurance System, or NYQAS, was developed and tested in 1986 as part of a HCFA-funded demonstration of case-mix reimbursement.[8]

The Resource Utilization Groups version II (RUGs-II), was used as the basis for the NYQAS surveillance process. RUGs-II collected individual assessment information necessary to assign residents to one of the 16 RUG categories. To gather this information, a data collection instrument, the Patient Review Instrument (PRI), was developed and tested. The PRI assessed approximately 20 different factors that had been found to be indicative of the need for specific types of medical, nursing, or rehabilitative care. This instrument was used to assess all residents every 6 months, regardless of payer (i.e., Medicare, Medicaid, or private payer). Each resident's individual PRI score was used to calculate the facility's weighted average, or the "case-mix index." This statistic became the multiplier used to determine each facility's rate, which could be adjusted twice a year as service requirements changed to reflect changes among the facility's residents.

A major shortcoming of the PRI was that it had been developed specifically to measure and predict resource consumption. It was not a source of clinical information for care planning. Thus, while these data were available to rate setters and the state's surveyors, they were virtually useless for determining what was being done for individual residents. The NYQAS survey process was intended to protect nursing home residents from financial incentives for substandard care, but it was too crude to capture the specifics of poor care in all but the most egregious cases.

Despite their imperfections, RUGs and NYQAS were important prototypes of what could be done when patient-level data were grouped. Their development, coinciding with the passage of the Nursing Home Reform Law and its requirement that information systems be developed based on the minimum data set, encouraged HCFA to expand the concept of case-mix payment to the Medicare program. HCFA, however, wanted to improve the payment system by correcting some of the shortcomings discovered during the initial RUGs and NYQAS demonstrations. The result was the HCFA-funded Multistate Nursing Home Case-Mix and Quality Demonstration. This demonstration used assessment information from the Minimum Data Set+ (MDS+, an enhanced version of the MDS, which became the prototype for MDS-2) to develop and implement a case-mix classification system. This system provided the basis for Medicaid and Medicare reimbursement for nursing home care and yielded better information about the impact of case-mix payment on quality of care. The following case vignette demonstrates some of the issues just discussed.

Case Vignette: Mrs. Jones and Mrs. Smith were admitted on the same day to Acme Nursing Home (ANH), a 100-bed skilled nursing facility. Mrs. Jones chose ANH in part because she was lonely following the death of her husband and in part because she no longer had someone to drive her to appointments and other errands. She was quite disabled by arthritis and could not ambulate independently. Mrs. Smith was more disabled. She was diabetic, with both renal and neurologic complications, and had Alzheimer's disease, which had reached the stage where Mrs. Smith was incontinent, wandered continually and was combative when personal care was being provided.

If ANH was in a state where Medicaid paid on a per diem basis (i.e., paid a fixed amount for any person admitted *regardless of individual characteristics) the nursing home would receive $10,000 per day [i.e., the number of residents in the facility (100) times $100 per resident per day]. If, on the other hand, ANH was in a "case-mix" state, all of the residents would be assessed using the MDS+ and, based on the results, the facility would receive a weighted score, or case-mix index (CMI), reflecting the proportion of heavy-care versus light-care residents in the nursing home on the day of the assessment (sometimes called "the full house sweep"). Thus, if ANH admitted a large proportion of patients like Mrs. Smith, its CMI would be relatively high, for example, 1.5. To calculate its payment level, ANH would multiply its CMI, 1.5 in this example, by the Medicaid per diem of $100/day and then multiply that product by the number of occupied beds, in this case 100, to arrive at a daily payment of $15,000. If ANH tended to admit people like Mrs. Jones, who are mildly to moderately physically disabled but otherwise cognitively intact, its CMI would be lower, about 0.8. The facility's payment rate would be only $8,000/day ($100/day $\times$ 0.8 $\times$ 100 occupied beds) because the number of care-provider hours required per resident would be lower and thus, less costly for the facility to provide.*

QUALITY ASSURANCE

In the preceding sections, we discussed how patient assessment information provides a historical record, a communication link among health-care team members, and a basis for predicting patient-service use, which, in turn, can be used to determine reimbursement rates. In this section, the ways in which documented assessment data are being used for quality assurance purposes is described.

Critics of quality measurement often assert that poor medical records reflect only the quality of documentation, not the quality of the care provided. In *The Criteria and Standards of Quality*, however, Donabedian reviewed several studies that explored the relationship between good record keeping and overall quality of care, using a variety of criteria.[9] He concluded that, in fact, there is an association between quality of record keeping and quality of care because, with good documentation, the record is complete enough to provide a reasonably accurate picture of what has happened to the patient, particularly when supplemented with observational studies and interviews of caregivers and patients.

In light of this finding, the results of patient-level assessments are being gathered and analyzed as a way of not only assessing care outcomes but also of enhancing the understanding of care pocesses. The better and more complete the documentation, the more accurately the composite picture reflects the actual processes of care delivery. Health care providers can use this information to monitor patients, assess quality of care, compare their practices to those of their peers, or to evaluate how close they are to reaching a professionally recognized benchmark.

Pattern Analysis

How health care providers order services and tests, perform procedures, or make suggestions to patients and their families regarding long-term-care services, may appear to follow logically from the facts available. Research shows, however, that service provision varies depending on geography and the type of health care provider. Using techniques such as small area variation analysis, it has become clear that what drives utilization of services is more highly variable than is generally believed. This conclusion, however, is difficult to discern if medical records are reviewed only by one individual.[10]

Starting in the 1970s, Wennberg began to use claims data to obtain population-based measures which, through epidemiologic techniques, could be used to understand resource allocation, service use, and outcomes of health care.[11] The findings, showing significant variations among physicians and between geographic regions, spawned an entire new science of medical investigation called small area variation analysis. For example, Wennberg found wide variations in the rates of hysterectomy in different communities in Maine, with the number of gynecologists in a community highly related to the number of hysterectomies performed.

Since then, several research studies have demonstrated, using small area variation analysis, that practice patterns and patient outcomes across geographic areas or between health care providers cannot be used to make inferences about the appropriateness and quality of care being delivered.

Quality Indicators

Claims files and billing data have also been used to identify the types of services provided, to infer patient conditions from these claims, and to examine outcomes (e.g., readmission rates, mortality rates, etc.) as indicators of quality of care. There are benefits to using such databases. For instance, the databases include large, population-based samples across broad geographic regions; they represent longitudinal records, so that groups can be tracked over time; the data have already been collected and, thus, are available at low cost; and the data are gathered and arrayed in such a way that defining sampling frames is relatively easy. At the same time, there has been considerable controversy over using these types of data for monitoring quality and measuring outcomes because the data lack important diagnostic and prognostic information that can be found only in the medical record.

In nursing homes, there is less need to rely on insurance data for quality assessment because the MDS will provide resident-specific clinical data. HCFA intends to use MDS data to prepare a profile of each facility that includes a resident census with a demographic breakdown as well as a list of quality indicator conditions that represent specific areas of concern. The quality indicators, developed in 1997 through a systematic process of interdisciplinary input, empirical analyses, and extensive field testing for validity and reliability, cover 12 domains that provide both resident- and facility-level information, describe findings not only as prevalence rates but also incidence rates, and facilitate an examination of both the processes and outcomes of care. Among the quality improvement (QI) indicators are conditions such as unanticipated weight loss, pressure ulcers, and dehydration. For each quality indicator, the HCFA report will note both the number and the percentage of residents with the condition as well as the percentage of residents in all facilities within the state with the condition. The report will give a percentile ranking of the facility on each quality indicator. In determining the presence or absence of a quality indicator, the report will not consider a resident's initial MDS but only MDSs conducted annually or after a significant change or, alternatively, changes noted on quarterly evaluations. By eliminating the initial MDS, the report will reflect care provided in the facility rather than conditions present at admission.

HCFA also prepares a resident-level summary using data from the initial MDS assessments. This summary notes whether the facility identified residents at high and low risk for each quality indicator. Surveyors use this report to pre-select the required case-mix stratified sample. Adjustments to the sample can be made after the survey begins based on the availability of residents. The selection process for the case-mix-stratified sample will not change from current practice. The sample includes both residents who require heavy care and those who require light care; it also includes residents who are capable of responding to interviews and those who are not. During the survey, the survey team evaluates the accuracy of resident assessments completed by facility staff. Specifically, surveyors examine the resident assessment instruments (RAIs) for thoroughness; evaluate the use of RAPs for identifying risk factors and causes of problem conditions; assess care needs, care planning, and implementation of care plans; and evaluate the actual care provided.

Standardized assessment instruments have been federally mandated for use only in the nursing home industry, but a growing number of other health care providers, including home- and community-based services, are adopting such instruments (see Chapter 8). One such tool is the Outcomes and Assessment Information Set (OASIS), which is being developed for use in home care. Like the MDS, OASIS will capture a wealth of clinical and psychosocial information, paying special attention to elements that are unique to home-based care. How often and by whom this information will be gathered is still being tested and discussed.

As more and more facilities use principles of total quality management (TQM) or continuous quality improvement (CQI), information gathered from medical records is expected to become the basis for assessing quality of care and measuring improvement. At present, however, administrative databases may be the only electronic tool available to monitor the care delivered by home-care agencies, day-care facilities, and other supportive services.

For all the enthusiasm currently shown for analysis of large databases, some caution should be exercised. Critics of large databases who examine medical records to learn about appropriate care, quality, and outcomes, believe that the only way to do so is to randomly assign patients to different treatment groups, medical plans, or other clusters, monitor their care, and then measure the outcomes. Some investigators contend that data from insurance claims forms, pharmacy records, and even medical records are so severely biased that the information may be all but unusable to measure outcomes. They also refute claims that the data can be adjusted using statistical methods to get around any biases. Despite these criticisms, many databases that were developed for one purpose (e.g., reimbursement) are being manipulated for another purpose (e.g., to yield information about patients' illnesses, physicians' practice patterns, and hospitals' success rates).

Report Cards

Aggregate data also are being used to prepare report cards that inform the public about the quality of specific services. For example, a booklet titled *Cardiac Surgery in New York State,* published by the New York State Department of Health, presents information about the performance of New York's surgeons and hospitals with respect to a number of cardiac operations.[12] The outcome of a collaborative, voluntary effort between the Department of Health and the state's Cardiac Advisory Committee (CAC), the booklet is the result of compiling data and using a risk-adjustment formula to analyze this information in a way that permits comparisons among surgeons and hospitals. The process began by collecting precise, meaningful data about patients and the outcomes of their surgery. The risk-adjustment formula was agreed on jointly, and the results were shared among the hospitals, the surgeons, and the Health Department. This process opened the way for quality improvement. Because such information could help patients and their families make informed choices about their own care, it was made available to the public in a small pamphlet, which not only presented the data but carefully explained how it had been gathered and what it meant.

Such report cards will undoubtedly become more commonplace as health care providers, including hospitals, health plans, physicians, and nursing homes, realize that consumers want to know about quality of care. In particular, managed care organizations, which are starting to target elders in large numbers, say that report cards similar to New York's cardiac surgery report will become a major marketing strategy for competing on demonstrated quality. Consumer choice is already considered vitally important in health care, but it cannot be exercised in any meaningful way in an information vacuum. That vacuum is rapidly being filled as information from medical records finds its way into large databases, where it can be analyzed to view care from a myriad of perspectives.

Performance reports vary in content. Some include clinical data, reporting process measures such as immunization rates and screening mammography rates; others include outcome measures such as infant mortality rates. For chronically ill patients, rates for readmission and the incidence of exacerbation of a given condition, such as asthma attacks, are useful measures of care effectiveness. Several states, including New York, Pennsylvania, and California, have developed report cards that rate hospitals and surgeons based on mortality rates following coronary artery bypass surgery.

Report cards have been used not only by the government but also by the private sector. The National Committee for Quality Assurance (NCQA), in collaboration with employers and health plans, developed the Health Plan Employer Data and Information Set (HEDIS). The most recent version presents performance indicators pertaining to quality, access to and satisfaction with care, membership, use of services, finance, and management. Of these indicators, few focus directly on quality of care. Most measure preventive services. As managed care organizations attempt to enroll Medicare beneficiaries, HEDIS undoubtedly will be updated to include performance measures that are more applicable to older patients. It should be noted that because HEDIS is so administratively oriented, there have been concerns and considerable controversy about its utility as a meaningful report card for plan quality. Nevertheless, in the absence of a better tool, most managed care organizations have incorporated HEDIS into their quality assessment activities.

Some managed care organizations have begun to develop their own report cards. US HealthCare, for example, spends considerable effort monitoring user satisfaction with physicians and services. This information is fed back to the physicians as a way of encouraging improvement. The value of this measure of satisfaction as an indicator of quality is questionable. Unfortunately, the capacity of managed care organizations to collect and analyze data for quality or other purposes is highly variable. Moreover, there is little standardization among plans in the data elements themselves, the definitions used, the accuracy of collection, or even the data systems employed. For the elder trying to decide among plans, the information in a plan's report card can be confusing or even misleading because it may appear that quality can be compared across plans when, in fact, it cannot be. In addition, the information needs of individuals, is different from that of institutional customers, for which much of the report card data was originally developed. For all of these reasons, the utility of report cards currently available to patients is being debated.

Although the foregoing developments directly impact services used by the elders, they were not driven primarily by an interest in programs used by older adults. Recent developments in the field of assessment and data collection, however, should have a profound impact on helping elders access appropriate services while assuring them the best quality of service once enrolled or admitted to a program. For example, the Joint Commission on Accreditation of Healthcare Organizations (JCAHO) has developed ORYX, a system for collecting standardized quality indicators, which will eventually allow comparison between and among providers. The ORYX system is currently in the early stages of implementation. Information on every Medicare-certified nursing home is now available on the internet. Accessing the *"nursing home compare"* category, one can obtain information from the last survey report for any certified nursing home in the United States. The information available includes the facility's ownership type, number of beds, and date of last inspection. Also reported is the total number of deficiencies for the selected nursing home as well as the average number and range of health deficiencies for nursing homes in that state. All deficiencies can be listed with the date of correction as well as the scope and severity assigned to the problem. Additional information explains the regulatory definitions of scope and severity. A drawback to this website presentation is its complexity. The person not familiar with health care terminology will find the information difficult to understand.

Benchmarking

Another use for aggregated patient assessment data is the development of benchmarks for quality care. Different definitions have been used for benchmarking. Some use it to describe the current situation, the starting point for further QI activities. Others see benchmarking as the establishment of a gold standard, or best practice, which health care providers should strive to achieve. For the latter definition, the best performers for a particular condition or practice must first be identified, and then their strategies for achieving superior results must be understood.

One of the biggest problems facing health care providers is difficulty obtaining credible information against which to compare themselves. For those in long-term care, the difficulty is that measurement techniques for quality improvement are not yet widely used. Some of the new long-term care databases can help correct this problem because they will be capable of providing comparable data across a number of outcome domains.

Quality Improvement Strategies

Another challenge facing those who assess the quality of health care is the need to replace inefficient and ineffective methods for monitoring quality with other techniques that not only better identify quality issues, but also do so in a way that leads to improvements. Through establishment of the Health Care Quality Improvement Program (HCQIP), HCFA changed the direction of Peer Review Organizations (PROs) from sole reliance on utilization review to evaluate quality to collaborative quality improvement projects. Another quality assurance method being promoted by HCFA, through the PROs and the Agency for Health Care Policy and Research (AHCPR), is the adoption of explicit criteria and standards, commonly in the form of clinical practice guidelines. The guidelines are developed by groups of experts using consensus-building techniques, which increases the reliability of quality judgments. Within hospitals, collaborative efforts have resulted in the development of clinical pathways or care maps as part of an ongoing quality improvement effort. Each pathway or map, which focuses on a specific medical condition or process, is developed by a multi-disciplinary team, consisting of representatives of all disciplines involved in the provision of patient care for that condition. The resulting pathway or care map improves delivery of patient care through standardization of processes and reduction in variance. An incidental benefit has been increased cost effectiveness and cost reduction in the acute-care setting. Its value in long-term care is still unknown.

COMPUTERIZED MEDICAL RECORDS

In the past, medical records consisted only of notes written by hand or transcribed from dictation, handwritten checklists and flow sheets, and laboratory values. When done well and written legibly, the chart was a rich source of information. Unfortunately, each health care provider maintained his or her own medical records system, so information from all sources, such as the hospital, physician's office, nursing home, and home health agency, rarely, if ever, came together. In the best case scenario, the same health care providers in an area took care of the patient so that continuity could be maintained. Medical record keeping is now changing rapidly in response to efforts to use electronic tools to document, track, synthesize, and monitor patient care. For example, on January 1, 1999, HCFA began requiring nursing homes and skilled nursing facilities to electronically submit MDS information for each of their residents. Starting in July 1999, surveyors could access this data prior to conducting a facility's recertification survey.

Given the trend toward an epidemiologic approach to quality improvement, the ability to gather information accurately and efficiently is critical. A major reason that variation analysis and practice profiling has had to rely on administrative databases is that they are built from information, such as billing data, that is already routinely collected electronically. By contrast, clinical data must be abstracted from the medical record, which exists only in hard copy, and then entered into a computer, a process that requires expertise in coding information.

A computer-based electronic patient record system has many advantages over paper systems. Such systems are specifically designed to support users by providing access to complete and accurate data; they can be programmed to issue alerts and reminders; and they can be adapted to clinical-decision support systems or otherwise linked to medical knowledge.[13] These systems also can provide universal, timely access to lifetime health data collected and maintained across the continuum of care. For chronically ill and elderly patients, whose conditions are complex and long-term and for whom care is likely to be fragmented, such a system has enormous clinical utility.

A computerized medical record system also can facilitate the use of patient-level data for continuous quality improvement efforts. Moreover, immediate access to clinical-level data not only supports administrative systems but also is invaluable for clinical practice, education, and research. In addition, an electronic record-keeping system is ideally suited for health status documentation and disease prevention. Finally, the system can promote quality care and also can enable an organization to better respond to the multiplying demands for data from outside agencies, such as managed care plans and HCFA.

Some work has already been done to incorporate clinical practice guidelines into computer-based patient records (CPR). This technique entails imbedding decisional algorithms into the program as it is written so that health care providers are prompted when certain information is entered. For example, as particular laboratory values or clinical findings are entered, the computer presents a series of questions to ensure that providers do not overlook appropriate follow-up services or treatments. Following a protocol may, in essence, streamline standards of care and reduce variability in practice behavior. The terminology for these computerized systems can be confusing, so some definitions are in order, even though they are in flux and not always adhered to universally. The American Health Information Management Association's (AHIMA) optical storage-based document imaging technology has three components: electronic filing cabinets (EFCs); electronic patient records (EPR) systems; and computer-based patient record (CPR) systems. There are many examples of fully automated CPRs in use today; however, there is no standardization of systems. Facilities or health care providers who use a computerized medical record may have difficulty in transferring information between systems. It should also be noted that getting such a system fully operational is a *very* complex undertaking for health care organizations, one that directly impacts physicians and other health care providers, who traditionally have been a reluctant group of computer users. The leadership in a facility must make a significant organizational and professional commitment to computerizing patient information as a component of its long-range strategy, particularly since the start-up effort will divert a portion of the resources currently supporting existing operations.

As with any new technology, the industry creating these systems is still defining its own direction, hence data formats, definitions, structures, and codes are yet to be standardized among the many vendors. For clinicians and health-care administrators, this state of affairs makes choosing a computerized medical record system a high stakes gamble because the one selected may not perform as promised or may prove to be incompatible with other systems to which it must link. With rapid cycles of obsolescence the rule in the electronics industry, system cost calculations should take into account the need for constant upgrading.

Despite these problems and concerns, it appears that electronic record keeping will continue to grow. Because such systems can potentially improve care for elders, health care providers involved in long-term care should actively participate in crafting the best systems possible. Too frequently, computerized medical record systems are designed for hospital use, rarely addressing the types of linkage and tracking needed to ensure coverage and compatibility across a variety of health care settings.

SUMMARY

Assessment, which begins the interaction between the health care provider and patient and serves to initiate the delivery of services, is also the means to measure what is being accomplished. Assessments generate information that, if carefully recorded and collected, becomes the basis for information systems that can help health care providers do their jobs better. Government's role is to ensure that assessment information is returned to those who generate it in order to educate them about their performance and to alert them to ways of improving care. This cycle of information will benefit patients as well as strengthen the entire health care system.

REFERENCES

1. Institute of Medicine. *Improving the Quality of Care in the Nursing Home.* National Academy Press; 1986. Washington, DC.
2. *Using Clinical Practice Guidelines to Evaluate Quality of Care.* Agency for Healthcare Policy and Research. AHCPR 95-0045. March; 1995. AHCPR Publications Clearinghouse, Silver Spring, MD.
3. Donabedian A. *Explorations in Quality Assurance and Monitoring. The Definition of Quality and Approaches to its Assessment,* vol. 1, Ann Arbor, MI: Health Administration Press; 1980.
4. Campion EW. The value of geriatric interventions. *N Eng J Med.* 1995;332:1376–1378.
5. Arling G, Karon SL, Sainfort F, Zimmerman DR, Ross R. Risk adjustment of nursing home quality indicators. *Gerontologist.* 1997; 37(6):757–766.

6. Fries BE, Schneider D, Foley WJ, et al. Refining a case-mix measure for nursing homes: resource utilization groups (RUG III). *Med Care.* 1994;32:668–680.

7. Kane RL. Paying nursing homes for better care. *J Commun Health.* 1976;2(1):1–4.

8. Koren M. Quality assurance in New York State: resident-centered protocols-the basis. *Provider.* December; 1998. Vol 12.

9. Donabedian A. *Explorations in Quality Assurance and Monitoring. The Definition of Quality and Approaches to its Assessment,* vol. 2. Ann Arbor, MI: Health Administration Press; 1982.

10. Park RE, Brook RH, Kosecoff J, et al. Explaining variations in hospital death rates: randomness, severity of illness, quality of care. *JAMA.* 1990;264(4):484–490.

11. Wennberg JE, Freeman JL, Shelton RM, Bubolz TA. Hospital use and mortality among Medicare beneficiaries in Boston and New Haven. *New Engl J Med.* 1989;321(17):1168–1173.

12. Green J, Wintfeld N. Report cards and cardiac surgeons: assessing New York's approach. *N Engl J Med.* 1995;332(18):1229–1232.

13. Institute of Medicine. *Study on Improving the Patient Record.* National Academy Press, Washington, DC, 1991.

APPENDIX 1
Activities of Daily Vision Scale

The following activities include those that some patients with visual problems find difficult. For each activity, I will ask you if you can do it, and then will ask you to rate the degree of visual difficulty you have. Think of how difficult each activity is with both eyes open and your glasses on if you wear them.

THE FOLLOWING QUESTIONS ARE RELATED TO <u>DRIVING:</u>

1a.) Have you ever driven a car?

1 ___ YES(to 1a)   2 ___ NO(to 3a)
(**If the patient has never driven, skip to question #3a)

1a) During the past 3 months, have you driven at night?

1 ___ YES(to 1b)   2 ___ NO(to 1c)

1b) Would you say that you drive at night with: (PLEASE CHECK ONLY ONE ANSWER)
1 ___ No difficulty at all (to 1d)
  ___ A little difficulty (to 1d)
3 ___ Moderate difficulty (to 1d)
4 ___ Extreme difficulty (to 1d)

1c) Is it because of your visual problems that you are unable to drive at night?
1 ___ Yes   2 ___ No
 (to 2a)   (to 2a)

1d) How difficult does seeing moving objects such as people or other cars make driving at night for you?
1 ___ Not difficult at all
2 ___ A little difficult
3 ___ Moderately difficult
4 ___ Extremely difficult
5 ___ So difficult, I no longer drive for this reason

1e) How difficult do oncoming headlights or street lights make driving at night for you?
1 ___ Not difficult at all
2 ___ A little difficult
3 ___ Moderately difficult
4 ___ Extremely difficult
5 ___ So difficult, I no longer drive for this reason

2a) During the past 3 months, have you been able to drive a car during the day?
1 ___ YES (to 2b)   2 ___ NO(to 2c)

2b) Would you say that you drive during the day with: (PLEASE CHECK ONLY ONE ANSWER)
1 ___ No visual difficulty at all
2 ___ A little difficulty because of vision
3 ___ Moderate difficulty because of vision
4 ___ Extreme difficulty because of vision

2c) Is it because of <u>visual problems</u> that you are unable to drive during the day?
1 ___ YES   2 ___ NO
 (to 3a)   (to 3a)

2d) During the past 3 months, have you been able to drive a car in unfamiliar areas?
1 ___ YES (to 2e)   2 ___ NO (to 2f)

2e) Would you say that you drive in
unfamiliar areas with:
(PLEASE CHECK ONLY ONE ANSWER)
₁ ___ No difficulty at all (3a)
₂ ___ A little difficulty (to 3a)
₃ ___ Moderate difficulty (to 3a)
₄ ___ Extreme difficulty (to 3a)

2f)Is it because of <u>visual</u>
<u>problems</u> that you are unable to
drive in unfamiliar areas?
₁ ___ YES   ₂ ___ NO
(to 3a)   (to 3a)

THE FOLLOWING ACTIVITIES REQUIRE <u>DISTANCE OR FAR VISION</u>:

3a) During the past three months, have you tried to read street signs at night either when driving or when you are a passenger in a car?
₁ ___ YES (to 3b)   ₂ ___ NO (to 3c)

3b) Would you say that you read
street signs at night with:
(PLEASE CHECK ONLY ONE ANSWER)
₁ ___ No difficulty at all
₂ ___ A little difficulty
₃ ___ Moderate difficulty
₄ ___ Extreme difficulty

3c) Is it because of <u>visual</u>
<u>problems</u> that you do not read
street signs at night?
₁ ___ YES   ₂ ___ NO
(to 4a)   (to 4a)

4a) During the past 3 months, have you tried to read street signs in daylight?
₁ ___ YES (to 4b)   ₂ ___ NO (to 4c)

4b) Would you say that you read
street signs in the daylight with:
(PLEASE CHECK ONLY ONE ANSWER)
₁ ___ No difficulty at all
₂ ___ A little difficulty
₃ ___ Moderate difficulty
₄ ___ Extreme difficulty

4c) Is it because of <u>visual</u>
<u>problems</u> that you do not read
street signs in daylight?
₁ ___ YES   ₂ ___ NO

5a) During the past 3 months, have you used public transportation?
₁ ___ YES (to 5b)   ₂ ___ NO (to 5c)

5b) Would you say that you use
public transportation with:
(PLEASE CHECK ONLY ONE ANSWER)
₁ ___ No visual difficulty at all
₂ ___ A little difficulty because of vision
₃ ___ Moderate difficulty because of vision
₄ ___ Extreme difficulty because of vision

5c) Is it because of <u>visual</u>
<u>problems</u> that you do not use
public transportation?
₁ ___ YES   ₂ ___ NO
(to 6a)   (to 6a)

6a) During the past 3 months, have you tried to walk down steps without handrails or help during daylight?
₁ ___ YES (to 6b)   ₂ ___ NO (to 6c)

6b) Would you say that you walk down steps with:
(PLEASE CHECK ONLY ONE ANSWER)
₁ ___ No apprehension (or fear) at all (to 6s)
2 ___ A little apprehension (or fear) (to 6s)
₃ ___ Moderate apprehension (or fear) (to 6s)
₄ ___ Extreme apprehension (or fear) (to 6s)

6c) Is it because of <u>visual</u>
<u>problems</u> that you are unable to
walk down steps without handrails
(to 7a)   (to 7a)or help?
₁ ___ YES   ₂ ___ NO

7a) During the past 3 months, have you tried to walk down steps
without handrails or help in dim light (or at dusk)?

1 ___ YES (to 7b)

2 ___ NO (to 7c)

7b) Would you say that you walk down steps
in dim light with:
(PLEASE CHECK ONLY ONE ANSWER)
1 ___ No apprehension (or fear) at all (to 8a)
2 ___ A little apprehension (or fear) (to 8a)
3 ___ Moderate apprehension (or fear) (to 8a)
4 ___ Extreme apprehension (or fear) (to 8a)

7c) Is it because of <u>visual</u>
<u>problems</u> that you are unable to
walk down steps in dim light
without handrails or help?
1 ___ YES   2 ___ NO
(to 8a)   (to 8a)

8a) During the past 3 months, on a bright sunny day, can you see peoples' faces from across the street?
1 ___ YES (to 8b)

2 ___ NO (to 8c)

8b) Would you say that you see faces in bright
sunlight with:
(PLEASE CHECK ONLY ONE ANSWER)
1 ___ No difficulty at all
2 ___ A little difficulty
3 ___ Moderate difficulty
4 ___ Extreme difficulty

8c) Is it because of <u>visual</u>
<u>problems</u> that you are unable to
see faces in bright sunlight?
1 ___ YES   2 ___ NO
(to 9a)   (to 9a)

THE FOLLOWING ACTIVITIES REQUIRE <u>NEAR VISION</u>:

9a) During the past 3 months, have you watched television?
1 ___ YES (to 9b)

2 ___ NO (to 9c)

9b) Would you say that you are able to see
television with :
(PLEASE CHECK ONLY ONE ANSWER)
1 ___ No difficulty at all (to 9d)
2 ___ A little difficulty (to 9d)
3 ___ Moderate difficulty (to 9d)
4 ___ Extreme difficulty (to 9d)

9c) Is it because of <u>visual</u>
<u>problems</u> that you are unable to
watch television?
1 ___ YES   2 ___ NO
(to 10a)   (to 10a)

9d) Can you read numbers on the television screen?
1 ___ YES (to 9e)

2 ___ NO (to 9f)

9e) Would you say that you are able to read
numbers with:
(PLEASE CHECK ONLY ONE ANSWER)
1 ___ No difficulty at all (to 10a)screen?
2 ___ A little difficulty (to 10a)
3 ___ Moderate difficulty (to 10a)
4 ___ Extreme difficulty (to 10a)

9f) Is it because of <u>visual</u>
<u>problems</u> that you are unable
to read numbers on the television
1 ___ YES   2 ___ NO
(to 10a)   (to 10a)

10a) During the past 3 months, have you tried to read the ordinary print in newspapers?
1 ___ YES (to 10b)

2 ___ NO (to 10c)

10b) Would you say that you read the ordinary
print in newspapers with:
(PLEASE CHECK ONLY ONE ANSWER)
1 ___ No difficulty at all
2 ___ A little difficulty
3 ___ Moderate difficulty
4 ___ Extreme difficulty

10c) Is it because of <u>visual</u>
<u>problems</u> that you cannot read
the ordinary print in newspapers?
1 ___ YES   2 ___ NO
(to 11a)   (to 11a)

11a) During the past 3 months, have you tried to read the directions on medicine bottles?

₁ ___ YES (to 11b)   ₂ ___ NO (to 11c)

11b) Would you say that you read the
directions on medicine bottles with:
(PLEASE CHECK ONLY ONE ANSWER)
₁ ___ No difficulty at all (to 12a)
₂ ___ A little difficulty (to 12a)
₃ ___ Moderate difficulty (to 12a)
₄ ___ Extreme difficulty (to 12a)

11c) Is it because of <u>visual</u>
<u>problems</u> that you cannot read
the directions on medicine bottles?
₁ ___ YES   ₂ ___NO
(to 12a)   (to 12a)

12a) During the past 3 months, have you tried to read the ingredients on cans of food?
₁ ___ YES (to 12b)   ₂ ___ NO (to 12c)

12b) Would you say that you read the
ingredients on cans of food with:
(PLEASE CHECK ONLY ONE ANSWER)
₁ ___ No difficulty at all
₂ ___ A little difficulty
₃ ___ Moderate difficulty
₄ ___ Extreme difficulty

12c) Is it because of <u>visual</u>
<u>problems</u> that you have not read
the ingredients on cans of food?
₁ ___ YES   ₂ ___ NO
(to 13a)   (to 13a)

13a) During the past 3 months, have you been able to write checks without help?
₁ ___ YES (to 13b)   ₂ ___ NO (to 13c)

13b) Would you say that you write
checks with:
(PLEASE CHECK ONLY ONE ANSWER)
₁ ___ No visual difficulty at all (to 14a)
₂ ___ A little difficulty because of vision (to 14a)
₃ ___ Moderate difficulty because of vision (to 14a)
₄ ___ Extreme difficulty because of vision (to 14a)

13c) Is it because of <u>visual</u>
<u>problems</u> that you cannot write
checks without help?
₁ ___ YES   ₂ ___ NO
(to 14a)   (to 14a)

14a) During the past 3 months, have you tried to use rulers, yard sticks or tape measures?
₁ ___ YES (to 15b)   ₂ ___ NO (to 15c)

15b) Would you say that you use
rulers, yard sticks or tape
measures with:
(PLEASE CHECK ONLY ONE ANSWER)
₁ ___ No visual difficulty at all (to 16a)
₂ ___ A little difficulty because of vision (to 16a)
₃ ___ Moderate difficulty because of vision (to 16a)
₄ ___ Extreme difficulty because of vision (to 16a)

15c) Is it because of <u>visual</u>
<u>problems</u> that you do not
use rulers, yard sticks or tape
measures?
₁ ___ YES   ₂ ___ NO
(to 16a)   (to 16a)

16a) During the past 3 months, have you tried to use a screwdriver?
₁ ___ YES (to 16b)   ₂ ___ NO (to 16c)

16b) Would you say that you use
a screwdriver with:
(PLEASE CHECK ONLY ONE ANSWER)
₁ ___ No visual difficulty at all (to 17a)
₂ ___ A little difficulty because of vision (to 17a)
₃ ___ Moderate difficulty because of vision (to 17a)
₄ ___ Extreme difficulty because of vision (to 17a)

16c) Is it because of <u>visual</u>
<u>problems</u> that you do not
use a screwdriver?
₁ ___ YES   ₂ ___NO
(to 17a)   (to 17a)

17a) During the past 3 months, have you prepared meals?
1___ YES (to 17b)

2___ NO (to 17c)

17b) Would you say that you
prepare meals with:
(PLEASE CHECK ONLY ONE ANSWER)
1 ___ No visual difficulty at all
2 ___ A little difficulty because of vision
3 ___ Moderate difficulty because of vision
4 ___ Extreme difficulty because of vision

17c) Is it because of <u>visual problems</u> that you do not prepare meals?
1 ___ YES   2___ NO
(to 18a)   (to 18a)

18a) During the past 3 months, have you tried to play cards?
1___ YES (to 18b)

2___ NO (to 18c)

18b) Would you say that you
play cards with:
(PLEASE CHECK ONLY ONE ANSWER)
1 ___ No visual difficulty at all (to 19a)
2 ___ A little difficulty because of vision (to 19a)
3 ___ Moderate difficulty because of vision (to 19a)
4 ___ Extreme difficulty because of vision (to 19a)

18c) Is it because of <u>visual problems</u> that you do not play cards?
1 ___ YES   2___ NO
(to 19a)   (to 19a)

19. How would you rate your overall vision, with your glasses or contacts on and both eyes open:
1 ___ blind
2 ___ poor vision
3 ___ fair vision
4 ___ good vision
5 ___ excellent vision

20. How would you rate your <u>current</u> vision with both eyes open and your glasses on, if 100 is excellent vision and 0 is blindness?_____ points

21.) <u>If you worked during the past year</u>, to what extent did your vision interfere with your ability to do your job?
1 ___ No difficulty working because of vision
2 ___ A little difficulty working because of vision
3 ___ Moderate difficulty working because of vision
4 ___ Extreme difficulty working because of vision
5 ___ Unable to work because of vision
0 ___ Unable to work because of other reasons.
0 ___ Retired from work.

22a. Do you use a magnifying glass for any visual activities?
1___ YES (to 21b)   2___ NO (23)

22b. IF YES, which activities?
1 ___ reading the newspaper
2 ___ reading books
3 ___ looking up numbers in the phone book.
4 ___ other
        please describe: _____
                         _____

23a. Do you use other visual aids for any visual activities?
1___ YES (to 21b)   2___ NO (23)

23b. IF YES, which activities?

1 ___ reading the newspaper

2 ___ reading books

3 ___ looking up numbers in the phone book.

4 ___ other

Please describe: _____

_____

24a.) Do you have difficulty with color vision?

1 ___ YES (to 21b)   2 ___ NO (23)

24b.) If yes, please describe:

_____

_____

_____

25a.) Are there other visual activities that you have difficulty with that were not included in the questions above?

If so, please describe:

_____

_____

Subscale Contents

Night driving score:	Questions 1a-e and 3a-c
Day driving score:	Questions 2a-f and 4a-c
Far vision score:	Questions 3a-7c and 9a-c
Near vision score:	Questions 11-19
Glare disability score:	Questions 1e, 8a-c, 10a-c, and 19
Overall ADVS score:	Questions 1-19

Score <80 indicates a problem requiring investigation; >80 may still be associated with silent conditions (e.g., Glaucoma)

Example: Glare Disability Score:

1e) How difficult do oncoming headlights or street lights make driving at night for you?

5 ___ Not difficult at all
4 ___ A little difficult
3 ___ Moderately difficult
2 ___ Extremely difficult
1 _X_ So difficult, I no longer drive for this reason

8a) During the past 3 months, on a bright sunny day, can you see peoples' faces from across the street?

_X_ YES (go to 8b)   ___ NO (go to 8c)

8b) Would you say that you see faces in bright sunlight with:

5 ___ No difficulty at all
4 ___ A little difficulty
3 _X_ Moderate difficult
2 ___ Extreme difficulty

8c) Is it because of *visual problems* that you are unable to see faces in bright sunlight?

1 ___ YES   ___ NO

10a) Can you read numbers on the television screen?

_X_ YES (go to 10b)   ___ NO (go to 10c)

10b) Would you say that you are able to read numbers with:

5 ___ No difficulty at all
4 _X_ A little difficulty
3 ___ Moderate difficulty
2 ___ Extreme difficulty

10c) Is it because of *visual problems* that you are unable to read numbers on the television screen?

1 ___ YES   ___ NO

19a) During the past 3 months, have you tried to play cards?

___ YES (go to 19b)   _X_ NO (go to 19c)

19b) Would you say that you play cards with:

5 ___ No visual difficulty at all
4 ___ A little difficulty because of vision
3 ___ Moderate difficulty because of vision
2 ___ Extreme difficulty because of vision

19c) Is it because of *visual problems* that you do not play cards?

1 ___ YES   _X_ NO*

In this example the glare disability score is created from questions 1, 8, 10, and 19.

*Note: The response to question 19 is excluded from the overall glare score because the patient does not participate in the activity for reasons other than visual difficulty.

Formula:

Mean: $\dfrac{\text{(Score for each item subject performs)}}{\text{Total number of items subject performs}} = \text{Mean}$

Example:

$\dfrac{(1 + 3 + 4)}{3} = 2.67$

0-100 Conversion: (Mean − 1) × 25 = sub-scale score

(2.67 − 1) × 25 = 42 points

ASSESSMENT OF LIVING SKILLS AND RESOURCES (ALSAR)

ALSAR TASKS	SKILLS (Individual accomplishes or procures task) Independent - 0 Partially Independent - 1 Dependent - 2 Record SKILL level	TASK RISK SCORE Combined Skill + Resource Level 3 or 4 = High 2 = Moderate 0 or 1 = Low			RESOURCES (Support for task completion extrinsic to individual) 0 - Consistently Available 1 - Inconsistently Available 2 - Not Available or in Use Record RESOURCE level
Telephoning	Locates phone numbers, dials, sends and receives information				Resources for telephoning
Reading	Reads and uses written information				Resources for reading
Leisure	Plans and performs satisfying leisure activities				Resources for satisfying leisure activities
Medication Management	Procures and takes medicine as ordered				Resources for managing medications
Money Management	Manages finances or procures financial services				Resources for managing finances
Transportation	Walks, drives or procures rides				Resources for transportation
Shopping	Lists, selects, buys, orders, stores goods				Resources for shopping
Meal Preparation	Performs all aspects of meal preparation or procures meals				Resources for meal preparation
Laundering	Performs or procures all aspects of doing laundering				Resources for laundering
Housekeeping	Cleans own living space or procures housekeeping service				Resources for housekeeping
Home Maintenance	Performs or procures home maintenance				Resources for home maintenance

"R" SCORE ⬯ (sum of 11 TASK RISK SCORES)

Name: _____ Interviewer: _____

Date: _____ Information Source: _____

©1991 ALSAR-Revised Format, TJK Drinka; JH Williams; M Schram; J Farrell-Holtan; R Euhardy: VAMC, Madison, WI

SUGGESTED SKILLS QUESTIONS	TASKS	SUGGESTED RESOURCES QUESTIONS

A. TELEPHONING (Using the phone to send and receive information)

--How often do you use the phone?
--Do you make calls or only use the phone if someone calls you?
--Can you hear the phone ringing?
--Can you hear what is being said?
--What number would you dial for an emergency?

--How many phones do you have? (location)
--Can you get to the phone if its ringing?
--Any special devices on your phone?   amplified headset?
  large scale numbers on dial?
--Are emergency phone numbers listed by each phone?

B. READING (Using written information)

--Do you have any difficulty reading?
--What do you usually read?
--Can you read newspaper size print, mail, medicine bottles?
--Can you read dials on the TV, thermostat, appliances?

--Do you wear glasses?   last vision exam?
--Do you have any low vision aids?   magnifier?
  large print materials?   talking books?
--Does someone read things for you?

C. LEISURE (Using time not spent for work, sleep, or self care)

--What do you do in your spare time (for fun)?
--Do you have any hobbies/pastimes?
--Are you active in any clubs or organizations?
--Are there any activities that you have given up recently?

--Is there a senior center near you?
--How do you keep in touch with friends and family?
--How often do you see them?   talk to them?
--Are there any activities you would like to begin?

D. MEDICATION MANAGEMENT (Taking medicine as ordered)

--Do you take any medications? How many? How often?
--What are they for?
--How often do you forget to take your medications?
--How do you renew your prescriptions?

--Does anyone help you take your medicine or re-order medicine?
--Do you have a system for taking medications?
--Do you have insurance to cover medications?
--Any medications you don't take because you can't pay for them?

E. MONEY MANAGEMENT (Managing finances)

--How do you manage your finances?   pay the bills?
--Do you use a checking account?
--How do you do your taxes?
--Can you live within your income?

--Does anyone help you with finances?
--Do you bank in person or by mail?
--Do you have a power of attorney?

F. TRANSPORTATION (Walking, driving, and using public transit)

--Do you drive?   at night?
--Do you drive out of town, or only in town?
--Are there restrictions on your license?
--Do you use public transportation?
--Do you arrange for your own transportation?

--How do you get around?
--Do you have a person drive you?
--Are your methods of transportation reliable?

G. SHOPPING (Listing, selecting, carrying, and storing items)

--Do you do your own shopping?
--Do you carry your purchases?
--How often do you go shopping?
--Do you ever shop by mail or phone?

--Does someone shop for you?
--Is that person available when you need them?
--Are there stores located near you?
--Do you use anything to carry your purchases?

H. MEAL PREPARATION (Food planning, storage, cooking, and serving)

--Do you cook your meals?
--Do you prepare your own snacks, breakfast or lunch?
--What do you do when your regular system for meals is not
  available?

--Are there restaurants or meal sites that you use?
--Does someone cook for you?
--Are your kitchen appliances adequate?

I. LAUNDRY (Carrying, washing, drying, and putting away clothing)

--Do you do your laundry?
--Do you do sorting?   carrying?   folding?   putting away?
--How often is laundry done?
--Do you arrange for laundry service?

--Does someone do the laundry?
--Where is the washer/dryer located?
--What do you use to carry the laundry?
--Are the laundry facilities adequate?

J. HOUSEKEEPING (Keeping dishes washed, pathways clear, rooms clean)

--Do you do the housekeeping?
--Do you do light work such as dishwashing, dusting, vacuuming?
--How often do you do the housekeeping?
--Do you arrange for housekeeping services?

--Does someone do your housekeeping?   how often?
--Are these services adequate?
--Could you afford housekeeping services?

K. HOME MAINTENANCE (Controlling temperature, clearing walks, and mowing lawn)

--What type of house do you live in?
--How do you do the outdoor work?   lawn?   walks?   windows?
--How do you do major (eg., fix leaking faucet) or minor
  (eg., change lightbulb) repairs?
--How do you control the temperature of your home?

--Does someone maintain your home for you?
--What equipment do you have for home upkeep (eg., tools, ladder,
  lawn mower)?
--Are maintenance supports readily available and reliable?

Instructions on use of the Assessment of Living Skills and Resources (ALSAR)

The Assessment of Living Skills and Resources, ALSAR, is an instrument developed to help health professionals assess Instrumental Activities of Daily Living in community dwelling elders. It can be administered by any professional discipline. It focuses on accomplishment of tasks rather than potential capabilities. Tasks were selected irrespective of traditional gender roles because elderly persons of both genders must accomplish the same IADLs to live independently.

The ALSAR is unique in that it measures task accomplishment by evaluating the interaction of skills (rated 0-2) and resources (rated 0-2) for each of the 11 tasks: Telephoning, Reading, Leisure, Medication Management, Money Management, Transportation, Shopping, Meal Preparation, Laundering, Housekeeping, and Home Maintenance.

On the ALSAR, the 11 IADL tasks are listed along the left side of the form. Skills and resources for each task are in separate columns. For each task, skills and resources are rated separately using three levels: (0) for independent; (1) for partially independent; and (2) for dependent. The scoring for each task is done as follows: enter the appropriate skill level for the task; enter the appropriate resource level for the task; add the two numbers. The resulting number is the risk score for that task. This task risk score is entered in the Risk Box for the appropriate task. The task risk score ranges from zero to four. A score of zero or 1 represents a low risk for not accomplishing that task. Two is moderate risk, and three or four is a high risk. These task risk scores help the clinician to prioritize patient care. The sum of the 11 task risk scores, known as the R-Score, is entered in the circle at the bottom of the form.

Skill is defined as accomplishment of a task by the older person. Skills relate to either performance or procurement by the older person. Procurement (task accomplished by another person) can substitute for independent performance only if *the patient takes responsibility* for procurement. A rating of (0) means that the person is independent in either performance or procurement whenever the task needs to be accomplished. A rating of (1) means partial performance or procurement. A rating of (2) means that the patient takes no responsibility for task performance or procurement. The patient may be dependent for motivational, cognitive, or physical reasons. If the patient claims to perform or procure accomplishment of a task but appearances suggest otherwise, a rating of (2) is assigned to reflect the incongruity and the need for further evaluation. To assess skills, focus only on the task you are assessing.

Resources are assessed separately from skills. Resource is defined as a support for task accomplishment that is extrinsic to the patient and may be human or technical, formal or informal. Resources include but are not limited to persons, equipment, services, and agencies. Resources are rated according to the level of availability and consistency of use. A rating of (0) is given if a resource is consistently available when the resource is needed. A rating of (1) is given if a clinician determines that a needed resource is unstable, inconsistent, or unreliable, or the caregiver provides resources for a task but is evidencing strain. A rating of 2 means that resources are insufficient for task accomplishment; available resources are not being used; safety is a factor; or that loss of the resource is imminent.

Example of scoring: An older person lives alone and cannot locate phone numbers. She asks a friend to come in once a day to help her with her calls. The friend agreed to come in every day but sometimes does not show up, thus the skill is partially independent (1) and the resource is inconsistently available (1). The task risk score for the task of telephoning is (2). For the task of home maintenance, the individual has never performed the skills of home maintenance and is totally dependent. However, the person consistently procures home maintenance services as needed so the skill score for the task of home maintenance is (0). Home maintenance resources are adequate and consistently available so the resource score for home maintenance is (0). The task risk score for home maintenance is (0).

The ALSAR was developed and tested through the collaborative efforts of a group of health professionals from different disciplines. The development and testing of the ALSAR was reported in *The Gerontologist* (Vol. 31:1, pp. 84-91). This revised format presents the ALSAR on the front side of the page and suggested questions relative to the eleven tasks on the reverse side. For more information contact Theresa Drinka, Ph.D., (715) 258-0741 or Jean Farrell-Holtan OTR, (608) 256-1901 Two one-half inch videotapes, "Overview of IADL Assessment" and "Administration of the ALSAR" are also available from the Madison VA GRECC (608) 262-7089.

APPENDIX 3
Assisted Living Center Tool

STATE OF CALIFORNIA - HEALTH AND WELFARE AGENCY   DEPARTMENT OF SOCIAL SERVICES

PHYSICIAN'S REPORT FOR RESIDENTIAL CARE FACILITIES FOR THE ELDERLY(RCFE)

I. FACILITY INFORMATION *(To be completed by the licensee/designee)*:

1. NAME OF FACILITY:	2. TELEPHONE:

3. ADDRESS: NUMBER: STREET:	CITY:	ZIP CODE:

4. LICENSEE'S NAME:	5. TELEPHONE:	6. FACILITY LICENSE NUMBER:

II. RESIDENT INFORMATION *(To be completed by the resident/resident's responsible person/licensee)*:

1. NAME:	2. SOCIAL SECURITY NUMBER:	3. BIRTH DATE/AGE:

4. AUTHORIZATION FOR RELEASE OF MEDICAL INFORMATION *(To be completed by resident/resident's legal representative)*

I hereby authorize release of medical information in this report to the facility named above.

5. SIGNATURE OF RESIDENT AND/OR RESIDENT'S LEGAL REPRESENTATIVE	6. ADDRESS	7. DATE

III. PATIENT'S DIAGNOSIS *(To be completed by the physician)*:

NOTE TO PHYSICIAN: The person named above is either a resident or prospective resident of a residential care facility for the elderly licensed by the Department of Social Services. The license requires the facility to provide primarily non-medical care and supervision to meet the needs of that person. THESE FACILITIES DO NOT PROVIDE SKILLED NURSING CARE. The information that you provide about this person is required by law to assist in determining whether the person is appropriate for care in this non-medical facility. It is important that all questions be answered. *(Please attach separate pages if needed.)*

1. DATE OF EXAM:	2. SEX:	3. HEIGHT:	4. WEIGHT:	5. BLOOD PRESSURE:

6. TUBERCULOSIS EXAMINATION RESULTS: ☐ Active ☐ Inactive ☐ No Evidence of Disease	7. DATE/TYPE OF TB TEST:

8. TB TREATMENT USED, IF APPLICABLE:

9. PRIMARY DIAGNOSIS:	10. TREATMENT/MEDICATION (TYPE AND DOSAGE)/EQUIPMENT:	11. CAN PATIENT MANAGE OWN TREATMENT/MEDICATION/EQUIPMENT? IF NOT, WHAT TYPE OF MEDICAL SUPERVISION IS NEEDED?
12. SECONDARY DIAGNOSIS(ES):	13. TREATMENT/MEDICATION (TYPE AND DOSAGE)/EQUIPMENT:	14. CAN PATIENT MANAGE OWN TREATMENT/MEDICATION/EQUIPMENT? IF NOT, WHAT TYPE OF MEDICAL SUPERVISION IS NEEDED?
15. CONTAGIOUS/INFECTIOUS DISEASE:	16. TREATMENT/MEDICATION (TYPE AND DOSAGE)/EQUIPMENT:	17. CAN PATIENT MANAGE OWN TREATMENT/MEDICATION/EQUIPMENT? IF NOT, WHAT TYPE OF MEDICAL SUPERVISION IS NEEDED?
18. ALLERGIES:	19. TREATMENT/MEDICATION (TYPE AND DOSAGE)/EQUIPMENT:	20. CAN PATIENT MANAGE OWN TREATMENT/MEDICATION/EQUIPMENT? IF NOT, WHAT TYPE OF MEDICAL SUPERVISION IS NEEDED?
21. OTHER CONDITIONS:	22. TREATMENT/MEDICATION (TYPE DOSAGE)/EQUIPMENT:	23. CAN PATIENT MANAGE OWN TREATMENT/MEDICATION/EQUIPMENT? IF NOT, WHAT TYPE OF MEDICAL SUPERVISION IS NEEDED?

LIC 602A (10/92)

24. PHYSICAL HEALTH STATUS:	YES	NO	ASSISTIVE DEVICE:	COMMENTS:
a. Auditory Impairment				
b. Visual Impairment				
c. Wears Dentures				
d. Special Diet				
e. Substance Abuse Problem				
f. Bowel Impairment				
g. Bladder Impairment				
h. Motor Impairment				
i. Requires Continuous Bed Care				

25. MENTAL CONDITION:	YES	NO	COMMENTS:
a. Confused/Disoriented			
b. Unable to follow Instructions			
c. Depressed			
d. Unable to Communicate Own Needs			
e. Unable to Leave Facility Unassisted			

26. CAPACITY FOR SELF-CARE:	GOOD	FAIR	POOR	COMMENTS:
a. Ability to Care for All Personal Needs				
b. Ability to Bathe Self				
c. Ability to Dress Self				
d. Ability to Feed Self				
e. Ability to Care for Own Toileting Needs				
f. Ability to Walk without Equipment or Other Assistance				

27. MEDICATION MANAGEMENT:	YES	NO	COMMENTS:
a. Can Administer Own Medications			
b. Can Store Own Medications			

28. AMBULATORY STATUS:

* **"Nonambulatory":** means persons who are unable to leave a building unassisted under emergency conditions because: 1) they are unable, or are likely to be unable, to physically and mentally respond to a sensory signal approved by the State Fire Marshal, or an oral instruction relating to fire danger; or 2) they depend upon mechanical aids such as crutches, walkers, and wheelchairs. **(NOTE:** A person who uses a cane is not considered nonambulatory.)

** **"Bedridden":** means persons who are unable to leave a building unassisted under emergency conditions and who also require assistance in turning and repositioning in bed.

a. This person is considered: ☐ Ambulatory ☐ Nonambulatory* ☐ Bedridden**

b. If resident is bedridden, what is the cause? *(Check one and describe nature of illness, surgery or other cause)*

EXPLANATION:

☐ Temporary Illness_____

☐ Recovery from Surgery_____

☐ Other_____

c. How long is bedridden status expected to persist? _____ days

29. PHYSICAL HEALTH STATUS: ☐ Good ☐ Fair ☐ Poor

30. COMMENTS:

31. PHYSICIAN'S NAME AND ADDRESS (PRINT):	
32. PHYSICIAN'S SIGNATURE:	33. DATE:
34. TELEPHONE: ( )	35. LENGTH OF TIME RESIDENT HAS BEEN UNDER YOUR CARE:

APPENDIX 4
The Barthel Index

Activity:

Bowels

    0 = Incontinent (or needs to be given enemas)

    5 = Occasional accident

    10 = Continent

Bladder

    0 = Incontinent, or catheterized and unable to manage alone

    5 = Occasional accident

    10 = Incontinent

Grooming

    0 = Needs help with personal care

    5 = Independent face/hair/teeth/shaving (implements provided)

Toilet Use

    0 = Unable

    5 = Needs some help, but can do something alone

    10 = Independent (on and off, dressing, wiping)

Feeding

    0 = Unable

    5 = Needs help cutting, spreading butter, etc., or requires modified diet

Transfers (bed to chair and back)

    0 = Unable

    5 = Major help (one or two people, physical), can sit

    10 = Minor help (verbal or physical)

    15 = Independent

Mobility (on level surfaces)

    0 = Immobile or <50 yards

    5 = Wheelchair independent, including corners, >50 yards

    10 = Walks with help of one person (verbal or physical) >50 yards

    15 = Independent (but may use any aid, for example, stick) >50 yards

Dressing

    0 = Dependent

    5 = Needs help but can do about half unaided

    10 = Independent (including buttons, zips, laces, etc.)

Stairs

    0 = Unable

    5 = Needs help (verbal, physical, carrying aid)

    10 = Independent

Bathing

    0 = Dependent

    5 = Independent (or in shower)

References: Mahoney F and Barthel DW. Functional Evaluation: The Barthel Index. MD State Med J., 14:61-65; 1965.

BECK DEPRESSION INVENTORY—1973 REVISION

Instructions: This is a questionnaire. On the questionnaire are groups of statements. Please read the entire group of statements in each category. Then pick out the one statement in that group which best describes the way you feel today, that is, right now? Circle the number beside the statement you have chosen. If several statements in the group seem to apply equally well, circle each one.

Be sure to read all the statements in each group before making your choice.

A. (Sadness)
0 I do not feel sad
1 I feel sad
2 I am sad all the time and I can't snap out of it
3 I am so sad or unhappy that I can't stand it

B. (Pessimism)
0 I am not particularly discouraged about the future
1 I feel discouraged about the future
2 I feel I have nothing to look forward to
3 I feel that the future is hopeless and that things cannot improve

C. (Sense of Failure)
0 I do not feel like a failure
1 I feel I have failed more than the average person
2 As I look back on my life all I can see is a lot of failures
3 I feel I am a complete failure as a person

D. (Dissatisfaction)
0 I get as much satisfaction out of things as I used to
1 I don't enjoy things the way I used to
2 I don't get real satisfaction out of anything anymore
3 I am dissatisfied or bored with everything

E. (Guilt)
0 I don't feel particularly guilty
1 I feel guilty a good part of the time
2 I feel quite guilty most of the time
3 I feel guilty all of the time

F. (Sense of Punishment)
0 I don't feel I am being punished
1 I feel I may be punished
2 I expect to be punished
3 I feel I am being punished

G. (Self-Dislike)
0 I don't feel disappointed in myself
1 I am disappointed in myself
2 I am disgusted with myself
3 I hate myself

H. (Self-Accusations)
0 I don't feel I am any worse than anybody else
1 I am critical of myself for my weaknesses or mistakes
2 I blame myself all the time for my faults
3 I blame myself for everything bad that happens

I. (Self-Harm)
0 I don't have any thoughts of killing myself
1 I have thoughts of killing myself but I would not carry them out
2 I would like to kill myself
3 I would kill myself if I had the chance

J. (Crying Spells)
0 I don't cry any more than usual
1 I cry more now than I used to
2 I cry all the time now
3 I used to be able to cry but now I can't cry even though I want to

K. (Irritability)
0 I am no more irritated now than I ever am
1 I get annoyed or irritated more easily than I used to
2 I feel irritated all the time now
3 I don't get irritated at all by the things that used to irritate me

L. (Social Withdrawal)
0 I have not lost interest in other people
1 I am less interested in other people than I used to be
2 I have lost most of my interest in other people
3 I have lost all of my interest in other people

M. (Indecisiveness)

0 I make decisions about as well as I ever could

1 I put off making decisions more than I used to

2 I have greater difficulty in making decisions than before

3 I can't make decisions at all any more

N. (Self-Image Change)

0 I don't feel I look any worse than I used to

1 I am worried that I am looking old or unattractive

2 I feel that there are permanent changes in my appearance that make me look unattractive

3 I believe that I look ugly

O. (Work Difficulty)

0 I can work about as well as before

1 It takes extra effort to get started at doing something

2 I have to push myself very hard to do anything

3 I can't do any work at all

P. (Sleep Disturbance)

0 I can sleep as well as usual

1 I don't sleep as well as I used to

2 I wake up 1–2 hours earlier than usual and find it hard to get back to sleep

3 I wake up several hours earlier than I used to and cannot get back to sleep

Q. (Fatigability)

0 I don't get any more tired than usual

1 I get tired more easily than I used to

2 I get tired from doing almost anything

3 I am too tired to do anything

R. (Anorexia)

0 My appetite is no worse than usual

1 My appetite is not as good as it used to be

2 My appetite is much worse now

3 I have no appetite at all any more

S. (Weight Loss)

0 I haven't lost must weight, if any, lately

1 I have lost more than 5 pounds

2 I have lost more than 10 pounds

3 I have lost more than 15 pounds

I am purposely trying to lose weight by eating less

Yes _____

No _____

T. (Somatic Preoccupation)

0 I am no more worried about my health than usual

1 I am worried about physical problems such as aches andpains; or upset stomach; or constipation

2 I am very worried about physical problems and it's hard to think of much else

3 I am so worried about my physical problems, I cannot think about anything else

U. (Loss of Libido)

0 I have not noticed any recent change in my interest in sex

1 I am less interested in sex than I used to be

2 I am much less interested in sex now

3 I have lost interest in sex completely

The descriptive title of each item, printed here in parentheses, is not generally included in the form of the scale given to the patient.

Braden Scale for Predicting Pressure Sore Risk

Patient's Name _____ Evaluator's Name _____ Date of Assessment _____

	1	2	3	4
SENSORY PERCEPTION — ability to respond meaningfully to pressure-related discomfort	**1. Completely Limited:** Unresponsive (does not moan, flinch, or grasp) to painful stimuli because of diminished level of consciousness or sedation. OR limited ability to feel pain over most of body surface.	**2. Very Limited:** Responds only to painful stimuli. Cannot communicate discomfort except by moaning or restlessness. OR has a sensory impairment that limits the ability to feel pain or discomfort over ½ of body.	**3. Slightly Limited:** Responds to verbal commands, but cannot always communicate discomfort or need to be turned. OR has some sensory impairment that limits ability to feel pain or discomfort in 1 or 2 extremities.	**4. No Impairment:** Responds to verbal commands. Has no sensory deficit that would limit ability to feel or voice pain or discomfort.
MOISTURE — degree to which skin is exposed to moisture	**1. Constantly Moist:** Skin is kept moist almost constantly by perspiration, urine, etc. Dampness is detected every time patient is moved or turned.	**2. Very Moist:** Skin is often, but not always moist. Linen must be changed at least once a shift.	**3. Occasionally Moist:** Skin is occasionally moist, requiring an extra linen change approximately once a day.	**4. Rarely Moist:** Skin is usually dry, linen only requires changing at routine intervals.
ACTIVITY — Degree of physical activity	**1. Bedfast:** Confined to bed	**2. Chairfast:** Ability to walk severely limited or nonexistent. Cannot bear own weight and/or must be assisted into chair or wheelchair.	**3. Walks Occasionally:** Walks occasionally during day, but for very short distances, with or without assistance. Spends majority on each shift in bed or chair.	**4. Walks Frequently:** Walks outside the room at least twice a day and inside room at least once every 2 hours during waking hours.
MOBILITY — ability to change and control body position	**1. Completely Immobile:** Does not make even slight changes in body or extremity position without assistance.	**2. Very Limited:** Makes occasional slight changes in body or extremity position but unable to make frequent or significant changes independently.	**3. Slightly Limited:** Makes frequent though slight changes in body or extremity position independently.	**4. No Limitation:** Makes major and frequent changes in position without assistance.
NUTRITION — *usual* food intake pattern	**1. Very Poor:** Never eats a complete meal. Rarely eats more than ⅓ of any food offered. Eats 2 servings or less protein (meat or dairy products) per day. Takes fluids poorly. Does not take a liquid dietary supplement. OR is NPO and/or maintained on clear liquids or IVs for more than 5 days.	**2. Probably Inadequate:** Rarely eats a complete meal and generally eats only about ½ of any food offered. Protein intake includes only 3 servings of meat or dairy products per day. Occasionally will take a dietary supplement. OR receives less than optimum amount of liquid diet or tube feeding.	**3. Adequate:** Eats over half of most meals. Eats a total of 4 servings of protein (meat, dairy products) each day. Occasionally will refuse a meal, but will usually take a supplement if offered. OR is on a tube feeding or TPN regimen that probably meets most of nutritional needs.	**4. Excellent:** Eats most of every meal. Never refuses a meal. Usually eats a total of 4 or more servings of meat and dairy products. Occasionally eats between meals. Does not require supplementation.
FRICTION AND SHEAR	**1. Problem:** Requires moderate to maximum assistance in moving. Complete lifting without sliding against sheets is impossible. Frequently slides down in bed or chair, requiring frequent repositioning with maximum assistance. Spasticity, contractures, or agitation leads to almost constant friction.	**2. Potential Problem:** Moves feebly or requires minimum assistance. During a move skin probably slides to some extent against sheets, chair, restraints, or other devices. Maintains relatively good position in chair or bed most of the time but occasionally slides down.	**3. No Apparent Problem:** Moves in bed and in chair independently and has sufficient muscle strength to lift up completely during move. Maintains good position in bed or chair at all times.	

Total Score _____

©Copyright Barbara Braden and Nancy Bergstrom, 1988. Reproduced by permission.

NOTE: IVs = intravenous feedings; NPO = nothing by mouth; TPN = total parenteral nutrition. For additional information on administration and scoring refer to the following: Braden BJ, Bergstrom N. Clinical utility of the Braden Scale for predicting pressure sore risk. *Decubitus.* 1989;2(3):44-51.

APPENDIX 7
CES-D Scale

NAME _____ AGE _____ SEX _____ DATE _____

WING _____ ROOM _____ PHYSICIAN _____ ASSESSOR _____

INSTRUCTIONS FOR QUESTIONS: Below is a list of the ways you might have felt or behaved.
Please tell me how often you have felt this way during the past week.

Score: *0 = Rarely or none of the time (less than 1 day)*   *1 = Some or little of the time (1–2 days)*
       2 = Occasionally or a moderate amount of time (3–4 days)   *3 = most or all of the time (5–7 days)*

During the past week:

_____   1. I was bothered by things that usually don't bother me.

_____   2. I did not feel like eating; my appetite was poor.

_____   3. I felt that I could not shake off the blues even with help from my family or friends.

_____   4. I felt that I was just as good as other people.

_____   5. I had trouble keeping my mind on what I was doing.

_____   6. I felt depressed.

_____   7. I felt that everything I did was an effort.

_____   8. I felt hopeful about the future.

_____   9. I thought my life had been a failure.

_____ 10. I felt fearful.

_____ 11. My sleep was restless.

_____ 12. I was happy.

_____ 13. I talked less than usual.

_____ 14. I felt lonely.

_____ 15. People were unfriendly.

_____ 16. I enjoyed life.

_____ 17. I had crying spells.

_____ 18. I felt sad.

_____ 19. I felt that people dislike me.

_____ 20. I could not get "going."

Although not designed for clinical diagnosis, the CES-D scale is based on symptoms of depression as seen in clinical cases. Seventy percent of patients with known depressions, but only 21% of the general population, scored at or above an arbitrary cutoff score of 16.

Adapted from: Radloff LS. The CES-D scale: A self-report depression scale for research in the general population. *Applied Psychological Measurement.* Summer 1977:1:385–401.

APPENDIX 8
Clock Drawing Test

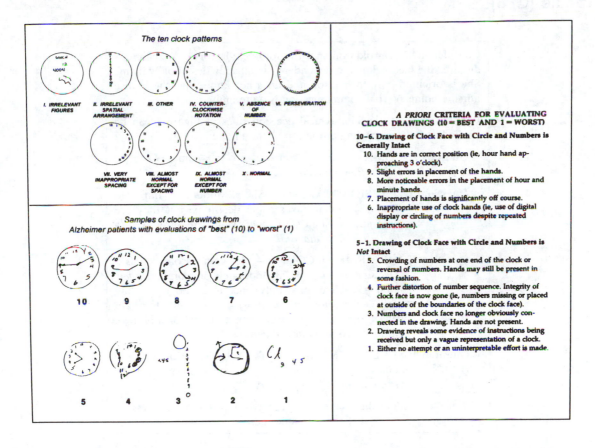

The ten clock patterns

I. IRRELEVANT FIGURES · II. IRRELEVANT SPATIAL ARRANGEMENT · III. OTHER · IV. COUNTER-CLOCKWISE ROTATION · V. ABSENCE OF NUMBER · VI. PERSEVERATION

VII. VERY INAPPROPRIATE SPACING · VIII. ALMOST NORMAL EXCEPT FOR SPACING · IX. ALMOST NORMAL EXCEPT FOR NUMBER · X. NORMAL

Samples of clock drawings from Alzheimer patients with evaluations of "best" (10) to "worst" (1)

10   9   8   7   6

5   4   3   2   1

A PRIORI CRITERIA FOR EVALUATING CLOCK DRAWINGS (10 = BEST AND 1 = WORST)

10–6. Drawing of Clock Face with Circle and Numbers is Generally Intact

10. Hands are in correct position (ie, hour hand approaching 3 o'clock).
9. Slight errors in placement of the hands.
8. More noticeable errors in the placement of hour and minute hands.
7. Placement of hands is significantly off course.
6. Inappropriate use of clock hands (ie, use of digital display or circling of numbers despite repeated instructions).

5–1. Drawing of Clock Face with Circle and Numbers is Not Intact

5. Crowding of numbers at one end of the clock or reversal of numbers. Hands may still be present in some fashion.
4. Further distortion of number sequence. Integrity of clock face is now gone (ie, numbers missing or placed at outside of the boundaries of the clock face).
3. Numbers and clock face no longer obviously connected in the drawing. Hands are not present.
2. Drawing reveals some evidence of instructions being received but only a vague representation of a clock.
1. Either no attempt or an uninterpretable effort is made.

The upper left drawing constitutes one scoring method. The bottom left and text on right side constitute another. The clock figures are from Wolf-Klein GP, Silverstone FA, Levy AP, et al. Screening for Alzheimer's Disease by Clock Drawing. J Am Geriatr Soc, 37(8):730–734, 1989, and Sunderland, T, Hill JL, Hellow, AM, et al. Clock Drawing in Alzheimer's disease: A Novel Measure of Dementia Severity. J Am Geriatr Soc, 37(8):725–729, 1989. Normative data are available in Clock Drawing: A Neuropsychological Analysis by Freedman, M, Leach, L, Kaplan, E, et al. Oxford University Press, 1994.

Consider an 87-year-old woman with a four-year history of Alzheimer's disease. She has declined to dependency in all activities of daily living. She is oriented only to her son and does not know that she is in a nursing home. Verbal communication is quite limited.

For this resident, the hierarchical decision rules in Figure 1 can be applied as follows, starting at the top of the Figure:

Question 1: COMA — No, the woman is not in a coma. *Go to the Left in flow diagram.*

Question 2: DECISION MAKING — She is Moderately Impaired (Code 2) — she makes some decisions, but they are poor, and constant staff supervision is required. *Go to the Left in flow diagram.*

Question 3: IMPAIRMENT COUNT — Her count score equals 3 (*Decision making* = 2, Moderately impaired; *Understood* = 2, able to make only concrete requests regarding basic needs: *Short-term memory* = 1, not able to retain new information for more than a couple of minutes). *Go to the Right in flow diagram.*

Question 4: SEVERE IMPAIRMENT COUNT — Count score equals 2 (*Decision making* = 2, and *Understood* = 2). *Go to the final CPS category.*

For this resident the final CPS category is: **Level 4, Moderately Severe Imapirment.**

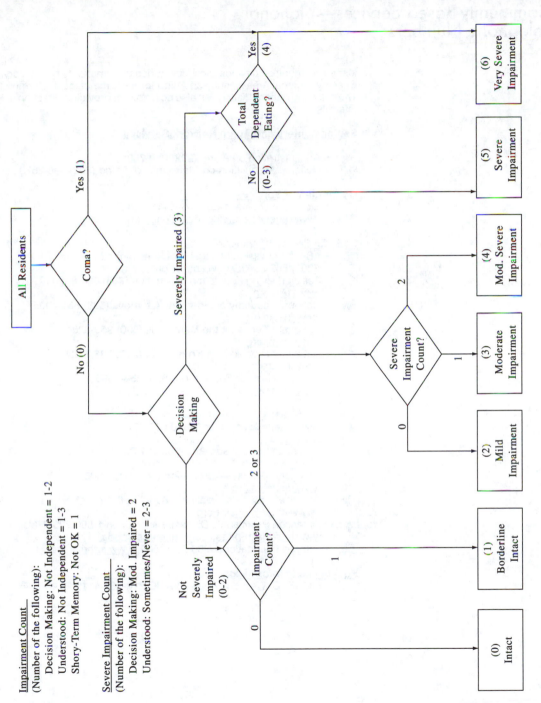

Impairment Count
(Number of the following):
Decision Making: Not Independent = 1-2
Understood: Not Independent = 1-3
Shory-Term Memory: Not OK = 1

Severe Impairment Count
(Number of the following):
Decision Making: Mod. Impaired = 2
Understood: Sometimes/Never = 2-3

All Residents

Coma?

No (0)

Yes (1)

Decision Making

Severely Impaired (3)

Total Dependent Eating?

No (0-3)

Yes (4)

(6) Very Severe Impairment

(5) Severe Impairment

Not Severely Impaired (0-2)

Impairment Count?

0

1

2 or 3

(0) Intact

(1) Borderline Intact

Severe Impairment Count?

0

1

2

(2) Mild Impairment

(3) Moderate Impairment

(4) Mod. Severe Impairment

APPENDIX 10
Community-Based Services—National Telephone Numbers

Many communities develop local directories to community-based services. Check your local Area Agency on Aging for a source of local referral listing. The following national listing can also be helpful in providing direction to local referrals.

Senior Centers and Aging Network Services

- Administration on Aging (202) 619-7501
- National Association on State Units of Aging (202) 898-2578

Continuum of Services

- Eldercare Locater 1-800-677-1116
  www.ageinfo.org/elderloc/elderlo.html

Specific Senior Services
- ABA Commission of Legal Problems of the Elderly
  (202) 662-8690. www.abanet.org
- Assisted Living Federation of America (703) 691-8100
  www.alfa.org
- National Academy of Elder Law Attorneys (520) 881-4005
  www.naela.org
- National Alliance for the Mentally III (800) 950-6264
  www.nami.org
- National Association of Home Care (202) 547-7424
  www.nahc.org
- National Hospice Foundation (800) 658-8898
  www.nho.org

Specific Diseases
- Alzheimer's Association 1-800-621-0379
  www.alz.org
- American Cancer Society 1-800-227-2345
  www.cancer.org
- American Diabetes Association (800) 342-2383
  www.diabetes.org
- American Heart Association 1-800-242-8721
  www.americanheart.org
- American Parkinson's Disease Association 1-800-223-2732
  www.the-health-pages.com/resources/apda
- Arthritis Foundation 1-800-283-7800 www.arthritis.org

Pocket Guide Information
- GRECC, West Los Angles VAMC 310-268-4110

APPENDIX 11
Community-Based Services—Referral Definitions With Payer Source and Telephone Reference

HOME SERVICES

 –**Emergency Response Systems** A system installed in the home which accesses a dispatcher for police, fire and paramedic services when they cannot reach the phone. PP, SL, NC

 – **Home Delivered Meals** A program sponsored by Area Agency on Aging (AAA). Nutrition services to provide meals for homebound seniors, frequently called Meals on Wheels. May provide special diets. SL PP

 – **Home Health Care** Time limited skilled nursing care with potential for improvement, a focus on rehabilitation provided by multiple disciplines. M, MC, HMO, VA

 – **Home Health Aide** - Personal care (bathing) by level of nurses aide. Rehabilitation services by interdisciplinary health team. Can be provided when receiving Home Health Care. M, MC, HMO

 – **Homemaker/Companion Services** assistance with light housekeeping, shopping, cooking, some companionship and personal care needs (IHSS provides or done by private providers). PP, SL, VA

– **Home Repair Services** Home repair provided by qualified individuals at no cost or at a sliding scale fee. (IHSS can provide) PP, SL

– **Hospice Care** Provides special interdisciplinary services and palliative care to the terminally ill. Predominantly for persons with cancer but available for all conditions where aggressive treatment is considered futile. Recommended for last six months of life. M, MC, HMO, VA

– **Telephone Reassurance/Friendly Visitor** service available for socially isolated elders to monitor their well being. PP, SL, NC

743

RESIDENTIAL SERVICES

– **Assisted Living** Professionally managed personal and health care services in a group setting, in addition to providing board and care services that supplement individual assistance with personal care. PP, MC (some states)

– **Continuing Care Retirement Community** One housing project that offers living arrangements ranging from independent to congregate living to intermediate care and skilled care facilities. PP

– **Nursing Homes** provide skilled nursing care and custodial care in an institutional setting on a 24 hour basis. Some are locked or secured to accommodate behavioral care needs and geropsychiatric patients. M, MC, VA, PP, PI

– **Residential Care Facilities for Elderly** (Board and Care) provide meals, housekeeping services and medication management in settings ranging from single family home to larger institutional facility. PP, SSI

– **Senior Citizen Apartments (Section 8)** provides affordable subsidized housing for elders spending over one-third of their income towards rent. PP, SSI

– **Shared Housing** Matches elder with person who can provide services in the home in exchange for room and board. PP

COMMUNITY SERVICES:

Adult Day Care – Social model day program designed for persons with a cognitive impairment. Hours vary but may provide up to 8 hours a day. PP, SL

– **Adult Day Health Care** – Socialization and rehabilitation program provided by health professionals for functionally impaired elderly. Hours vary. PP, MC, VA

 – **Congregate Meals** – Daily affordable nutritionally balanced noon time meal served at neighborhood community center such as a senior center, church, or synagogue. Provided by AAA. SL

See Table 26-4 for an explanation of the abbreviations.

– **Exercise Programs** – Physical activity programs – some with disease-specific focus, i.e., Twinges in the Hinges for arthritis. PP, SL, NC

 – **Information and Referral** – Referrals to local programs and agencies that provide senior services. VA, NC

 – **Legal Services** – Assistance with wills, durable power health care conservatorship, as well as legal advocacy. PP, SL

 – **Outpatient Mental Health** – M, MC, HMO, VA

– **Protective Services** – A government funded program that advocates appropriate care for elderly and dependent individuals living at home. Ombudsman services exist to preserve the rights of persons living in institutional settings.

– **Public Guardian** – Provides guardianship services for chronically ill individuals who are a public responsibility.

 – **Recreation** – Programs of activity provided at City Community or Senior Centers. NC

– **Respite Care** Services designed to provide relief for primary caregivers of persons with serious physical or mental impairment who are still living at home. PP, SL, VA

– **Senior Center** Services can vary from a neighborhood center offering social activities and meals for seniors during the day to a multipurpose senior center which provides information and referral, home visits, case management, home delivered meals, transportation, housing information, and legal services. NC

– **Support Groups** Assist patient and their caregivers to cope with the transitions and changes often accompanying a chronic illness. NC

–**Transportation** Travel by automobile or specialized vans to and from community resources and service providers. PP, SL

APPENDIX 12
The Confusion Assessment Method (CAM) Diagnostic Algorithm

Feature 1: Acute Onset and Fluctuating Course	This feature is usually obtained from a family member or nurse and is shown by positive responses to the following questions: Is there evidence of acute change in mental status from the patient's baseline? Did the abnormal behavior fluctuate during the day, that is, tend to come and go, or increase and decrease in severity?
Feature 2: Inattention	This feature is shown by a positive response to the following question: Did the patient have difficulty focusing attention, for example, being easily distractible, or having difficulty keeping track of what was being said?
Feature 3: Disorganized Thinking	This feature is show by a positive response to the following question: Was the patient's thinking disorganized or incoherent, such as rambling or irrelevant conversation, unclear or illogical flow of ideas, or unpredictable switching from subject to subject?
Feature 4: Altered Level of Consciousness	This feature is shown by any answer other than "alert" to the following question: Overall, how would you rate this patient's level of consciousness? (alert [normal], vigilant [hyperalert], lethargic [drowsy, easily aroused], stupor [difficult to arouse], or coma [unarousable])

The diagnosis of delirium by CAM requires the presence of features and 1 and 2 and either 3 or 4

APPENDIX 13
Cornell Scale for Depression
in Dementia

NAME_____ AGE _____ SEX _____ DATE _____

WING _____ ROOM _____ PHYSICIAN _____ ASSESSOR _____

Ratings should be based on symptoms and signs occurring during the week before interview. No score should be given if symptoms result from physical disability or illness.

SCORING SYSTEM

a = Unable to evaluate   0 = Absent   1 = Mild to intermittent   2 = Severe

a	0	1	2	**A. MOOD-RELATED SIGNS**
				1. Anxiety: anxious expression, rumination, worrying
				2. Sadness: sad expression, sad voice, tearfulness
				3. Lack of reaction to present events
				4. Irritability: annoyed, short tempered

a	0	1	2	**B. BEHAVIORAL DISTURBANCE**
				5. Agitation: restlessness, hand wringing, hair pulling
				6. Retardation: slow movements, slow speech, slow reactions
				7. Multiple physical complaints (score 0 if gastrointestinal symptoms only)
				8. Loss of interest: less involved in usual activities (score only if change occurred acutely, i.e., in less than one month)

a	0	1	2	**C. PHYSICAL SIGNS**
				9. Appetite loss: eating less than usual
				10. Weight loss (score 2 if greater than 5 pounds in one month)
				11. Lack of energy: fatigues easily, unable to sustain activities

a	0	1	2	**D. CYCLIC FUNCTIONS**
				12. Diurnal variation of mood: symptoms worse in the morning
				13. Difficulty falling asleep: later than usual for this individual
				14. Multiple awakening during sleep
				15. Early morning awakening: earlier than usual for this individual

a	0	1	2	**E. IDEATIONAL DISTURBANCE**
				16. Suicidal: feels life is not worth living
				17. Poor self-esteem: self-blame, self-depreciation, feelings of failure
				18. Pessimism: anticipation of the worst
				19. Mood congruent delusions: delusions of poverty, illness or loss

SCORE _____	Score greater than 12 = Probable Depression

Notes/Current Medications: _____

_____

_____

Instructions for use:
(Cornell Dementia Depression Assessment Tool)

1. The same CNA (certified nursing assistant) should conduct the interview each time to assure consistency in response.

2. The assessment should be based on the patient's normal weekly routine.

3. If uncertain of answers, questioning other caregivers may further define the answer.

4. Answer all questions by placing a check in the column under the appropriately numbered answer. (a = unable to evaluate, 0 = absent, 1 = mild to intermittent, 2 = severe).

5. Add the total score for all numbers checked for each question.

6. Place the total score in the "SCORE" box and record any subjective observation notes in the "NOTES/CURRENT MEDICATIONS" section.

7. Scores totaling twelve (12) points or more indicate probable depression.

APPENDIX 14
Epworth Sleepiness Scale

Name:_____

Today's date: _____ Your age (years): _____

Your sex (male = M; female = F): _____

How likely are you to doze off or fall asleep in the following situations, in contrast to feeling just tired? This refers to your usual way of life, in recent times. Even if you have not done some of these things recently, try to work out how they would have affected you. Use the following scale to choose the *most appropriate number* for each situation:

> 0 = would *never* doze
> 1 = *slight* chance of dozing
> 2 = *moderate* chance of dozing
> 3 = *high* chance of dozing

Situation	Chance of dozing
Sitting and reading	_____
Watching TV	_____
Sitting, inactive in a public place (e.g. a theater or a meeting)	_____
As a passenger in a car for an hour without a break	_____
Lying down to rest in the afternoon when circumstances permit	_____
Sitting and talking to someone	_____
Sitting quietly after a lunch without alcohol	_____
In a car, while stopped for a few minutes in the traffic	_____

Reprinted with permission from American Sleep Disorder Association and Sleep Research Society. Sleep, 16(6): 540–545; 1991.

FIM (motor)	FIM (cognitive)
Self-care	**Communication**
A. Self care	N. Comprehension
B. Grooming	O. Expression
C. Bathing	**Social cognition**
D. Dressing upper body	P. Social integration
E. Dressing lower body	Q. Problem solving
F. Toileting	R. Memory

Self-care

- A. Self care
- B. Grooming
- C. Bathing
- D. Dressing upper body
- E. Dressing lower body
- F. Toileting

Sphincter control

- G. Bladder management
- H. Bowel management

Mobility

Transfer:

- I. Bed, chair, wheelchair
- J. Toilet
- K. Tub, shower

Locomotion

- L. Walk/wheelchair
- M. Stairs

FIM (cognitive)

Communication

- N. Comprehension
- O. Expression

Social cognition

- P. Social integration
- Q. Problem solving
- R. Memory

FIM Scoring:

Independence:
- 7 — complete independence (timely, safely)
- 6 — modified independence (device used)

Modified dependence:
- 5 — supervision
- 4 — minimal assistance (subject performs >75% of task)
- 3 — moderate assistance (subject performs 50-74% of task)

Complete dependence:
- 2 — maximal assistance (subject performs 25-49% of task)
- 1 — total assistance (subject performs <25% of task)

Modified from Grander CV, Hamilton BB. The Uniform Data System for Medical Rehabilitation report on first admissions for 1991. Am J Phys Med & Rehabil 1993;72:33–38.

APPENDIX 16
Geriatric Depression Scale
(Short Version)

1. Are you basically satisfied with your life?

*2. Have you dropped many of your activities and interests?

*3. Do you feel that your life is empty?

*4. Do you often get bored?

5. Are you in good spirits most of the time?

*6. Are you afraid that something bad is going to happen to you?

7. Do you feel happy most of the time?

*8. Do you often feel helpless?

*9. Do you prefer to stay at home, rather than going out and doing new things?

*10. Do you feel you have more problems with memory than most?

11. Do you think it is wonderful to be alive now?

*12. Do you feel pretty worthless the way you are now?

13. Do you feel full of energy?

*14. Do you feel that your situation is hopeless?

*15. Do you thing that most people are better of than you are?

*"Yes" answers indicating depression, otherwise "no" answers indicate depression.

The GDS can be a self-rating or observer-rated inventory.

Cut off: Normal (0–5).

Yesavage JA. Geriatric depression scale. Psychopharmacol Bull 1988;24:709.

APPENDIX 17
Geriatric Pain Assessment

Date:_____   Medical Record Number_____

Patient's Name_____

Problem List: Medications:

_____   _____
_____   _____
_____   _____
_____   _____

                        Pain Description:

Pattern: Constant   Intermittant   Pain Intensity:
Duration:_____   0 1 2 3 4 5 6 7 8 9 10
Location:_____   None   Moderate   Severe
Character:
Lancinating   Burning   Stinging Radiating   Worst Pain in Last 24 hours:
Shooting   Tingling   0 1 2 3 4 5 6 7 8 9 10
                                                None   Moderate   Severe
Other Descriptors:
                                        Mood:_____
_____
_____   Depression Screening Score: _____
_____
                                        Gait and Balance Score: _____
Exacerbating Factors: Impaired Activities:

_____   _____
_____   _____
                                        _____
Relieving Factors:
                                        Sleep Quality:_____
_____   Bowel Habits:_____
_____
                                        _____

Other Assessments or Comments: _____
_____
_____

Most Likely Cause of Pain_____

Plans:_____
_____
_____
_____

Printed with permission from American Geriatric Society Panel on Chronic Pain in Older Persons: The management of chronic pain in older persons. J Am Geriatr Soc, 46:635–651, 1998.

APPENDIX 18
Geriatric Screen for Impairment in the Ambulatory Elderly

Name _____ Date _____ / _____ / _____

Did the patient bring in the bottles or a list of all of his/her medicines? (if they take any)   Yes_____   No_____

1. NUTRITION
Weigh patient: <100 lbs_____   >100 lbs_____
Ask: Have you lost 10 lbs over the past six months without trying to do so?   Yes_____   No_____

Positive screen: Yes or weight < 100 lbs.

2. HEARING
Right Ear _____   _____   Left Ear _____   _____
          1000-Hz   2000-Hz   1000-Hz   2000-Hz

Positive screen: Patient unable to hear the 1000-Hz or the 2000-Hz frequency in <u>both</u> ears OR patient unable to hear the 1000-Hz and the 2000-Hz frequency in <u>one</u> ear (or any combination of two negative responses).

3. VISION
Ask: "Do you have difficulty driving or watching television or reading or doing any of your daily activities because of your eyesight?" (even while wearing glasses)   Yes_____   No_____
Positive screen: Yes
IF POSITIVE SCREEN HAVE PATIENT COMPLETE SNELLEN EYE CHART
          Right Eye_____   Left Eye_____

4. MENTAL STATUS
Instruct: "I am going to name 3 objects: pencil, truck, book. I will ask you to repeat their names now and then again a minute from now. Please try to remember them."
          RECORD THIS AFTER ASKING QUESTION ON AADL-IADL-ADL (ITEM 7)

All 3 objects named?   Yes_____   No_____
Positive screen: No.

5. URINARY INCONTINENCE
Ask: "In the last year, have you ever lost your urine and gotten wet?"   Yes_____   No_____

IF ANSWER IS NO THEN SKIP TO ITEM 6.
IF ANSWER IS YES THEN ASK THE FOLLOWING:
"Have you lost urine at least 6 separate days?"   Yes_____   No_____
Positive screen: Yes to both questions.

6. DEPRESSION
Ask: "Do you often feel sad or depressed?"   Yes_____   No_____
Positive screen: Yes.

7. AADL-IADL-ADL
Ask: "Are you <u>able</u> to..."
Do strenuous activities like fast walking or bicycling?   Yes_____   No_____

Do heavy work around the house, like washing windows, walls or floors?   Yes_____   No_____

Go shopping for groceries or clothes?   Yes_____   No_____

Get to places out of walking distance? (drive, take a bus)   Yes_____   No_____

Bathe, either a sponge bath, tub bath or shower?   Yes_____   No_____

Dress, like putting on a shirt, buttoning and zipping, or putting on shoes?   Yes_____   No_____
Positive screen (for each): Unable to do or able to do with help or supervision from another person.

          REMEMBER TO HAVE PATIENT COMPLETE 3 ITEM RECALL ABOVE

8. <u>MOBILITY</u>

Using a watch, time in seconds while observing the patient after asking:
"Rise from the chair, walk 20 feet, turn, walk back to the chair and sit down."
The patient should walk at a rapid, but comfortable pace.
Positive screen: >15 seconds to complete task.

≤15 sec_____   >15 sec_____

APPENDIX 19
Geriatric Screening in Primary Care:
Guide for Use of Appendix 18

Problem	Screening Measure	Positive Screen	Supporting Data
Vision	Two parts: Ask: "Do you have difficulty driving or watching television or reading or doing any of your daily activities because of your eyesight?" If yes, then: Test each eye with Snellen chart while patient wears corrective lenses (if applicable).	Yes to question and inability to read greater than 20/40 on Snellen chart.	Question: derived from some of the most reliable items on the Boston Activities of Daily Vision Scale; test-retest reliability is 0.8; Snellen chart: gold standard.
Hearing	Use audioscope set at 40 dB. Test hearing using 1000 and 2000 Hz.	Inability to hear 1000 or 2000 Hz in both ears; or inability to hear frequencies in either ear.	In physicians' offices: sensitivity = 0.94; specificity = 0.72.
Leg mobility	Time the patient after asking: "Rise from the chair. Walk 20 feet briskly, turn, walk back to the chair and sit down."	Unable to complete task in 15 seconds.	Modified version of the "Up & Go"; inter-rater and test-retest reliability = 0.99; good correlations with other measures of gait and balance (0.6 to 0.8).
Urinary incontinence	Two parts: Ask: "In the past year, have you ever lost your urine and gotten wet?" If yes, then ask: "Have you lost urine on at least 6 separate days?"	Yes to both questions.	83% agreement between patient response and urologic assessment.
Nutrition, weight loss	Two parts Ask: "Have you lost 10 lbs. over the past 6 months without trying to do so?" Weigh the patient.	Yes to the question or weight < 100 lb.	Question: relative risk of death = 2.0 (NHEFS); weight: PPV of malnutrition = 0.99.
Memory	Three-item recall.	Unable to remember all three items after 1 minute.	Likelihood ratios for dementia: recalls all 3 = 0.06; recalls 2 = 0.5; recalls < 2 = 3.1.
Depression	Ask: "Do you often feel sad or depressed?"	Yes to the question.	Sensitivity = 0.78; specificity = 0.87.
Physical disability	Six questions: "Are you able to . . . "do strenuous activities like fast walking or bicycling?" "do heavy work around the house like washing windows, walls, or floors?" "go shopping for groceries or clothes?" "get to places out of walking distance?" "bathe, either a sponge bath, tub bath, or shower?" "dress, like putting on a shirt, buttoning and zipping, or putting on shoes?"	Yes to any of the questions.	Coefficient of reproducibility 0.96; test-retest reliability 0.88; good correlation with other measures of physical function 0.63–0.89.

NHEFS = National Health Epidemiologic Follow-up Study. PPV = positive predictive value.

SOURCE: Adapted with permission from Moore AA, Siu AL. Screening for common problems in ambulatory elderly: clinical confirmation of a screen instrument. *Am J Med*. 1996;100(4):440 (with personal communication from Tamara B. Harris, MD). Reprinted with permission from Excerpta Medica, Inc.

APPENDIX 20
Global Deterioration Scale (GDS)

<table>
<tr><td>COMPOUND</td></tr>
<tr><td>STUDY</td></tr>
<tr><td>FORM GDS</td></tr>
<tr><td>PAGE _____ OF _____</td></tr>
</table>

SUBJECT I.D. _____
SUBJECT NO. |__|__|__|__|
STUDY DAY
DATE |___|___|___|
     Mo.   Day   Yr.

Rate the subject's level of cognitive functioning.

1 **No cognitive decline**	No subjective complaints of memory deficit. No memory deficit evident on clinical interview.
2 **Very mild cognitive decline**	Subjective complaints of memory deficit, most frequently in following areas: (a) forgetting where one has placed familiar objects; (b) forgetting names one formerly knew well. No objective evidence of memory deficit on clinical interview. No objective deficits in employment or social situations. Appropriate concern with respect to symptomatology.
3 **Mild cognitive decline**	Earliest clear-cut deficits. Manifestations in more than one of the following areas: (a) patient may have gotten lost when traveling to an unfamiliar location; (b) co-workers become aware of patient's relatively poor performance; (c) word and name finding deficits become evident to intimates; (d) patient may read a passage or a book and retain relatively little material; (e) patient may demonstrate decreased facility in remembering names upon introduction to new people; (f) patient may have lost or misplaced an object of value; (g) concentration deficit may be evident on clinical testing. Objective evidence of memory deficits obtained only with an intensive interview. Decreased performance in demanding employment and social settings. Denial begins to become manifest in patient. Mild to moderate anxiety accompanies symptoms.
4 **Moderate cognitive decline**	Clear-cut deficit on careful clinical interview. Deficit manifest in following areas: (a) decreased knowledge of current and recent events; (b) may exhibit some deficit in memory of one's personal history; (c) concentration deficit elicited on serial subtractions; (d) decreased ability to travel, handle finances, etc. Frequently no deficit in following areas: (a) orientation to time and person; (b) recognition of familiar persons and faces; (c) ability to travel to familiar locations. Inability to perform complex tasks. Denial is dominant defense mechanism. Flattening of affect and withdrawal from challenging situations occur.
5 **Moderately severe cognitive decline**	Patient can no longer survive without some assistance. Patient is unable during interview to recall a major relevant aspect of current life: e.g., an address or telephone number of many years, the names of close family members (such as grandchildren), the name of the high school or college from which patient graduated. Frequently some disorientation to time (date, day of week, season, etc.) or to place. An educated person may have difficulty counting back from 40 by 4s or from 20 by 2s. Persons at this stage retain knowledge of many major facts regarding themselves and others. They invariably know their own names and generally know their spouse's and children's names. They require no assistance with toileting and eating, but may have some difficulty choosing the proper clothing to wear.
6 **Severe cognitive decline**	May occasionally forget the name of the spouse upon whom they are entirely dependent for survival. Will be largely unaware of all recent events and experiences in their lives. Retain some knowledge of their past lives but this is very sketchy. Generally unaware of their surroundings, the year, the season, etc. May have difficulty counting from 10, both backward and sometimes, forward. Will require some assistance with activities of daily living, e.g., may become incontinent, will require travel assistance but occasionally will display ability to travel to familiar locations. Diurnal rhythm frequently disturbed. Almost always recall their own names. Frequently continue to be able to distinguish familiar from unfamiliar persons in their environment. Personality and emotional changes occur. These are quite variable and include: (a) delusional behavior, e.g., patients may accuse their spouse of being an impostor, may talk to imaginary figures in the environment, or to their own reflection in the mirror; (b) obsessive symptoms, e.g., person may continually repeat simple cleaning activities; (c) anxiety symptoms, agitation, and even previously nonexistent violent behavior may occur; (d) cognitive abulia, i.e., loss of willpower because an individual cannot carry a thought long enough to determine a purposeful course of action.
7 **Very severe cognitive decline**	All verbal abilities are lost. Frequently there is no speech at all—only grunting. Incontinent of urine; requires assistance toileting and feeding. Loses basic psychomotor skills, e.g., ability to walk. The brain appears to no longer be able to tell the body what to do. Generalized and cortical neurologic signs and symptoms are frequently present.

Enter rating here

[ ]

© Barry Reisberg, M.D.

APPENDIX 21
Hamilton Psychiatric Rating Scale for Depression

Patient's Name _____

Date _____

Comments _____

_____

ITEM	RATING
1. Depressed Mood Sadness, hopelessness, gloomy pessimistic, weeping, worthless Behavior. Faces, posture, weeping voice.	
2. Guilt Feelings Pathologic guilt, non-rationalizing self-blame, feelings of self-reproach	
3. Suicide Recurrent thoughts of death; life is empty, not worth living, isolation, suicide gestures, threats, or attempts.	
4. Initial Insomnia Difficulty getting to sleep after going to bed.	
5. Middle Insomnia Difficulty staying asleep.	
6. Delayed Insomnia Early-morning awakening.	
7. Work and Interest Apathy, loss of pleasure and interest in work, hobbies, social activities, recreation, inability to obtain satisfaction, decreased performance in work and in home duties. (Do not rate fatigue or loss of energy)	
8. Retardation Psychomotor: Slowing of thoughts, speech and movement	
9. Agitation Psychomotor: Fidgeting, restlessness or pacing, clenching fists, kicking feet, wringing hands, biting lips, pulling hair, gesturing with arms, picking at hands and clothes.	

ITEM	RATING
10. Anxiety (Psychologic) Tense, unable to relax, irritable, easily startled, worrying over trivia. Phobic symptoms, apprehensive of impending doom, fear of loss of control, panic episodes.	
11. Anxiety (Somatic) Physiologic concomitants of anxiety. Effects of autonomic overactivity, "butterflies", indigestion, stomach cramps, belching, diarrhea, palpitations, hyper-ventilation, paresthesia, sweating, flushing, tremor, headache, urinary frequency.	
12. Loss of Appetite	
13. Anergia Fatigability feels tired or exhausted, loss of energy, heavy or dragging feelings in arms or legs.	
14. Loss of Libido Impairment of sexual performance.	
15. Hypochondriasis Morbid preoccupation with real or imagined bodily symptoms or functions.	
16. Weight Loss Since onset of illness or since last visit.	
17. Loss of insight Denial of "nervous" illness, attributes illness to visits, over work, climate or physical symptoms. Does not recognize symptoms are "nervous" in origin.	

17-ITEM SUB-TOTAL ☐

ITEM	RATING
18. Diurnal Variation Change in mood.	
19. Hypersomnia (More Time Spent in Bed) Retires earlier and/or rises later than usual, not necessarily sleeping longer.	
20. Hypersomnia (Oversleeping) Sleeping more than usual.	
21. Hypersomnia (Napping) Naps, excessive daytime sleepi-ness.	
22. Increased Appetite Change in appetite marked by increased food intake or excessive cravings.	
23. Weight Gain Since onset of illness or since last visit.	
24. Psychic Retardation Slowness of speech and thought processes, inhibition of well or feeling as if thought processes are paralyzed.	
25. Motor Retardation Slowness of movements and affective expression.	

25-ITEM SUB-TOTAL ☐

APPENDIX 22
Hearing Handicap Inventory for Elderly-Screening (HHIE-S)*

Instructions: The purpose of this scale is to identify the problems your hearing loss may be causing you. Answer Yes, Sometimes, or No for each question. <u>Do not skip a question if you avoid a situation because of your hearing loss.</u> It is important that you answer all questions. If you use a hearing aid, please answer the way you hear <u>without</u> the hearing aid.

E   S

(E1) Does a hearing problem cause you to feel embarrassed when meeting new people?

4 __   Yes

2 __   Sometimes

0 __   No

(E2) Does a hearing problem cause you to feel frustrated when talking to members of your family?

4 __   Yes

2 __   Sometimes

0 __   No

(S3) Do you have difficulty when someone speaks in a whisper?

4   __   Yes

2   __   Sometimes

0   __   No

(E4) Do you feel handicapped by a hearing problem?

4 __   Yes

2 __   Sometimes

0 __   No

(S5) Does a hearing problem cause you difficulty when visiting friends, relatives, or neighbors?

4   __   Yes

2   __   Sometimes

0   __   No

(S6) Does a hearing problem cause you to attend religious services less often than you would like?

4   __   Yes

2   __   Sometimes

0   __   No

(E7) Does a hearing problem cause you you to have arguments with family members?

4 __   Yes

2 __   Sometimes

0 __   No

(S8) Does a hearing problem cause you difficulty when listening to a TV or radio?

4   __   Yes

2   __   Sometimes

0   __   No

(E9) Do you feel that any difficulty with your hearing limits or hampers your personal or social life?

4 ___   Yes

2 ___   Sometimes

0 ___   No

(S10) Does a hearing problem cause you difficulty when in a restaurant with relatives or friends?

4 ___   Yes

2 ___   Sometimes

0 ___   No

___   Emotional Subscale Total

___   Social Subscale Total

_____   **Total Score**

Remember to answer <u>all of the questions</u> and if you wear a hearing aid answer the way you hear <u>without</u> the hearing aid.

* Reprinted with permission of the author, from Ventry, I. & Weinstein, B. The Hearing Handicap Inventory for the Elderly: A new tool. <u>Ear and Hear.</u>, 83, 128-134 (1982).

Key:
S = Social Subscale Question E = Emotional Subscale Question
Yes = 4 Points
Sometimes = 2 Points
No = 0 Points

The range of results for total score are:
0-8 No Hearing Handicap
9-24 Mild to Moderate Hearing Handicap
25-40 Severe Hearing Handicap

Safety Item	Yes	No	Comment
1. Are emergency numbers kept by the phone and regularly updated?			
2. Do family members and other caregivers know how to report an emergency?			
3. Are patient, family, and caregivers aware of the dangers of smoking, especially in bed?			
4. If oxygen is used, do patient and caregivers know correct use of equipment, how to operate and clean it correctly?			
5. Are firearms stored unloaded and locked up?			
6. Are all poisons (medications, detergents, insecticides, cleaning fluids, polishes, etc.) kept out of reach of children and discarded when no longer needed?			
7. Is there a fire alarm and extinguisher? Do patient and caregivers know how to use it?			
8. Do the family and caregivers have an escape plan in case of fire or other disaster?			
9. Are throw rugs eliminated or fastened down?			
10. Are all electrical cords in working order, in the open, and not run under rugs or carpets or wrapped around nails?			
11. Are non-slip mats placed in bathtubs and showers?			
12. Are banisters or railings placed along stairways?			
13. Are stairs, halls, and doorways free of clutter?			
14. Are all steps and sidewalks clear of tools, toys, and other articles?			
15. Does adaptive or medical support equipment function adequately?			

Safety Item	Yes	No	Comment
16. Do patient and caregivers know safe and effective use of equipment?			
17. Do patient and caregivers know procedures to follow if equipment malfunctions?			

SOURCE: Ferrell BA. Home care. In: Cassel CK, Cohen HJ, Larson EB, et al., eds. *Geriatric Medicine*. 3rd ed. New York: Springer Verlag; 1997:115. Reprinted with permission.

APPENDIX 24
Physical Activities of Daily Living (ADL)

This form may help you assess the functional capabilities of your older patients. The data can be collected by a nurse from the patient, or from a family member or other caregiver.

I = Independent   *A = Assistance required*   *D = Dependent*

Obtained from: Patient	Informant	Activity	Guidelines for Assessment
I A D	I A D	**Bathing** *(sponge, shower, tub)*	I = Able to bathe completely or needs help with only a single body part A = Needs help with more than one body part, getting in/out of tub or special tub attachments D = Completely unable to bathe self
I A D	I A D	**Dressing/Undressing**	I = Able to pick out clothes, dress/undress self, manage fasteners/braces; tying shoes excluded A = Need assistance as remains partially undressed D = Completely unable to dress/undress self
I A D	I A D	**Personal Grooming**	I = Able to comb hair/shave without help A = Needs help to comb hair, shave D = Completely unable to care for appearance
I A D	I A D	**Toileting**	I = Able to get to, on and off toilet, arrange clothes, clean organs of excretion; uses bedpan only at night A = Needs help getting to and using toilet; uses bedpan/commode regularly D = Completely unable to use toilet
I A D	I A D	**Continence**	I = Urination/defecation self-controlled A = Partial or total urine/stool incontinence or control by enemas, catheters, regulated use of urinals/bedpans D = Uses catheter or colostomy
I A D	I A D	**Transferring**	I = Able to get in/out of bed/chair without human assistance/mechanical aids A = Needs human assistance/mechanical aids D = Completely unable to transfer; needs lifting
I A D	I A D	**Walking**	I = Able to walk without help except from cane A = Needs human assistance/walker, crutches D = Completely unable to walk; needs lifting
I A D	I A D	**Eating**	I = Able to completely feed self A = Needs help with cutting, buttering bread, etc. D = Completely unable to feed self or needs parenteral feeding

SOURCE: Reprinted with permission from *Modules in Clinical Geriatrics.* Copyright ©1997 by Blue Cross and Blue Shield Association and the American Geriatrics Society.

APPENDIX 25
Instrumental Activities of Daily Living (IADL)

This form may help you assess the functional capabilities of your older patients. The data can be collected by a nurse from the patient, or from a family member or other caregiver.

I = Independent   *A = Assistance required*   *D = Dependent*

Obtained from: Patient	Informant	Activity	Guidelines for Assessment
I A D	I A D	**Using Telephone**	I = Able to look up numbers, dial, receive and make calls without help A = Able to answer phone or dial operator in an emergency but needs special phone or help in getting number, dialing D = Unable to use the telephone
I A D	I A D	**Traveling**	I = Able to drive own car or travel alone on buses, taxis A = Able to travel but needs someone to travel with D = Unable to travel
I A D	I A D	**Shopping**	I = Able to take care of all food/clothes shopping with transportation provided A = Able to shop but needs someone to shop with D = Unable to shop
I A D	I A D	**Preparing Meals**	I = Able to plan and cook full meals A = Able to prepare light foods but unable to cook full meals alone D = Unable to prepare any meals
I A D	I A D	**Housework**	I = Able to do heavy housework, i.e., scrub floors A = Able to do light housework but needs help with heavy tasks D = Unable to do any housework
I A D	I A D	**Taking Medicine**	I = Able to prepare/take medications in the right dose at the right time A = Able to take medications but needs reminding or someone to prepare them D = Unable to take medications
I A D	I A D	**Managing Money**	I = Able to manage buying needs, i.e., write checks, pay bills A = Able to manage daily buying needs but needs help managing checkbook, paying bills D = Unable to handle money

SOURCE: Reprinted with permission from *Modules in Clinical Geriatrics.* Copyright © 1997 by Blue Cross and Blue Shield Association and the American Geriatrics Society.

<u>LSNS Original 10 item scale</u>

1. How many relatives do you see or hear from at least once a month?
   Response options and scoring:
   - 0 = none
   - 1 = one
   - 2 = two
   - 3 = 3 or 4
   - 4 = 5 - 8
   - 5 = nine or more

2. How often do you see or hear from relative with whom you have the most contact?
   Response options and scoring:
   - 0 = less than monthly
   - 1 = monthly
   - 2 = 2-3 times a month
   - 3 = weekly
   - 4 = 2-3 times a week
   - 5 = daily

3. How many relatives do you feel at ease with that you can talk about private matters?
   Response options and scoring:
   - 0 = none
   - 1 = one
   - 2 = two
   - 3 = 3 or 4
   - 4 = 5 - 8
   - 5 = nine or more

4. How many friends do you see or hear from at least once a month?
   Response options and scoring:
   - 0 = none
   - 1 = one
   - 2 = two
   - 3 = 3 or 4
   - 4 = 5 - 8
   - 5 = nine or more

5. How often do you see or hear from friend with whom you have the most contact?
   Response options and scoring:
   - 0 = less than monthly
   - 1 = monthly
   - 2 = 2-3 times a month
   - 3 = weekly
   - 4 = 2-3 times a week
   - 5 = daily

6. How many friends do you feel at ease with that you can talk about private matters?
   Response options and scoring:
   - 0 = none
   - 1 = one
   - 2 = two
   - 3 = 3 or 4
   - 4 = 5 - 8
   - 5 = nine or more

7. When you have an important decision to make do you have someone to talk to about it?
    Response options and scoring:
    5 = always
    4 = very often
    3 = often
    2 = sometimes
    1 = seldom
    0 = never

8. When other people have an important decision to make, do they talk to you about it?
    Response options and scoring:
    5 = always
    4 = very often
    3 = often
    2 = sometimes
    1 = seldom
    0 = never

9. How often do you help your family, friends, or neighbors....?
    Response options and scoring:
    5 = always
    4 = very often
    3 = often
    2 = sometimes
    1 = seldom
    0 = never

10. Do you live alone or with others?
    Response options and scoring:
    5 = lives with spouse
    4 = lives with friends or other relatives (not spouse)
    2 = lives with paid helper only
    0 = lives alone

A clinical cut-off point of 20 or less has been suggested as a marker of social isolation.

PATIENT'S NAME: _____   DATE: _____

	NONE	MILD	MODERATE	SEVERE
THROBBING	0) ____	1) ____	2) ____	3) ____
SHOOTING	0) ____	1) ____	2) ____	3) ____
STABBING	0) ____	1) ____	2) ____	3) ____
SHARP	0) ____	1) ____	2) ____	3) ____
CRAMPING	0) ____	1) ____	2) ____	3) ____
GNAWING	0) ____	1) ____	2) ____	3) ____
HOT-BURNING	0) ____	1) ____	2) ____	3) ____
ACHING	0) ____	1) ____	2) ____	3) ____
HEAVY	0) ____	1) ____	2) ____	3) ____
TENDER	0) ____	1) ____	2) ____	3) ____
SPLITTING	0) ____	1) ____	2) ____	3) ____
TIRING-EXHAUSTING	0) ____	1) ____	2) ____	3) ____
SICKENING	0) ____	1) ____	2) ____	3) ____
FEARFUL	0) ____	1) ____	2) ____	3) ____
PUNISHING-CRUEL	0) ____	1) ____	2) ____	3) ____

NO PAIN ├──────────────────────────────────┤ WORST POSSIBLE PAIN

PPI

0	NO PAIN	____
1	MILD	____
2	DISCOMFORTING	____
3	DISTRESSING	____
4	HORRIBLE	____
5	EXCRUCIATING	____

Note: Descriptors 1-11 represent the sensory dimension of pain experience and 12-15 represent the affective dimension. Each descriptor is ranked on an intensity scale of 0-3. The present pain intensity (PPI) and visual analog scale are also included to provide overall pain intensity scores.

Source: Melzack R, Katz J: The McGill Pain Questionnaire: Appraisal and current status. In Turk DC, Melzack R (Eds), New York, Guildford Press, 1992.

MY MEDICAL DIRECTIVE

This Medical Directive shall stand as a guide to my wishes regarding medical treatments in the event that illness should make me unable to communicate them directly. I make this Directive, being 18 years or more of age, of sound mind, and appreciating the consequences of my decisions.

SITUATION A

If I am in a coma or a persistent vegetative state and, in the opinion of my physician and two consultants, have no known hope of regaining awareness and higher mental functions no matter what is done, then my goals and specific wishes — if medically reasonable — for this and any additional illness would be:

☐ prolong life; treat everything
☐ attempt to cure, but reevaluate often
☐ limit to less invasive and less burdensome interventions
☐ provide comfort care only
☐ other (*please specify*): _____

Please check appropriate boxes:

	I want	I want treatment tried. If no clear improvement, stop.	I am undecided	I do not want
1. Cardiopulmonary resuscitation (chest compressions, drugs, electric shocks, and artificial breathing aimed at reviving a person who is on the point of dying).		*Not applicable*		
2. Major surgery (for example, removing the gallbladder or part of the colon).		*Not applicable*		
3. Mechanical breathing (respiration by machine, through a tube in the throat).				
4. Dialysis (cleaning the blood by machine or by fluid passed through the belly).				
5. Blood transfusions or blood products.		*Not applicable*		
6. Artificial nutrition and hydration (given through a tube in a vein or in the stomach).				
7. Simple diagnostic tests (for example, blood tests or x-rays).		*Not applicable*		
8. Antibiotics (drugs used to fight infection).		*Not applicable*		
9. Pain medications, even if they dull consciousness and indirectly shorten my life.		*Not applicable*		

1) Copyright 1990 by Linda L. Emanuel and Ezekiel J. Emanuel. The authors of this form advise that it should be completed pursuant to a discussion between the principal and his or her physician, so that the principal can be adequately informed of any personal medical information, and so that the physician can be appraised of the intentions of the principal and the existence of such a document which may be made part of the principal's medical records.

2) This form was originally published as part of an article by Linda L. Emanuel and Ezekiel J. Emanuel, "The Medical Directive: A New Comprehensive Advance Care Document" in *Journal of the American Medical Association*, June 9, 1989:261:3290. It does not reflect the official policy of the American Medical Association.

Initials & Date: _____

Instructions Circle yes, not sure, or no to indicate whether you agree with each statement. If you do <u>not</u> agree with the "always" statements, this could mean that you agree with these statements some of the time, but not always. You can use the space at the bottom of the page to explain and clarify your beliefs.

Personal and spiritual beliefs

Many people have special personal or spiritual beliefs that they want respected in decision making about life-sustaining treatments. What are yours?

I believe that it is <u>always</u> wrong to withhold (not start) treatments that could keep me alive.	Yes	Not sure	No
I believe that it is <u>always</u> wrong to withdraw (stop) treatments that could keep me alive after they've been started.	Yes	Not sure	No
I believe it is wrong to withhold (not provide) nutrition and fluids given through tubes, even if I am terminally ill or in a permanent coma.	Yes	Not sure	No
I do not wish to receive a blood transfusion or any blood products, such as plasma or red blood cells.	Yes	Not sure	No
I would like to have my pastor, priest, rabbi, or other spiritual advisor consulted regarding any difficult health care decision that must be made on my behalf.	Yes	Not sure	No

(write in name) _____

I believe in other forms of treatment, such as healing through prayer, acupuncture, or herbal remedies. I want the following treatments included in my care:	Yes	Not sure	No

_____

I believe that controlling pain is very important, even if the pain medications might hasten my death.	Yes	Not sure	No
I believe that my loved ones should take their own interests into consideration, as well as mine, when making health care decisions on my behalf.	Yes	Not sure	No
I believe that it is acceptable to consider the financial burden of treatment on my loved ones when making health care decisions on my behalf.	Yes	Not sure	No
I believe that my loved ones should follow my directions as closely as possible.	Yes	Not sure	No

Additional beliefs and/or explanations for my beliefs:

_____

_____

Initials & Date: _____

What makes your life worth living?

Life like this would be:

Instructions This exercise will help you think about and express what really matters to you. For each row, check (✔) one answer to express how you would feel if this factor by itself described you.	difficult, but acceptable	worth living, but just barely	not worth living	can't answer now
a. I can no longer walk but get around in a wheelchair.				
b. I can no longer get outside—I spend all day at home.				
c. I can no longer contribute to my family's well being.				
d. I am in severe pain most of the time.				
e. I have severe discomfort most of the time (such as nausea, diarrhea, or shortness of breath).				
f. I rely on a feeding tube to keep me alive.				
g. I rely on a kidney dialysis machine to keep me alive.				
h. I rely on a breathing machine to keep me alive.				
i. I need someone to help take care of me all of the time.				
j. I can no longer control my bladder.				
k. I can no longer control my bowels.				
l. I live in a nursing home.				
m. I can no longer think clearly—I am confused all the time.				
n. I can no longer recognize family/friends.				
o. I can no longer talk and be understood by others.				
p. My situation causes severe emotional burden for my family (such as feeling worried or stressed all the time).				
q. I am a severe financial burden on my family.				
r. I cannot seem to "shake the blues."				
s. Other (write in):				

Instructions To help others make sense out of your answers, think about the following questions and be sure to explain your answers to your loved ones and health care providers.

If you checked "worth living, but just barely" for more than one factor, would a combination of these factors make your life "not worth living?" If so, which factors?

If you checked "not worth living," does this mean that you would rather die than be kept alive?

If you checked "can't answer now," what information or people do you need to help you decide?

Severe Dementia

Imagine you have severe dementia (see pg. 29 for details). This means you:
- cannot think or talk clearly, are confused and no longer recognize family members
- seem uninterested in what's happening around you
- are not in any pain
- are able to walk, but get lost without supervision
- need help with getting dressed, bathing, and bowel and bladder functions

Part A: Feelings about quality of life

Check the answer that best describes how you would feel about having severe dementia for the rest of your life.	Life like this would be difficult, but acceptable	Life like this would be worth living, but just barely	Life like this would <u>not</u> be worth living
	☐	☐	☐

Part B: Preferences for different life-sustaining treatments

Imagine that while you have this dementia, you develop a life-threatening illness. The doctors feel that no matter what treatment you receive, you will remain demented, but the treatment will keep you from dying.

Check an answer for each treatment that best reflects what you would want.	I would want to receive this treatment	I would rather die naturally and not have this treatment	I don't know/can't answer right now
Antibiotics			
CPR			
Feeding tube: for a short time			
for the rest of my life			
Dialysis: for a short time			
for the rest of my life			
Mechanical ventilator: for a short time			
for the rest of my life			
Comfort care	✔		
Other treatments: (fill in)			

Part C: Reasons for my decisions or other comments

Would your answers be different if you seemed happy most of the time? **Yes** **No**

Would your answers be different if you seemed unhappy most of the time? **Yes** **No**

How?

APPENDIX 29
The Annotated MiniMental State Examination (AMMSE)

MiniMental LLC

NAME OF SUBJECT_____ Age _____

NAME OF EXAMINER _____ Years of School Completed ____

Approach the patient with respect and encouragement.   Date of Examination _____
Ask: "Do you have any trouble with your memory?" ☐ Yes ☐ No
"May I ask you some questions about your memory?" ☐ Yes ☐ No

SCORE	ITEM

5 ( )   TIME ORIENTATION

Ask:

"What is the year_____ (1), season_____ (1),

month of the year_____ (1), date_____ (1),

day of the week _____ (1)"?

5 ( )   PLACE ORIENTATION

Ask:

"Where are we now? What is the state_____ (1), city_____ (1),

part of the city_____ (1), building_____ (1),

floor of the building_____ (1)?"

3 ( )   REGISTRATION OF THREE WORDS

Say: "Listen carefully. I am going to say three words. You say them back after I stop.
Ready? Here they are... PONY (wait 1 second), QUARTER (wait 1 second), ORANGE (wait one
second). What were those words?"

_____ (1)

_____ (1)

_____ (1)

Give 1 point for each correct answer, then repeat them until the patient learns all three.

5 ( )   SERIAL 7s AS A TEST OF ATTENTION AND CALCULATION

Ask: "Subtract 7 from 100 and continue to subtract 7 from each subsequent remainder
until I tell you to stop. What is 100 take away 7 ?"_____ (1)

Say:

"Keep Going."_____ (1), _____ (1),

_____ (1), _____ (1).

3 ( )   RECALL OF THREE WORDS

Ask:

"What were those three words I asked you to remember?"

Give one point for each correct answer._____ (1),

_____ (1), _____ (1).

2 ( )   NAMING

Ask:

"What is this?" (show pencil) _____ (1). "What is this?" (show watch)_____ (1).

O V E R

MiniMental LLC

1 ( ) **REPETITION**

Say:

"Now I am going to ask you to repeat what I say. Ready? 'No ifs, ands, or buts.'
Now you say that." _____ (1)

3 ( ) **COMPREHENSION**

Say:

"Listen carefully because I am going to ask you to do something:
Take this paper in your left hand (1), fold it in half (1), and put it on the floor." (1)

1 ( ) **READING**

Say:

"Please read the following and do what it says, but do not say it aloud." (1)

Close your eyes

1 ( ) **WRITING**

Say:

"Please write a sentence." If patient does not respond, say: "Write about the weather." (1)

_____

_____

1 ( ) **DRAWING**

Say: "Please copy this design."

TOTAL SCORE _____   Assess level of consciousness along a continuum

Alert	Drowsy	Stupor	Coma

	YES	NO
Cooperative:		
Depressed:		
Anxious:		
Poor Vision:		
Poor Hearing:		
Native Language:		

	YES	NO
Deterioration from previous level of functioning:		
Family History of Dementia:		
Head Trauma:		
Stroke:		
Alcohol Abuse:		
Thyroid Disease:		

FUNCTION BY PROXY

Please record date when patient was last able to perform the following tasks.
Ask caregiver if patient independently handles:

	YES	NO	DATE
Money/Bills:			
Medication:			
Transportation:			
Telephone:			

Median Mini–Mental State Examination Score by Age and Educational Level

	Education				
	0–4y	5–8y	9–12y	≥12y	Total
18–24	23	28	29	30	29
25–29	25	27	29	30	29
30–34	26	26	29	30	29
35–39	23	27	29	30	29
40–44	23	27	29	30	29
45–49	23	27	29	30	29
50–54	22	27	29	30	29
55–59	22	27	29	29	29
60–64	22	27	28	29	28
65–69	22	27	28	29	28
70–74	21	26	28	29	27
75–79	21	26	27	28	26
80–84	19	25	26	28	25
≥ 85	20	24	26	28	25
Total	22	26	29	29	29

SOURCE: Adapted from Crum RM, Anthony JC, Bassett SS, et al. Population-based norms for the Mini–Mental State Examination by age and educational level. *JAMA*. 1993;269:2386–2391. Copyright 1993, American Medical Association. Reprinted with permission.

Mini Nutritional Assessment

Last Name: _____ First Name: _____ M.I. _____ Sex: _____ Date: _____

Age: _____ Weight (kg): _____ Height (cm): _____ Knee Height (cm): _____

Complete the form by writing the numbers in the boxes. Add the numbers in the boxes and compare the total assessment to the Malnutrition Indicator Score.

Anthropometric Assessment

1. Body Mass Index (BMI) (weight in kg)/(height in m^2)
  a. BMI< 19 = 0 points
  b. BMI 19 to < 21 = 1 point
  c. BMI 21 to < 23 = 2 points
  d. BMI >23 = 3 points

2. Mid-arm circumference (MAC) in cm
  a. MAC < 21 = 0.0 points
  b. MAC 21 ≤ 22 = 0.5 points
  c. MAC > 22 = 1.0 points

3. Calf circumference (CC) in cm
  a. CC < 31 = 0 points
  b. CC ≥ 31 = 1 point

4. Weight loss during last 3 months
  a. weight loss greater than 3 kg (6.6 lb) = 0 points
  b. does not know = 1 point
  c. weight loss between 1 and 3 kg = 2 points
  d. no weight loss = 3 points

General Assessment

5. Lives independently (not in a nursing home or hospital)
  a. no = 0 points   b. yes = 1 point

6. Takes more than 3 prescription drugs per day
  a. yes = 0 points   b. no = 1 point

7. Has suffered psychological stress or acute disease in the past 3 months
  a. yes = 0 points   b. no = 1 point

8. Mobility
  a. bed or chair bound = 0 points
  b. able to get out of bed/chair but does not go out = 1 point
  c. goes out = 2 points

9. Neuropsychological problems
  a. severe dementia or depression = 0 points
  b. mild dementia = 1 point
  c. no psychological problems = 2 points

10. Pressure sores or skin ulcers
  a. yes = 0 points   b. no = 1 point

Dietary Assessment

11. How many full meals does the patient eat daily?
  a. 1 meal = 0 points
  a. 2 meals = 1 point
  a. 3 meals = 2 points

12. Selected consumption markers for protein intake
  • At least one serving of dairy products (milk, cheese, yogurt) per day ☐ Yes ☐ No
  • Two or more servings of legumes or eggs per week ☐ Yes ☐ No
  • Meat, fish, or poultry every day ☐ Yes ☐ No
  a. 0 or 1 yes = 0.0 points
  b. 2 yes = 0.5 points
  c. 3 yes = 1.0 points

13. Consumes two or more servings of fruits or vegetables per day
  a. no = 0 points   b. yes = 1 point

14. Has food intake declined over the past 3 months due to loss of appetite, digestive problems, chewing or swallowing difficulties?
  a. severe loss of appetite = 0 points
  b. moderate loss of appetite = 1 point
  c. no loss of appetite = 2 points

15. How much fluid (eg, water, juice, coffee, tea, milk) is consumed per day? (1 cup = 8 oz.)
  a. less than 3 cups = 0.0 points
  b. 3 to 5 cups = 0.5 points
  c. more than 5 cups = 1.0 points

16. Mode of feeding
  a. unable to eat without assistance = 0 points
  b. self-fed with some difficulty = 1 point
  c. self-fed without any problem = 2 points

Self-Assessment

17. Do they view themselves as having nutritional problems?
  a. major malnutrition = 0 points
  b. do not know or moderate malnutrition = 1 point
  c. no nutritional problem = 2 points

18. In comparison with other people of the same age, how do they consider their health status?
  a. not as good = 0.0 points
  b. do not know = 0.5 points
  c. as good = 1.0 points
  d. better = 2.0 points

Assessment Total (max. 30 points)

MALNUTRITION INDICATOR SCORE

≥ 24 points = well-nourished   17 to 23.5 points = at risk of malnutrition   < 17 points = malnourished

Vellas B, Guigoz Y, Garry PJ. Nutrition, 1999, 15(2):116–122.

APPENDIX 31
Morse Fall Scale

1. History of falling .... no 0 ___
                                                  yes 25 ___

2. Secondary diagnosis .... no 0 ___
                    yes 15 ___

3. Ambulatory aid
   - none/bedrest/nurse assist .... 0 ___
   - crutches/cane/walker .... 15 ___
   - furniture .... 30 ___

4. Intravenous therapy/heparin lock .... no 0 ___
                               yes 20 ___

5. Gait
   - normal/bedrest/wheelchair .... 0 ___
   - weak .... 10 ___
   - impaired .... 20 ___

6. Mental Status
   - oriented to own ability .... 0 ___
   - overestimates/forgets limitations .... 15 ___
                                     Total ___

Morse JM, Morse RM, Tylko SJ. Development of a scale to identify the fall-prone patient. Canadian Journal on Aging. 1989;8:366-377.

Definitions for the Morse Fall Scale

History of falling
Yes (scored 25) if a previous fall is recorded during the present admission or if there is immediate history of physiological falls (i.e. from seizures, impaired gait) prior to admission.

Secondary diagnosis
Yes (15) if more than one medical diagnosis is listed on the patient chart.

Ambulatory aids
Scored 0 if patient walks without a walking aid even if assisted by a nurse, or is on bed rest.
Scored 15 if ambulatory with crutches, cane or walker.
Scored 20 if clutches onto furniture for support.

Intravenous therapy
Scored 20 if has an IV apparatus or heparin lock.

Gait
Normal gait scored 0 if patient is able to walk with head erect, arms swinging freely at the side, and strides without hesitation. Weak gait scored 10 if patient is stooped, but able to lift head while walking. Furniture support may be sought, but isof feather-weight touch, almost for reassurance. Steps are short and the patient may shuffle.
Impaired gait scored 20 if patient is stooped may have difficulty rising from the chair, attempts to rise by pushing on the arms of the chair and/or by "bouncing". The patient's head is down and because balance is poor the patient grasps onto the furniture, a person, or walking aid for support and cannot walk without assistance. Steps are short and the patient shuffles. If patient is wheelchair bound, the patient is scored according to the gait s/he uses when transferring from the wheelchair to the bed.

Mental Status
The patient is asked if s/he is able to go to the bathroom alone or if s/he needs assistance, or if s/he is permitted up. If the patient's response is consistent with the orders for ambulation, the score is 0.
If the response is not consistent with the orders, or if the patient's assessment is unrealistic, the score is 15.

The authors suggest each institution determine its own cutoff for high risk.

APPENDIX 32
Norton Scale for Assessing Risk of Pressure Ulcers

		Physical Condition	Mental Condition	Activity	Mobility	Incontinent	
		Good 4 Fair 3 Poor 2 Very bad 1	Alert 4 Apathetic 3 Confused 2 Stupor 1	Ambulant 4 Walk/help 3 Chairbound 2 Bed 1	Full 4 Slightly Limited 3 Very limited 2 Immobile 1	Not 4 Occasional 3 Usually/urine 2 Doubly 1	Total Score
Name	Date						

The Norton Scale uses five criteria to assess patients' risk for pressure ulcers. Scores of 14 or less indicate liability to ulcers; scores of <12 indicate very high risk.

Doreen Norton, Rhoda McLaren and A N Exton-Smith, An investigation of Geriatric Nursing Problems in Hospital, National Corporation for the Care of Old People (now Centre for Policy on Ageing), London, 1962.

The Warning Signs of poor nutritional health are often overlooked. Use this checklist to find out if you or someone you know is at nutritional risk.

Read the statements below. Circle the number in the yes column for those that apply to you or someone you know. For each yes answer, score the number in the box. Total your nutritional score.

DETERMINE YOUR NUTRITIONAL HEALTH

	YES
I have an illness or condition that made me change the kind and/or amount of food I eat.	2
I eat fewer than 2 meals per day.	3
I eat few fruits or vegetables, or milk products.	2
I have 3 or more drinks of beer, liquor or wine almost every day.	2
I have tooth or mouth problems that make it hard for me to eat.	2
I don't always have enough money to buy the food I need.	4
I eat alone most of the time.	1
I take 3 or more different prescribed or over-the-counter drugs a day.	1
Without wanting to, I have lost or gained 10 pounds in the last 6 months.	2
I am not always physically able to shop, cook and/or feed myself.	2
TOTAL	

Total Your Nutritional Score. If it's —

0-2   **Good!** Recheck your nutritional score in 6 months.

3-5   **You are at moderate nutritional risk.** See what can be done to improve your eating habits and lifestyle. Your office on aging, senior nutrition program, senior citizens center or health department can help. Recheck your nutritional score in 3 months.

6 or more   **You are at high nutritional risk.** Bring this checklist the next time you see your doctor, dietitian or other qualified health or social service professional. Talk with them about any problems you may have. Ask for help to improve your nutritional health.

These materials developed and distributed by the Nutrition Screening Initiative, a project of:

 AMERICAN ACADEMY OF FAMILY PHYSICIANS

THE AMERICAN DIETETIC ASSOCIATION

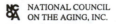 NATIONAL COUNCIL ON THE AGING, INC.

Remember that warning signs suggest risk, but do not represent diagnosis of any condition. Turn the page to learn more about the Warning Signs of poor nutritional health.

APPENDIX 34
Items From the Patient History Relevant to the Older Driver

1. Do you now drive a car? _____ Yes _____ No
2. During the past week, how many days did you drive?
3. What percentage of your total driving time was spent:
   a. Driving at night _____%
   b. Driving on the freeways _____%
   c. Driving during rush hour _____%
   d. Driving to complete essential errands (for example, to buy food, go to the bank or cleaners) _____%
4. a. In the past year, have you changed your driving patterns? _____ Yes _____ No
   b. If yes, how? (Check all that apply)
      1. _____ Do not drive at night
      2. _____ Do not drive on freeways
      3. _____ Do not drive in rain/fog and so forth
      4. _____ Do not drive during rush hour
      5. _____ Do not drive as far
      6. _____ Drive only when absolutely necessary (e.g., to buy food, go to the bank or cleaners)
      7. _____ Do not drive when someone else is available to drive
      8. _____ Do not drive when I am tired or feel ill
5. In the past year, have you had any accidents or "near-misses" while driving? _____ If yes, how many? _____
6. Do you have any of the following problems?
   a. _____ Loss of vision
   b. _____ Hearing loss
   c. _____ Memory problems
   d. _____ Parkinson's disease
   e. _____ Stroke
   f. _____ Diabetes mellitus
   g. _____ Coronary heart disease or chest pain
   h. _____ Extra heart beats
   i. _____ Arthritis, what joints _____
   j. _____ Falling
7. List the medications that you are taking

Name	Strength (dose)	How often it is taken
_____	_____	_____
_____	_____	_____
_____	_____	_____
_____	_____	_____
_____	_____	_____
_____	_____	_____
_____	_____	_____

8. During the past week, how many drinks containing alcohol did you consume? _____

Clinical Features	Score
Motor deficit in arm	
Grade 5	0
Grade 4	0.4
Grade 3	0.8
Grade 1-2	1.2
Grade 0	1.6
Proprioception (eyes closed)	
Locates affected thumb:	
Accurately	0
Slight difficulty	0.4
Finds thumb via arm	0.8
Unable to find thumb	1.2
Balance	
Walks 10 feet without help	0
Maintains standing position	0.4
Maintains sitting position	0.8
No sitting balance	1.2
Cognition	
Mental Test Score 10	0
Mental Test Score 8-9	0.4
Mental Test Score 5-7	0.8
Mental Test Score 0-4	1.2

Total Score = 1.6 + motor + proprioception + balance + cognition

Interpretation: Low scores at admission are associated with better outcomes in rehabilitation.

Reprinted with permission from Kalra L, Crome P. The role of prognostic scores in targeting stroke rehabilitation in elderly patients. J Am Geriatr Soc 1993; 41:396–400.

APPENDIX 36
Performance-Oriented Mobility Assessment (POMA)

BALANCE

Chair

Instructions: Place a hard armless chair against a wall. The following maneuvers are tested.

1. Sitting down
   - 0 = unable without help *or* collapses (plops) into chair *or* lands off center of chair
   - 1 = able and does not meet criteria for 0 or 2
   - 2 = sits in a smooth, safe motion *and* ends with buttocks against back of chair and thighs centered on chair
2. Sitting balance
   - 0 = unable to maintain position (marked slide forward or leans forward or to side)
   - 1 = leans in chair slightly or slight increased distance from buttocks to back of chair
   - 2 = steady, safe, upright
3. Arising
   - 0 = unable without help or loses balance or requires > three attempts
   - 1 = able but requires three attempts
   - 2 = able in ≤ two attempts
4. Immediate standing balance (first 5 seconds)
   - 0 = unsteady, marked staggering, moves feet, marked trunk sway or grabs object for support
   - 1 = steady but uses walker or cane *or* mild staggering but catches self without grabbing object
   - 2 = steady without walker or cane or other support

Stand

5a. Side-by-side standing balance
   - 0 = unable *or* unsteady *or* holds ≤ 3 seconds
   - 1 = able *but* uses cane, walker, or other support *or* holds for 4–9 seconds
   - 2 = narrow stance without support for 10 seconds
5b. Timing ___ ___ . ___ seconds
6. Pull test (subject at maximum position attained in #5, examiner stands behind and exerts mild pull back at waist)
   - 0 = begins to fall
   - 1 = takes more than two steps back
   - 2 = fewer than two steps backward and steady
7a. Able to stand on right leg unsupported
   - 0 = unable *or* holds onto any objects *or* able for < 3 seconds
   - 1 = able for 3 or 4 seconds
   - 2 = able for 5 seconds
7b. Timing ___ ___ . ___ seconds
8a. Able to stand on left leg unsupported
   - 0 = unable *or* holds onto any object *or* able for < 3 seconds
   - 1 = able for 3 or 4 seconds
   - 2 = able for 5 seconds
8b. Timing ___ ___ . ___ seconds
9a. Semitandem stand
   - 0 = unable to stand with one foot half in front of other with feet touching *or* begins to fall *or* holds for ≤ 3 seconds
   - 1 = able for 4 to 9 seconds
   - 2 = able to semitandem stand for 10 seconds
9b. Timing ___ ___ . ___ seconds

10a. Tandem stand

    0 = unable to stand with one foot in front of other *or* begins to fall *or* holds for ≤ 3 seconds

    1 = able for 4 to 9 seconds

    2 = able to tandem stand for 10 seconds

10b. Timing ___ ___ . ___ seconds

11. Bending over (to pick up a pen off floor)

    0 = unable *or* is unsteady

    1 = able, but requires more than one attempt to get up

    2 = able and is steady

12. Toe stand

    0 = unable

    1 = able but < 3 seconds

    2 = able for 3 seconds

13. Heel stand

    0 = unable

    1 = able but < 3 seconds

    2 = able for 3 seconds

GAIT

Instructions: Person stands with examiner. Walks down 10-foot walkway (measured). Ask the person to walk down walkway, turn, and walk back. The person should use customary walking aid.

Bare Floor (flat, even surface)

1. Type of surface: 1 = linoleum or tile; 2 = wood; 3 = cement or concrete; 4 = other _____ [not included in scoring]

2. Initiation of gait (immediately after told to "go")

    0 = any hesitancy or multiple attempts to start

    1 = no hesitancy

3. Path (estimated in relation to tape measure). Observe excursion of foot closest to tape measure over middle 8 feet of course.

    0 = marked deviation

    1 = mild or moderate deviation *or* uses walking aid

    2 = straight without walking aid

4. Missed step (trip or loss of balance)

    0 = yes, and would have fallen *or* more than two missed steps

    1 = yes, but appropriate attempt to recover *and* no more than two missed steps

    2 = none

5. Turning (while walking)

    0 = almost falls

    1 = mild staggering, but catches self, uses walker or cane

    2 = steady, without walking aid

6. Step over obstacles (to be assessed in a separate walk with two shoes placed on course 4 feet apart)

    0 = begins to fall at any obstacle *or* unable *or* walks around any obstacle *or* > two missed steps

    1 = able to step over all obstacles, but some staggering and catches self *or* one to two missed steps

    2 = able and steady at stepping over all four obstacles with no missed steps

Scoring – 19 or less = high risk of falling; 20–25 intermediate; more than 25 no unusual risk.

SOURCE: Courtesy of Mary E. Tinetti, MD. Adapted with permission.

APPENDIX 37
Pressure Ulcer Scale for Healing
(PUSH) Tool 3.0

Patient Name:_____   Patient ID#:_____

Ulcer Location: _____   Date:_____

DIRECTIONS:
Observe and measure the pressure ulcer. Categorize the ulcer with respect to surface area, exudate, and type of wound tissue. Record a sub-score for each of these ulcer characteristics. Add the sub-scores to obtain the total score. A comparison of total scores measured over time provides an indication of the improvement or deterioration in pressure ulcer healing.

Length	0	1	2	3	4	5	
	0 cm^2	<0.3 cm^2	0.3-0.6 cm^2	0.7-1.0 cm^2	1.1-2.0 cm^2	2.1-3.0 cm^2	
x Width		6	7	8	9	10	Sub-score
		3.1-4.0 cm^2	4.1-8.0 cm^2	8.1-12.0 cm^2	12.1-24.0 cm^2	>24.0 cm^2	
Exudate Amount	0	1	2	3			Sub-score
	None	Light	Moderate	Heavy			
Tissue Type	0	1	2	3	4		Sub-score
	Closed	Epithelial Tissue	Granulation Tissue	Slough	Necrotic Tissue		
							Total Score

Length x Width: Measure the greatest length (head to toe) and the greatest width (side to side) using a centimeter ruler. Multiply these two measurements (length x width) to obtain an estimate of surface area in square centimeters (cm2). Caveat: Do not guess! Always use a centimeter ruler and always use the same method each time the ulcer is measured.

Exudate Amount: Estimate the amount of exudate (drainage) present after removal of the dressing and before applying any topical agent to the ulcer. Estimate the exudate (drainage) as none, light, moderate, or heavy.

Tissue Type: This refers to the types of tissue that are present in the wound (ulcer) bed. Score as a "4" if there is any necrotic tissue present. Score as a "3" if there is any amount of slough present and necrotic tissue is absent. Score as a "2" if the wound is clean and contains granulation tissue. A superficial wound that is reepithelializing is scored as a "1". When the wound is closed, score as a "0".

4 - Necrotic Tissue (Eschar): black, brown, or tan tissue that adheres firmly to the wound bed or ulcer edges and may be either firmer or softer than surrounding skin.

3 - Slough: yellow or white tissue that adheres to the ulcer bed in strings or thick clumps, or is mucinous.

2 - Granulation Tissue: pink or beefy red tissue with a shiny, moist, granular appearance.

1 - Epithelial Tissue: for superficial ulcers, new pink or shiny tissue (skin) that grows in from the edges or as islands on the ulcer surface.

0 - Closed/Resurfaced: the wound is completely covered with epithelium (new skin).

Version 3.0: 9/15/98
©National Pressure Ulcer Advisory Panel

PRESSURE ULCER HEALING CHART
(To Monitor Trends in PUSH Scores Over Time)
<small>(use a separate page for each pressure ulcer)</small>

Patient Name:_____ Patient
ID#:_____

Ulcer Location: _____
Date:_____

Directions: Observe and measure pressure ulcers at regular intervals using the PUSH Tool. Date and record PUSH Sub-scale and Total Scores on the Pressure Ulcer Healing Record below.

	PRESSURE ULCER HEALING RECORD												
DATE													
Length x Width													
Exudate Amount													
Tissue Type													
Total Score													

Graph the PUSH Total Score on the Pressure Ulcer Healing Graph below.

PUSH Total Score	PRESSURE ULCER HEALING GRAPH									
17										
16										
15										
14										
13										
12										
11										
10										
9										
8										
7										
6										
5										
4										
3										
2										
1										
Healed 0										
DATE										

PUSH Tool Version 3.0: 9/15/98

Instructions for Using the PUSH Tool

To use the PUSH Tool, the pressure ulcer is assessed and scored on the three elements in the tool:

> •Length x Width --> scored from 0 to 10
> •Exudate Amount ---> scored from 0 (none) to 3 (heavy)
> •Tissue Type ---> scored from 0 (closed) to 4 (necrotic tissue)

In order to insure consistency in applying the tool to monitor wound healing, definitions for each element are supplied at the bottom of the tool.

Step 1: Using the definition for length x width, a centimeter ruler measurement is made of the greatest head to toe diameter. A second measurement is made of the greatest width (left to right). Multiple these two measurements to get square centimeters and then select the corresponding category for size on the scale and record the score.

Step 2: Estimate the amount of exudate after removal of the dressing and before applying any topical agents. Select the corresponding category for amount & record the score.

Step 3: Identify the type of tissue. Note: if there is ANY necrotic tissue, it is scored a 4. Or, if there is ANY slough, it is scored a 3, even though most of the wound is covered with granulation tissue.

Step 4: Sum the scores on the three elements of the tool to derive a total PUSH Score.

Step 5: Transfer the total score to the **Pressure Ulcer Healing Graph**. Changes in the score over time provide an indication of the changing status of the ulcer. If the score goes down, the wound is healing. If it gets larger, the wound is deteriorating.

Pre-Visit Questionnaire: Initial Visit

Today's date: _____

1. **Name:** _____

2. **Address:** _____
   street address/   apt. number

   _____
   city/state   zip

3. **Phone:** (___) _____

4. **What is your date of birth?** _____/_____/_____
   month   day   year

5. **Sex**:1)___Male

   2)___Female

6. **Who filled out this form?**_____

   *Relationship, if other than patient _____

7. **Who has been your previous primary doctor?**

    Name: _____

    Address: _____

    _____

    Phone number: _____

8. **Do you plan to continue to be followed by this doctor?**

    1)___NO

    2)___YES

    3)___Not sure

PAST MEDICAL HISTORY

9. Which medical conditions do you have or have you had in the past?

(Check all that apply)

I.   EYE & EAR PROBLEMS

a)____Cataracts

b)____Glaucoma

c)____Macular degeneration of the eye

d)____Hearing loss/hearing aid

e)____Other, specify_____

II.   HEART PROBLEMS

a)____Heart attack: ____year

c)____Heart failure

d)____High blood pressure

e)____Irregular heart beats

f)____Other, specify_____

III.   LUNG PROBLEMS

a)____Asthma

b)____Bronchitis

c)____Emphysema

d)____Other, specify_____

IV.   BONE & JOINT PROBLEMS

a)____Arthritis

b)____Osteoporosis

c)____Fractured hip, wrist or spine (circle which one)

d)____Gout

e)____Other, specify_____

V.   GLAND PROBLEMS

a____Diabetes

b____Thyroid overactive (high)

c)____Thyroid underactive (low)

d)____Other, specify_____

VI.   KIDNEY & URINARY TRACT PROBLEMS

a)____Kidney disease

b)____Prostate disease

c)____Frequent bladder or kidney infections

d)____Other, specify_____

VII.   GASTROINTESTINAL PROBLEMS

a)___Ulcers

b)___Heartburn/Hiatal hernia

c)___Diverticulosis

d)___Liver disease/Cirrhosis

e)___Hepatitis

f)___Polyps

g)___Gallbladder disease

h)___Other, specify_____

VIII.   NERVOUS SYSTEM PROBLEMS

a)___Stroke

b)___Dementia/Alzheimer's

c)___Parkinson's Disease

d)___Epilepsy/Seizures

e)___Other, specify_____

IX.   OTHER HEALTH PROBLEMS

a)___Anemia

b)___Hernia

c)___Thrombosis (blood clots)

d)___Cancer, of what_____?

e)___Depression

f)___Sexual function problems,   specify_____

_____

g ___Other, specify_____

_____

_____Check if you do not now or did not have any of these problems

10. List Surgeries (Operations). Use back of page, if needed.

DATE	SURGERY (OPERATIONS)

11. List Other Hospitalizations. Use back of page, if needed.

DATE	REASON

12. Do you have any drug allergies?

1)____NO

2)____YES.→ If YES, specify below ⌐

NAME OF DRUG	REACTION

13. **Gather all your prescription and non-prescription medicines** (pills, capsules, eye drops, nasal sprays, ointments for your skin, aspirin, laxatives, calcium, supplements, vitamins, etc.), **everything that you used at least twice in the last year**. Separate those that you use regularly (even once a week) from those that you use only as needed. **Bring all medications with you when you come for your visit.**

___Check here if you did not use **any** medicine during the past year.

I.   List all medicines that you use regularly **at this time.**

Current medications used **regularly**	What strength?	How do you use it? (How many? How many times a day?)
Example: Tylenol	500 mg.	1 pill 3 times a day

II.   List medicines that you used "as needed" **at least twice in the last year.** (Any medicines used daily or even weekly should be listed above.)

Medications used "as needed" at least twice **in the last year**.	How often? (weekly? monthly?)	What strength?	How do you use it? (How many? How many times a day?)

SOCIAL HISTORY

14. With whom do you live? (check one)
   1)__Alone
   2)__With spouse or partner
   3)__With child or other family
   4)__Others, not family
   5)__Other, specify_____

15. Which of the following best describes your residence? (check one)
   1)__Own house or condo
   2)__Rent house, condo or apartment
   3)__Live with other in their home, condo or apartment
   4)__Retirement hotel
   5)__Board and care/residential care facility
   6)__Other, specify_____

16. Are you currently (check one)
   1)__Married
   2)__Divorced/Separated
   3)__Widowed
   4)__Single/Never married

17. Are you currently (check one)
   1)_____Retired
   2)_____Working at least part-time
   3)_____Looking for work

18. **What has been your principal occupation?**

   _____

19. **How much school did you complete? (check one)**

   1)____Less than 6th grade

   2)____Less than high school graduate

   3)____High school graduate

   4)____Some college

   5)____College graduate

   6)____More than college graduate

20. **Do you <u>employ</u> someone to provide care or help you in your home?**

   1)____NO

   2)____YES.→ If YES, **How many hours a day and how many days**

   a week is your paid helper available for you?

   _____ hours a day and_____days a week

21. **Is this sufficient to meet your needs?**

   1)____NO

   2)____YES

22. **Do you get help from a family member or friend in your home?**

   1)____NO

   2)____YES.→If YES, **How many hours a day and how many days a week**

   is your family member or friend available for you?

   _____ hours a day and_____days a week

23. **Is this sufficient to meet your needs?**

   1)____NO

   2)____YES

24. Do you provide care for a family member?

    1)____NO

    2)____YES

25. Do you drink alcohol, including beer and wine? (check one)

    1)____Daily

    2)____Greater than 3 times a week

    3)____1 to 3 times a week

    4)____Less than 1 time a week

    5)____Never

26. Have you ever smoked cigarettes?

    1)____NO

    2)____YES.→ If YES, **Are you now smoking?**

        a)____no. If no,

            1. How many years ago did you quit?_____

            2. For how many years did you smoke?____

            3. How much did you smoke?___packs per day

       b)____yes. If yes,

            1. How many years have you smoked?_____

            2. How much do you smoke?____packs per day

FAMILY HISTORY

27. Have any members of your family had any of the following conditions? check all that apply)

    1)____Dementia or Alzheimer's Disease

    2)____Cancer, of what?_____

    3)____Heart disease

    4)____Stroke

    5)____Diabetes

    6)____Depression

    7)____None of these

28.　　We want to know if you need help with any of the following, and who helps you. Fill out for each task.

TASK	DON'T NEED HELP	NEED HELP	IF YOU NEED HELP, WHO HELPS? (Name and Relationship)
Feeding yourself			
Getting from bed to chair			
Getting to the toilet			
Getting dressed			
Bathing			
Using the telephone			
Taking your medicines			
Preparing meals			
Managing money/financial affairs/checkbook			
Doing laundry			
Doing house work			
Shopping for groceries			
Driving			
Doing 'handyman' work			
Climbing a flight of stairs			
Getting to places beyond walking distance			

29. To be certain that we've covered everything, during <u>the last three months</u>, have you had any of the following symptoms or problems? (check all that apply)

I. GENERAL PROBLEMS
- a)_____Weight loss
- b)_____Weight gain
- c)_____Fevers
- d)_____Chills
- e)_____Sweats

II. EYES
- a)_____Trouble seeing
- b)_____Eye pain

III. EAR, NOSE, MOUTH, THROAT
- a)_____Trouble hearing
- b)_____Ear pain or itching
- c)_____Sinus problems
- d)_____Nose bleeds
- e)_____Sore throat
- f)_____Teeth problems

III. HEART PROBLEMS
- a)_____Chest pain or tightness
- b)_____Rapid or irregular heart beat
- c)_____Swelling of feet

IV. LUNG PROBLEMS
- a)_____Persistent cough
- b)_____Difficulty breathing or shortness of breath

V. DIGESTION PROBLEMS
- a)_____Dental problems
- b)_____Difficulty swallowing
- c)_____Frequent indigestion or stomach ache
- d)_____Frequent nausea or vomiting
- e)_____Change in bowel habits
- f)_____Black bowel movement or bleeding from rectum
- g)_____Frequent diarrhea
- h)_____Persistent constipation

VI. BONE AND JOINT PROBLEMS
- a)_____Leg pain on walking
- b)_____Back or neck pain
- c)_____Joint pain or stiffness
- d)_____Foot problems
- e)_____Falls

VII. BRAIN AND NERVOUS SYSTEM PROBLEMS
- a)_____Frequent headaches
- b)_____Frequent dizzy spells
- c)_____Passing out or fainting
- d)_____Paralysis, leg or arm weakness
- e)_____Numbness or loss of feelings
- f)_____Serious problem with memory or difficulty thinking
- g)_____Tremor or shaking
- h)_____Problem with sleep

VIII MOOD/SADNESS PROBLEMS
- a)_____Depression
- b)_____Anxiety

IX. GYNECOLOGY PROBLEMS
- a)_____Vaginal bleeding after you stopped having your periods
- b)_____Breast lumps or discomfort
- c)_____Vaginal discharge

X. KIDNEY & URINARY TRACT PROBLEMS
- a)_____Urination at night
- b)_____Frequent urination
- c)_____Painful urination
- d)_____Difficulty starting or stopping urination
- e)_____Loss of urine or getting wet

XI. SKIN PROBLEMS
- a)_____Rash
- b)_____sores
- c)_____itching

XII. GLAND PROBLEMS
- a)_____Excessive thirst
- b)_____Feel too hot or too cold

_____Check here if you have not had any of these problems during the last 3 months.

PLANNING FOR FUTURE HEALTH CARE

30. Do you have a medical Durable Power of Attorney?

    1)____NO

    2)____YES

31. Do you have a living will?

    1)____NO

    2)____YES

HEALTH MAINTENANCE

32. Have you ever had an examination of your bowel with a scope (sigmoidoscopy or colonoscopy)?

    1)____NO

    2)____YES.→ If YES, When did you have your most recent sigmoidoscopy or colonoscopy?___(year)

33. In the past 12 months, have you had a test for blood in your stool (three cards at home)?

    1)____NO

    2)____YES

34. Have you ever had the Pneumovax vaccine (a shot to prevent pneumonia)?

    1)____NO

    2)____YES→ If YES, In what year did you have your last pneumovax vaccine?_____(year).

35. Have you ever had a tetanus shot?

    1)____NO

    2)____YES.→ If YES, In what year did you have your last tetanus booster?_____(year)

36. Have you had a flu shot this season, (October-February)?

    1)____NO

    2)____YES

    3)____Not applicable (March-September)

37. Do you always wear a seatbelt when you ride in a car?

    1)____NO

    2)____YES

38. Do you currently participate in any regular activity or program designed to improve or maintain your physical fitness? (either on your own or in a formal class)

    1)____NO

    2)____YES.→ If YES, **Check what you do currently.**

      a)____Walking

      b)____Swimming

      c)____Aerobics or exercise classes

      d)____Dancing

      e)____Jogging

      f)____Bicycling or stationary bike

      g)____Tennis

      h)____Golf

      i)____Bowling or boccie

      j)____None of the above

      k)____Other: specify_____

QUESTION FOR MEN ONLY

(After completing question 40 please go to question 44)

39. **Have you ever had a prostate exam (rectal exam)?**

    1)____NO

    2)____YES.→ If YES, **When did you have your most recent prostate exam?**____(year)

40. **Have you ever had a blood test to look for cancer of the prostate (PSA)?**

    1)____NO

    2)____YES.→ If YES, **When did you have your most recent blood test to look for prostate cancer?**
    _____(year)

QUESTIONS FOR WOMEN ONLY

41. **Do you perform breast self-exam (BSE) once a month?**

    1)____NO

    2)____YES

42. **Have you ever had a mammogram?**

    1)____NO

    2)____YES.→ If YES, **Have you had a mammogram within the last 2 years?**

    a)____no

    b)____yes, month_____ year_____

43. **Have you had a hysterectomy (surgical removal of the uterus)?**

    1)____YES (go to question 44)

    2)____NO.→ If NO, **Have you ever had a Pap smear/pelvic examination?**

    a)____no (go to question 44)

    b)__yes → If yes, **When was your last Pap smear?**

    month_____year__

44. **Do you have any other health problems that you would like your doctor to know about before your visit?**

THANK YOU FOR COMPLETING THIS FORM.

APPENDIX 39
Screening Questionnaire for Sleep Apnea

Are you sometimes sleepy in the daytime? In the following situations do you often find yourself fighting to stay awake or falling asleep?

1. Sitting in a theater, lecture, or meeting?	NO _____	YES _____
2. Watching television, for only 20 min?	NO _____	YES _____
3. Reading a book for only 15 min?	NO _____	YES _____
4. After driving for 30 min?	NO _____	YES _____
How many times each week do you take a nap that was not planned?	0-1 _____	2-3 _____
		4-7 _____
Has your spouse or roommate complained about your loud snoring?	NO _____	YES _____
Do you sometimes wake up in the morning with a headache?	NO _____	YES _____
Do you usually still feel groggy and unrefreshed 30 min after morning awakening?	NO _____	YES _____
Do you frequently sweat during your sleep, even when the room is not too hot for most people?	NO _____	YES _____
As an adult, have you ever awakened from sleep gasping, choking, or having wet the bed?	NO _____	YES _____
Have you been told that you move excessively during sleep, or have you awakened finding yourself sitting up or getting out of bed?	NO _____	YES _____
Which of the following forms of insomnia have you experienced at least 3 nights every week, for at least 2 months?		
Wake up three or more times and cannot get back to sleep for at least 5 min?	NO _____	YES _____
Wake up too early in the morning before you have had a decent night's sleep?	NO _____	YES _____
Wake up too early in the morning before you have had a decent night's sleep?	NO _____	YES _____
Lie in bed awake for at least 2 h during the night?	NO _____	YES _____
Because of your sleep problems, do you feel too exhausted or irritable to manage your full daily schedule, or to do mental work like learning something new or writing an important letter?	NO _____	YES _____

If you answered yes to any question, or reported that a behavior occurred more than once a week, you might benefit from further evaluation of your sleep-related symptoms. Ask your physician.

Reprinted with permission from Karger

SF-36 QUESTIONNAIRE ITEMS

1. In general, would you say your health is:

    (Circle One Number)

Excellent	1
Very good	2
Good	3
Fair	4
Poor	5

2. **Compared to one year ago**, how would you rate your health in general **now**?

    (Circle One Number)

Much better now than one year ago	1
Somewhat better now than one year ago	2
About the same	3
Somewhat worse now than one year ago	4
Much worse now than one year ago	5

The following items are about activities you might do during a typical day. Does **your health now limit you** in these activities? If so, how much?

(Circle One Number on Each Line)

		Yes, Limited a Lot	Yes, Limited a Little	No, Not Limited at All
3.	**Vigorous activities,** such as running, lifting heavy objects, participating in strenuous sports	1	2	3
4.	**Moderate activities**, such as moving a table, pushing a vacuum cleaner, bowling, or playing golf	1	2	3
5.	Lifting or carrying groceries	1	2	3
6.	Climbing **several** flights of stairs	1	2	3
7.	Climbing **one** flight of stairs	1	2	3
8.	Bending, kneeling, or stooping	1	2	3
9.	Walking **more than a mile**	1	2	3
10.	Walking **several blocks**	1	2	3
11.	Walking **one block**	1	2	3
12.	Bathing or dressing yourself	1	2	3

During the **past 4 weeks**, have you had any of the following problems with your work or other regular daily activities **as a result of your physical health**?

(Circle One Number on Each Line)

	Yes	No
13. Cut down the **amount of time** you spent on work or other activities	1	2
14. **Accomplished less** than you would like	1	2
15. Were limited in the **kind** of work or other activities...................	1	2
16. Had **difficulty** performing the work or other activities (for example, it took extra effort)	1	2

During the **past 4 weeks,** have you had any of the following problems with your work or other regular daily activities **as a result of any emotional problems** (such as feeling depressed or anxious)?

(Circle One Number on Each Line)

	Yes	No
17. Cut down the **amount of time** you spent on work or other activities	1	2
18. **Accomplished less** than you would like	1	2
19. Didn't do work or other activities as **carefully** as usual...............	1	2

20. During the **past 4 weeks,** to what extent has your physical health or emotional problems interfered with your normal social activities with family, friends, neighbors, or groups?

(Circle One Number)

Not at all 1
Slightly 2
Moderately 3
Quite a bit 4
Extremely.. 5

21. How much **bodily** pain have you had during the **past 4 weeks**?

(Circle One Number)

None 1
Very mild.. 2
Mild.. 3
Moderate... 4
Severe 5
Very severe 6

22. During the **past 4 weeks,** how much did **pain** interfere with your normal work (including both work outside the home and housework)?

(Circle One Number)

Not at all 1
A little bit 2
Moderately 3
Quite a bit 4
Extremely.. 5

These questions are about how you feel and how things have been with you **during the past 4 weeks.** For each question, please give the one answer that comes closest to the way you have been feeling.

How much of the time during the **past 4 weeks** . . .

(Circle One Number on Each Line)

	All of the Time	Most of the Time	A Good Bit of the Time	Some of the Time	A Little of the Time	None of the Time
23. Did you feel full of pep?	1	2	3	4	5	6
24. Have you been a very nervous person?............	1	2	3	4	5	6
25. Have you felt so down in the dumps that nothing could cheer you up?.....................	1	2	3	4	5	6
26. Have you felt calm and peaceful?....................	1	2	3	4	5	6
27. Did you have a lot of energy?...........................	1	2	3	4	5	6
28. Have you felt downhearted and blue?	1	2	3	4	5	6
29. Did you feel worn out?...................................	1	2	3	4	5	6
30. Have you been a happy person?	1	2	3	4	5	6
31. Did you feel tired?	1	2	3	4	5	6

32. During the **past 4 weeks,** how much of the time has your **physical health or emotional problems** interfered with your social activities (like visiting with friends, relatives, etc.)?

(Circle One Number)

All of the time 1
Most of the time 2
Some of the time 3
A little of the time 4
None of the time....................................... 5

How TRUE or FALSE is <u>each</u> of the following statements for you.

(Circle One Number on Each Line)

	Definitely True	Mostly True	Don't Know	Mostly False	Definitely False
33. I seem to get sick a little easier than other people...	1	2	3	4	5
34. I am as healthy as anybody I know.	1	2	3	4	5
35. I expect my health to get worse.	1	2	3	4	5
36. My health is excellent.	1	2	3	4	5

STEP 1: RECODING ITEMS

ITEM NUMBERS	Change original response category [a]	To recoded value of:
1,2,20,22,34,36	1 ----------- >	100
	2 ----------- >	75
	3 ----------- >	50
	4 ----------- >	25
	5 ----------- >	0
3,4,5,6,7,8,9,10,11,12	1 ----------- >	0
	2 ----------- >	50
	3 ----------- >	100
13,14,15,16,17,18,19	1 ----------- >	0
	2 ----------- >	100
21,23,26,27,30	1 ----------- >	100
	2 ----------- >	80
	3 ----------- >	60
	4 ----------- >	40
	5 ----------- >	20
	6 ----------- >	0
24,25,28,29,31	1 ----------- >	0
	2 ----------- >	20
	3 ----------- >	40
	4 ----------- >	60
	5 ----------- >	80
	6 ----------- >	100
32,33,35	1 ----------- >	0
	2 ----------- >	25
	3 ----------- >	50
	4 ----------- >	75
	5 ----------- >	100

[a] Precoded response choices as printed in the questionnaire.

STEP 2: AVERAGING ITEMS TO FORM SCALES

Scale	Number Of Items	After Recoding Per Table 1, Average The Following Items:
Physical functioning	10	3 4 5 6 7 8 9 10 11 12
Role limitations due to physical health	4	13 14 15 16
Role limitations due to emotional problems	3	17 18 19
Energy/fatigue	4	23 27 29 31
Emotional well-being	5	24 25 26 28 30
Social functioning	2	20 32
Pain	2	21 22
General health	5	1 33 34 35 36

APPENDIX 41
Short Portable Mental Status Questionnaire (SPMSQ)

1. What is the date today? (month/day/year) [all 3 correct score]
2. What day of the week is it?
3. What is the name of this place? [any correct description]
4. What is your telephone number? [street address if no phone]
5. How old are you?
6. When were you born? (month/day/year) [all 3 correct to score]
7. Who is the President now?
8. Who was the President just before him?
9. What is your mothers maiden name?
10. Subtract 3 from 20 and keep subtracting three from each new number all the way down. [whole series to score]

Potential Error Score: 10
Adjustments to error score: allow one error if not educated beyond grade school; allow one less error if educated beyond high school.

Error Score:
0-2 Intact intellectual function
3-4 Mild intellectual impairment
5-7 Moderate intellectual impairment
8-10 Severe intellectual impairment

Source: Pfeiffer E. A short portable mental status questionnaire for the assessment of organic brain deficit in elderly patients. J Am Geriatr Soc. 1975;23: 433-441.

APPENDIX 42
Sleep Log

Please fill out this Sleep Log every morning about 30 minutes after getting up. Guess the approximate times. Do not worry if your figures are not absolutely correct. We are interested in your opinion of how you slept. Date the night when it started, not when you fill it out (for example, if you filled the log out on Wednesday morning, Oct. 5, the date of the night is Tuesday, Oct. 4).

	SUN	MON	TUES	WED	THURS	FRI	SAT
DATE							
Did you take naps yesterday? If yes, give total length of sleep In minutes.							
Did you take any sleeping medication? Give time and amount.							
When did you turn out your lights, actually trying to sleep?							
How many minutes did it take you to fall asleep last night?							
How often did you awaken last night?							
How many minutes were you awake during last night? Do not Count the time it took you to fall asleep initially.							
When did you wake up for the last time this morning?							
How many hours did you actually sleep last night?							
When did you get out of bed for the last time this morning?							
Compared with your own avg. over the last month, how well did you sleep last night? Choose one from the list below, left.							
Overall, how refreshing and restorative was your sleep? Choose one from the list below, right.							

1. Much worse than my average
2. Slightly worse than my average
3. Fairly typical for me

4. Slightly better than my average
5. Much better than my average

1. Not at all restorative-derived no benefit from my time in bed
2. Some slight restorative value
3. Restorative, but not adequately so

4. Relatively satisfactory
5. Very satisfactory-feel completely refreshed and ready for the day

Reprinted by permission from Hauri & Linde, 1990

APPENDIX 43
Social Support Network-Clinical
Screening Instrument (SSN-CSI) Scale

<u>(6 LSNS-A items plus 3 RAND SSS items)</u> *alpha = .84

1. How many relatives do you see or hear from at least once a month?
2. How many relatives do you feel close to that you can call on them for help?
3. How many relatives do you feel at ease with that you can talk about private matters?
4. How many friends/neighbors do you see or hear from at least once a month?
5. How many friends/neighbors do you feel close to that you can call on them for help?
6. How many friends/neighbors do you feel at ease with that you can talk about private matters?
7. How often do you have someone to love?
8. How often does someone show love and affection to you?
9. How often do you have someone to share worries?

Response options and scoring:
(Same as those listed for LSNS-A and SSS-A respectively.)

*Cronbach alphas from analyses run on data drawn from a random sample of 200 Non-Hispanic White Elderly (65 years plus) living in Los Angeles County. Interviewed in their homes by trained interviewers from UCLA's Survey Research Center as part of a NIA funded study. For more information on this study, see:

1. Villa, V.M., Wallace, S.P., Moon, A. & Lubben, J.E. (1997), A Comparative Analysis of Chronic Disease Prevalence Among Older Koreans and non-Hispanic Whites, *Journal of Family and Community Health*, 20(2): 1-12.
2. Moon, A. Lubben, J.E. & Villa, V.M. (1998), Awareness and Utilization of Community Long Term Care Services by Elderly Korean and non-Hispanic White Americans, *The Gerontologist*, 38: 309-316.

DEPARTMENT OF VETERANS AFFAIRS

VA ADVANCE DIRECTIVE:
Living Will and Durable Power of Attorney for Health Care

This form is a tool to document or capture a patient's wishes regarding a designated health care agent and their future treatment preferences. This form is a tool, not an end in itself. The form does not substitute for comprehensive dialogue with the patient. It is expected that the health care professional assisting the patient will bring up for discussion other possible end stage scenarios, as appropriate. Supplemental pages may be appended as necessary.

I, _____ write this document as a directive
(print or type patient's name and social security number)
regarding my health care. I have put my initials by the choices I want.

Part I. - Durable Power of Attorney for Health Care (DPAHC)

initials	I appoint this person to make decisions about my health care if there ever comes a time when I cannot make those decisions myself.

Name
Street Address
City, State and ZIP Code
Work Telephone Number with Area Code	Home Telephone Number with Area Code

If the person above cannot or will not make decisions for me, I appoint this person:

Name
Street Address
City, State and ZIP Code
Work Telephone Number with Area Code	Home Telephone Number with Area Code

initials	I have notified the individuals listed above of my decision.
initials	I have not appointed anyone to make health care decisions for me in this or any other documents.

Part II. - Living Will

These are my, _____ wishes for my future
(print or type patient's name and social security number)
health care if there ever comes a time when I can't make these decisions for myself. I want
the person I have appointed as my Health care Agent (HCA), my doctors, my family and
others to be guided by the decisions I have made below.

A. Life-Sustaining Treatments

initials

If I should have an incurable or irreversible condition that will cause my death, or
am in a state of permanent unconsciousness from which, to a reasonable degree of
medical certainty there can be no recovery, it is my desire that my life not be
artitificially prolonged by administration of "life-sustaining" procedures. If, at that
time, I am unable to participate in decisions regarding my medical treatment, I direct
my physician to withhold or withdraw procedures that merely prolong the dying
process and are not necessary to my comfort or freedom from pain.

B. Treatment Preferences/Other Directions

initials

You have the right to be involved in all decisions about your health care. If you
have wishes not covered in other parts of this document, please indicate them here.
Treatments or situations you may wish to consider include, but are not limited to:
Transfusion, dialysis, CPR, artificial nutrition and hydration, mechanical breathing,
pain medications, antibiotics, and a time-limited trial of a given therapy.

_____

_____

_____

_____

_____

_____

_____

_____

Part III. - Signatures

A. **Your signature** — By my signature below I show that I understand the purpose and the effect of this document.

Signature	Social Security Number	Date
Name (Printed or Typed)		
Street Address		
City, State and ZIP Code		

B. **Your Witnesses' Signatures**

I am not, to the best of my knowledge, named in the person's will.
I am not the person appointed as Health Care Agent (HCA) in this advance directive.
I am not a health care provider (or an employee of the health care provider), or financially responsible, now or in the past, for the care of the person making this advance directive. *(Exception: where other witnesses are not reasonably available, employees of the Chaplain Service, Psychology Service, Social Work Service, or nonclinical employees such as Voluntary Service or Environmental Management Service may serve as witnesses.)*

Witness #1: I personally witnessed the signing of this advance directive.

Signature	Date
Name (Printed or Typed)	
Street Address	
City, State and ZIP Code	

Witness #2: I personally witnessed the signing of this advance directive.

Signature	Date
Name (Printed or Typed)	
Street Address	
City, State and ZIP Code	

APPENDIX 45
Visual Analog Scale

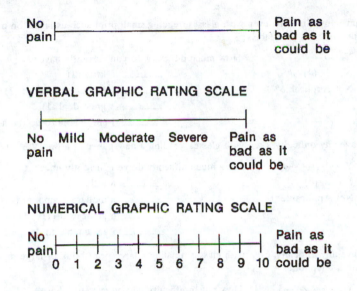

No pain ├────────────────────────────────┤ Pain as bad as it could be

VERBAL GRAPHIC RATING SCALE

├────────────────────────────────┤

No pain   Mild   Moderate   Severe   Pain as bad as it could be

NUMERICAL GRAPHIC RATING SCALE

No pain ├─┼─┼─┼─┼─┼─┼─┼─┼─┼─┤ Pain as bad as it could be
     0 1 2 3 4 5 6 7 8 9 10

Note: Examples of visual analog scales with word or number anchors. Visual-analog scales are usually constructed on horizontal or vertical lines, 100 millimeters in length. Subjects are asked to indicate pain intensity on the line. Pain is usually scored on a 0-100 scale by measuring the distance in millimeters from the zero end of the line.

1. Do you have any difficulty, even with glasses, reading small print such as labels on medicine bottles, a telephone book, or food labels?

    _____ Yes ------------>   How much difficulty do you currently have?

    _____ No   (4)   _____ a little (3)

    _____ Not Applicable*   _____ a moderate amount (2)

                                      _____ a great deal (1)

                                      _____ I am unable to do the activity (0)

2. Do you have any difficulty, even with glasses, reading a newspaper or a book?

    _____ Yes ------------>   How much difficulty do you currently have?

    _____ No   (4)   _____ a little (3)

    _____ Not Applicable*   _____ a moderate amount (2)

                                        _____ a great deal (1)

                                      _____ I am unable to do the activity (0)

3. Do you have any difficulty, even with glasses, reading a large print book or large print newspaper or numbers on a telephone?

    _____ Yes ------------>   How much difficulty do you currently have?

    _____ No   (4)   _____ a little (3)

    _____ Not Applicable*   _____ a moderate amount (2)

                                      _____ a great deal (1)

                                      _____ I am unable to do the activity (0)

4. Do you have any difficulty, even with glasses, recognizing people when they are close to you?

    _____ Yes ------------>   How much difficulty do you currently have?

    _____ No   (4)   _____ a little (3)

    _____ Not Applicable*   _____ a moderate amount (2)

                                      _____ a great deal (1)

                                      _____ I am unable to do the activity (0)

5. Do you have any difficulty, even with glasses, seeing steps, stairs or curbs?

    _____ Yes ------------>   How much difficulty do you currently have?

    _____ No   (4)   _____ a little (3)

    _____ Not Applicable*   _____ a moderate amount (2)

                                      _____ a great deal (1)

                                      _____ I am unable to do the activity (0)

* See Introduction to Respondent

6. Do you have any difficulty, even with glasses, reading traffic signs, streeet signs or store signs?

    _____ Yes ------------>   How much difficulty do you currently have?
    _____ No   (4)   _____ a little (3)
    _____ Not Applicable*   _____ a moderate amount (2)
                                       _____ a great deal (1)
                                       _____ I am unable to do the activity (0)

7. Do you have any difficulty, even with glasses, doing fine handwork like sewing, knitting, crocheting or carpentry?

    _____ Yes ------------>   How much difficulty do you currently have?
    _____ No   (4)   _____ a little (3)
    _____ Not Applicable*   _____ a moderate amount (2)
                                         _____ a great deal (1)
                                       _____ I am unable to do the activity (0)

8. Do you have any difficulty, even with glasses, writing checks, or filling out forms?

    _____ Yes ------------>   How much difficulty do you currently have?
    _____ No   (4)   _____ a little (3)
    _____ Not Applicable*   _____ a moderate amount (2)
                                         _____ a great deal (1)
                                       _____ I am unable to do the activity (0)

9. Do you have any difficulty, even with glasses, playing games such as bingo, dominos, card games, or mah jong?

    _____ Yes ------------>   How much difficulty do you currently have?
    _____ No   (4)   _____ a little (3)
    _____ Not Applicable*   _____ a moderate amount (2)
                                         _____ a great deal (1)
                                       _____ I am unable to do the activity (0)

10. Do you have any difficulty, even with glasses, taking part in sports like bowling, handball, tennis, or golf?

    _____ Yes ------------>   How much difficulty do you currently have?
    _____ No   (4)   _____ a little (3)
    _____ Not Applicable*   _____ a moderate amount (2)
                                         _____ a great deal (1)
                                       _____ I am unable to do the activity (0)

    * See Introduction to Respondent

11. Do you have any difficulty, even with glasses, cooking?

      _____ Yes ------------>   How much difficulty do you currently have?

      _____ No   (4)

      _____ Not Applicable*

                                          _____ a little (3)

                                          _____ a moderate amount (2)

                                          _____ a great deal (1)

                                          _____ I am unable to do the activity (0)

12. Do you have any difficulty, even with glasses, watching television?

      _____ Yes ------------>   How much difficulty do you currently have?

      _____ No   (4)

      _____ Not Applicable*

                                          _____ a little (3)

                                          _____ a moderate amount (2)

                                          _____ a great deal (1)

                                          _____ I am unable to do the activity (0)

13. Do you currently drive a car?

            _____ **Yes** (skip to 14)

            _____ **No** (go to 13A)

13A. Have you ever driven a car?

            _____ **Yes** (go to 13B)

            _____ **No** (Stop here; end of questionnaire)

13B. Why did you stop driving? (Select most important reason)

            _____ Because of my vision. (Stop here; end of questionnaire)

            _____ Because of another illness. (Stop here; end of questionnaire)

            _____ For another reason. (Stop here; end of questionnaire)

14. How much difficulty do you have driving during the day because of your vision? Do you have:

            _____ No difficulty? (4)

            _____ A little difficulty? (3)

            _____ A moderate amount of difficulty? (2)

            _____ A great deal of difficulty? (1)

            _____ I am unable to or don't drive during the day. (0)

15. How much difficulty do you have driving at night because of your vision? Do you have:

            _____ No difficulty? (4)

            _____ A little difficulty? (3)

            _____ A moderate amount of difficulty? (2)

            _____ A great deal of difficulty? (1)

            _____ I am unable to or don't drive during the day. (0)

Scoring of the VF-14: Scores for each item ranged from 4 when "no difficulty" was reported to 0 when "unable to do" was reported. An item was not included when the person did not do the activity for a reason other than vision. Scores of all activities that were performed or were not performed because of difficulty with vision were then averaged. The average score was then multiplied by 25, resulting in a possible final score ranging between 0 (unable to do because of vision) and 100 (able to do all items without difficulty).

* See Introduction to Respondent

Steinberg EP, Tielsch JM, Schein OD, et al. The VF-14: An index of functional impairment in patients with cataract. Arch Ophthalmol 1994;112:630–638.

APPENDIX 47
Zarit Caregiver Burden Scale

CAREGIVER QUESTIONNAIRE

INSTRUCTIONS: THE FOLLOWING IS A LIST OF STATEMENTS, WHICH REFLECT HOW PEOPLE SOMETIMES FEEL WHEN TAKING CARE OF ANOTHER PERSON. AFTER EACH STATEMENT, CIRCLE HOW OFTEN YOU FEEL THAT WAY, NEVER, RARELY, SOMETIMES, FREQUENTLY, OR NEARLY ALWAYS. THERE ARE NO RIGHT OR WRONG ANSWERS.

	Never	Rarely	Sometimes	Frequently	Nearly Always
1. Do you feel that your relative asks for more help than he/she needs?	0	1	2	3	4
2. Do you feel that because of the time you spend with your relative that you don't have enough time for yourself?	0	1	2	3	4
3. Do you feel stressed between caring for your relative and trying to meet other responsibilities for your family or work?	0	1	2	3	4
4. Do you feel embarrassed over your relative's behavior?	0	1	2	3	4
5. Do you feel angry when you are around your relative?	0	1	2	3	4
6. Do you feel that your relative currently affects your relationship with other family members or friends in a negative way?	0	1	2	3	4
7. Are you afraid what the future holds for your relative?	0	1	2	3	4
8. Do you feel your relative is dependent upon you?	0	1	2	3	4
9. Do you feel strained when you are around your relative?	0	1	2	3	4
10. Do you feel your health has suffered because of your involvement with your relative?	0	1	2	3	4
11. Do you feel that you don't have as much privacy as you would like, because of your relative?	0	1	2	3	4
12. Do you feel that your social life has suffered because you are caring for your relative?	0	1	2	3	4
13. Do you feel uncomfortable about having friends over, because of your relative?	0	1	2	3	4
14. Do you feel that your relative seems to expect you to take care of him/her, as if you were the only one he/she could depend on?	0	1	2	3	4

	Never	Rarely	Sometimes	Frequently	Nearly Always
15. Do you feel that you don't have enough money to care for your relative, in addition to the rest of your expenses?	0	1	2	3	4
16. Do you feel that you will be unable to take care of your relative much longer?	0	1	2	3	4
17. Do you feel you have lost control of your life since your relative's illness?	0	1	2	3	4
18. Do you wish you could just leave the care of your relative to someone else?	0	1	2	3	4
19. Do you feel uncertain about what to do about your relative?	0	1	2	3	4
20. Do you feel you should be doing more for your relative?	0	1	2	3	4
21. Do you feel you could do a better job in caring for your relative?	0	1	2	3	4
22. Overall, how burdened do you feel in caring for your relative?	0	1	2	3	4

CAREGIVER'S NAME: _____

DATE: _____

Reference: Zarit, S. H., Reever, K.E., Bach-Peterson, J. (1980), Relatives of the impaired elderly; correlates of "feelings of burden." *The Gerontologist* 20:6, 649–655.

ISBN 0-07-134725-9

90000

9 780071 347259